# Handbook
# of Health Professions
# Education

Responding to New Realities
in Medicine, Dentistry, Pharmacy,
Nursing, Allied Health,
and Public Health

*Christine H. McGuire,*
*Richard P. Foley,*
*Alan Gorr, Ronald W. Richards,*
*and Associates*

# Handbook
# of Health Professions
# Education

Jossey-Bass Publishers

San Francisco • Washington • London • 1983

HANDBOOK OF HEALTH PROFESSIONS EDUCATION
*Responding to New Realities in Medicine, Dentistry, Pharmacy, Nursing, Allied Health, and Public Health*
by Christine H. McGuire, Richard P. Foley, Alan Gorr, Ronald W. Richards, and Associates

Copyright © 1983 by: Jossey-Bass Inc., Publishers
433 California Street
San Francisco, California 94104

&

Jossey-Bass Limited
28 Banner Street
London EC1Y 8QE

**Library of Congress Cataloging in Publication Data**

Main entry under title:

Handbook of health professions education.

  Includes bibliographies and indexes.
  1. Medical education.   2. Paramedical education.
I. McGuire, Christine H.
R735.H28    1983        610'.7'11        83-48160
ISBN 0-87589-579-4

Manufactured in the United States of America

The paper in this book meets the guidelines for permanence and durability of the Committee on Production Guidelines for Book Longevity of the Council on Library Resources.

JACKET DESIGN BY WILLI BAUM

FIRST EDITION

*Code 8326*

*A joint publication in*
The Jossey-Bass
Higher Education Series
*and*
The Jossey-Bass
Health Series

to

GEORGE E. MILLER, M.D.

physician, pioneer, scholar, provocateur,
scientist, builder, teacher

who inspired this work,
its author-editors,
many of its contributors,
and an entire generation
of health professions
educators around the globe

# Contents

# Tables

## Chapter 13

## Part Three

## Chapter 18

# Figures

# Preface

Some three years ago, a small group of faculty from the Center for Educational Development, at what was then called the University of Illinois at the Medical Center, invited a few colleagues from the professional colleges on that campus to join with them in planning a conference on health professions education. The conference was to be the center's contribution to the celebration of the one hundredth anniversary of the founding of the University of Illinois College of Medicine. As such, the initiating group—who subsequently became the author-editors of this *Handbook*—thought it fitting that the conference be dedicated to Dr. George E. Miller—founder of the center, pioneer in the science of medical education, peripatetic scholar, and visionary—whose hallmark question "What is the evidence?" haunted our deliberations.

Very soon the conference planning committee found itself deeply embroiled in what amounted to a very exciting seminar on policy directions for the eighties and nineties. Not surprisingly, we found that we could not talk sense about the next decade or so in the absence of an extensive data base about the evolution of health professions education over the last decade or so, its current status, and the findings from research conducted in recent years. Since no all-inclusive summary of trends in health professions education was available and no critical integration of research findings existed, the conference committee commissioned the leading scholar in each field to prepare a comprehensive background paper on the topic of his or her expertise. Together, these papers constitute a definitive statement of where we are and what we have learned from twenty years' experience and study; they form Parts One and Two of this volume and are prerequisite to understanding the future.

In the midst of our deliberations, the total ambiance in which we were working changed dramatically: new social, political, and economic forces—of which all health professions educators were subliminally aware, but which most had refused to allow to rise to consciousness—took command of our thinking in very explicit ways. Demands of the public for readily available, high-quality care at reasonable cost were heard in every quarter; funding sources that had talked very expansively throughout the sixties and most of the seventies began to take an ever more cautious, even pessimistic, stand; as the Reagan administration began to consolidate its power, it was clear that a new philosophy would guide political decisions about support of health care and health professions education; with the Gray Panthers and other groups crying "foul," it was equally clear that the debate about public policy in the health arena would be a lengthy and heated one—there were just too many social value issues to be resolved, the most compelling of which was the absolute necessity to find a way of eliminating the nuclear threat to all humanity. Nor were the value questions made easier by other technological revolutionism, which extended the capabilities of health providers but which also placed them in the midst of every controversy about who should benefit, for how long, at what cost, to whom, from each new discovery. Once again it became apparent that no one could talk sense about future directions of health professions education without a thorough understanding and systematic analysis of the new social context in which it and its products would operate. And once again the conference planning committee commissioned the experts in each field to prepare a series of position papers on the new realities; these comprise Part Three of this *Handbook*.

Only with a clear view of what we have learned from the past and what we may expect in the future can decision makers in health professions education give responsible consideration, to programmatic alternatives. In this consideration, the expectations of the public and the constraints on academic health science centers must be reconciled in a viable program of action; that dialogue constitutes Part Four of this *Handbook*.

Thus, this *Handbook* brings together for the first time a comprehensive, critical review and analysis, by leading scholars, of all the essential elements for rational decision making. As such, we believe that it can be useful to policy makers at all levels in educational institutions, in professional associations, and in governmental agencies.

Individual faculty members of policy committees—committees on curriculum, instruction, evaluation, and examinations—and educational administrators at all ranks in schools and colleges in the health professions will find in this book a rich source of ideas for improving educational programs, an authoritative description of innovations and directions in current practice—practice with regard to admissions, curriculum, instruction, and evaluation—a critical examination of what seems to work and why, a scholarly analysis of the new context in which professional education must function, and a thoughtful agenda for required reform and for the requisite research to support that reform.

Both staff of professional associations and members of their policy groups concerned with accreditation, licensure, certification, and continuing education will find here a convenient summary of the status and direction of training in their respective fields, of the implications of that training for entry into practice and for continued learning, and of the state-of-the-art with respect to certification and educational practice.

At the federal level, legislators, their staffs, members of governmental advisory committees, and agency personnel who implement the mandates of Congress and the recommendations of public groups will find in this book a discriminating discussion of the nature and results of prior governmental initiatives and a sophisticated guide to changing conditions in health care and health manpower that require consideration in formulating new policy. Both must be understood if we are to avoid the mistakes of the past and to provide realistically for the concerns of the future.

Finally, educational researchers who now work or who plan to work in health professions settings will find in this book a comprehensive guide to the literature, a meticulous inventory of what we have learned from twenty years of experimentation and study, and an enlightened enumeration of the questions and issues that now require investigation.

All participants in the health professions educational enterprise—students, faculty, practitioners, organizations, and agencies—will need to understand the logical argument and the evidence that have led inexorably to the recommendations to be found in the final section of this book. We hope the reader will find the journey there as exhilarating as have the authors.

## Acknowledgments

The author-editors of this book are grateful to the members of our Medical Center Advisory Committee: Dr. Thomas W. Beckham, formerly dean of the College of Associated Health Professions and new vice-chancellor for Academic Affairs, Dr. Helen K. Grace, formerly dean of the College of Nursing and now program director of the W. K. Kellogg Foundation; Dr. William J. Grove, formerly vice-chancellor for academic affairs and now program director of the W. K. Kellogg Foundation; Dr. Swailem S. Hennein, professor of community health sciences of the School of Public Health; Mrs. Isabel Martin, coordinator of graduate medical education at the University of Illinois Hospital; Dr. Lawrence M. Solomon, professor and head of dermatology; and Dr. William H. Young, director of continuing education and public service. Their cogent advice and stimulating participation in the on-going conference and seminar on health professions education that preceded the preparation of this volume were crucial in shaping the outcomes of our deliberations.

Nor was the assistance we received limited to the boundaries of our own institution. We were fortunate in being able to confer with an illustrious National Advisory Committee composed of Dr. Arthur S. Elstein, professor of medical education at Michigan State University; Dr. John G. Freymann, president of the National Fund for Medical Education; Dr. Tamas Fülöp, director of health manpower development of the World Health Organization; Dr. Alfred Gelhorn, visiting professor of health policy and management of the Harvard University School of Public Health; Dr. Hilliard Jason, director of the National Center for Faculty Development; Dr. Robert Knouss, formerly Staff of the U.S. Senate Committee on Labor and Human Resources; and Dr. Victor Neufeld, chairman of the M.D. program at McMaster University. To all of these, we are indebted for their forward-looking contributions and challenging reactions to our recommendations that are embodied in the portrayal of the future to be found in this text.

We are also grateful to our many colleagues from across the country—including especially the numerous panelists, small-group leaders, and rapporteurs—who joined with us in an intense three-day discussion of the new realities and their implications for health professions education that has contributed so greatly to our formulation of the issues and the alternatives.

Finally, without the skilled and creative support of Jane Whitener, director of conferences and institutes, and her dedicated assistants, and of Gladys Khan, administrative secretary of the Center for Educational Development, and her expert associates, this ambitious project could never have come to fruition.

*Chicago, Illinois*　　　　　　　　　　　　　　　　　Christine H. McGuire
*September 1983*　　　　　　　　　　　　　　　　　　　Richard P. Foley
　　　　　　　　　　　　　　　　　　　　　　　　　　　Alan Gorr
　　　　　　　　　　　　　　　　　　　　　　　　Ronald W. Richards

# The Authors

CHRISTINE H. McGUIRE is professor of health professions education in the Center for Educational Development at the Health Sciences Center of the University of Illinois at Chicago, where she has been a member of the faculty since 1961. She received the B.A. degree (1937) in literature from Muskingum College and the M.A. degree (1938) in education from Ohio State University. Subsequently (1938–1941), she did postgraduate study in economics at the University of Chicago, where she was member of the economics faculty from 1941 to 1961 and also chief examiner in social sciences from 1946 to 1961. She has served as consultant to a number of health professions educational institutions, professional associations, and governmental agencies both here and abroad and is currently consultant to the Division of Health Manpower of the World Health Organization. She was national chairman of the Group on Medical Education of the Association of American Medical Colleges (1974–1975), president of the National Council on Measurement in Education (1975–1976), and vice-president for education in the professions of the American Educational Research Association (1981–1983). She is a current or recent member of the editorial boards of a number of educational journals in the health professions.

Author or coauthor of several books and numerous articles on evaluation in health professions education, McGuire is perhaps best known for *Construction and Use of Written Simulations* (with Solomon and Bashook, 1976) and *Clinical Simulations—Problems in Patient Management* (with Solomon, 1971). Her current interests include continuing research on simulation in the evaluation of professional competence, program evaluation, and cross-national study of the relations between national health priorities and health manpower development.

RICHARD P. FOLEY is associate professor of health professions education and associate director for educational programs in the Center for Educational Development at the Health Sciences Center of the University of Illinois at Chicago. He received the B.A. degree (1965) in history from Roosevelt University and the Ph.D. degree (1976) in education from the University of Chicago.

Foley's main research activities have been in faculty development and educational degree programs for health professionals. As a result of his interest in improving the instructional skills of health professionals, he has developed a national and international reputation as a consultant on faculty development and has worked with the American Medical Association, the American Medical Record Association, the Medical Library Association, the American Psychiatric Association, and the World Health Organization. His experiences with these organizations led to his book, *Teaching Techniques: A Handbook for Health Professionals* (with J. Smilansky, 1980).

ALAN GORR is assistant professor of health professions education in the Center for Educational Development and assistant professor of health resources management in the School of Public Health at the Health Sciences Center of the University of Illinois at Chicago. He received the B.A. degree (1964) in philosophy from the University of Iowa, the M.A. degree (1967) in medieval studies from the University of Toronto, the Ph.D. degree (1971) in social foundations of education from the University of Iowa, and the M.P.H. degree (1977) from the University of Illinois.

Gorr's research efforts have centered on the relationship of curriculum to larger philosophical and social concerns. He is the editor of two volumes, *The School in the Social Setting* (1979) and *Problems in Today's Education* (1975). His current interests include public health education and development of curriculum materials for problem-based medical education.

RONALD W. RICHARDS is professor of health professions education and director of the Center for Educational Development at the Health Sciences Center of the University of Illinois at Chicago. He received the B.A. degree (1963) in political science from Miami University and the M.A. degree (1965) in education and the Ph.D. degree (1968) in higher education from Michigan State University.

Richards has concentrated on organization and management of health professions education, curriculum development, and primary care education. He has directed training programs for professionals interested in careers in medical education and serves as educational and management consultant to medical schools, professional associations, and international agencies.

Prior to joining the Center for Educational Development, Richards was the founding director of Michigan State University's Upper Peninsula Medical Education Program, a regionally based program whose goals included designing and implementing an undergraduate and graduate primary care curriculum through creating ambulatory-patient care/teaching centers at which students learn most of the basic sciences and clinical medicine. While at Michigan State he was also director of the Office of Medical Education Research and Development and professor of medical education.

WILLIAM E. BROWN, D.D.S., M.S., is dean of the University of Oklahoma College of Dentistry, Oklahoma City.

Margaret M. Bussigel, Dr. paed., is assistant professor of health professions education in the Center for Educational Development at the Health Sciences Center, University of Illinois at Chicago.

Richard M. Caplan, M.D., is associate dean for continuing medical education at the University of Iowa College of Medicine, Iowa City.

Charles W. Ford, Ph.D., is dean of the College of Health Sciences, University of New England, Biddeford, Maine.

Tamas Fülöp, M.D., Ph.D., M.P.H., is director of health manpower development in the World Health Organization, Geneva, Switzerland.

Helen K. Grace, R.N., Ph.D., F.A.A.N., is program director at the W. K. Kellogg Foundation, Battle Creek, Michigan.

Jack Hadley, Ph.D., is senior research associate at the Urban Institute, Washington, D.C.

Herbert E. Klarman, Ph.D., is professor emeritus of economics in the Graduate School of Public Administration, New York University, New York.

Milton Kotelchuck, Ph.D., M.P.H., is assistant professor of health policy in the Department of Social Medicine and Health Policy at Harvard Medical School and research associate at Children's Hospital Medical Center, Boston, Massachusetts.

August P. Lemberger, Ph.D., is dean and professor of pharmacy, the School of Pharmacy, University of Wisconsin at Madison.

Russell G. Mawby, Ph.D., is chairman and chief executive officer at the W. K. Kellogg Foundation, Battle Creek, Michigan.

Duncan Neuhauser, Ph.D., is professor of epidemiology and community health at Case Western Reserve University, Cleveland, Ohio.

Edmund D. Pellegrino, M.D., is John Carroll Professor of Medicine and Medical Humanities at Georgetown University Medical Center, Washington, D. C.

W. Ann Reynolds, Ph.D., is chancellor of the California State University system, Long Beach, California.

Agnes G. Rezler, Ph.D., is professor of health professions education at the Health Sciences Center, University of Illinois at Chicago.

Julius B. Richmond, M.D., is professor of health policy at Harvard Medical School and adviser on child health policy at Children's Hospital Medical Center, Boston, Massachusetts.

EDWIN F. ROSINSKI, Ed.D., is professor and director of the Office of Medical Education at the University of California at San Francisco.

HOWARD G. SACHS is associate provost of the Ohio State University, Columbus.

ALEXANDER M. SCHMIDT, M.D., is vice chancellor for health affairs at the University of Illinois at Chicago.

CECIL G. SHEPS, M.D., M.P.H., is Taylor Grandy Distinguished Professor of Social Medicine and professor of epidemiology at the University of North Carolina at Chapel Hill.

CHEVES McC. SMYTHE, M.D., is dean of the Aga Khan Hospital and Medical College, Karachi, Pakistan.

FRANK T. STRITTER, Ph.D., is a professor in the schools of medicine, education, and public health and director of the Office of Research and Development for Education in the Health Professions at the University of North Carolina at Chapel Hill.

RAYMOND R. SUSKIND, M.D., is director of the Institute of Environmental Health in the College of Medicine, University of Cincinnati, Ohio.

MARJORIE PRICE WILSON, M.D., is senior associate dean in the University of Maryland School of Medicine, Baltimore.

WARREN WINKELSTEIN, JR., M.D., M.P.H., is professor of epidemiology at the University of California at Berkeley.

# Handbook
of Health Professions
Education

Responding to New Realities
in Medicine, Dentistry, Pharmacy,
Nursing, Allied Health,
and Public Health

# Part One

---

## Trends and Priorities
## in Health Professions
## Education

# Introduction:

# Pressures, Concerns,

# and Responses

# of the Professions

## Christine H. McGuire

Looking backward without benefit of the methods of scientific inquiry is merely nostalgic indulgence; looking backward utilizing the procedures of rigorous analysis is a quintessential tool of science—indispensable to understanding, forecasting, controlling, and responding to events. In this first section of the *Handbook of Health Professions Education*, looking backward entails an analysis and critique of the innovations in health professions education that took place between 1960 and 1980. The authors' assessments of our current status are presented collectively as a necessary foundation on which policy for the future may be built.

Chapter One examines the political, social, and economic context in which the educational ferment of the sixties and seventies took place. Chapters Two through Eight detail and analyze the educational initiatives that each of the health professions—medicine, dentistry, pharmacy, nursing, allied health, public health, and graduate education in health sciences centers—has undertaken over the past two decades in response to pressures for change. The section concludes with a comparison and contrast of the stimulus, nature, and significance of curricular reform during that period.

In Chapter One, Richards and Bussigel highlight the major social forces of the sixties and seventies. They not only describe the general milieu, but also identify the salient factors that were of primary significance in conditioning the responses of educators in the health professions. Among these factors, they stress the importance of the belief in the unlimited expansion of both health services and health professions education that was prevalent in the early sixties. They argue that this optimism, combined with the growing turmoil of the youth culture and the politics of equality, conditioned the social strategy that was employed to bring health professions institutions into accord with social goals. Finally, they point to the growing disillusionment with purely technological and financial responses to health needs and expectations that brought the era to a close.

As the succeeding chapters reveal, it is clear that the educational reforms introduced in the sixties and seventies in each of the professions represent a perhaps overly enthusiastic, even overly successful, response to societal pressures and incentives for unrestrained growth. Efforts to bring about this growth were characterized by frenetic activity—activity to extend research capabilities, to augment the knowledge base, to enlarge health care facilities and modify their nature, to expand the numbers and types of health professionals, to increase the heterogeneity of the groups from which they were recruited, and to obtain greater diversity in their goals and in the settings in which they practiced their professions.

Heightened potential for both cooperation and conflict in defining and implementing professional roles, and the resulting nascent intergroup conflicts are clearly delineated, especially in Grace's description of the struggle for control in nursing (Chapter Two), Ford's concern with defining the field of "allied health" (Chapter Six), Sheps's documentation of the ever expanding arena of public health (Chapter Seven), and Sachs's and Reynolds's view of graduate education in the health sciences center as a "stepchild in the promised land" (Chapter Eight).

## Common Pressures

Beyond the perennial issues of professional education—"For what?" and "Controlled by whom?"—it is clear that during the sixties and seventies prior equilibria in many of the professions were disturbed by other common factors that generated similar experiments and innovations. These factors—and the responses they elicited—are discussed in the several chapters of Part One. Among the most striking are the following:

*Federal Initiatives.* The offers of dollars from Washington as a reward for expanding student capacity and research effort impinged strikingly on all health professions education. Wilson (Chapter Two) argues convincingly that new schools, larger classes, and new staffing patterns changed the character of undergraduate education, while the increased emphasis on research created further tension between research and teaching in academic medicine. Ford (Chapter Six) laments the vulnerability to which schools of allied health are now subject as a consequence of their earlier dependence on those dollars. Sachs and Reynolds (Chapter Eight) attribute the changing administrative structures, responsibilities, and loci of control in graduate education at health sciences centers in large part to the lures of the expanding research establishment.

*The "Knowledge Explosion."* Cliché or not, the accelerating rate of expansion of knowledge and of related changes in technology since World War II has impacted heavily on all health professions education, in particular on medicine, pharmacy, and dentistry. Wilson (Chapter Two) provides graphic evidence not only of the discovery of new knowledge but also of the creation of completely new and "hyphenated disciplines" that must somehow be accommodated in the medi-

cal curriculum and that have caused major realignments in the relative
significance of older disciplines. Lemberger (Chapter Four) argues that the post–
World War II revolution in our knowledge of drugs and their synthesis created the
pharmaceutical industry and changed forever the role of the pharmacist. Brown
(Chapter Three) regards the "overcrowding" of the dental curriculum, consequent
on the expanding knowledge base, as an urgent problem that must be addressed.

*The Settings of Professional Education.* Unlike medicine, dentistry, and
pharmacy for which all professional training occurs in a dedicated professional
school, training in nursing, allied health, and public health may take place in a
variety of settings. The first degree for nurses may be obtained in a hospital or in
an academic setting, and the length and nature of the program leading to entry
level varies considerably depending on the locus of training and the degree
awarded. According to Grace (Chapter Five) this creates serious problems in the
nursing profession, which are further compounded by separations between academia and practice. Ford (Chapter Six) reviews the history of on-the-job training in
allied health and compares the nature and prospects of current professional programs offered in a health science center with those offered in community colleges,
where many different kinds of affiliations must be undertaken to provide clinical
experience. Sheps (Chapter Seven) speaks feelingly of the situation in public
health, where a vast proportion of professional preparation occurs in academic
settings other than schools of public health. He makes clear that the problems
arising from this diversity in training settings are exacerbated by the heated debate
surrounding the role of field experience in any type of program.

*The Proliferation of Higher Degrees.* Sachs and Reynolds (Chapter Eight)
note that the greatly increased prestige of and opportunity for careers in research
in the biomedical sciences have stimulated the creation and expansion of new
graduate programs—both professional and research degree programs—at health
science centers across the country. They add that most of these programs were
engrafted onto existing structures with inadequate regard for the underlying nature of the basic organism, and all bring with them problems of control. Grace
(Chapter Five) poses the dilemma for nursing as a matter of higher education
versus apprentice training. She insists on the need to increase the numbers of
doctorally prepared nurses who are capable of conducting research in the discipline of nursing. Lemberger (Chapter Four) cites the debate within the pharmacy
profession surrounding the Doctor of Pharmacy degree and the difficulties that
program poses in accreditation. Ford (Chapter Six) alludes to the need for creating
opportunities for persons in allied health to obtain higher degrees in their fields,
and Sachs and Reynolds (Chapter Eight) point out the consequent problems with
regard to graduate faculty recruitment and status. Sheps (Chapter Seven) notes the
many different kinds and levels of degree programs in public health and raises
questions about the possibility of their integration into any coherent system.

In the absence of a clear rationale for the creation of new higher degrees—
especially research degrees—in the health professions some cynics argue that such
programs may, in fact, represent merely a response to pressure for increased status,
which will result in "over-professionalization" to a degree that threatens the
quality and availability of health care. Whether or not readers concur with this
particular criticism, they will recognize that the justifications for new degrees
offered by some of the authors in Part One reveal three important attitudes:

(1) continuing competition for control among members of the health care team, (2) ambivalence toward and even frustration with direct patient care in some professions, and (3) a failure to define the roles and functions of health personnel at a level that permits the society to project manpower needs and that enables educational planners to identify program goals.

Finally, Sachs and Reynolds (Chapter Eight) make it abundantly clear that the proliferation of higher degrees in all areas requires experimentation with new programs, demands extensive development of faculty and research resources, raises questions of both cost and quality, and creates problems of administration and control. And as many of the authors in Part One imply, the creation of new degrees revives the never ending argument about practice versus research orientations in the faculty and the role of research and research training in preparation for practice.

*Demands for Assuring Continued Competence.* Problems related to the responsibility of the professions and of academic health centers for assuring the continued competence of health practitioners are noted by virtually all the authors in Part One. Brown (Chapter Three) observes that in dentistry, as in most of the health professions, "once licensed, always licensed." He concludes that no satisfactory program for continuing education has yet been developed by professional schools. His challenging recommendations to remedy this situation are instructive for all professions. Wilson (Chapter Two) sees the development of the skills and motivation for lifetime learning as a major objective of undergraduate medical education. Sheps (Chapter Seven) argues that the universities should assume primary responsibility for continuing education.

## Academia's Response

Educational institutions in all of the health professions responded to the altered social priorities, the changing social and economic conditions of the sixties and seventies, and their own internal concerns by expanding their facilities for training health professionals. Despite the ensuing difficulties, that was in some ways the least significant of their responses. Perhaps of greater import in the long run were those responses that entailed changes in admission policies; modifications in instructional and evaluation methodologies; introduction of new subjects into programs; initiation of large curricular "experiments"; establishment of liaisons with ambulatory care centers, community hospitals, and other new instructional settings; creation of local units dedicated to educational research and development; and indulgence in a flurry of faculty development efforts to prepare researchers and clinicians to perform their educational roles more effectively.

The following are illustrative of the many innovations in each of the professions, as reported by the authors in Part One:

- The establishment of admissions programs designed to encourage and support minority enrollments
- Experimentation with modifications in the length of the programs for the professional degree and, in the case of medicine, integration of the professional degree program with preprofessional training and/or research training
- Greater use of educational objectives and introduction of competency-based programs

- Development of new areas of specialization and introduction of alternate tracks at the undergraduate level
- Earlier introduction to clinical experience and greater integration of the basic and clinical disciplines
- Development of problem-based or other forms of integrated rather than discipline-oriented curricula
- Reduction in laboratory experience and inclusion of the humanities and the social and behavioral sciences, either in professional training and/or in general education prerequisites
- Employment of more varied learning systems and instructional formats, including self-study, self-assessment, independent study, small-group discussion, expanded use of audiovisual aids, and introduction of new media, such as simulation and closed-circuit television
- Establishment of community-based and/or community-oriented programs combined with a generally greater emphasis on primary care

Though the exact form innovations took in different fields and institutions varied, the experiments and experience in each of them are instructive to all. What is notably absent, however, as Rosinski (Chapter Nine) forcibly points out, is any systematic attempt to evaluate the efficacy of these newer interventions in professional education. He adds that it is not clear whether failure to provide evidence on their value facilitated or inhibited innovation and encouraged or discouraged its more general adoption. In comparing and contrasting curricular reform in the several health professions, Rosinski argues persuasively that certain general trends affected all fields: First was the period of unbridled growth and rampant experimentation. This was followed by the emergence of various pressure groups—governmental, student, faculty, philanthropic, consumer and other interests—who lobbied for their own, often competing, reforms. Later curricular modification reflected a confluence of these forces, and "reform" in the late seventies could best be characterized as "accretion through cumulative additions of specific courses and activities." Rosinski's stimulating comparative analysis of the responses of the professions to this changing ambiance provides the basis for serious speculation about the direction which curriculum development and research can and should take in the future.

## Unique Concerns and Responses

While these were the general responses to the pressures of the times in which schools in all the health professions participated to some degree, priorities for reform during the sixties and seventies varied from one profession to another, depending on the unique constellation of concerns that characterized each. For the most part, medicine and dentistry, as reported by Wilson (Chapter Two) and Brown (Chapter Three), were expanding and were introducing curricular and instructional changes in response to student unrest on the one hand and to the growth of knowledge and technology on the other. Both were doing so in the context of a stable concept of the role and functions of the practitioners they trained. Educational reforms in these professions reflect only relatively minor modifications in practice (such as the use of flouride in dentistry and CT scanners in medicine); the reforms reveal no underlying concern or doubt about the basic nature of the profession, no anxiety about its status in or contribution to society, and no pressure for its fundamental restructuring.

In contrast, debate and reforms in both nursing and pharmacy education, as reported by Grace (Chapter Five) and Lemberger (Chapter Four), reflect not only deep discontent with the traditional role and status of practitioners but also increasingly urgent demands for more and different responsibilities that might ultimately require fundamental changes in the nature of the profession and the relations of its practitioners to other health professionals. As noted earlier, Grace argues for more academic preparation of nurses to "elevate" them from patient care into administrative and research roles; Lemberger urges expansion of the preparation of pharmacists to assume a newly developing clinical role and deep cutbacks in training for the traditional dispensing role; both authors envisage a restructuring of the health care team.

Still other concerns characterized the fields of allied health and public health, both of which appeared to be searching for an identity that would give unity to programs preparing individuals of diverse background and experience for highly disparate roles. Ford (Chapter Six) describes the problems of unifying what is actually a group of professions ranging from those with clear patient care responsibilities (such as occupational therapy) to those quite remote from the clinical setting (such as medical laboratory sciences). Sheps (Chapter Seven) limns a dramatic picture of almost revolutionary change in the nature of public health responsibilities, incredible diversity in the levels and functions for which individuals are trained and in the settings in which they practice their profession, increasing complexity and extreme variation in their interprofessional relations—all complicated by the heterogeneity of their students. As he observes, public health, unlike any of the other health professions, accepts students whose prior preparation ranges from an A.B. or B.S. program to a professional or graduate research degree and/or years of professional experience in any one of a number of possible fields. These dissimilar individuals—again unlike the situation in other health professions—do not enroll in a single standard program but pursue assorted programs preparing them for the multifaceted roles comprising the field of public health.

Finally, in the view of Sachs and Reynolds (Chapter Eight), the primary concerns facing graduate colleges in health sciences centers revolve around issues of administrative structure and organization, allocation of responsibility for and control of programs, and generation of funds and faculty to support them.

### Coda

Though there are special concerns and reactions to pressures that differ significantly among the several health professions, the experiences and responses of each, as described in Chapters Two through Nine, are instructive to all; and the problems and solutions of all must be understood by educators in each, if there is to be any hope of developing a coherent health care delivery system and a set of appropriate educational programs to support it. Comparison and contrast of developments, and assessments of current status in the several professions, can provide a sound platform from which we will be able to plan the future more rationally. Past innovation has, for the most part, been limited to manipulations of curricular content and of structural components of programs; there are far too few examples of basic rethinking and redesign of programs to bring them into better alignment with today's needs. What is required in planning for the future is, as Rosinski urges in Chapter Nine, to redefine our institutional objectives, to relate them more directly to the needs of society and the new roles of practitioners, to involve faculty more completely in change, and to evaluate the efficiency, effectiveness, and relevance of evolving educational programs.

*Ronald W. Richards*
*Margaret M. Bussigel*

# 1

# Adapting to Changing Social, Economic, and Political Conditions

Looking back on the 1960s frequently evokes a strong emotion in those who lived through it. The sixties was a period of turmoil, growth, and change, which at the time seemed to be shaping the future much more strongly than had other decades. The sixties seemed to be something special. Attempting to identify accurately, however, what that "something special" was is difficult. It was, for example, during this decade that significant civil rights legislation was passed, the first student uprisings took place, the Vietnam War reached its greatest escalation, Americans went to the moon, science became king, a great society was envisioned, medical coverage for the aged and the poor was legislatively ensured, scholastic aptitude test scores peaked, and the popularity of the Beatles spread throughout the world. The pattern of events was diverse, but for all the diversity there was one characteristic which seemed to epitomize the period—a near limitless confidence in the ability of the country to assure individuals equal opportunity in the pursuit of society's tangible and intangible riches.

The sixties was a decade of heightened perception on the part of both mainstream and minority Americans of the inequalities implicit in our social system. As the general wealth of the nation increased, so too did the hope that it was possible to afford all Americans equal access to the increasing luxuries and privileges, whether they be material goods, educational achievement, or health and well-being. The concept of equality was expanded considerably during this time to include equal access not only to material goods but also to a set of indefinable intangibles that determine the "quality of life." As a result of such changing attitudes, the sixties became a period of noteworthy social reform in the United States.

## Social Reform in the United States

The social reform of the 1960s followed a long-established pattern in the United States, in which both the goals and strategies are conservative in character. Neither revolutionary clashes between social classes to accomplish redistribution of power, wealth, and privilege nor socialist approaches entailing the replacement of private with governmental ownership of the means of production have received wide support. Social reform in the United States has been influenced by characteristic American enthusiasm and optimism. The basic political, economic, and social structures have been regarded as fundamentally sound, their weaknesses viewed as rectifiable within the existing system. But serious weaknesses were perceived by the social reformers of the sixties. In Goldman's words, "the reformer saw his problem as that of a country in which great extremes of wealth were the pattern, . . . and farmers, industrial workers, and the minorities were the gravely depressed groups" (Goldman, 1960, p. 334).

The predominant strategy for social change has been to call upon government to make a basically sound system work better. Over the years, it has become increasingly accepted that government can be a primary means for extending the opportunities of the American system to a larger number of people. Yet, with characteristic conservative leanings, the use of government, particularly the use of centralized federal government, is seen not as a replacement for capitalism but as a way of preserving and making capitalism work to the benefit of a larger proportion of society.

The political party system in the United States plays a part in shaping the basically conservative character of social reform. American political parties are pragmatic rather than ideological; they are local grass roots rather than national phenomena (Rossiter, 1960). They have but one objective—to win elections. White (1982) underscores the influence of the Democratic party in the social reform movement of the fifties, sixties, and seventies through its support for the enfranchisement of the disenfranchised. Motivated to win elections, Democrats sought to obtain the votes of a growing number of urban blacks migrating to northern cities from the South. This movement of blacks into the Democratic party provided incentive for the creation of federal social programs aimed at the needs of blacks and other minorities. In such ways, political parties in the United States tend to make the system adaptable and responsive. However, the local rather than national character of those parties limits modern social reform in the United States. Although the Democratic party has seen the federal government as an essential vehicle for accomplishing its reform purposes, the party's local character has tempered the nature and extent of governmental intervention.

As noted previously, the goal of social reform during the 1960s was to provide equal access for all members of society to material and nonmaterial riches. The causes of existing inequities were regarded as isolated social pathologies that led to poverty and discrimination by race, ethnic origin, or sex. It followed that the goal should be achieved by attacking those social pathologies using the existing structures of a fundamentally healthy system. Within this generally conservative framework, the government role took several forms. Legislation was passed declaring discriminatory practices to be illegal, and the federal government was empowered to prosecute offenders. The judiciary reviewed laws in light of modified interpretations of the U.S. Constitution. The government created new agencies for providing a myriad of social, educational, and economic services. Rules and regulations were promulgated to influence the way the transactional processes of the social system occurred. The existing systems were expanded, thereby making them able to serve large numbers of society's members. To some degree, all of these strategies demonstrated two dominant themes: the allocation of money to under-privileged individuals and organizations (allocative policies) and the withholding of money unless regulatory rules were followed (restrictive policies).

American faith in finding technological solutions to problems influenced the allocative strategy employed by the federal government. Those social pathologies that were seen to be inhibiting the extension of equal access were regarded as challenges to be overcome in the same manner that technological wizardry put spacecraft on the moon and nuclear weaponry under the ocean. Solving social problems called for social engineering. This implied a process in which barriers to equal opportunity were identified, and universities were called upon to conduct research, create solutions, and educate new professionals skilled in dealing with the problems at hand. Examples of programs resulting from this process are abundant. The programs addressed educational, health, and economic problems but failed to attack their roots. Landmark legislation such as the Civil Rights Act of 1964, for example, was frequently reduced to such simplistic forms of imple-mentation as the transfer of black children to better-equipped, formerly all-white schools. Similarly, the objectives of the Great Society were translated into build-ing new highways in Appalachia and new housing projects in New York.

In the late sixties and early seventies, the allocative approach to social reform was supplemented by a restrictive strategy. There were two reasons for this. In the early phases of the Great Society program there was government money to be spent and little hard data on what worked and what did not. Thus, almost any good idea—and some not-so-good ones—was supported. With experience and the expectation that government be somewhat accountable for results, guidelines, criteria, and outcome measures naturally followed. Another reason for the emer-gence of the restrictive approach was that by the late 1960s and early 1970s social services systems—be they education, welfare, or health care—had become heavily dependent on federal support. Under these circumstances, the government could influence behavior by threatening to withhold funding. The carrot approach—the government will make funds available if something desired by the government is done, was followed by the stick approach—the government will take funds away if something desired by the government is not done. Schools would not receive federal funds, for example, unless their affirmative action plans met governmental approval. Contractors would not receive the bid on government jobs unless they met certain minority employment quotas. Hospitals would not be reimbursed for computerized axial tonometry equipment unless the purchase had been approved by various health planning agencies. What began as a movement to extend oppor-tunity to all by expenditures of government funds turned restrictive.

However, both the allocative and restrictive techniques with which the federal government attempted to exert influence upon public policies came under increasing criticism during the 1970s because of their ineffectiveness and costli-ness. The reform strategies were aimed at decreasing the disparities in American society. Yet, in spite of governmental activities, the median income of black families in 1969 was still only 63 percent of white families' median income, up from 53 percent in 1960. Between 1960 and 1970 the ratio of black to white male unemployment rose from 1.83 to 1.97. During the same period, the ratio of teenage black to teenage white unemployment rose from 2.57 to 5.70 (U.S. Commission on Civil Rights, 1978, pp. 49, 30, 32). The reformers may have been sincere in their intentions, but their results were clearly unsatisfactory. Compounding the problem of ineffectiveness were changes on the economic front. During the 1960s there was broad-based public and political consensus not only that the federal government should move in new directions but also that the country could afford the financial cost. While the economic growth pattern of the sixties was capable of supporting an allocative strategy, seeds were sown that made major contributions to the economic decline of the following decade.

A few indicators of economic trends in the United States pertaining to health care and education demonstrate this relationship. Until the 1960s, the per capita growth in national health expenditures in the United States remained approximately in pace with the increase in the gross national product (GNP); between 1940 and 1960 the GNP increased by a factor of 5.1, from $100 billion to $506 billion, and per capita national health expenditures rose by a factor of 4.9, from $29.62 to $146.30. The rise from $4 billion to $26 billion in absolute health expenditures was somewhat sharper, so that the nation's health bill rose from 4 percent of the GNP in 1940 to 5.3 percent twenty years later. It took only ten more years, the sixties, to increase the portion of GNP expended on health to an impressive 7.6 percent, and by 1975 the figure had risen to 9 percent. The growth in GNP and in national health expenditures had clearly become out of step. By 1979, the GNP was 4.7 times larger than in 1960. National health expenditures had, however, increased much more rapidly, by a factor of 7.9, to some $212.2 billion or $942.94 per capita. Such changes in economic growth and expenditures were not limited to health. Costs for education, another sector receiving considerable federal interest, rose from 5.6 percent of the GNP in 1961 to 7.8 percent in 1971. During the 1970s, the perception grew that expenditures for social services were outstripping the nation's capacity to pay for them.

Thus, it was in a time of economic growth and overall prosperity that the extension of equal opportunity to pursue the riches of the nation became the goal of social reform. The federal government entered sectors that had previously been regarded as almost exclusively the domains of private interests or local government. In doing so, it chose strategies based on the belief in existing structures, in equality through social engineering, and in economic expansion. New professions were created and existing ones expanded in what has been called the professionalization of reform. This is nowhere more apparent than in the health sector, where the federal government had been content to play a relatively minor financial, non-decision-making role until the mid-1960s.

### Reform in the Health Sector

The massive health legislation passed by Congress in the mid-sixties, most notably the provision of Medicare and Medicaid, abruptly ended the minimal role of the federal government in health care. "The historical significance of what (the Eighty-ninth) Congress did will not be found in the details of the twenty-three laws it passed relating to health, but in the fact that this legislation taken in total established health care as a civil right and a matter of public policy" (Freymann, 1974, p. 103). As in other sectors, the heightened awareness of inequality and the new belief that equal access to a high quality of life was each individual's right motivated a major reform response. The resources made available to the existing system of health care increased without extensive prior review of the ability of that system to create the desired qualitative change in health care delivery. Instead of creating a new health care system capable of responding to tangible and intangible needs of modern society, the allocative strategy of reform served to entrench the traditional system of fragmented care. What happened in the health care sector is not a distinctive phenomenon; rather it is a microcosm of the American political system—a panoply of lobbying groups striking compromises that advance their self-interest. The influence of the health care lobbyists took the sharp edges off the reform proposals that might otherwise have restructured existing systems, and turned them to the advantage of the health care industry.

The growing consensus for governmental intervention on behalf of equal opportunity coincided with unparalleled public endorsement of the benefits of science. The counterpoint of social engineering at the general policy level for the Great Society was the scientification of medical care. Former Surgeon General Shannon claims that "the period 1945-1965 . . . will be viewed in retrospect as the time when U.S. science reached the summit of broad uncritical public support— what might be called the 'Augustan era' of American success" (Shannon, 1969, p. 770). One of the clearest indicators of this trend was the enormous growth of the National Institutes of Health (NIH) whose postwar budget increased rapidly, reaching $430 million in 1960 and more than doubling to $1 billion in 1965. A large portion of these funds supported medical research projects conducted outside of the NIH, most commonly in academic health centers. This provided financial incentives for basic biological and clinical research and lent further support to a traditional, Cartesian approach to medical science. Thus, the tendency to divide the human body into more and more specialized parts for the purposes of research contrasted sharply with the parallel demands for more primary care and a more holistic approach to health problems.

During the sixties, technological solutions coexisted uncomfortably with humanitarian concerns. By the 1970s technological inclinations and humanistic values spawned what Fox has called the medicalization of American society, placing upon medicine the responsibility to pay less homage to science and more to humanity: "The medicalization process entails the assertion of various individual and collective rights to which members of the society feel entitled and which they express as 'health,' 'quality of life,' and 'quality of death.' The process also involves heightened awareness of a whole range of imperfections, injustices, dangers, and afflictions that are perceived to exist in the society; a protest against them; and a resolve to take action that is more therapeutic than primitive" (Fox, 1977, p. 14). Yet, the attention paid by medicine to social ills was uneasy, for social problems were generally regarded as pathologies to be dealt with in the same way as acute illnesses—that is, through specialization and a curative focus. Thus, many of the social problems in the health sector were labeled and treated like biological malfunctions. Drug abuse, school behavioral problems, inability to keep a job, and even excessive gambling were medicalized for attention by an enlarged health care team within a health care delivery system which had experienced little structural change—again, a costly experiment in social engineering.

Data on government expenditures in the health sector furnish an interesting description of governmental activities in the sixties. In 1960, when the nation's health care bill was only $26.9 billion, private sources accounted for 75.3 percent of these expenditures. The public sector contributed only $6.6 billion, or 24.7 percent of the total bill. The public contribution rose slightly to 26.1 percent of total expenditures in 1965, and then zoomed up to 37.1 percent and $27.8 billion in 1970 (U.S. Department of Health and Human Services, 1980, p. 211). Two trends were occurring simultaneously, and, in fact, reinforcing each other: first, total health expenditures were rising at a very rapid rate; second, the public sector was becoming increasingly responsible for financing health expenses. But where did this increased funding go? The answer seems to be: mostly where it had always gone—there was just more of it. Medicare offers an excellent example of this generalization. Public per capita health expenditures for persons 65 and over rose from $142 in 1965 to $523 in 1970 and $1,047 in 1976. The proportion of these public expenditures going toward hospital care remained, however, virtually the same (approximately 60 percent) from 1965 to 1976 (U.S. Department of Health and Human Services, 1980, Table 73). So, while the per capita outlay of funds increased tremendously after the Medicare legislation, there seems to have been relatively little effect on the structure of the health care system serving the aged. Despite the special needs of this group, the funding emphasis remained on acute care in the hospital setting.

Whether or not it can be attributed to federal spending strategies, there was certainly a sharp increase in the consumer price index (CPI) for medical care, and particularly for hospital care after 1965. Clearly, rising costs in the medical care sector made a significant contribution to the generally high inflation rate the nation started to experience at this time. Between 1965 and 1970, the consumer price for medical care rose considerably more rapidly (34.7 percent)* than it did for all items together (23.1 percent) (U.S. Department of Health and Human Services, 1980, Table 73). To a large extent, the increases in the cost of medical care reflect the fact that the service sector in general began to become relatively more expensive than nonservice products during the 1960s. The distribution of CPI increases within the medical care sector is, therefore, probably of somewhat more interest to our analysis. Table 1 indicates that hospital costs had, indeed, been increasing more rapidly than other medical care costs even before 1965, but the period from 1965 to 1970 was significant for a number of reasons: (1) The CPI for a hospital room rose by an incredible 91.7 percent. Unlike other medical services, the rate of increase in the costs of a hospital room peaked between 1965 and 1970, remaining high but nonetheless declining after 1970. (2) Based on a CPI = 100 for 1967, the costs of a hospital room overtook the costs of other medical care services for the first time between 1965 and 1970. While it is clear that hospital costs would have increased rapidly in any case during the sixties and seventies, the analysis also indicates that, given the emphasis on hospital care in federal expenditures, simultaneously rising hospital costs consumed a large portion of the increased funding

---

*This figure reflects the change in combined costs of medical care services and medical care commodities.

Table 1. Consumer Price Index (1967 = 100) for All Medical Care Services,
Physician Services, and Hospital Room, 1960-1979.

| Service | 1960 | 1965 | 1970 | 1975 | 1979 | % Change | | | |
| | | | | | | 1960–1965 | 1965–1970 | 1970–1975 | 1975–1979 |
|---|---|---|---|---|---|---|---|---|---|
| All Medical Care Services | 74.9 | 87.3 | 124.2 | 179.1 | 258.3 | 16.6 | 42.3 | 44.2 | 44.3 |
| Physician Services | 77.0 | 88.3 | 121.4 | 169.4 | 245.5 | 14.7 | 37.5 | 39.5 | 44.9 |
| Hospital Room | 57.3 | 75.9 | 145.4 | 236.1 | 368.2 | 32.5 | 91.7 | 62.4 | 56.0 |

Source: Based on Table 63, U.S. Department of Health and Human Services, 1980.

without changing quality of care. The extent to which the increased funding provoked the increased costs remains a matter for debate.

The evidence shows that reform in the health sector followed the general pattern of reform based on social engineering strategies. The goal was equal access to health care for all people regardless of their ability to pay. A dual-class system of health care was to be replaced by a one-class system with the government paying the bill for the elderly and the poor. Our economic wealth was considered sufficient to expand the health care system at governmental expense.

In addition to paying the costs of health care delivery, the government supported the continuation of a traditional, Cartesian approach to progress in the medical sciences through its system of research funding. The storehouse of new knowledge produced by the massive, government-funded, basic biological research effort begun in the 1950s was to be integrated into the health care system in order to improve health and limit the consequences of illness. The outcome of this frenzy of governmental activity has been a larger, more costly, but fundamentally unchanged system for delivering health care. Whether society is healthier or, more modestly, whether health care is now more accessible to all remains a matter for debate. The evidence suggests, however, that whatever the benefits, the public is now convinced that we cannot afford the cost.

## Health Professions Education

The American inclination to professionalize reform led to the expansion of health professions schools and to the creation of new kinds of health professionals. More physicians, nurses, dentists, occupational therapists, pharmacists, public health workers, and others were needed if health care was to be more readily available to all individuals. In addition to quantitative manpower needs, it was determined that the benefits of scientific research in such areas as heart disease, cancer, and stroke should be disseminated through educational programs for practitioners. The strategies employed to provide society with more health professionals followed the dominant reform pattern of expanding existing schools, creating similar new schools, and applying new educational technology and expertise to the teaching/learning process.

Federal funds were made available not only to increase enrollment in health professions schools but also to support innovation in educational approaches. New schools were created with a wide variation in curricular patterns. In many programs a significant proportion of the students' training occurred in community hospitals where education and research functions are secondary to patient care. Students were given a greater degree of responsibility for their own learning through such innovations as early introduction to clinical work, more integrated teaching of biological sciences, considerable improvement in the systems by which students and programs were evaluated, a greater proportion of the total curriculum devoted to elective experiences, and independent study programs. Some curricular changes mirrored the societal interest in improving the quality of life. Courses such as Man and Society, Introduction to Behavioral Sciences, and the Social Context of Health Care found their way into the curricula of health sciences schools. One of the outgrowths of the expansionary period was national and international interest in applying the theories and research findings on teaching and learning to the process of educating health professionals. Units for educational research and development were established in many medical schools, as well as in some of the other health professions schools. This emergence of experts in the education of health professionals is consistent with the general pattern of applying science and technology to the solution of social problems and of the professionalization of reform.

Two factors, however, markedly limited educational innovation in health professions education during the 1960s and 1970s: (1) the subspecialization of basic science research and patient care services and (2) the character of the health care delivery system itself. Basic science research produced an ever-expanding body of scientific knowledge of different types that the faculty felt students needed to know. Humanistic inclinations and a social responsiveness had to contend with academe's formidable enthusiasm for biophysical, scientific views of medicine. In addition, federal support for health care through Medicare and Medicaid dramatically expanded the existing system with its primary orientation toward hospital care of episodic illness. Neighborhood health centers or rural clinics, for example, never entered the system's mainstream.

As in other policy areas, allocative strategies for expanding health professions education were followed by regulatory ones. Because government funds were freely available for expansion in the sixties, federal support came to represent a significant percentage of the operating budget of health professions schools, thereby increasing the government's influence enormously. In the 1970s, the government began to exercise its power by attaching more conditions to its funds. The early general goal of increasing the number of health practitioners evolved into such specific targeted programs as promotion of training for primary care practitioners for underserved rural and urban areas. In medicine, for example, it became necessary for a school to demonstrate that a certain percentage of its graduates chose primary care types of residency programs in order to remain eligible for government support.

By its appointment in 1970 of the Carnegie Commission on Higher Education, the Carnegie Foundation gave credence to the directions in which public policies were driving health professions education, much as it had in 1910 with its support of the Flexner study. The 1970 Carnegie Commission's report specified four components for better health care: "more and better health manpower; more and better health care facilities; better financing arrangements for the health care of the population; better planning for health manpower and health care delivery." Its objectives found their way into federal legislation when the Comprehensive Health Manpower Training Act of 1971 became law.

In a remarkably short period of time, however, the political consensus that brought about government support for health professions education began to come apart. For example, by 1974 the support for teacher training, initiated in the legislation of 1965 establishing Regional Medical Programs and supported in the Comprehensive Health Manpower Training Act of 1971, was dropped from subsequent legislation. By 1978, Joseph Califano, long-time spokesman for the Great Society, declared that the problem was too many physicians, not too few (Califano, 1979). The federal government had come full circle.

## Summary

A review of public policy with respect to health and the health professions from 1950 to 1980 reflects changing priorities. With the goal of improving health care through equal access to the health care system and through heightened levels of scientific knowledge, the federal government embarked on an expansionary path. Allocative strategies for research, medical care services, education, and training were implemented in the sixties, followed in the seventies by restrictive strategies intended to target the expansion toward an improvement in geographic and specialty distribution.

The policies of the sixties led to considerable expansion in both health care services and health professions education. There is, however, little evidence of basic change; although larger, both the educational and the delivery systems look very much as they did in 1960. The enthusiasm and sincere involvement of the 1960s gave the appearance of newness, but they reflected a misplaced optimism that the American social and economic system had limitless capacity for expansion and growth.

As long as new resources and privileges are being supported by growth, nontraditional recipients can be attended to, conflicting goals may be implemented, and traditional standards for monitoring the impact of new programs can be relaxed. However, in nongrowth periods, change requires a redistribution of resources and privileges, and will, therefore, confront much more resistance. By the early seventies, the United States was already moving from a period of rapid economic growth toward stagnation, although it took a long time to recognize the warnings and to realize how deeply this would impact on public policy. As Freymann (1974, p. 138) points out, "Incessant expansion became such a fixture of our national life that it inspired the infinity principle. Long after the frontier closed, faith in endless growth continued to dominate our thought. In fact, it dominated our thinking so completely that any limit on growth was inconceivable—until events broke upon us which could no longer be ignored."

## References

Califano, J. "The Government: Medical Education Partnership." *Journal of Medical Education*, 1979, *54*, 19–24.

Carnegie Commission on Higher Education. *Higher Education and the Nation's Health*. New York: McGraw-Hill, 1970.

Fox, R. "The Medicalization and Demedicalization of American Society." *Daedalus*, 1977, *106* (1), 9–22.

Freymann, J. *The American Health Care System: Its Genesis and Trajectory*. New York: Medcom, 1974.

Goldman, E. *Rendezvous with Destiny*. New York: Vintage Books, 1960.

Riska, E. "Social Reform and Reform in Medical Education." In A. D. Hunt and L. E. Weeks (Eds.), *Medical Education Since 1960: Marching to a Different Drummer*. East Lansing: Michigan State University Foundation, 1980.

Rossiter, C. *Parties and Politics in America*. New York: Cornell University Press, 1960.

Shannon, J. A. "Science and Social Purpose." *Science*, 1969, *163*, 769–773.

U.S. Commission on Civil Rights. *Social Indicators of Equality for Minorities and Women*. Washington, D.C.: U.S. Government Printing Office, 1978.

U.S. Department of Health and Human Services. *Health, United States, 1980*. Washington, D.C.: U.S. Government Printing Office, 1980.

White, T. H. *America in Search of Itself: The Making of the President, 1956–1980*. New York: Harper & Row, 1982.

# 2

*Marjorie Price Wilson*
*Cheves McC. Smythe*

# Medicine

Since 1960, indeed since the middle of the nineteenth century in America, medical education has been in a continuing state of ferment and adaptive change; this change has resulted from the compulsive tendency of the faculty to impart the best of what they know to the next generation of physicians. That knowledge is derived primarily from advances in medical science. This constant activity is modulated by opinion leaders both inside and outside academic medicine (Lee, 1965; Funkenstein, 1966; Cope and Zacharias, 1966; Turner, 1967; Jacobson, 1967). These leaders, appreciating the advances in medical knowledge that have resulted from scientific research, seeing our increased capacity to provide comprehensive care to patients, and perceiving the compelling needs of society, have provided a vision of the ultimate goals of medical education. These goals have remained remarkably stable during the period under review, 1960 to 1980.

## Opinion Leaders

In 1958, the Alan Gregg Memorial Lecture of the Association of American Medical Colleges (AAMC) was established to encourage the development of the classical literature of medical education. A review of those lectures not only reveals the values that undergird our medical education system but also provides a reflection of current societal issues. In 1960, for example, Joseph Wearn (1961) set forth three problems for attention: the adaptation of medical education to scientific knowledge, the delicate balance of research with teaching and patient care (and, one might add, of patient care with teaching and research), and the relation of university medical centers to medical care for the whole community. In his 1963 Alan Gregg lecture, Willard C. Rappleye said: "At the same time, we must retain the unifying principles of 'master generalizations' of medical science and the

20

concepts of the patient as a whole and the family as the basic unit of society—not those of disease and organ orientation only. . . . One of the responsibilities of medical education at all levels is to translate the new discoveries into the preparation of qualified physicians and the numerous other health workers whose duty is to apply advancing knowledge to the needs of patients and the community" (1963, pp. 902-903). In 1965, Ward Darley (1966) took up the issue of financing of medical education and the need for an increase in enrollment and additional new medical schools.

These and other spokesmen have repeatedly described what was perceived to be the appropriate response of medical education to the values and current needs of society. To the Gregg lectures can be added the annual AAMC Presidential Addresses, the papers from the Annual Congress on Medical Education, and the reports of the AAMC Teaching Institutes. The first six of these institutes, convened during the fifties, concerned the teaching of physiology, biochemistry, pharmacology, pathology, microbiology, immunology, genetics, anatomy, and anthropology (Comroe, 1954; Association of American Medical Colleges, 1955, 1956). Attention was then directed to clinical teaching (Gee and Richmond, 1959; Gee and Child, 1961), and the Eighth Teaching Institute concerned medical education and medical care (Sheps, Wolf, and Jacobsen, 1961). Julius Comroe's (1962) report of the Ninth Institute on research and medical education is a classic on the role of biomedical research in education. To be sure, these individuals have generally articulated a consensus (Hubbard, Gronvall, and DeMuth, 1970). Radical ideas are rare, divergent opinions exist and are sometimes noted, but these classical statements represent what emerged as the general consensus about trends, needs, qualities, and standards.

The 1966 Gregg lecturer, James A. Shannon (1967), after reviewing the development of biomedical research in the United States, proposed the involvement of medical education with four urgent issues: the need for an integrated process of graduate education pervaded by unified qualitative criteria, an immediate national examination of the feasibility of the expansion of classes of existing medical schools (which he said seemed unavoidable), an accelerating rate of professional obsolescence of physicians as an inescapable consequence of the advance of medical science (he suggested that every sixth year of the practicing physician's career should be spent in a formal educational process upon which continued licensure would be dependent), and, finally, a broader role for the behavioral sciences in medical education and an emphasis upon public responsibility of physicians. By the late 1960s then, the concept of the continuum of medical education, the emphasis on formal continuing education, the quantitative expansion of medical school classes, and the importance of the behavioral sciences had been recognized and embedded in our lore.

The Gregg lectures continued to elucidate the insights of the times. MacLeod in 1968, Gordon in 1970, and Heard in 1971 identified what was then our future and now our present. MacLeod told us that the principal issue was that schools were being called upon to expand their role in society. Gordon asserted that the relationship of a university's academic health center to health service reform should surely be a central concern to that institution's authorities. Heard's eloquent forecast of the present state of health affairs in "The Seamless Web of Health and Policy" also set forth appropriate guidance standards for public participation in health policy. He wisely cautioned that there is a limit somewhere to the productivity of a society and, consequently, on how much can be done and by how many, in all the realms for which we hold limitless ambition, including health. He cautioned that if the drive for increased consumption is endemic in the American ethos, increased labor and financial efficiency are a necessity, and that our social and political processes need to breed a rationalizing of expectations. He concluded by saying that "all health professionals would find that what they do and want to do are matters of public policy" and "their effective participation will be greatly influenced by their breadth of viewpoint and their understanding of the full society within which they function and of the processes of decision making that will ultimately determine what they do and their institutions are asked to do, permitted to do, or forced to do" (Heard, 1971, p. 932). We were enmeshed in the seamless web.

## Financial Incentives

The philanthropic organizations and the government, both federal and state, have been the sources of another type of major influence. Through the power of the purse, these organizations have often provided the wherewithal to implement change. Examples abound: construction of new medical schools, expansion of class size, shortening of the curriculum to three years, emphasis on primary care, the training of physicians' assistants, development of area health education centers, outreach of the educational programs to community sites, and admission of greater numbers of minority and disadvantaged students (Sanazaro, 1967; Cooper, 1976).

Federal legislation has followed the generally articulated view of what should happen; medical schools were frequently well on the way toward implementing a change when the government came along with the needed support (Wilson, 1972). Why then the feeling of misalignment with government initiatives in recent years? Undoubtedly, the sense of regimentation, the absence of innovation, the general pedestrian nature of the required response, and the restrictive nature of government terms and conditions have caused the concern. The academic enterprise prides itself on its diversity, but, rather than encouraging experimentation and creativity as it does in the biomedical research arena, government support for educational innovation has imposed a sameness. The government wrote the protocol for the educational projects and many foundations followed suit; unfortunately, such heavy-handed prescription does not engender the most creative solutions.

## Other Change Agents

We shall examine in some detail the critically important effects of new knowledge on the medical curriculum and will touch briefly on the influence of changing societal attitudes and priorities. Other significant forces driving changes in medical education include: the federal legislation aimed at expansion of medical schools, the Medicare/Medicaid legislation, and the growth of tertiary care and graduate medical education.

*The Health Professions Education Assistance Act of 1963 and Its Various Amendments.* In 1958, the first of a series of reports calling for forced draft expansion of medical schools appeared. In 1963, the first direct federal support of medical education was signed into law. From 1960 to 1980, the numbers of undergraduate medical students more than doubled, an increase made possible by the significant expansion of virtually all existing medical schools and the organization of over forty new schools. Whether this expansion has affected the actual content of the curriculum is unclear; it has, however, radically changed the environment for medical student learning. Larger classes mean different student-to-student and student-to-teacher dynamics (Sanazaro, 1966; Hubbard and Howard, 1967). Rapid expansion of faculty means large numbers of young recruits to the teaching ranks. New schools mean establishing teaching programs where none existed before. In summation, expansion lysed the status quo and induced readiness for change in many areas. New people brought in new ideas. Curricula were not so much changed because of expansion, but expansion decreased resistance to change (Sanazaro, 1967; Wilson, 1972; Cooper, 1976).

*Medicare-Medicaid.* It is virtually impossible to overstate the effects of the 1965 Medicare-Medicaid legislation on academic medical centers and their medical schools. The legislation has contributed to the decline of city-county hospitals as the prevailing site of medical education; changed the social contract between a patient and student-physician; promoted the expansion of medical schools by unleashing a tidal wave of pent-up demand; focused attention on the medical problems of minorities, the aged, and the disabled; altered the financing of faculty activity; and pushed faculties into a more direct role in patient care. By making all patients "private," Medicare-Medicaid has eased the way for educational programs in truly private patient settings. While this legislation has not directly affected the content of the curriculum, it has enhanced the readiness for change, and has had a direct impact on intern and residency training.

*Graduate Medical Education and Tertiary Care.* By 1960, the great majority of American medical graduates entered postgraduate training. The trend of referral of difficult cases to academic centers, established by the great university hospitals, was further strengthened by the appearance of sophisticated technology that made it possible to offer patients more advanced care than that available in many of their home communities. This same new knowledge and new technology stimulated development of specialties within specialties, the so-called subspecialties, which should more properly be called the superspecialties. Financial and other reward systems fostered their development. With these changes, the rotating internship gave way to the straight internship, which gave way to PGY-1. Three-year residency training programs became almost a minimum, with longer programs common. Clinical fellows or advanced clinical trainees were layered onto the residents. The most obvious impact of this growth was on fourth-year medical students who were squeezed out of their role in bedside care. This growth of many subspecialties was a significant factor in the emergence of the "elective" fourth year. Even more important was the change in patient populations to sicker and older patients who needed a level of attention requiring hours of physicians' time. This demand resulted in pressures for even more growth of house staff and a larger number of fellows. Concurrent expansion of medical school graduating classes generated the need for places where these graduates

could be trained. These and many other forces have literally transformed the
university teaching hospital of 1960 into the academic medical center of 1980—a
more crowded, more impersonal, more hurried, much larger, and much, much
more complex institution (Graduate Medical Education National Advisory
Committee, 1980).

As is true of many social changes, the swing toward specialization and the
accompanying rapid diminution in the training of general physicians produced a
situation which demanded its own correction. In addition, the specialty training
programs were undoubtedly successful in that highly qualified people were produced in such numbers that they sought practice opportunities in smaller and
smaller, and more and more dispersed communities. The result was that a higher
and more sophisticated level of care became available in these communities. This,
in turn, both highlighted the demand for general physicians and, with a lessened
flow of referred patients to academic medical centers, forced the latter's attention
on the surrounding communities. The overall net effect was a growing attractiveness of less specialized care, family medicine, and primary care. The pressure
became so intense that federal subsidies were mobilized to support the development of such training programs. The establishment of graduate training programs in primary care led to the demand for curriculum time, which led many
medical schools to introduce a required clerkship in family medicine.

## Change of Curricular Goals

At the risk of oversimplification, medical school teaching can be divided
into four distinct, if overlapping, thrusts. The first is the transmission of cognitive
*knowledge,* the facts, figures, and concepts on which modern Western scientific
medicine is built. This material has often been defined as the content of the
medical curriculum. The second thrust is the inculcation of *basic skills* which
medical students must acquire before they can perform as physicians. Obvious
examples are the physical examination, the medical history, and the ability
to perform effectively in collecting and interpreting information relative to a
patient's problems, which can be called clinical data gathering skills. The third is
the transference of a group of *attitudes and values* that are involved in the professionalization or socialization of an individual from a university student to a
junior physician. The fourth is more difficult to define, but it involves teaching
the student how to exploit and use the available sources of information and
imprinting *habits of lifelong learning or continuing scholarship.* In this chapter,
this fourth thrust is seen as derived from the teaching methodologies, means,
modalities, situations, and environments in all their rich complexity that the
modern North American medical school provides its students. As a further oversimplification, each of these four thrusts of medical teaching can be seen as driven
or modulated by a dominant change agent, though all are influenced by many
overlapping forces.

The cognitive knowledge presented to medical students is constantly impacted by new scientific discoveries, new concepts, new interpretations of existing
knowledge, and the growth of biomedical information. Between 1960 and 1980,
this growth was prodigious, and it was the research laboratory, the disciplined,
formal, organized acquisition of new knowledge that was the driving force of

change. The growth of knowledge is both theoretically and actually limitless (at least within the parameters of an individual student's capacity to master it), whereas curriculum time is very rigidly limited. Thus, the accelerating effectiveness of worldwide biomedical research efforts has exposed the curriculum to a host of inexorable pressures for change. This is by no means a new phenomenon, but what is different is its accelerating tempo and magnitude, which will continue in the next decades.

Though the skills expected of the young physician have not changed as much, the aggregate skills of all types of physicians have increased, and each is expected to be aware of what can be done by others. This fact permits the construction of a parallelism that relates skill and technology in a fashion analogous to the relation between cognitive content of the curriculum and effective biomedical research. In this context, technology has undergone impressive growth and evolution in the two decades in question, and it has had an impact on the medical curriculum, especially in its clinical and postgraduate phases.

New content and new technology undoubtedly have implications for attitudes and values (Ham, 1964; Fogarty International Center, 1970). Oral contraceptives and the intrauterine contraceptive devices are obvious examples. But even more definitive are changes in the society at large. The years between 1960 and 1980 have hardly been uneventful in terms of social upheaval, and the inhabitants of medical schools have been anything but isolated. Eichna's account of his second passage through medical school is a particularly poignant reflection of some of these changes (Eichna, 1980).

The forces affecting the fourth thrust of medical education, the environment in which learning occurs and the interaction within that environment, are not so easily isolated. Larger classes, the growth of tertiary care in major teaching hospitals, dependence upon affiliated hospitals, growth of faculty, influence of outside pressures, and sources of funds have all combined to change the environment of medical teaching and learning. Constantly hovering over all of this is the as yet unrealized potential of new communication and electronic data processing technology.

If these are the parameters in which changes may be examined, in the current milieu of constant flux one must also attempt to define when a change is a change rather than simply a variation. Is a shift in emphasis a change? Is the ablation of old information and its replacement by the new a change? Is the rearrangement and regrouping of existing material a change? Is the presentation of equivalent material in different formats, such as block as compared to integrated teaching, a change? Does the emergence of a new department or the creation of a new division, undoubtedly a considerable organizational change, equate to a curriculum change? This is a very small sample of some of the things continuously occurring in medical schools. We believe that since change is continuous, it is only feasible to examine the types of forces which produce change and provide brief illustrative vignettes rather than attempt to discriminate between the significant and nonsignificant elements of change.

### Structural Innovations

Because of the abundance of examples of innovations and modifications which occurred in the period between 1960 and 1980, they have been rather arbitrarily labeled as structural or content changes in order to sort out the principal categories of activity. Structural changes have to do primarily with the physical or temporal environment of learning. No changes, of course, were purely structural in the mechanical sense, and nearly all derived from the goal of improving the curriculum from an educational or learning standpoint.

*The Multidiscipline Laboratory.* The late fifties and early sixties saw the introduction and extensive adoption of the multidiscipline (MD) laboratory. A set of teaching laboratories for each major department required a great deal of expensive space, often utilized for only brief periods during the year and thus subject to great pressures for conversion to other purposes. The appearance of the multidisciplinary teaching laboratory of twenty years ago was a response to these sorts of pressures. Such labs required less space and permitted the acquisition of a higher order of instrumentation useful for many purposes. But the popularity of this adaptation has waned. Most of the new schools constructed in the sixties utilized this design, only to find that in the seventies, basic science laboratory experience for the student was being abandoned; it is only now being reintroduced (Harrell, 1964; Spilman, 1966; Baum and Koushanpour, 1967; Jaussi and others, 1971; Marchand and Steward, 1974). A comparison to the MD laboratory was the student study cubicle located near the laboratory or in or near the health sciences library (Harrell, 1964). Today we see students working in groups around the cathode-ray tube with audio and videotapes, filmstrips, and computer-assisted instruction modules.

*Early Clinical Experience and Integrated Instruction.* The early introduction of clinical medicine in the first, or at least the second, year of the curriculum was a popular innovation of the sixties, a time when students in higher education became preoccupied with relevance. The benefit of this concept is related as much to the socialization or professionalization of the student as to the specific content of medicine. Exposure to clinical medicine per se as an early or introductory experience has given way to reliance on correlative medicine directed at integrating the basic and clinical sciences, a sounder approach to preparation for specific clinical learning. There are also many examples of organ system and interdepartmental teaching, particularly in the basic sciences (Ham, 1962; Spilman, 1965; Robbins, 1968; Rossee, 1974; Association of American Medical Colleges, Council of Academic Societies, 1981).

*Curriculum Electives and Specialization.* The opening up of the curriculum and the introduction of electives was an advance in curricular development that permitted the student more independence in individualizing his own curriculum. A number of schools offer a tracking option that provides a specialty training continuum of at least one year prior to fulfilling the requirements for the M.D. degree. Nearly every medical school has experimented with at least one year, usually the fourth, that is completely elective, although we are seeing a return to greater structure in the senior year in some. One medical school with a completely elective curriculum has reinstituted controls which assure that no student can receive the M.D. degree without exposure to a balanced array of subject matter areas fundamental to the undergraduate preparation of the physician. Currently, ninety-four (or 74.6 percent) of the medical schools offer a combined M.D./Ph.D. program (*Association of American Medical Colleges Curriculum Directory*, 1981).

*Duration of the M.D. Curriculum.* The majority of medical schools have a four-year curriculum, and the majority of students complete four years of undergraduate work before entering medical school. However, there is considerable variation in this traditional sequence. *The AAMC Curriculum Directory, 1981–1982,* indicates that in 12 schools, students can be admitted to combined undergraduate-graduate programs after high school, in 8 after the second year of college, and 109 out of 126 schools admit students after the third year of college.

An important innovation was begun at Northwestern in 1961 with the admission of highly qualified students directly from secondary school to a special program that permitted them to complete work for the M.D. degree in six years (Cooper, 1976). Currently, nineteen medical schools report having programs combined with undergraduate studies that lead to the M.D. degree in six years or less. These programs have proved quite successful and have increased in number. For the most part, the students become undifferentiated from their peers traversing the more traditional route to the M.D. degree. Some studies have shown that they do as well or better than their peers on several measurable dimensions, such as examination, receipt of various awards and honors, and placement in Postgraduate Year–1 (PGY–1) positions (Campbell and DeMuth, 1976; Lanzoni and Kayne, 1976; Pritchard, 1976). Advantages of this approach to shortening the total time involved include decreased total financial expenditure for the student and the possibility of attracting very able students to medicine who might forego the opportunity because of time or cost. The principal benefit, however, seems to be the possibility that such a program curtails the excessive stress traditional students face in competing for admission to medical school and allows students to select more difficult undergraduate courses that might interest and benefit them or to vary their premedical preparation in a more liberal direction (Daubney, Wagner, and Rogers, 1981).

The wholesale introduction and then decline in the three-year medical curriculum presents a different picture. The rise and fall of the three-year curriculum stands as a model of the impact of opinion leaders and financial incentives on the medical education system in North America. The 1970 Carnegie Commission report, *Higher Education and the Nation's Health,* advocated a reduction in the medical curriculum from four to three years to reduce costs to students and institutions (Carnegie Commission on Higher Education, 1970). The pressure to increase the output of physicians had also crescendoed and, together with these ideas and recommendations, resulted in the Comprehensive Health Manpower Training Act of 1971, which provided federal capitation grant bonuses to schools introducing a three-year medical curriculum and/or enrollment increases. Prior to that time, support for curriculum shortening had been available only through special project grants.* It is significant that in 1981 no medical school offered only a regular three-year program. However, 104 offered a regular four-year program only, two schools offered a three-year program with option for four, and 14 offered a four-year program with option for three years (*Association of American Medical Colleges Curriculum Directory,* 1981).

---

*For a thorough review of the three-year curriculum in U.S. medical schools in the first half of the 1970s, see Beran and Kriner, 1978.

In the early 1970s, the medical schools were propelled toward the three-year curriculum primarily because of the federal financial incentive; when the specific support disappeared, so did the programs (Beran, 1979). The principal disadvantage to the students was the bias against them in competition for PGY-1 positions. The basic science faculty felt the pressure of compression of the subject material as severely as did the students. For the most part, although the time was shortened and the hours devoted to each discipline decreased, much of the same material was included. The process did motivate the faculty to analyze the curriculum thoroughly and, as the reconversion to four years began, some of the useful adaptations were retained. This sociology lesson bears witness to the influence that external forces can have on medical education. The study of the process of this modification reveals that educational objectives were essentially absent in the initial conversion and still played a minor role in the reversion to the traditional time frame. Also, as it turned out, the funds available from the federal government never matched the promised levels (Kettel and others, 1979; Trzebiatowski and Peterson, 1979).

### Changes in Curriculum Content: The Basic Sciences

Anatomy, biochemistry, physiology, pharmacology, microbiology, pathology, and the introduction to clinical medicine are all taught in all North American medical schools, often in that sequence in the first two years of the curriculum. However, there are many variations in sequence, emphasis, and methodology (Wagner, 1962; Behal, 1973; Levy, Bresnik, and Williams, 1973; Bowers and Purcell, 1974; Spilman and Spilman, 1975).

*Anatomy.* Gross human anatomy has not changed nor has knowledge of it, but what has changed is the knowledge of ultrastructure. Electron microscopy is commonplace, and the extraordinary growth of a dazzling array of labeling techniques has led to greatly increased appreciation of cellular mechanisms. As a result, the research done in anatomy departments has become increasingly difficult to distinguish from that done by biochemists or cellular physiologists. Linked to this is the virtual disappearance of the formally trained gross anatomist of generations past. Thus the course in gross anatomy, undoubtedly a significant body of knowledge for physicians, has tended to become a course taught by those whose primary interests and rewards lie elsewhere. One experienced basic science department chairman suggests that the objective of today's anatomy or physiology faculties is not to teach medical students to be physiologists or anatomists, but to transmit to them the principles, concepts, and facts necessary to permit and promote understanding of medical phenomena. If this be true, the average medical student need not develop great facility as a physiologist or anatomist or biochemist. These attitudes have tended to mold medical school courses into what can be characterized as highly sophisticated survey courses through which, in the undergraduate university analogy, a student must progress to qualify for his or her major. For the large majority of students the "major" will be the study of some clinical specialty or subspecialty of applied medicine where facility is not only expected, but demanded (American Association of Anatomists, 1966; Harris, Sorlie, and Stolpe, 1973; Kahn, Conklin, and Glover, 1973).

Anatomy illustrates the negative side of what might be called the underside of change. When the amount of time available is fixed and new material is added, then old material must be subtracted. Gross anatomy, with not so very many hours of lecture and many, many hours of dissection, and microscopic anatomy (histology), with few hours of lecture and many hours of peering through microscopes, have been compressed as other material has grown. The anatomic sciences also illustrate another type of change: a whole array of models is readily available to permit three-dimensional demonstration of anatomy without the necessity for a cadaver; superb photographs readily displayed on a variety of screens provide excellent illustrations; plastic replicas of bones and three-dimensional models of the eye, ear, heart, pelvis, lung, and the reproductive, urinary, and gastrointestinal structures are ubiquitous. In addition, extraordinary advances in radiography have created both a need for better understanding of anatomic relationships and a new breed of clinical anatomists able and willing to teach, using their extraordinary technology as the vehicle for their demonstrations.

*Neuroanatomy and the Neurosciences.* The neuroanatomy course of yesteryear was a mix of gross central nervous system anatomy, some neurohistology, and rudiments of neurophysiology. It was often a short course at the end of a regular anatomy course. The great strides in understanding and appreciating the complexity of the nervous system, the technologies used in unraveling some of that complexity, changing ideas about modes of neurotransmission, and rapid evolution of what might be called hormonal aspects of central nervous system function have all forever transformed that minor course. One now hears of neurosciences or neurobiology, an amalgam of neuroanatomy, central nervous system ultrastructure, neurophysiology, neurochemistry, neuropharmacology, and behavioral determinants of disease. In some institutions this grouping has been formalized in a departmental structure or nearly autonomous substructure; the result is a potential for curricular offerings of great richness.

An interesting side issue of this kind of development is the medical students' perceptions of the material, the successful passage of which represents their initiation as junior physicians. For years, anatomy with its mass of detail, its insistence on command of material by rote memory, its written and practical exams, and its demand for timely completion of dissections, was seen as the hurdle at the front door of medicine that had to be cleared. Then, as anatomy waned and biochemistry waxed, the latter became the rite of passage. At least in some institutions, neuroscience, in all its glorious complexity, is taking on that role. No interpretation of these perceptions of medical students is offered beyond evidence that their sense of the relative density of the material provided them is a reaction to the beliefs of the faculty about the actual and eventual importance of that material.

*Biochemistry and Molecular Biology.* Between 1960 and 1980, molecular biology appeared and achieved phenomenal growth. This same period has seen the elucidation of countless biochemical mechanisms. The successful identification of the exact defect in sickle-cell disease and the ability to explain the manifestations of that common and protean disorder on the basis of a single molecular defect dramatized the concept of disease as a molecular disorder. Today's well-based assumption is that all disease can eventually be described in molecular terms; what is wanting is the time, effort, and research support to achieve that goal. We could not begin to describe the countless achievements of biochemistry and their impact on curricular content. In addition, medical schools now enjoy the benefit of students, much better prepared in chemistry and biology, who are the survivors of a vigorous selection process. The problem for the designer of a course in biochemistry is what to teach, at what level, in how much depth, and what to exclude. Biochemistry, in contrast to anatomy, must deal with wide variations in what can be called the chemical literacy of the students, which varies from those who struggled through the required two undergraduate courses to those who have concentrated on science in college and are prepared to handle quite sophisticated chemistry (Kolata, 1979; "Molecular Biology . . . ," 1979; Kornberg, 1980; Stoker, 1980).

These issues evolve into old and unanswerable questions of how much chemistry students should be expected to master before they go on to other studies. How much chemistry is essential to the practice of medicine? And of what sort of medicine? How much is necessary for understanding disease mechanisms? How much is necessary for the physician to be able to ask or to see the right questions about disease mechanisms? And how much to be able to enter preparation for a research career? Obviously, each step requires greater command of the language of modern biochemistry. But should all students be expected to perform at some median level? Should the least strong be evaluated in relationship to a cohort of the strongest? There are no answers. But, since biochemistry has undoubtedly become the *lingua franca* of scientific medicine, these are and will be questions which all medical school biochemistry faculties will have to face for some time. Once again, it is the limitless growth of knowledge being driven against the limited time available and the limited capacity of the individual students to absorb in that time, that produces the conflicts out of which come these unanswerable questions (Wagner, 1962).

*Genetics.* Although there are artificialities in separating molecular biology from biochemistry and as many or more in separating that from microbiology, genetics is a special case which warrants some emphasis. Certainly, growth of knowledge in genetics has been linked with the growth of molecular biology. However, the latter seldom appears listed in the curriculum as a separate discipline or course. Occasionally, the label appears in a compound department such as biochemistry and molecular biology. Molecular biology is not a separate unit because, to a large extent, it grew out of biochemistry and microbiology. Also, its concepts and techniques are now integral parts of the armamentarium of many advanced, biologically oriented research disciplines. The same has been more or less true of genetics. Easily traced to the Watson and Crick description of the structure of deoxyribonucleic acid, but really going further back than that, genetics has zoomed from a bit player on the medical curricular stage to a major influence. The realization of the role of genetics not only in determining the course of human disease but also its role in conditioning the emergence of many disorders has enormously stimulated interest in its clinical applicability. Genetics and the ingenious techniques that have evolved for its study place it in the forefront of the so-called new biology. The growth of genetics exemplifies all of the following:

•   The impact of the new biology on medical thinking
•   The tendency of powerful new aggregates of knowledge to coalesce into a

discipline that first demands and then gets organizational recognition, first of its existence and later of its autonomy

- The conflict between new knowledge and old, with the new eventually displacing the old in the curriculum—for example, more genetics and less dissection in anatomy
- The dilemma of selection of how much or what to teach and in what depth, from an abundantly rich lodé
- The relation of new knowledge to attitudes, values, and, finally clinical practices—for example, the relevance of prenatal diagnosis to abortion

Genetics has earned what will presumably be a growing place in the undergraduate medical curriculum and will be part of that curriculum for the foreseeable future (Childs, Huether, and Murphy, 1981; Fraser, 1980; Teplitz, 1980; Hecht, 1981; McKusick, 1981; Simpson and others, 1981).

*Physiology.* Physiology emerged as a separate major preclinical medical discipline over a hundred years ago. As the study of function, physiology compiled a brilliant record in its elucidation of organ function, of mechanisms through which organ function is integrated, and of how disease produces distortions in these functions—the so-called pathophysiology or physiology of disease. As understanding of disease and research shifted to cellular and then subcellular and molecular levels, the classic physiology found itself somewhat in the same position as anatomy. Its subject matter was of high relevance to physicians but of little moment to the cutting edge of physiological research. At the same time, brilliant advances in instrumentation allowed observations in virtually any intensive care unit, heretofore possible only in experimental animals. As the scientific base of medical practice expanded and training improved, a wide array of physicians became both skilled and literate practicing clinical physiologists, most often only in their own fields of special interest. This has had an enormous impact on who teaches physiology, where in the curriculum, where in the academic medical center, and with what subjects.

Other forces have combined to make the mammalian physiological experiments and laboratories for medical students anachronistic. It must be remembered that such laboratories became widespread in American medical school teaching about sixty or seventy years ago. The laboratory slows the transmission of concepts, giving those more comfortable with objects and more capacity to learn through their hands a more even footing with those very adept at acquiring purely symbolic logic. It imparts an idea of the difficulty of acquiring data, a sense of the necessity of evaluating all data, and some ability to do so. It also furnishes students with what has been called a feel for, or appreciation of, the limits of working with living tissues. In today's jargon, the laboratory was very much a "hands-on" experience closely related to what the neophyte physician saw his mentors doing.

Then both knowledge and technology advanced enormously. Costs soared. The cost of animal experiments for much larger classes became anything but a trivial item in the face of higher standards of care for the animals and startling increases in the costs of procuring and maintaining them. Even more impressive has been the growing expense and sophistication of the instrumentation used in

hospital laboratories for physiological and biochemical observations. The research done at medical school levels requires an instrumentation far beyond that
necessary to get across to medical students important but relatively simple concepts, such as glomerular filtration or the forces leading to the formation of
edema. This does not imply that the capacity to examine urine and to draw
conclusions from a blood film or a stained sputum smear is no longer important.
But what medical school can afford an amino acid analyzer or a scintillation
counter for classroom use, and what investigator would lend one to the inexperienced except under rigidly controlled circumstances? The result has been an
evolution away from long hours in the laboratory for large numbers of students.
Other inhibiting forces include the frequent impossibility of expanding laboratories to accommodate larger classes and the general unwillingness to adapt schedules for their use by subgroups of classes.

Further, if the objective of medical school teaching is to impart principles,
concepts, and facts that promote understanding of physiological phenomena,
then there is no necessity for students to develop facility as physiologists and
therefore less need for laboratory exposure. More material, more emphasis on
concept than skill, and larger classes have all crowded the medical student back
into the lecture hall in a period during which the lecture is roundly denounced as
archaic, passive learning at its worst, and far inferior to other forms of interactive
teaching and learning, or to the use of a variety of new media for teaching.

Parallel events in the clinical years also impact the issue. Larger classes,
multiple hospital affiliations, geographic dispersion of clinical teaching, and
different requirements for time allocation by the great variety of clinical specialties fragment the clinical classes. The growth of clinical faculty has mitigated the
manpower problem and abolished dependence on a few reliable lecturers. Thus,
classwide formal lecture series have almost disappeared from clinical curricula,
but that change has generated pressures to crowd lecture material back into the
first two years. What emerges is more dependence on lectures and less on demonstration in the preclinical years, with the reverse true in the clinical years. Teaching methodologies may not have changed but have shifted.

These phenomena are described under the subheading of physiology but
are by no means restricted to this discipline, though it is especially illustrative.
Also, not so subtle signs of the physiologists' shifting focus to cellular and subcellular events are found in such descriptors as "physiology and cellular biology" as
a department name. If, for instance, this means that physiology is concerned with
the fundamental topic of mechanisms of contractility in cardiac muscle cells, who
is responsible for the more mundane but equally vital topic of hemodynamics and
cardiac output? And where should that material be taught? This is illustrative of
the forces producing integrated teaching and the ever shifting and blurring of
lines of demarcation between clinical and preclinical science.

*Microbiology.* Bacteriology and virology have been among the most active
participants in building the new biology. Theirs has always been a cellular and,
for many years now, a subcellular world. In addition, there is obvious relevance of
the material covered to the realities of clinical medicine. Changes include less
emphasis on public health, less emphasis on bacteriological techniques, more
emphasis on mechanisms of bacterial action and metabolism, a great expansion of
virology, and exploration of the basis of pathogenesis of infection and the interre-

lation of bacteriology and the use of antibiotics. There has also been shifting emphasis as disease incidence has changed, for example, away from tuberculosis toward a variety of gram-negative organisms.

*Immunology.* Advances in microbiology, virology, molecular biology, and genetics have combined to produce not only dramatic increases in knowledge of immunology but also, more importantly, a different conceptualization of the place of immunological phenomena in biology. The recognition of, defense against, and reactions produced by normal, abnormal, overactive, underactive, controlled, and uncontrolled responses to the invasion of what is perceived as foreign agents is now understood as a system as intricate, complex, beautiful, and vital to the economy of the organism as the cardiovascular system. This has modified our ideas about the nature of disease. All of this is of obvious importance to the physician, but where and how does it find expression in the curriculum? Immunologically oriented enclaves can be found in departments of bacteriology, pharmacology, pathology, medicine, surgery, pediatrics, obstetrics-gynecology, and in groups concerned with transplantation and cancer research and treatment. Curricular offerings correspondingly vary from organized independent courses presented by autonomous departments to excerpted material related to any or all of the above fields. It is reasonable to assume that there will be continuous development in immunology and that it, like neurobiology and genetics, will become a more or less permanent major discipline until, at some unknown time in the future, it is displaced by a new wave of scientific discovery.

*Pharmacology.* Because of the advances which have occurred in pharmacology over the past twenty-five years, it has assumed an important place as an interface between the basic sciences and the clinical sciences. Most of the modern pharmacology is wholly removed from the classical methods previously employed and utilizes state-of-the-art methods which are equally applied in other basic sciences. But pharmacology goes further in that it provides a stronger link between basic and clinical medicine than ever before. This is especially apparent as immunology and genetic engineering impact on pharmacology to identify sites of drug action, develop new drugs, and deliver them to sites of action. The more fundamental understanding of the physical and chemical properties of therapeutic agents obtained through modern molecular pharmacology makes it possible to devise new ways of analyzing their effects on biological systems and to introduce new modalities and reevaluate old ones still in use. New experimental techniques and understanding of physiological and biophysical properties permit the identification in both animals and humans of specific targets of drug action heretofore unknown.

Growth in the number, specificity, and potency of drugs has greatly increased the skills required for their efficacious use in humans and has reinforced the strength of pharmacology and its hold on a significant place in the curriculum. As empirical knowledge has given way to elegant understanding of how and why drugs exert their action, this new material has appeared in the curriculum. The link between basic pharmacology and clinical pharmacology has also been strengthened so that subjects ranging from the molecular basis of drug action to the way drugs should be used in practice are covered. Topics including pharmacokinetics, clinical toxicology, drug reactions and interactions, clinical trials, and relevant statistics are taught by clinical pharmacologists who may reside in either the basic science or clinical departments. In fact, clinical pharmacology is being promoted by some as a new medical specialty. Advocates suggest the separation of diagnosis from treatment of the patient, with the clinical pharmacologist assuming the responsibility for the treatment phase much like diagnostic and therapeutic radiology are divided. Indeed, an American Board of Clinical Pharmacology has already been established and initiated a program of certification. Whatever future organizational arrangements may be, with the interest and confidence in the development of new and effective drugs as high as it is, pharmacology will maintain a major place in the medical curriculum (Csaky, 1976; Yates, 1979; Dollery, 1978; Dreux, 1979; Spector, Roberts, and Vesell, 1981).

*Pathology.* The great change in pathology has been the displacement of the light microscope as the instrument on which the discipline depends. This has led to less emphasis on acquisition of skill in its use and less emphasis on gross pathology and autopsy pathology, accompanied by extraordinary growth in clinical pathology. These changes are a reflection of growth of knowledge, growing technological sophistication, and the capacity of clinical pathologists and their instruments to gather data about disease and, therefore, to gain insight into disease mechanisms. With these changes, pathology has shifted away from seeing itself as a preclinical discipline and insisted that it is a clinical science. Moreover, in the Western Reserve model of integrated system teaching, pathology has tended to be diffused through the curriculum. Also in the organ system model, well-trained clinical subspecialists have, as in the case of physiology, become expert in the pathology of their areas of interest and ready, willing, and able to teach it. As a result, pathology has become a less singularly prominent force in the curriculum.

Pathology and its teaching have also been brushed by the capacity of the discipline to generate literally rivers of clinical data. Who is responsible for its interpretation, storage, use, and integration with other data? Who should teach medical students how to manage not a paucity but an overabundance of information? Whose problem is it to formulate some approach to distinguishing the significant from the insignificant? Who teaches the appropriate use of all the information gained? These questions remain unanswered but manifest themselves in the appearance of curriculum material variously labeled as clinical logic or clinical problem solving.

These changes have been accompanied by a decline in the importance of the autopsy in the curriculum and the place of gross pathology in teaching medical students about disease. The reason is simply that these time-honored and at one time critically important disciplines have been displaced by a more powerful technology (Brinkhous, 1980; Stasney, 1980; Mitchell and others, 1981; Lundberg, 1981; Mistry and Davis, 1981).

*Other Courses.* Parasitology, epidemiology, radiation biology, toxicology, medical jurisprudence, biostatistics, and what can be called computer literacy—all have their advocates. All are important. All are taught with varying emphasis. All remain, however, minor or secondary courses in the basic science curricula of the North American medical schools. Despite cogent reasons to the contrary, the impressive intellectual power and the compelling and awesome beauty of the new biology exemplified by immunology, genetics, virology, and neurobiology will dominate changes in the medical basic science curriculum for the immediately foreseeable future (Abelson, 1980; Davis, 1980).

## Changes in Curriculum Content: The Clinical Sciences

*Introduction to Clinical Medicine.* For many years, physical diagnosis came at the end of the second preclinical year. This course was designed to drill students in the acquisition of the skills necessary to gather clinical data from the examination of the patient. In 1960, the patients often resided in the wards of public hospitals or chronic disease hospitals. Departments of medicine carried the major burden of the instruction. Classes were small, usually two to four students to a preceptor. The Medicare-Medicaid legislation had a drastic effect on the relationship of physicians to patients and on attitudes of patients toward physicians: The "social contract" between the indigent patients and the young physicians who serve them changed, the pattern of diseases found in city hospitals changed, and class size and heterogeneity increased dramatically. In addition, the role of physical diagnosis was modified by the accuracy, ease, effectiveness, and ubiquity of many of the new technologies. Further, the preparation and background of many new instructors differed greatly from that of their predecessors. Appreciation of the need to introduce more awareness of the behavioral aspects of illness and the desire to have the students acquire more precise interviewing skills have also had their effects. These changes, combined with the increasingly vocal student demand for an earlier introduction to clinical medicine, had their impact on the courses which introduced students to clinical medicine (Barondess, 1979).

In principle, faculties were receptive to change. Part of their response has been the introduction of the integrated organ system curriculum, with first- and second-year material presented by clinicians. Other responses include exposing beginning medical students to patients in a variety of arrangements, in such roles as observer or interviewer. Students are usually introduced to abnormal human behavior, the role of behavior in disease, the interactions between illness and behavior, and the social determinants of disease in some form of lecture or seminar courses during the first two years, when they are given the opportunity to acquire some experience in patient interviewing skills. There are many variations in how this teaching is done. Trained models, imaginative use of television, two-way mirrors, and contact with chronically ill patients in chronic disease hospitals have all been tried at various medical schools, with the success of the teaching modality as much related to the enthusiasm of the innovator as to the inherent qualities of the technique. Students now come to the clinical years with more exposure to the clinical aspects of medicine; it is somewhat harder to document whether they come with more actual experience with patients. This is a change in which immediate teaching objectives have been broadened, teaching techniques have changed, and the personnel involved (both the instructors and the patients) are different. However, the overall objective of a vitally important course has remained the same—for the students to acquire skills of clinical data gathering and observation as a prelude to their full clinical experience.

*Third Year: Clinical Clerkships.* If the major teaching objective of the first two years in medical school is to have the students acquire the cognitive knowledge and symbolic logic necessary to comprehend illness as it occurs in Western industrialized societies, and if the objective of the transition course described above is to have them acquire the skills necessary to gather clinical data, then the objective of the third-year clinical clerkships is to give the students the opportunity to practice and perfect their recently acquired skills.

In terms of objectives and goals, setting and focus, the third year of medical school has changed relatively little over the twenty years in question. However, the sequence of clerkships and the time devoted to them, the kinds of hospitals in which they occur, and the backgrounds of the people responsible for the instruction vary from school to school. Long rotations on medicine and surgery and somewhat shorter exposure to pediatrics, obstetrics, gynecology, and psychiatry are characteristic. The emphasis on inpatient experience, usually with very ill people, is essentially unchanged. However, the sorts of patients, their diseases, the technology available for their care, the numbers of house officers and fellows, and the role of the attending staff have all changed. Virtually all teaching is now the responsibility of full-time, salaried, clinical faculty, with only a minority of volunteer instructors carrying the load—a distinct shift from the situation in 1960. These faculty bring to their interactions with students different experiences, different training, different values, and different reward systems; as a result, they furnish a role model quite different from their immediate postwar predecessors.

The new community-based medical schools, which have nearly all appeared in the last two decades, are an even more striking illustration of change in clinical teaching (Hunt and Weeks, 1979). These institutions have in common a more tenuous link with parent universities, relatively loose ties with other forms of graduate scientific education, less emphasis on bench scientific research, and no primary teaching hospital controlled by a full-time faculty. More importantly, they do have strong commitments to the communities in which they are located, emphasis on preparation of their students for primary care and less specialized forms of practice, virtually total dependence on existing hospitals in their communities for clinical teaching, a much larger role for volunteer and partially salaried physicians practicing in these hospitals (both in terms of their involvement in teaching and for access to their patients), and a more behaviorally oriented and less disease model dominated approach to illness. These institutions do represent a change—a real change. In terms of support, they serve a distinctly definable constituency to whose needs and beliefs they should be and are responsive. As such, they must be more locally oriented. They have neither the benefits nor the problems involved in responsibilities for a major teaching hospital. Though they teach the same science as the orthodox medical schools, they reflect significantly different attitudes and values. Their very existence reaffirms the intuitively obvious but not always experientially realized fact that there is more than one way to educate a physician (Stokes, 1967; Sweeney and Mitchell, 1971; Gellhorn and Scheuer, 1978).

*Fourth Year.* With the virtual disappearance of the view that the medical schools should prepare the student for the direct practice of medicine, the place of the fourth year in the medical school forever changed. With adoption of the view that it is the responsibility of a medical school to prepare its graduates to enter some form of postgraduate or residency training, the fourth-year student is caught between the needs of the clinical clerks below and the responsibilities of the junior residents above. Relieved of the senior-year rotation through the outpatient clinics, characteristic of the pre-sixties, students find themselves in teaching environments increasingly crammed with expanding varieties of trainees. From

July to January, the student's psychic energy is drained into selecting both the field and location of postgraduate training, decisions vitally important to a future career and justifiable causes for anxiety. From January to March, the student waits in feverish and anguished expectation to learn where fate will next deposit him or her. From March to graduation, the student languishes in relieved and relaxed preparation for a move to bigger and better things. Though some schools have reintroduced more structure, the real business of the fourth year—now called the elective or selective year—is covered in most schools with a varyingly polished veneer of noninvolvement and sometimes limited intellectual discipline.

Obviously, this distinctly jaundiced viewpoint is an overstatement of the case. Through World War II some medical students did enter practice directly upon graduation or after a year's rotating internship. Medical schools were responsible for preparing these students for direct and often unsupervised responsibility for patients. Thus, the fourth year had to be a practicum or subinternship. Reflections of this need are seen in some of the older courses, such as Bandaging and Splinting or Minor Surgery. The most obvious modern holdover of this need is found in the high prominence midwifery retains in the modern medical curriculum. This anachronism is a derivative of the time when all physicians were expected to attend women in labor and to care for the newborn. Given the obvious social value of good infant and maternal care and the enormous, very tragic cost of unnecessary maternal and fetal loss, sound practical training in at least normal obstetrics was mandatory. Contrast that with the practices of contemporary industrial society, where intrahospital delivery by a small cadre of highly trained obstetricians is the norm. Although this is changing again with the advent of alternative childbirth settings, normal obstetrics for more physicians is no more or less mandatory a skill than the ability to set a fracture or to extract a cataract. Though the old requirement of a stated minimum number of deliveries has disappeared, the required clerkship in obstetrics remains, whereas one in diagnostic radiology—a skill used by virtually all physicians—is not required. These facts illustrate the interplay between the conservatism and protectionism of faculties and changing social needs. They also illustrate the fact that while the content of the curriculum may indeed be voted upon and approved by the faculty, in the final analysis many forces, almost all of them largely external to the individual medical schools, exert inexorable pressures toward some conformity.

The pressures of expanded bodies of knowledge and different forms of practice do play upon the relation between third and fourth years. In general, the usual five required clerkships have been increased to include experiences in family medicine and/or ambulatory care and often some minimal requirements in at least a sample of the surgical specialties and sometimes neurology. These required clerkships encompass fifty or more weeks and therefore must occupy some time in the fourth year. Elective or selective periods characteristically total twenty-four to twenty-eight weeks. Interestingly, a demanding academic requirement such as a thesis or completion of a comprehensive final examination is rare, although a significant number of schools require the National Board Examinations for graduation.

In short, the absence of clearly defined objectives and structure imposes on the fourth year the diffuseness characteristic of it in many medical schools. Many students wisely take advantage of this and enter acting internships or sign up for electives at other institutions to learn new ways of doing things and to help toward difficult decisions about field and location of postgraduate training. However, one must wonder whether this low-demand period—coming between the very demanding initial years of medical school and the equally demanding rigors of the early postgraduate years—is a necessary and healthy adaptation or diastole (Johns and Smith, 1973; Barbee and Dinham, 1977; Geertsma and others, 1977; Korst, 1977).

## Continuing Curricular Concerns

*Public Expectations.* As the power of modern scientific medicine has increased, as the power of its major institutions has grown, and as the resources flowing to it have expanded, interests and pressures have emerged to bring new, additional, or differently focused subject material before medical students. Characteristically, those who advocate the introduction of this material feel it should be required, whereas those responsible for managing the curriculum, already frantic about pressures from many other sources, often resist the introduction of new material. Examples include emphasis on humanistic or holistic medicine (Glick, 1981); more and better teaching of the social sciences in general in medical schools; recognition of the fact that the family is the basic unit of society and that medicine should be addressed to this unit rather than only to the individual or disease; pressure for recognition that the primary care needs of a large part of the population are not met; insistence that preventive medicine is, in the best sense of the term, the only cost-effective medicine; demands that medicine cope with the growing elderly population; insistence on attention to cost containment; non-Western medicine; and concern about nutrition, the role of exercise in health, and, finally, human sexuality. These sorts of things are joined by demands that more attention be given to the problems of the ubiquity of skin diseases and the needs of the handicapped and the mentally retarded (Straus, 1965; Hamburg, 1979; Jonas, 1979; Gallagher and Vivian, 1979; Friedman, 1979; Praiss and Gjerde, 1980).

*Humanities and Social Sciences.* Medicine is as much based in sociology or the nature of human-to-human interactions as it is in the natural sciences with their concentration on molecular or submolecular interactions. The last two decades, 1960 to 1980, have seen major social changes and changing attitudes toward many health-related beliefs. Nutrition, human sexuality, exercise, non-Western medicine, escalating concern for costs, growing concern about ethics, the impact of changes in family structure, the origins of the wave of malpractice suits, attempts to understand the changing relationships of medicine and organized religion, perceptions of the impact of behavior and life-style on disease, profound concern about the needs of growing numbers of old people, the sources of epidemic drug abuse, and single parenting—all are examples of issues whose various proponents demand the attention of the medical curriculum. None of these is trivial; all are examples of what has been called the medicalization of social problems. To a greater or lesser extent, all are of potential concern to physicians, and all touch upon problems dealt with daily by many physicians, especially those in primary care fields. Concern about overemphasis on the disease model or the lack of emphasis on behavioral determinants, not of disease but of sickness, represent value judgments. The amount of time, concentration, and seniority of teachers presenting these topics represent the collective belief of a faculty about human illness, which is expressed in what the professors profess to their students. The variations from school to school are enormous. There is little debate about the actual importance of the sciences that deal with the sociological and behavioral aspects of human dysfunction and misery; the debate is about their *relative* importance. For a few centuries, natural science has presented an irresistible force, and it will, no doubt, continue to be the dominant change agent in the medical curriculum.

Over 80 percent of the medical schools now list courses which commonly identify the behavioral sciences per se; less often, the humanities, medical sociology, medicine and society, and ethics are specified. These course offerings reflect the goal of transmitting to students information about the societal factors impinging upon medical practice and the interaction between the patient and the physician or the physician and other health care workers. The probability is that if the content of the material presented by each school were analyzed, the variation between schools listing such courses and those that do not would not be very significant. There has undoubtedly been an increase in the amount of attention given these topics, but it has in no way lessened the dominance of natural science in the medical school curriculum. Whether the current structure represents a real change or an adaptation of the ever-shifting interface between medicine and the society it serves is a matter of judgment.

*Primary Care, Family Medicine, and Ambulatory Care.* At the risk of offending those who have written not just chapters, but books, about primary care or family medicine or ambulatory care, we boldly lump them together, not to imply that they represent a single discipline but to illustrate one of the most significant changes that has occurred in the medical curriculum in the past ten years—that is, the orientation toward primary, comprehensive, and continuing medical care of the patient in the context of the family (Pelligrino, 1966; Wood, Mayo, and Marsland, 1975).

Primary care is presented to medical students as either a required or an elective clerkship in virtually all medical schools (Giacolone and Hudson, 1977). The locale of this experience is widely varied—from model family clinics to large-scale clinic operations managed by the medical schools or teaching hospitals, to preceptorships in practitioners' offices in neighboring towns. For years, medical students have been taught in outpatient settings as a part of their internal medicine, obstetrics, or pediatrics rotations. Indeed, a frequent pattern was to have either the third- or fourth-year clerks assigned to the outpatient, with the other group assigned to the inpatient service. However, the focus of that care was characteristically in relation only to the specialty involved. The objective of the new programs is first contact care, a willingness to address all of a patient's problems, and long-term care, not care related only to a single episode of illness. It is also the explicitly stated intent of these programs to recruit students to careers in primary care, to create training situations that will prepare residents for such careers, and often to place trainees in practice situations where there is a perceived need.

Established faculties did not accept these programs readily. There were problems in identifying and recruiting a teaching faculty, providing an adequate setting, determining the appropriate place in their clinical training for students to be introduced to such care, and, as with clinical teaching in ambulatory settings, financing the whole operation. Numerous incentives were offered both at federal and state levels to stimulate the growth of these programs. Their decline upon the withdrawal of these subsidies might be predicted, but they have done so very well and are now so firmly established that it is much more likely that family medicine or primary care will join medicine, surgery, pediatrics, obstetrics, and psychiatry in a clerkship required of all students for graduation.

*The Rise and Fall and Rise Again of Preventive Medicine.* Prevention of infectious diseases—by sanitation, improved living environment, better nutrition, immunization, control of vectors, and education of the public—has been one of the health success stories of the past one hundred years. The desire to apply the lessons learned from this experience and the knowledge that many degenerative diseases could be delayed in onset and reduced in frequency, if not prevented altogether, have reawakened interest in preventive medicine. Saward and Sorensen (1978) believe that the heightened interest in preventive medicine stems from the progressive disillusionment with curative medicine. They point out that improvements in health status have not been commensurate with advances in the scientific and technological base of medical practice.

Despite our knowledge about the causes of disease, we are still at a loss to know how to prevent many illnesses. Physicians and their patients are beginning to understand the limits of medical care and to appreciate that personal preventive measures relating to life-style and behavioral change are critical factors in prevention. There is a great distance, however, between understanding and implementing effective measures in a democratic society. Though the recent eradication of smallpox throughout the world is a dramatic example of the power of prevention, failure to implement what we know about the use of seat belts, speed limits, and helmets for motorcyclists is more typical.

Epidemiology is the fundamental basic science of preventive medicine, and, as in biomedical knowledge, there has been a virtual explosion of knowledge in this area in the last two to three decades. Improved analytical methods and the use of the computer have empowered preventive medicine with a new capability. One of the major contributions of the clinical epidemiologist is expertise in the design, execution, and analysis of clinical trials, health care evaluation, and etiological studies. The curricular content of preventive medicine encompasses medical epidemiology, biostatistics, behavioral sciences, environmental or occupational medicine, and health or medical administration. Preventive medicine, public health, community medicine, and occupational medicine focus on the conquest of chronic disease; their domain is the full natural history of disease from etiology through prevention and rehabilitation. Community medicine looks at the health of populations or groups of people. In all these, the focus is on identifying and reducing the risk factors involving individuals, whole communities, or groups of employees. The future holds the possibility of preventive strategies aimed at reducing occupational and environmental risk factors. Holmes (1980) describes these possibilities in "Prevention: An Idea Whose Time Has Come?" He emphasizes that the scope of prevention relates to such major categories of concern as geriatrics, maternal and child health, and the prevention of alcohol and drug abuse.

It has finally been appreciated that prevention of the major degenerative diseases of the late twentieth century depends upon three actions: (1) control of many environmental factors, (2) a great deal of public education, and (3) persuasion of target populations that each individual through control of personal habits has the largest role to play in the prevention of these diseases. Students are now learning, by both their own personal experience and encounters with their patients, that each physician must urge good health habits on every patient. Control of smoking, the identification of alcoholism, the so-called epidemic of exercise, the wide success of efforts to control hypertension, the publicity given to the bad effects of the use of drugs—all are examples of popular acceptance of concepts about preventive medicine. Thus, in terms of getting its messages across to large segments of both the population at large and physicians, preventive medicine is a success. It is now time for preventive medicine to assume once again a more prominent role in the curriculum, through discrete courses and the integration of the rich array of teaching and learning materials that it is developing throughout the curriculum (Langmuir, 1964; Shepard and Roney, 1964; Makover, 1965; Barker, 1976; Lilienfeld and Lilienfeld, 1977; Shindell, 1978; Jonas, 1979; Hamburg, 1979; Foege, 1981; Moore, 1981; Segall and others, 1981).

*Topics of Special Interest.* The last two decades have seen human sexuality as a topic of polite conversation move from the bedroom to the living room, and from there to the pages of newspapers and widely distributed family magazines. The same thing has happened both in medical schools and in the interaction between physicians and patients. A survey of the course headings or curricular offerings of medical schools for 1981–1982 reveals that "Sexuality" appears as a heading in 12 percent of the listings (*Association of American Medical Colleges Curriculum Directory*, 1981). This, of course, tells us nothing of the content or quality of offerings, nor the teaching skills or attitudes of the faculty providing the instruction. However, medical school faculties can be assumed to be aware of the frequency of sexual dysfunction and the unhappiness related to it. Physicians are daily confronted with the many behavioral and social problems related to single parenting, illegitimate births, teenage pregnancies, rampant venereal disease, homosexuality, and divorce. In addition, physicians find that they must be prepared to cope with patients, especially younger ones, who are not only open about and very willing to bring their sexual concerns to physicians but also expect some help. Whether the medical schools are leaders or followers in the American "sexual revolution" is beside the point. Physicians, especially those in primary care, are expected to know something about human sexuality and to be able to deal with sexuality in a nonjudgmental fashion. How the topic is best taught is a more difficult question, on which there is no consensus. There is also great variation in who teaches it—whether psychologist, therapist, family practitioner, gynecologist, urologist, or psychiatrist will depend more than anything else on those who are most interested and concerned at each institution. This area is inescapably a significant addition to the content of the curriculum.

Cost control, non-Western medicine, nutrition, aerobic exercise, and medical jurisprudence are lumped together, not because their content has anything in common, but because all are of interest to growing segments of the public who seek answers to their many questions about such topics from physicians, who in turn generate pressure to have a variety of topics covered in the curriculum.

Medical jurisprudence is taught in all schools, frequently as a required course. Cost control is talked about in all schools, but effective courses are rare. Non-Western medicine might be described as a conversation piece or curiosity in most schools. Aerobics is a fad. While all of these are legitimate topics of concern and relevance to contemporary medicine, they must compete with other material that is judged to be more important. Medical faculties are often criticized for their conservatism and inertia. To the enthusiast, impatient because his favorite topic is not accepted, this inertia is seen as wrongheaded and obstructionist; to someone who takes the longer view, the inertia of medical faculties is seen as in the best interests of the society they serve. A profession that has seen phrenology, Fletcherism, phlogiston, bloodletting, autointoxication, and the more extreme examples of Freudian psychiatry come and go, knows that more of today's enthusiasms are transient than permanent. The profession's behavior is based on the conviction that it is better to be skeptical than uncritical.

## Agenda for the Future

One thing is certain—physicians must comprehend an overwhelming quantity of information drawn together from the natural sciences, the social sciences, and the humanities in the treatment of each patient. We have commented on many changes that have occurred over the past two decades. There are as many and more which we have omitted, not for lack of significance but for lack of time and space (Matlack, 1972).*

We have asserted that the expansion of our understanding of biological phenomena and knowledge of the natural sciences has been the single most potent force for lasting curricular change in this period. It will continue to be so. However, during this same period, medicine has come to appreciate that the environment and the patient's own behavior and life-style have an important impact on the etiology of disease and illness and on the outcome of any therapy. The very nature of some of our scientific explorations has led us to the kind of ethical issues that literally surround the beginning and end of life (Lesse, 1980).

What does all this mean to medical educators, to the faculty? What we have observed in most medical schools is not radical change. Not surprisingly, even the more innovative programs of the new medical schools of the past two decades slowly but surely evolve toward a more traditional curriculum. What is often missing is a clear set of objectives that derive from a consensus about what it really means to educate a physician (Geschwind, 1979). What manner of physician does the faculty want to represent its educational product in the world (Mellinkoff, 1977; Vouri, 1979; Moy, 1979; Tosteson, 1979; Challoner, 1980)? Nearly all faculties, when faced with the rapidly expanding body of scientific knowledge, would rather substitute the new for the old or add it to the curriculum (Salzman, Donovan, and Allen, 1972; Shapiro and others, 1974). In cramming in all the scientific

*Case Histories of Ten Medical Schools, published by the Josiah Macy, Jr., Foundation (Lippard and Purcell, 1972), and Medical Education Since 1960: Marching to a Different Drummer (Hunt and Weeks, 1979), published by the W. K. Kellogg Foundation and Michigan State University, chronicled this twenty-year period of change and the development of new medical schools during the period. The reader is referred to these volumes for illuminating case histories not touched on here.

knowledge possible, the faculty must remember that students graduate knowing only today's science, even though it may represent the cutting edge. But students must be prepared to practice their profession for thirty years or more, well beyond the year 2000. Anderson and Graham (1980), in their study of comparative information loads in various disciplines, estimate that medical students in the basic sciences must assimilate twenty-four new facts/concepts per hour! They conclude from their studies that to give students time for reading and development of special skills, as well as other academic activities and free time, an accepted learning rate should be about four to six facts/concepts per hour.

Because of their conviction that our academic institutions are ill-prepared to apply effectively the modern technology available to help them and their desire to develop a blueprint of the requisite steps for remedying that situation, Wilson and Smythe have been studying for the past two years the management of information in medicine. A particularly important dimension for medical educators is the requirement that medical students become computer literate (Virgo and Hody, 1976). (See Chapter Twenty-One for an extended discussion of the implications of the computer revolution for medical education.) The application of electronic data processing in medicine and in our daily lives will quicken in the near future to a pace almost as rapid as the development of the new biology. Our lives and the attendant information overload have reached an almost intolerable level of complexity (Weed, 1981). We must discover ways to simplify our work, to reduce the amount of information—particular facts—that we must carry in our memories, and without slowing the pace of scientific and technological development, to modulate the frenetic activity currently required to keep abreast. The mind must be less burdened with facts and freed to understand and elaborate the conceptual frameworks of bodies of knowledge. Medical students must understand that they are making a commitment to a lifetime of learning if they are to maintain their intellectual and moral integrity as physicians charged with the care of others. The faculty is obliged to guide them in the understanding and learning of the conceptual frameworks, along with a sensible loading of the facts, and to guide them in becoming skilled in the use of modern technology that can assist them in extending their memories and in continuing their learning.

The physician must, in some way, manage to maintain command of a rapidly changing scientific field in which he or she specializes. What medical education must also assure is that physicians have an understanding of human beings as individuals and as members of society as they relate to their families and to their environment, in the home, the community, and the workplace. The quality of an individual's life, and therefore health and well-being, is as much dependent on adequate functioning in these roles as it is on knowledge of the cause, nature, and cure of disease.

We have suggested that the classical literature of medical education has frequently been the bellwether of the next scenario. Another Alan Gregg lecture illustrated the point that if we as medical educators will only listen (as we admonish our students to do in caring for their patients), we can understand and see what must be done. Tosteson (1981) in the 1980 Gregg lecture, *Science, Medicine, and Education,* examined human beings as organisms, as social beings, and as individuals, and eloquently elaborated the scenario we prescribe for the future. In an earlier address on the same subject to the Council of Deans, he reminded us that each of us is born alone and dies alone, and it is the role of the physician to help the individual along that way. He concluded, "Our growing understanding makes us humble before the vast complexity of our being but also proud of our greater power to influence our lives. As physicians, let us use this power to deepen and strengthen our caring and learning in medicine" (p. 15). The medical curriculum of the future essentially serves the same purpose the curriculum has always served—to educate and nurture a sensitive, intuitive, compassionate human being, educated and knowledgeable in the best of modern science and dedicated to supporting the human struggle for survival in a complex world.

## References

Abelson, J. "A Revolution in Biology." *Science*, 1980, *209* (4463), 1319-1321.

American Association of Anatomists, Educational Affairs Committee. "Curriculum, Faculty, and Training in Anatomy." *Journal of Medical Education*, 1966, *41*, 956-964.

Anderson, J., and Graham, A. "A Problem in Medical Education: Is There an Information Overload?" *Medical Education*, 1980, *14*, 4-7.

Association of American Medical Colleges. "The Teaching of Pathology, Microbiology, Immunology, Genetics: Report of the Second Teaching Institute." *Journal of Medical Education*, 1955, *30*, Part 2.

Association of American Medical Colleges. "The Teaching of Anatomy and Anthropology in Medical Education: Report of the Third Teaching Institute." *Journal of Medical Education*, 1956, *31*, Part 2.

Association of American Medical Colleges, Council of Academic Societies. *Integrated Teaching of Basic Medical and Clinical Sciences.* Resource draft compiled for discussion groups. Washington, D.C.: Association of American Medical Colleges, 1981.

*Association of American Medical Colleges Curriculum Directory, 1981-1982.* Washington, D.C.: Association of American Medical Colleges, 1981.

Barbee, R. A., and Dinham, S. M. "Student Decision-Making and Performance in a Flexible Time Curriculum." *Journal of Medical Education*, 1977, *52*, 882-887.

Barker, W. H. *Preventive and Community Medicine in Primary Care.* U.S. Department of Health, Education, and Welfare Publication no. 76-879. Washington, D.C.: U.S. Government Printing Office, 1976.

Barondess, J. A. "The Training of the Internist." *Annals of Internal Medicine*, 1979, *90*, 412-417.

Baum, J. H., and Koushanpour, E. "Establishment and Organization of a Multidisciplinary Laboratory." *Journal of Medical Education*, 1967, *42*, 752-756.

Behal, F. J. "A View of the Comprehensive Role of the Basic Sciences in Medical Education." *Journal of Medical Education*, 1973, *48* (2), 166-170.

Beran, R. L. "The Rise and Fall of the Three-Year Medical School Programs." *Journal of Medical Education*, 1979, *54* (3), 248-249.

Beran, R. L., and Kriner, R. E. *A Study of Three-Year Curricula in U.S. Medical Schools.* Washington, D.C.: Association of American Medical Colleges, 1978.

Bowers, J. Z., and Purcell, E. F. (Eds.). *Teaching the Basic Medical Sciences:*

*Human Biology.* Report of Macy Conference held November 26–29, 1973. New York: Josiah Macy, Jr., Foundation, 1974.

Brinkhous, K. M. "Pathology." *Journal of the American Medical Association,* 1980, *243* (21), 2205–2207.

Campbell, C., and DeMuth, G. R. "The University of Michigan Integrated Premedical-Medical Program." *Journal of Medical Education,* 1976, *51* (4), 290–295.

Carnegie Commission on Higher Education. *Higher Education and the Nation's Health: Policies for Medical and Dental Education.* New York: McGraw-Hill, 1970.

Challoner, D. R. "Dilemmas Posed by the New Biology for the Future of Medical Education: A Medical School Perspective." Paper presented to 91st Meeting of Group on Institutional Planning, October 26, 1980. Washington, D.C.: Association of American Medical Colleges, 1980.

Childs, B., Huether, C. A., and Murphy, E. A. "Human Genetics Teaching in U.S. Medical Schools." *American Journal of Human Genetics,* 1981, *33* (1), 1–10.

Comroe, J. H., Jr. (Ed.). "Research and Medical Education: Report of the Ninth Teaching Institute." *Journal of Medical Education,* 1962, *37,* Part 2.

Comroe, J. H., Jr., and others. "The Teaching of Physiology, Biochemistry, Pharmacology: Report of the First Teaching Institute." *Journal of Medical Education,* 1954, *29,* Part 2.

Cooper, J. A. D. "Undergraduate Medical Education." In J. Z. Bowers and E. F. Purcell (Eds.), *Advances in American Medicine: Essays at the Bicentennial.* Vol. I. New York: Josiah Macy, Jr., Foundation, 1976.

Cope, O., and Zacharias, J. *Medical Education Reconsidered: Report of the Endicott House Summer Study on Medical Education, July 1965.* Philadelphia: Lippincott, 1966.

Csaky, T. Z. "Is There an Identity Crisis in Medical School Pharmacology?" *Journal of Medical Education,* 1976, *51* (11), 935–937.

Darley, W. "Medical School Financing and National Institutional Planning: Eighth Annual Alan Gregg Memorial Lecture." *Journal of Medical Education,* 1966, *41* (2), 97–109.

Daubney, J. H., Wagner, E. E., and Rogers, W. A. "Six-Year B.S./M.D. Programs: A Literature Review." *Journal of Medical Education,* 1981, *56* (6), 497–503.

Davis, B. D. "Frontiers of the Biological Sciences." *Science,* 1980, *209* (4452), 78–89.

Dollery, C. T. "Clinical Pharmacology and Therapeutics in the 1980s." *British Journal of Clinical Pharmacology,* 1978, *6,* 379.

Dreux, C. "Fundamental Research in Biology and Tomorrow's Pharmacology." *Methods and Findings in Experimental Clinical Pharmacology,* 1979, *1* (1), 11–21.

Eichna, L. W. "Medical School Education, 1975–1979: A Student's Perspective." *New England Journal of Medicine,* 1980, *303* (13), 727–734.

Foege, W. B. "Prevention and World Health: The Next Two Decades." Katharine Boucot Sturgis Lecture. *Preventive Medicine,* 1981, *10,* 112–117.

Fogarty International Center. *Reform of Medical Education: The Role of Research in Medical Education.* Number 7. Washington, D.C.: U.S. Government Printing Office, 1970.

Fraser, F. C. "The Role of Genetics in Medicine." *Birth Defects,* 1980, *16* (5), 1–6.

Friedman, E. "Changing the Course of Things: Costs Enter Medical Education." *Hospitals,* 1979, *53* (9), 82–85.

Funkenstein, D. H. "Current Changes in Education Affecting Medical School Admissions and Curriculum Planning." *Journal of Medical Education,* 1966, *41* (5), 401–423.

Gallagher, C. R., and Vivian, V. M. "Nutrition Concepts Essential in the Education of the Medical Student." *American Journal of Clinical Nutrition,* 1979, *32* (6), 1330–1333.

Gee, H. H., and Child, C. G., III (Eds.). "Report of the Second Institute on Clinical Teaching: Report of the Seventh Teaching Institute." *Journal of Medical Education,* 1961, *36,* Part 2.

Gee, H. H., and Richmond, J. B. (Eds.). "Report of the First Institute on Clinical Teaching: Report of the Sixth Teaching Institute." *Journal of Medical Education,* 1959, *34,* Part 2.

Geertsma, R. H., and others. "An Independent Study Program Within a Medical Curriculum." *Journal of Medical Education,* 1977, *52* (2), 123–132.

Gellhorn, A., and Scheuer, R. "The Experiment in Medical Education at the City College of New York." *Journal of Medical Education,* 1978, *53,* 574–582.

Geschwind, N. "Even Homer Sometimes Nods: Can We Avoid Cerebral Technological Obsolescence?" Unpublished paper presented at the Harvard Medical School Educational Workshop, June 1979.

Giacalone, J. J., and Hudson, J. I. "Primary Care Education Trends in U.S. Medical Schools and Teaching Hospitals." *Journal of Medical Education,* 1977, *52* (12), 971–981.

Glick, S. "Humanistic Medicine in a Modern Age." *New England Journal of Medicine,* 1981, *304* (17), 1036–1037.

Gordon, L. "A Healthy University in a Sick Society?—Alan Gregg Memorial Lecture." *Journal of Medical Education,* 1970, *45* (11), 847–853.

Graduate Medical Education National Advisory Committee. *Final Report to Patricia Harris, Secretary, Department of Health and Human Services.* September 30, 1980, Vol. 1. Washington, D.C.: U.S. Government Printing Office, 1980.

Hagstad, H. V. "Preventive Medicine in Today's Curriculum." *Journal of Veterinary Medicine Association,* 1979, *174,* 384–386.

Ham, T. H. "Medical Education at Western Reserve University: A Progress Report for the Sixteen Years, 1946–1962." *New England Journal of Medicine,* 1962, *267,* 868–874, 916–923.

Ham, T. H. "The Training of the Physician: Research in the Teaching-Learning Process—Two Experimental Modules." *New England Journal of Medicine,* 1964, *271,* 1042–1046.

Hamburg, D. A. "Disease Prevention: The Challenge of the Future." *American Journal of Public Health,* 1979, *69* (10), 1026–1033.

Harrell, G. T. "Student Study Cubicles." *Journal of Medical Education,* 1964, *39,* 32–39.

Harrell, G. T., Hamilton, J. M., and Butt, A. "A Multidiscipline Student Teaching Laboratory: Incorporation in a Simple Building Design." *Journal of Medical Education,* 1964, *39,* 828–837.

Harris, J. A., Sorlie, W. E., and Stolpe, S. G. "Independent Study Curriculum in Gross Anatomy." *Journal of Medical Education*, 1973, *48* (11), 1023-1025.

Heard, A. "The Seamless Web of Health and Policy—Alan Gregg Memorial Lecture, 1971." *Journal of Medical Education*, 1971, *46* (11), 927-932.

Hecht, F. "Teaching Medical Genetics and Alice in Wonderland." *American Journal of Human Genetics*, 1981, *33* (1), 138-139.

Holmes, C. "Prevention: An Idea Whose Time Has Come?" *Western Journal of Medicine*, 1980, *132*, 471-473.

Hubbard, W. N., Jr., and Howard, R. B. "The Educational Environment in the Large Medical School." *Journal of Medical Education*, 1967, *42*, 633-641.

Hubbard, W. N., Jr., Gronvall, J. A., and DeMuth, G. R. (Eds.). "The Medical School Curriculum." *Journal of Medical Education*, 1970, *45*, Part 2.

Hunt, A. D., and Weeks, L. E. (Eds.). *Medical Education Since 1960: Marching to a Different Drummer.* Battle Creek: W. K. Kellogg Foundation and Michigan State University, 1979.

Jacobson, E. D. "Revolution in the Medical Curriculum." *Journal of Medical Education*, 1967, *42*, 1081-1086.

Jaussi, J. R., and others. "Evaluation and Proposed Modifications of Multidisciplinary Laboratories." *Journal of Medical Education*, 1971, *46* (10), 869-875.

Johns, C. E., and Smith, R. D. "An Independent Study Program in Medical School." *Journal of Medical Education*, 1973, *48* (8), 732-738.

Jonas, S. "Health-Oriented Physician Education: There's HOPE for the Future." *Journal of Community Health*, 1979, *4* (4), 259-266.

Kahn, R. H., Conklin, J. L., and Glover, R. A. "A Self-Instructional Program in Microscopic Anatomy." *Journal of Medical Education*, 1973, *48* (9), 859-863.

Kettel, L. J., and others. "Arizona's Three-Year Medical Curriculum: A Postmortem." *Journal of Medical Education*, 1979, *54* (3), 210-216.

Kolata, G. B. "Developmental Biology: Where Is It Going?" *Science*, 1979, *206* (4416), 315-316.

Kornberg, A. "Biochemistry Evolving." *Canadian Journal of Biochemistry*, 1980, *58* (2), 93-96.

Korst, D. R. "The Independent Study Program at the University of Wisconsin Medical School." *Journal of Medical Education*, 1977, *52*, 404-412.

Langmuir, A. D. "The Training of the Physician: Education and Training in Preventive Medicine and Public Health." *New England Journal of Medicine*, 1964, *271*, 772-774.

Lanzoni, V., and Kayne, H. L. "A Report on Graduates of the Boston University Six-Year Combined Liberal Arts/Medical Program." *Journal of Medical Education*, 1976, *51* (4), 283-289.

Lee, P. V. "Experimentation in Medical Education: The Student, the Patient, and the University." *Annals of the New York Academy of Science*, 1965, *128*, 532-543.

Lee, P. V., and Bamburger, J. W. "Multidiscipline Student Laboratories: University of Southern California School of Medicine." *Journal of Medical Education*, 1964, *39*, 846-856.

Lesse, S. "Ethics and the Future Health Sciences: The Need for a New Code." *American Journal of Psychotherapy*, 1980, *34* (2), 149-152.

Levine, R. J. "The Future of Clinical Research." *New England Journal of Medicine*, 1979, *301* (23), 1295-1296.

Levy, M., Bresnick, E., and Williams, W. L., Jr. "A Student Feedback Model Designed to Elicit Data for Effective Curricular Modification in Basic Sciences." *Journal of Medical Education,* 1973, *48* (12), 1148–1150.

Lilienfeld, D. E., and Lilienfeld, A. M. "Corner of History. Teaching Preventive Medicine in Medical Schools: An Historical Vignette." *Preventive Medicine,* 1977, *6,* 469–471.

Lippard, V. W., and Purcell, E. (Eds.). *Case Histories of Ten New Medical Schools.* New York: Josiah Macy, Jr., Foundation, 1972.

Lundberg, G. D. "Contempo '81 Pathology." *Journal of the American Medical Association,* 1981, *245* (21), 2212–2213.

McKusick, V. A. "The Last Twenty Years: An Overview of Advances in Medical Genetics." *Progress in Clinical Biological Research,* 1981, *45,* 127–144.

MacLeod, C. M. "Society Challenges the Medical Schools: Tenth Annual Alan Gregg Memorial Lecture." *Journal of Medical Education,* 1968, *43* (4), 425–432.

Makover, H. B. "Preventive Medicine in the American Medical School." *Annals of New York Academy of Science,* 1965, *128,* 607–611.

Marchand, E. R., and Steward, J. P. "Trends in Basic Medical Science Instruction Affecting Role of Multidiscipline Laboratories." *Journal of Medical Education,* 1974, *49* (2), 171–175.

Matlack, D. R. "Changes and Trends in Medical Education." *Journal of Medical Education,* 1972, *47,* 612–619.

Mellinkoff, S. M. "The Physician of Tomorrow." *Journal of the American Medical Association,* 1977, *237* (18), 1952–1953.

Mistry, F. D., and Davis, J. S. "Teaching Efficient and Effective Utilization of the Clinical Laboratory." *Journal of Medical Education,* 1981, *56* (4), 356–358.

Mitchell, F. L., and others. "The Impact of Technology on Medicine: The Impact of Technology on Clinical Pathology over the Last Twenty-Five Years." *Journal of Medical Engineering Technology,* 1981, *5* (1), 13–21.

"Molecular Biology: Suffering from Shock." *Nature,* 1979, *278* (5705), 587.

Moore, G. "Preventive Medicine Redefined." *Journal of Medical Education,* 1981, *56,* 358–360.

Moy, R. H. "Critical Values in Medical Education." *New England Journal of Medicine,* 1979, *301* (13), 694–697.

Pelligrino, E. D. "Generalist Function in Medicine." *Journal of the American Medical Association,* 1966, *198,* 541–545.

Praiss, I., and Gjerde, C. "Cost Containment Through Medical Education." *Journal of the American Medical Association,* 1980, *244* (1), 53–55.

Pritchard, H. N. "The Lehigh-Medical College of Pennsylvania Six-Year B.A.-M.D. Program." *Journal of Medical Education,* 1976, *51* (4), 296–298.

Rappleye, W. C. "The Expanding Functions of Medical Education: The Alan Gregg 1963 Memorial Lecture." *Journal of Medical Education,* 1963, *38,* (11), 899–905.

Robbins, F. C. "Revision at Reserve." *Harvard Medical Alumni Bulletin,* Spring 1968, 17–18.

Rossee, C. "Integrated Versus Discipline Oriented Instruction in Medical Education." *Journal of Medical Education,* 1974, *49* (10), 445–459.

Salzman, L. F., Donovan, J. C., and Allen, P. Z. "A Study of Curricular Change: The Acquisition and Retention of Factual Knowledge." *Journal of Medical Education,* 1972, *47* (8), 631–636.

Sanazaro, P. J. "Class Size in Medical School." *Journal of Medical Education,* 1966, *41,* 1017–1029.

Sanazaro, P. J. "Innovations in Medical Education: Social and Scientific Determinants." *Archives of Neurology,* 1967, *17,* 484–493.

Saward, E., and Sorensen, A. "The Current Emphasis on Preventive Medicine." *Science,* 1978, *200,* 889–894.

Segall, A., and others. "A General Model for Preventive Intervention in Clinical Practice." *Journal of Medical Education,* 1981, *56,* 324–333.

Shannon, J. A. "The Advancement of Medical Research: A Twenty-Year View of the Role of the National Institutes of Health—Ninth Annual Alan Gregg Memorial Lecture." *Journal of Medical Education,* 1967, *42* (2), 97–108.

Shapiro, A., and others. "The Impact of Curricular Change on Performance on National Board Examinations." *Journal of Medical Education,* 1974, *49* (12), 1113–1118.

Shepard, W. P., and Roney, J. G. "The Teaching of Preventive Medicine in the United States." *Millbank Memorial Fund Quarterly,* 1964, *42* (4), Part 2.

Sheps, C. G., Wolf, G. A., and Jacobsen, C. (Eds.). "Medical Education and Medical Care—Interactions and Prospects: Report of the Eighth Teaching Institute." *Journal of Medical Education,* 1961, *36,* Part 2.

Shindell, S. "Past President's Address. Thirty-Fourth Annual Meeting of Association of Teachers of Preventive Medicine." *Journal of Community Health,* 1978, *3* (4), 289–291.

Simpson, J. L., and others. "Genetic Counseling and Genetic Services in Obstetrics and Gynecology: Implications for Educational Goals and Clinical Practice." *American Journal of Obstetrics and Gynecology,* 1981, *140,* 70–80.

Spector, R., Roberts, R., and Vesell, E. S. "Clinical Pharmacology: A New Specialty." *American Journal of Medicine,* 1981, *7,* 221–222.

Spilman, E. L. "The Administration of a Coordinated Teaching Curriculum." *Journal of Medical Education,* 1965, *40,* 1049–1057.

Spilman, E. L. "Some Advantages and Disadvantages of Multidiscipline Laboratories." *Journal of Medical Education,* 1966, *41,* 143–149.

Spilman, E. L., and Spilman, H. W. "A Pair Comparison Study of the Relevance of Nine Basic Science Courses." *Journal of Medical Education,* 1975, *50* (7), 667–671.

Stasney, J. "The Future Challenge for Anatomic Pathology." *Journal of Environmental Pathology and Toxicology,* 1980, *4* (5–6), 313–316.

Stoker, M. "New Medicine and New Biology." *British Medical Journal of Clinical Research,* 1980, *281,* 1678–1682.

Stokes, J., III. "Innovations in Medical Education–Developing Schools." *Federal Bulletin,* 1967, *54,* 188–197.

Straus, R. "Behavioral Science in the Medical Curriculum." *Annals of the New York Academy of Science,* 1965, *128,* 599–606.

Sweeney, G. D., and Mitchell, D. L. M. "An Introduction to the Study of Medicine: Phase I of the McMaster M.D. Program." *Journal of Medical Education,* 1971, *50* (1), 70–77.

Teplitz, R. L. "Genetics." *Journal of the American Medical Association,* 1980, *243* (21), 2186–2188.

Tosteson, D. C. "Learning in Medicine." *New England Journal of Medicine,* 1979, *301* (13), 690–694.

Tosteson, D. C. "Science, Medicine, and Education." *Journal of Medical Education,* 1981, *56* (1), 8–15.

Trzebiatowski, G. L., and Peterson, S. "A Study of Faculty Attitudes Toward Ohio State's Three-Year Medical Program." *Journal of Medical Education,* 1979, *54* (3), 205–209.

Turner, T. B. "The Medical Curriculum in Evolution." *Journal of Medical Education,* 1967, *42*, 926–929.

Virgo, J. A., and Hody, G. L. "Computer-Based Instruction and the Health Sciences Library." *Journal of Medical Education,* 1976, *51* (8), 644–647.

Vouri, H. "Education and the Quality of Health Services." *Health Policy and Education,* 1979, *1*, 67–69.

Wagner, R. R. "The Basic Medical Sciences, the Revolution in Biology, and the Future of Medical Education." *Yale Journal of Biological Medicine,* 1962, *35*, 1–11.

Wearn, J. T. "Immediate Problems for Medical Educators: Third Alan Gregg Memorial Lecture." *Journal of Medical Education,* 1961, *36* (2), 113–118.

Weed, L. L. "Physicians of the Future." *New England Journal of Medicine,* 1981, *304*, 903–907.

Wilson, M. P. "Medical Schools in the Planning Stage: Are More Schools Needed?" *Journal of Medical Education,* 1972, *47*, 677–689.

Wood, J., Mayo, F., and Marsland, D. "A Systems Approach to Patient Care, Curriculum, and Research in Family Practice." *Journal of Medical Education,* 1975, *50* (12), 1106–1112.

Yates, F. E. "Integrative Pharmacology—Beyond Structure-Activity Relationships into Pharmacolinguistics." *American Journal of Physiology,* 1979, *237*, R251–R253.

*William E. Brown*

# 3

# Dentistry

In the early days of the United States, dentists learned their skills through an apprenticeship system. Formal dental education began only with the founding of the Baltimore College of Dental Surgery in 1840, which marked the turning point in separating dental and medical education. The first university-sponsored dental school was established at Harvard in 1867, an event that ultimately led to the recognition of dentistry as a learned and scholarly profession. Until 1929, however, dental education was primarily technically oriented and was predominantly conducted by private, proprietary schools.

### Milestones in the Evolution of Dental Education*

The Flexner report in 1910 provided the initial stimulus for the move away from proprietary medical education that occurred in the ensuing years. Over the next fifty years, medical education was guided by Flexner's recommendations that it become a university function, that it be scientifically based and research oriented, that higher admissions standards be employed, and that full-time faculty committed to teaching and research be recruited.

The Gies' report in 1926 is the dental equivalent of the Flexner report. By recommending two years of predental education followed by a three-year dental curriculum, greater application of the basic sciences to clinical dentistry, and improved teaching facilities and equipment, it hastened the integration of dental education into the university.

---

*The following brief history of major studies of dental education is based on the summary compiled by Santangelo (1981).

Numerous studies made in the years following the Gies' report have contributed to the present status of dental education. L. E. Blauch's 1935 report brought some degree of standardization to dental curricula and made the recommendation that the dental curriculum be four years in length preceded by two years of college study. The 1940 study by the Council on Dental Education of the American Dental Association (ADA) resulted in the adoption of the *Requirements for the Approval of a Dental School,* which stipulated two years of preprofessional education followed by four years of dental education; required courses to be included in the dental curriculum were prescribed, and the specified number of clock hours of instruction was limited to no less than 3,800 and no more than 4,400.

Major studies over the past fifteen years have focused on the nature and integration of curricula as actually implemented in U.S. dental schools. In 1967–1968, the Council on Dental Education published a report of the results of a survey of dental curricula, which contained an analysis of the status and variation in clock hours of instruction. In 1976, the council and the American Association of Dental Schools reported the results of a joint curriculum study, the most comprehensive review of dental curricula ever undertaken. The data in that study provided the necessary baseline for future comparative studies of curricula. A special committee representing the higher education community reviewed the 1976 curriculum study and published a critique in 1980, which stressed the importance of ongoing improvement in the continuum of dental education, from preprofessional through professional to lifetime learning, and which emphasized the need for dental education to become more fully integrated into the university and academic health center (American Dental Association, Council on Dental Education, 1980). The most recent study on advanced dental education, carried out by the American Association of Dental Schools (AADS) in concert with the Council on Dental Education, identified new directions for postdoctoral programs and their relations to the full spectrum of dental education.

### Changing Dental Manpower Requirements

Following several years of debate on health manpower needs, the Congress in 1963 passed the Health Professions Education Assistance Act. It provided aid to build new schools, replace and remodel existing facilities, and support students through a program of direct loans. This act was amended in 1965, 1968, 1971, and in later years to provide a broad spectrum of assistance to dental schools and other health professions education institutions in the additional form of general institutional support, student aid, financial distress grants, special project grants, and grants for advanced training. During these years, this money induced schools to admit more students, reduce curriculum time, develop new learning methods (especially self-instruction), establish extramural learning systems, recruit minority students, improve the geographic distribution of dental manpower, and train expanded-duty auxiliaries. Although the intent of Congress was laudable and many of the projects came to fruition, it is doubtful that anyone intended for increased federal support to result, as it did, in a surplus of dentists, higher operating costs, higher tuitions, and fiscal uncertainties in the dental schools (Bruce, 1981).

In 1960, there were 3,616 first-year dental students in the United States; by 1980, that number had risen to 6,030 (American Dental Association, 1981a). However, as capitation funds were phased out, predoctoral enrollments declined, at least to some extent. The number of dental auxiliary students has also increased substantially, as has that of general practice residents, while the figure for dental specialty students has remained almost constant since 1971. Over the past twenty years, this expansion in programs, student enrollments, and numbers of graduates has been accompanied in a number of states by the assignment of additional functions to dental hygienists and dental assistants. The stimulus for enlarging the functions of these dental auxiliaries was the projected need to respond to increasing demands for services required by a rapidly growing population and financed by an anticipated national health insurance program.

The U.S. Department of Health and Human Services has recently predicted a surplus of dentists within the next decade. Dentists claim that an overall surplus now exists, especially in some regions, and many schools are already reducing student enrollment. It appears that more dental graduates are establishing practices in underserved communities, that larger numbers seek a year of residency prior to practice, and that fewer are establishing independent practices immediately following graduation. The typical 1980 graduate was approximately $20,000 in debt upon graduation (American Association of Dental Schools, 1982, p. 8). This factor, together with the projected surplus of dentists, is producing career decisions that differ from those made as recently as 1975.

*Characteristics of Dental Practice.* Since 1950, dental practice has changed significantly, as has the delivery of services. New equipment (most notably the air-driven hand piece), more effective anesthetics and other drugs to ensure patient comfort, new esthetic filling materials, and a host of preventive agents and methods have all served to upgrade the oral health of the public. There is substantial evidence to indicate that, despite increasing information available to the public on plaque control, the prevalence of periodontal disease has not changed significantly over the past decade, while the prevalence of dental caries has decreased. The decrease in dental caries is undoubtedly due to the use of fluoride in drinking water and its application topically or orally. Vaccine for caries is currently under study, and researchers predict an effective one will be available within the next twenty years (American Dental Association, 1982, p. 11). By the year 2000, a higher proportion of the dentist's time is likely to be spent on problems relating to supporting tissues and to an aging population. Hopefully, these changes in the characteristics of dental practice will be reflected in revised dental curricula, and, ideally, curricular changes will precede those occurring in practice.

*Licensure of Dentists.* A dentist must be licensed in the jurisdiction in which he or she practices. While there is no national licensure or reciprocity, there are four regional examining boards, national written examinations accepted by all but the state of Delaware, and licensure in several states through a credentialing process. The National Dental Board Examinations consist of two parts: One covers the basic sciences and is usually taken toward the end of a student's second year; the other assesses knowledge of the clinical sciences and is taken in the senior year. Applicants for regional board examinations, which consist of written and clinical components, must have passed Parts I and II of the National Dental Board

Examinations. Upon successful completion of a regional board examination, a dentist is eligible for licensure in all the states in the region. Licensure is granted after the applicant successfully completes an interview with the board and passes a written examination on the state's dental practice act.

Foreign dental graduates are not numerous in the United States. It is difficult for them to become licensed, since only fifteen states accept them as candidates for licensure unless they have also earned a degree from a U.S. dental school. Furthermore, the failure rate among foreign graduates in the fifteen states which do examine them is very high: In 1979, 681 of 917 candidates (73.5 percent) failed, according to the records of the American Dental Association.

However, once licensed, always licensed; reexamination is not required of anyone. Thus, assurance of continuing professional competence is a national concern of dental organizations. For this reason, ten states now require a certain number of hours of continuing education credit as a condition for renewal of the license (American Dental Association, Council on Dental Education, 1980). The effect of this requirement upon a dentist's competency is not known; the profession is struggling to evaluate the system, to improve the quality of continuing education, and to find new and more effective methods to ensure lifelong competency.

### Educational Personnel

*Admission and Retention of Students.* In 1967, 56 percent of all first-year dental students had a baccalaureate or master's degree; by 1980-81, this figure had risen to 83.6 percent. Between 1970 and 1980, first-year enrollment increased by 32 percent, total enrollment by 38 percent, and the number of graduates by 43 percent (American Dental Association, 1981a). In 1970, women comprised only 1.4 percent of total enrollment and minority students only 5 percent (American Dental Association, 1971). In 1980-81, these figures had increased to 17 percent and 11.5 percent, respectively (American Dental Association, 1981a). However, since 1975, the size of the applicant pool has decreased by over 40 percent and the ratio of applicants to first-year class positions has fallen from 2.5:1 to 1.4:1, a ratio comparable to that prevailing in 1960, just prior to the federal government's involvement in health professions education (Powell, 1981). Nonetheless, the continuing decline is a serious matter because it results from such persistent factors as the costs of dental education and of establishing a practice, the lure of such other careers as engineering, and, perhaps, an increasing tendency for dentists to discourage prospective students about a career in dentistry because of the current market.

Admission criteria are similar in most U.S. dental schools. They include the predental academic record, Dental Aptitude Test scores, recommendations from preprofessional counselors, an interview in some schools, and career choice/motivation questionnaires in a few schools. Since 1973, the attrition rate for first-year students has remained constant at 3.5 percent, almost evenly divided between personal and academic reasons (American Dental Association, 1981b).

Stimulated by the increasing numbers of dentists entering the work force and the changing migration patterns of the population, some schools have recently expanded student counseling services to include advice about career decisions and practice locations. The National Health Professions Placement Network (NHPPN) sponsored by the American Dental Association Health Foundation and the W. K. Kellogg Foundation attempted to match dentists and locations or employers. For dentists, its services included finding associateships with existing practices, identifying salaried professional positions, locating practices for sale, and establishing practices in underserved communities. For the employer or community, NHPPN assisted in identifying new associates for existing practices, employing salaried professionals, disposing of professional practices, and recruiting professionals for communities. Because the results of this project were not as great as had been anticipated, funding was terminated in November 1982.

*Faculty and Staffing.* Though exact personnel information is not available for the early sixties, it is clear that the number of faculty members and nonacademic staff has increased significantly over the last twenty years. Several factors help to explain this increase. First, institutional expectations of a faculty member's role have changed markedly. In 1960, it was not unusual for a full-time clinical faculty member to spend eight to ten half-days per week with students; that figure has now fallen to four to five. Currently, faculty members at most institutions have multiple responsibilities that must be met if they are to progress effectively through the ranks of academia. Although the responsibilities vary among institutions, departments, and academic ranks, they generally include—in addition to teaching in various settings, research, and creative writing—direct patient care, service on college and university committees, and service to professional groups and community agencies. Also, there is a growing trend toward continuing self-development and toward earning such necessary credentials as advanced degrees and specialty board certificates. With these expanded roles of faculty members, it is clear that more faculty personnel are required to do the job for the same number of students than was the case in 1960 (Brown, 1981).

The evaluation of faculty performance has been a concern at many institutions and is receiving increasing attention as fiscal resources dwindle and student enrollment falls. In the June 1977 issue of the *Journal of Dental Education* devoted to faculty evaluation, Chambers (1977, p. 299) reviewed in detail the purposes of evaluation of faculty, the sources of information to do so, evaluation subjects, and the methods required to implement a system. He commented on the political realities surrounding evaluation but affirmed that "faculty evaluation is also a scientific process, or at least one capable of being greatly improved by rigorous, empirical study, which has yet to be performed." Mackenzie (1977, pp. 302–306) outlined the components of a faculty evaluation program and stated that effective faculty development efforts should accompany evaluation. He discussed the serious conflict between improving teaching skills and performing creative activities more closely related to promotion, salary increases, and tenure. He recommended that a faculty evaluation system be developed by cooperation between evaluation specialists and faculty, that it be based on a broad spectrum of data to reduce bias and subjectivity, and that standards, criteria, and operational guidelines be given to each participant. He cautioned that the cost of such a system not exceed its benefits. Guild (1977), in reviewing the deficiencies of faculty assessment and reward systems, described recent developments in the behavioral sciences that could improve them. He suggested both new procedures and new criteria but warned that they are more difficult to apply than those currently in

### Table 1. Personnel in U.S. Dental Schools in 1980.

|  | Range |
|---|---|
| Number of full-time basic science faculty | 0–134 |
| Number of full-time clinical faculty | 23–97 |
| Number of part-time clinical faculty | 3–338 |
| Number of full-time equivalents (FTE) | .8–81.2 |
| Undergraduate student/clinical faculty ratio | .90–10.54 |
| Total student/clinical faculty ratio | 1.62–11.65 |
| Number of FTE basic science support personnel | 3–129 |
| Number of FTE clinical science support personnel | 16–204 |

*Source:* American Dental Association, 1980a.

### Table 2. Average Student Contact Hours Per Week—Full-Time Faculty.

|  | 1959–1960* | 1976** |
|---|---|---|
| Basic science faculty | 11.5 |  |
| Clinical faculty | 29.0 |  |
| Professors, clinical science |  | 16 |
| Associate professors, clinical science |  | 18 |
| Assistant professors, clinical science |  | 20 |

*Source:* Hollingshead, 1961.
**Source:* American Dental Association, 1977.

use. He predicted that if they are not applied, mediocre instruction and diversion to more rewarding academic activities will occur.

Given the fiscal restraints facing dental education during the eighties, the increasing competition for patients from the private sector, the cost of buying property, and the likelihood of reduced enrollments, it is probable that the number of faculty positions will decline, that fewer faculty members will choose to relocate, and that more dentists will be interested in academic/research careers. In such an event, the pool of good potential faculty members will grow, and schools will undoubtedly become more selective in recruiting faculty to the few positions that become available. More schools will require advanced training and M.S. or Ph.D. degrees. Qualitative research experience and formal training in educational methods will become crucial criteria to those seeking faculty positions. More schools will establish formal faculty development programs, and meaningful creativity by the faculty member will be required for advancement in rank and tenure. Faculty performance before and after tenure will be more precisely measured at regular intervals. Under these circumstances, dental education will be able to take another step forward, unless there is continuing erosion of fiscal support for preparing new teachers and researchers (Brown, 1981).

In contrast, in the absence of a fiscal disaster and/or substantial reduction in the numbers of students, it is unlikely that support staff will be cut. Increases in the numbers of such personnel were originally occasioned by expansion and modernization of facilities (for example, multiple smaller clinics instead of one large clinic, use of the instrument-tray system, more effective management of sterilization, and an in-house dental laboratory) and by numerous programmatic changes (for example, Dental Assistant Utilization [D.A.U.] and Training in Expanded Auxiliary Management [TEAM] programs, prevention and recall programs, improved patient management), all of which increased the amount of required logistical support. These requirements are not likely to change in the near term.

## Curriculum

Dentistry, like other medical sciences, has added an immense body of new knowledge since 1950. Dental curricula have become packed and intense, and faculty and students alike are concerned about the learning environment, which often appears hurried, stressful, and, sometimes, antithetical to learning. This problem was exacerbated during the early 1970s when, in response to federal financing incentives, fifteen schools changed their curricula from four academic years to three calendar years. Today, only one school (University of the Pacific) retains the three-year curriculum.

According to *Dental Education in the United States, 1976* (American Dental Association, 1977) ten schools reported total clock hours ranging between 4,000 and 4,499, twenty-one schools reported totals ranging between 4,500 and 4,999, and fifteen between 5,000 and 5,499. In 1981, Harvard reported clock hours in the 7,000 range for a five-year curriculum, the first four years of which are traditional, with the fifth year being devoted to electives either in a biomedical research or a public health track. From these data it is evident that dental students commonly spend in excess of thirty-five hours per week in a classroom, laboratory, or clinic. In addition, outside study time is substantial, especially in the first two years (Brown, 1981). Even superior students report that there is not enough time to study all materials thoroughly. Hence, students become selective and often tend to concentrate on the pressure points or on high-risk subjects and take their chances on other subject areas. Preclinical and clinical courses often compete with basic science courses for the student's time, and in the third and fourth years at many institutions, the pressure of clinical requirements and accompanying outside laboratory effort may get in the way of almost everything else.

*Overcrowding.* Although few faculty or students disagree that the curriculum is overcrowded, there is little agreement on the effects of overcrowding, on possible solutions to the problem, or even if solutions are required. At the very least, questions need to be asked about the effects of the curriculum on students' physical and mental health; what they learn and retain; their attitudes toward the institution, faculty, and patients; their development of interpersonal skills, especially with patients; and their interest in continuing education. These and other questions should stimulate studies of significant merit and assistance to dental schools.

At present, several possible solutions to the overcrowding problem are under active discussion in the dental community. These include changed admissions and residency requirements, lengthening of the curriculum, and greater selectivity in course content, as described in the following paragraphs (Brown, 1981).

*Require some or all of the basic science courses as prerequisites for admission.* This has been discussed by many and tried by a few institutions. If all the basic science courses were taught prior to dental school admission, about 20 percent of the curriculum would be freed up. The disadvantages of such a solution include the costs of mounting these courses at feeder schools, the uneven quality of these courses among institutions, the diminished opportunity for predental students to gain a liberal education, and the lack of correlation between the basic and the clinical sciences.

*Require a one-year residency prior to licensure.* In 1981, there were over 800 residency positions for approximately 5,200 graduates. It is estimated that about 2,500 graduates applied for these positions. Consequently, the American Association of Dental Schools (1980) has recommended that the number of residency places be increased to accommodate approximately half the graduates each year. Over the long range, this is an attractive solution to the overcrowding problem because it would provide a bridging year between school and practice, enable the graduate to gain speed and confidence, and provide a broader experience with patient problems. However, this may be the wrong time to implement such a program. Federal support for dental residencies is being reduced or eliminated, and an additional year of study might further reduce an already declining applicant pool.

*Increase the curriculum to five years.* Theoretically, increasing curricular time should be beneficial to the learning process and the quality of the graduates. However, this would add substantially to the cost of dental education and would cause the student to lose an additional year's income from practice. Further, there is no reliable evidence that lengthening the curriculum would result in improved health of the public. Indeed, there is always the danger that course materials and clinical requirements would simply be expanded to fill the additional time. Given the state of the economy and the declining applicant pool, this would be a difficult option to implement.

*Select course content more precisely.* Given current fiscal restraints, this may be the only viable alternative immediately available; certainly curricular efficiency and effectiveness make sense under any circumstances. However, to develop the appropriate curriculum it is necessary to know precisely what is now done in practice, to predict the future of dental practice within reasonable limits, to develop a strategy for continued learning and continued competence through the lifetime of practice, and to determine the minimum curricular essentials that will ensure competency. While it will be difficult to make these determinations, their study is well worth support. Through the collaboration of the Council on Dental Education of the ADA and the AADS, a prospectus has, in fact, been developed and is being used as a vehicle to explore funding to find out what is being done in practice.

*Basic Science Instruction.* Since the times of Flexner and Gies, dental education has endeavored to correlate the basic and clinical sciences so that basic science instruction is perceived as relevant and not merely as an educational hurdle to be overcome. In 1979–1980, nineteen dental schools had their own basic science departments, at twenty-eight schools departments were shared between medicine and dentistry, at nine schools they were located in the medical school, and at four schools they were in an independent division. Although one might expect better correlation and increased learning at the schools with their own departments, no evidence to support this contention is available. Many schools have worked at improving the correlation between the basic and clinical sciences by establishing departments of oral biology that teach oral basic sciences, by appointing basic science faculty members with both D.D.S. and Ph.D. degrees, by using dental examples in basic science courses, by utilizing clinical faculty to teach basic science courses, and by introducing patient history seminars that incorporate basic science–related information. The Florida modular system (Shreve and others, 1980), for example, is designed to achieve integration of clinical, basic, behavioral, and dental sciences by use of (1) a multidisciplinary team approach for modular instruction, (2) clinical modules containing correlative basic science information taught by basic scientists, (3) student presentations of patients that include review of the basic biological aspects of managing the patient, (4) behavioral sciences faculty to observe and reinforce students' interpersonal skills with patients, and (5) clinical evaluation of students with respect to their fulfillment of clinical terminal objectives for dental biomaterials. Shreve states that student reaction to this format is positive.

Mackenzie (1980) describes six ways in which a health professional can profit from a knowledge of the basic sciences and suggests that these be used to organize basic science instruction. He argues that in order to facilitate transfer of knowledge, the curriculum should associate present learning of biology with future clinical situations, require active processing of information during learning, use advanced organizers to provide frameworks for new learning, teach and test for understanding rather than facts, analyze clinical tasks for decisions requiring biological information, and require practice in biologically based intellectual skills involving thinking, judgment, and decisions.

*The Place of Behavioral and Social Sciences.* The behavioral and social sciences have become common in dental curricula since about 1960. The courses in this area are generally intended to help students learn about themselves and their patients, to recognize the signs of abnormal behavior and ways of dealing with it, to identify the characteristics of special population groups with particular problems, and to be aware of the role of the dentist in community health. In addition, these courses often address social and political issues of interest to the dentist, questions of ethics and jurisprudence, and concerns about practice administration and the appropriate utilization of dental auxiliaries. However, the correlation of the behavioral and social sciences with the clinical sciences has not been accomplished to any great extent. Many clinical faculty are not yet sensitive to this more humanistic approach, and it is difficult for them to find time in the clinical setting to demonstrate the principles in work with individual patients. Additionally, students may not be motivated toward the behavioral sciences, probably because they do not have full responsibility for their patients and do not see the importance of the interpersonal relations; that becomes clear only when graduates enter the increasingly competitive world of practice. Finally, though there is some evidence that dentists who have had clinical experience with handicapped or otherwise clinically compromised patients are generally willing to treat them in practice, the effects of adding the behavioral and social sciences to the curriculum on performance and attitudes of dentists are not known in detail.

*The Role of Curriculum Committees.* Other questions that need to be asked about curriculum and course content include: Who decides on course content? How can reasonable decisions be made without taking away faculty rights? How can curriculum committees become effective? It is doubtful that anyone has valid answers to these questions, but answers are important, if the overcrowding problem is to be solved.

Although their roles will vary significantly, curriculum committees are common to all dental schools. Some are creative and stimulate review and improvements; others are passive and do little, and some may even impede progress. It is doubtful that many curriculum committees really know the content of their own curriculum. Unnecessary repetition, outdated or irrelevant material, and the omission of new information are likely results of ineffective curricular reviews. There is a need to define the role of curriculum committees and to develop a logical system to monitor and assess curricula. Ideally, curriculum committees should be granted the authority to review curricula thoroughly and critically and make whatever changes are indicated in a timely fashion. For example, each department or teaching area might be required to review its teaching programs every other year and make changes, based on a critical review of the current literature and an understanding of the contemporary and predicted practice of dentistry. Following the review by individual teaching units, clusters of departments and teaching areas with related programs might be required to meet to review proposed changes and to identify any omissions and duplications. The final document could then be submitted to the curriculum committee, which would have ultimate authority, subject only to the approval of the dean.

## Learning Systems

Over the past decade, dental educators have devoted an enormous amount of time and effort to learning systems. Clinical dental education and audiovisual learning systems, which include almost every conceivable piece of equipment and software package, are inseparable. The "hands-on" preclinical experiences and the small size of the oral cavity are major reasons why audiovisuals are so important.

A significant component of the 1976 curriculum study (American Dental Association, 1977) concerned collecting and analyzing data on learning systems. Those conducting the study anticipated much more variety than was actually reported. It was found that between 1965 and 1975, there had been a general reduction in laboratory instruction in basic science courses. Most schools reported some laboratory instruction in the anatomical sciences, microbiology and immunology, general pathology, and physiology; fewer than half reported any laboratory instruction in biochemistry and pharmacology. The traditional sequence of lecture-laboratory-clinic instruction still prevailed in the clinical sciences, although the data revealed a slight shift from lectures to small group sessions and self-instruction. Self-instructional materials were used more widely in the clinical sciences than in the basic sciences, with some self-instruction reported by twenty-two schools in the field of periodontics, fifteen schools in general pathology, and only eight in anatomical science. The curriculum study concluded that "a learning system is really a composite of several subsystems, that traditional learning methods still have merit, and that the best one for each school will be the one which most effectively manages existing resources to meet existing needs." It stated further that "self-pacing requires guideposts for student progress. The student must know what he is expected to accomplish within a given period of time. The self-pacing concept also requires faculty dedication and special managerial skills to insure that students are effectively utilizing this learning system" (American Dental Association, 1977, quoted in Brown, 1981, p. 629).

*Project ACORDE.* Project ACORDE (MacIntyre, 1977; Shugars, Trent, and Heymann, 1979; Kress, Silversin, and Colenback, 1979) was a nationwide, cooperative effort to design, develop, evaluate, and distribute preclinical teaching materials that were acceptable to most dental schools and dental auxiliary programs. It was funded by the Division of Dentistry of the U.S. Public Health Service. It resulted in the production of twenty-six learning packages which, after field tests and revisions, were made widely available. By 1977, twenty-six dental schools and ninety dental auxiliary programs were using ACORDE materials.* Users have been generally pleased with the efficiency and quality of the materials; nonusers have cited cost, differences in techniques, and problems in incorporating the materials into established programs as reasons for not participating. The cost of Project ACORDE was substantial, and, given the declining federal resources and the cost of travel, a comparable project is not likely to be mounted in the near future. Displays of audiovisual materials at the annual meeting of the American Association of Dental Schools verify that an enormous quantity of learning materials has been developed in recent years. However, it appears that there is limited sharing of these materials among dental schools and that the philosophy of reinventing the wheel still persists. Fiscal restraints in the eighties may have significant impacts on the production, use, and sharing of learning materials (Brown, 1981).

Although difficult to document, it appears that enthusiasm for revising learning materials diminishes after the initial development. Lack of time and absence of rewards are often cited as reasons. If usage of audiovisual materials were quantified, it would probably be found that $2 \times 2$ slides are employed far more than any other method. They are inexpensive, easily replaced by new slides, and simple to transport.

*Self-Instruction.* During the 1970s, self-instruction attracted much attention with two schools, the University of Florida and the University of Texas at Houston, relying exclusively on a system of self-instruction and self-pacing. These institutions appear to be generally pleased with this system and intend to continue to employ it. In reporting on six years of experience with the flexible, modular curriculum at Florida, Allen and Collett (1978) cite as advantages that it permits student self-pacing; allows modification of the curriculum based upon the validation process; increases communication among educators, students, and instructional design personnel; permits inclusion of clinical activities at appropriate levels in the curriculum; increases the validity and reliability of evaluation procedures; requires the faculty to clarify those competencies and skills required for graduation; facilitates a logical, planned, and integrated approach to the pro-

---

*The materials are being marketed by the Quercus Corporation of Castro Valley, California.

fessionalization of the student; encourages cooperation among dental schools by having instructional materials in convenient units to increase the potential for sharing; provides a mechanism for review and remedial instruction; and takes into consideration the students' background of knowledge, skills, and attitudes and allows them to progress accordingly. They cite as disadvantages that it requires reorientation and retraining of faculty, involvement of faculty members in all disciplines in planning and designing the curriculum, development of a more advanced evaluation scheme, monitoring the needs of the student for effective scheduling, greater expense than the traditional approach, and more faculty effort from all disciplines. Allen and Collett state that revision of the modules is feasible and, in their opinion, easier to bring about than revisions of traditional curricula. They estimate the cost of revising materials to be approximately $15,000 per year, not including faculty time.

Williams (1981) reviewed the dental literature concerning self-instruction from 1960 to 1980 and reported that compared to traditional instructional methods, effective self-instruction is capable of increasing cognitive knowledge in a shorter period of time with greater student satisfaction but has little effect on psychomotor skills. Williams further reported that student requests for peer and faculty interaction appear to limit the effectiveness of curricula that are entirely self-instructional. He lamented the loss of role model when faculty members have limited interaction with students. He suggested that self-instruction, augmented and evaluated by small group peer interaction and supplemented by presentations by faculty members, may provide the correct balance of these three elements. He asked a number of questions, some of which suggest important studies: How does one measure the true effectiveness of learning systems—by knowledge acquisition (short-term gain) and/or by knowledge retention (how much and after what length of time)? Why does a promising program appear in the literature only one time? What happens to it? What are the components and principles of self-instruction that make the difference in learning effectiveness?

## Learning Objectives

The Commission on Dental Accreditation requires that objectives for all courses be available for review for accreditation site visits. It is the impression of the commission that since initiating this requirement several years ago, courses are, at the very least, better organized, and students know in advance what they are expected to learn. The 1976 curriculum study surveyed extensively the use of instructional objectives by the nation's dental schools (American Dental Association, 1977). In the section entitled "Conclusions and Recommendations on Instructional Objectives," the report stated: "In a relatively brief timespan, a number of internal and external factors have acted to produce a widespread acceptance of instructional objectives by the dental schools. Yet despite the reports of acceptance and use, two elements may act to render instructional objectives less than optimally useful. First, faculty may merely pay lip service to instructional objectives in order to comply with mandates necessary for accreditation. Second, and at the opposite end of the spectrum, faculty may become so wedded to instructional objectives that their teaching is restricted to these objectives. Furthermore, nearly half of the students responded that goals and objectives were reported orally or not at all" (American Dental Association, 1977, p. 41).

If indeed the concept of instructional objectives is to be effective, communication is necessary at all levels of the educational process. This vital communication between faculty and administration, between faculty and other faculty, and between faculty and students appears too often to be either infrequent or inefficient. Consequently, the curriculum study (American Dental Association, 1977, p. 42) recommended that: (1) Administrators should develop overall objectives for the institution; these objectives should then serve as guidelines for the more specific objectives developed for individual instructional areas by the faculty associated with those areas. (2) Instructional objectives should be disseminated by faculty in written form to students and all other faculty, regardless of the teaching responsibilities of those faculty. (3) Instructional objectives should be monitored and, when necessary, updated by the combined efforts of the department head, departmental clusters, and curriculum committees in order to coordinate effectively the objectives for all courses offered by the school. (4) The administration should act to orient faculty to the view that, while written instructional objectives are useful tools, they cannot form the sole focus of instruction. Certain attitudes or refined levels of knowledge and skills do not often lend themselves to the development of written objectives but should be included within a faculty member's goals. A study of objectives—how they are used, if they are used, student responses and attitudes toward objectives—might shed new light.

### Evaluation of Students

The dental literature has not included much on testing, at least in recent years. At present, there is no precise information about the number and types of tests given in dental schools; it is assumed that most tests are multiple choice to conform to National Dental Board Examinations, to enable rapid scoring, and to eliminate grader subjectivity. Test question banks, computer-regulated testing (Howell, 1979), and tips on taking these examinations (Geller and Shemesh, 1979) are parts of the present testing scene. Data about the effectiveness of multiple-choice examinations in assessing higher levels of learning and about "test-wiseness" are not available in the literature.

The teaching and evaluation of clinical judgment are important components of the dental curriculum but difficult to perform with precision. Judgment is generally associated with maturation and experience. Mackenzie and others (1977) reviewed the complexities of developing clinical judgment and expressed the view that most curricula do not emphasize the learning of the judgmental process. In their analysis, they divided the judgmental process into three components—input, mediation, and output—and made suggestions about ways these components could be employed in four instructional phases—introductory, initial guidance, application, and feedback. It is not clear how judgment is now taught, except by conversation between a student and an instructor about a patient's problems. At some schools judgment is measured and graded as either plus, minus, or neutral at each patient appointment. As the student progresses through the curriculum, the judgment factor becomes a larger component of the student's grade for a course. It is, however, a subjective call by the faculty member.

Dental education might improve the learning system by defining judgment and the criteria against which it is measured more precisely and by calibrating the faculty members who will be evaluating judgment.

The 1976 curriculum study (American Dental Association, 1977) included recommendations urging (1) the development of objective criteria for the evaluation of student clinical performance; (2) calibration of all clinical faculty in the evaluation process; (3) feedback to students in a manner to provide information that can be used to assess progress or difficulties, plan remediation, and assess effectiveness of instruction; (4) the use of both criterion-referenced and norm-referenced assessment to maximize the accuracy of student evaluation, with the criterion-referenced method used primarily to evaluate clinical performance; and (5) the development and implementation of mechanisms that facilitate qualitative judgments about the adequacy of both the procedures and the final products.

### New Directions and Recommendations

The report, *Advanced Dental Education: Recommendations for the '80s* (American Association of Dental Schools, 1980), included eleven recommendations that were intended to stimulate discussion throughout the dental profession and to result in definitive action. In December 1980, the Council on Dental Education reviewed these recommendations and took action on several which the council perceived to be within its purview. Among those approved were the following:

*Recommendation 1: A five-year review and analysis of predoctoral dental education.* The council believes that future curriculum studies should be incorporated in the *Annual Survey* and should focus on documenting trends. These studies should be limited to such curricular areas as clock hours of instruction, changes in curricular emphasis, and the scope and content of didactic versus nondidactic instruction in the basic sciences, preclinical and clinical dental sciences, and the behavioral sciences. In fact, in 1981 for the first time each dental school reported curricular clock hours in the basic, behavioral, and clinical sciences according to their respective modes of instruction. The council also proposed that a major comprehensive study of the general practice of dentistry be done, in cooperation with the American Association of Dental Schools and the American Association of Dental Examiners, to focus on an analysis of the current practice of general dentistry and to identify projected trends. A primary goal of this study is to relate general practice and the predoctoral curriculum so that curricular decisions are based on as much data as possible about what practitioners do in the field.

*Recommendation 4: Review the purpose of specialty recognition and accomplish the most effective structuring of those areas deserving specialty recognition.* The council believes that the criteria for recognition of special areas of dental practice should be studied and revised, if necessary, and that a study should be conducted to determine the functions, procedures, and techniques that characterize the practice of each of the recognized specialties. A committee has begun work on this project and has prepared a preliminary report for the council's December 1981 meeting.

*Recommendation 11: Create an independent Commission on Advanced Education in Medicine and Dentistry.* The Council believes that this recommendation should be postponed until data resulting from the implementation of the other recommendations are available for analysis and review.

The status of the other eight recommendations is unclear at this time. They concern increasing the number of positions for advanced training in general practice, decreasing the number of first-year clinical dental specialty positions, developing and evaluating model programs for advanced education programs, providing stipends for all dentists in advanced general practice residency programs, and increasing both individual and institutional financial support for advanced education programs preparing dentists for careers in education and research. Most of these recommendations would be costly and would require external funding. With the current patterns of budgetary cutbacks by the federal executive and the Congress, one cannot be optimistic about their implementation, at least in the near future. If, however, the decision makers agree that they represent sound policy, then the longer range may produce more opportunities for residency training and the preparation of teachers and researchers (Brown, 1981).

Like the other health professions, dentistry and dental education have entered a period of serious reassessment and planning for the future. Oversupply of manpower, geographic and specialty maldistribution, high cost of services, changes in the characteristics of dental practice due to the use of fluorides and other preventive measures, and the ever-increasing knowledge requirements are probably the major forces presently driving dental education. Dental education has changed substantially since 1960, and the changes have generally been positive—for example, improved facilities, faculties, curricula, and learning methods. Yet, much remains to be done, and the following recommendations for future studies may produce additional advances:

- Survey present dental practices in order to detail their characteristics and, based on the status of research in prevention and trends in the mode of practice, predict the characteristics of dental practices in 1990 and 2000. Then adjust dental education programs to prepare graduates for practice as it will actually occur.
- Develop effective ways to monitor and evaluate curricula and courses to avoid unnecessary duplication, identify omissions, and explore ways to introduce new information without further extending the curriculum.
- Develop and evaluate methods to reduce crowding in the curriculum.
- Identify and validate those factors in the dental education environment that result in negative attitudes on the part of some dental students.
- Evaluate the effectiveness of the various learning systems used in dental education.
- Develop and assess improved methods to evaluate the clinical performance of students, courses, and teachers.
- Study and validate methods to improve the correlation of basic, clinical, and behavioral sciences.
- Examine the use of course objectives and the attitudes of faculty and students toward their employment.
- Develop and validate methods to assure continuing competency of the practicing professional.

**References**

Allen, D. L., and Collett, W. K. "A Progress Report on Six Years' Experience with a Flexible, Modular Dental Curriculum." *Journal of Dental Education*, 1978, *42*, 290–295.

American Association of Dental Schools. *Advanced Dental Education: Recommendations for the '80s.* Washington, D.C.: American Association of Dental Schools, 1980.

American Association of Dental Schools. *Survey of Dental Seniors.* Washington, D.C.: American Association of Dental Schools, 1982.

American Dental Association. *Annual Report on Dental Education, 1970–71.* Chicago: American Dental Association, 1971.

American Dental Association. *Dental Education in the United States, 1976.* Chicago: American Dental Association, 1977.

American Dental Association. *Dental Faculty Information: Annual Report, 1979–1980, Supplement 10.* Chicago: American Dental Association, 1980a.

American Dental Association. *Report of the Special Higher Education Committee to Critique the 1976 Dental Curriculum Study.* Chicago: American Dental Association, 1980b.

American Dental Association. *Annual Report on Dental Education, 1980–81.* Chicago: American Dental Association, 1981a.

American Dental Association. *Dental Student Attrition, 1980–81.* Supplement to the *Annual Report on Dental Education, 1980–81.* Chicago: American Dental Education, 1981b.

American Dental Association. *Interim Report of the Special Commission on the Future of Dentistry.* Chicago: American Dental Association, 1982.

American Dental Association, Council on Dental Education. *Continuing Dental Education Requirements.* Chicago: American Dental Association, 1980.

Brown, W. E. "The Present Status of U.S. Dental Education." *Journal of Dental Education*, 1981, *45*, 628–634.

Bruce, H. W., Jr. "The Impact of Federal Legislation and Declining Financial Resources on Dental Education." *Journal of Dental Education*, 1981, *45*, 646–651.

Chambers, D. W. "Faculty Evaluation: Review of the Literature Most Pertinent to Dental Education." *Journal of Dental Education*, 1977, *41*, 290–300.

Eversole, L. R. "Programmed Instruction in General Pathology: Evaluation of Performance in Comparison to Conventional Instruction and Scholastic Achievement." *Journal of Dental Education*, 1979, *43*, 214–216.

Geller, L. M., and Shemesh, M. "Analysis of Answer Changes by Dental Students on Multiple-Choice Tests in Pathology: Attack on an Educational Myth." *Journal of Dental Education*, 1979, *43*, 159–164.

Guild, R. E. "Faculty Behavior: Appraisal and Rewards." *Journal of Dental Education*, 1977, *41*, 307–319.

Hollingshead, B. S. *The Survey of Dentistry.* Washington, D.C.: American Council on Education, 1961.

Howell, B. E. "Computer-Regulated Testing Procedures in a Self-Paced Modular Curriculum Employing Microfiche as Test Storage Medium." *Journal of Dental Education*, 1979, *43*, 349–350.

Kress, G. C., Jr., Silversin, J. B., and Colenback, P. R. "A Study of the Impact of Project ACORDE on Dental Education in the United States." *Journal of Dental Education*, 1979, *43*, 204–209.

MacIntyre, M. L. "Project ACORDE: A Historical Review." *Journal of Dental Education*, 1977, *41*, 545–553.

Mackenzie, R. S. "Essential Features of a Faculty Evaluation Program." *Journal of Dental Education*, 1977, *41*, 301–306.

Mackenzie, R. S. "Curriculum Considerations for Correlating Basic and Clinical Sciences." *Journal of Dental Education*, 1980, *44*, 248–256.

Mackenzie, R. S., and others. "Teaching Clinical Judgment in Periodontics." *Journal of Dental Education*, 1977, *41*, 537–544.

Powell, R. A. "The Impact of a Declining Pool of Applicants on Dental Education." *Journal of Dental Education*, 1981, *45* (10), 652–656.

Santangelo, M. V. "The History and Development of Dental Education in the United States." *Journal of Dental Education*, 1981, *45*, 619–627.

Shreve, W. B., and others. "Integration of the Basic, Behavioral, and Biomaterials Sciences with the Clinical Curriculum." *Journal of Dental Education*, 1980, *44*, 76–79.

Shugars, D. A., Trent, P. J., and Heymann, H. O. "Effectiveness of Project ACORDE Materials: Applied Evaluative Research in a Preclinical Technique Course." *Journal of Dental Education*, 1979, *43*, 510–514.

Williams, R. E. "Self-Instruction in Dental Education: 1960–1980." *Journal of Dental Education*, 1981, *45*, 290–299.

# 4

*August P. Lemberger*

# Pharmacy

---

Evolution in pharmaceutical education in the period 1960–1980 has been so rapid that, had it not occurred in an orderly fashion, it would have been labeled revolution. Profound discoveries in the pharmaceutical sciences and innovative additions to the pharmacist's role as a health care provider combined to produce an evolutionary wave that swept through pharmaceutical education with an irresistible force.

## Historical Perspective

The seeding of this phenomenon can be traced to the scientific revolution in pharmacy spawned by World War II and the discovery of penicillin. Never before had a therapeutic agent of such delicate chemistry been developed for mass use; never before had the full capacity of science been brought to bear on the formulation of drug delivery systems capable of converting a laboratory curiosity into a useful drug product. Thus was the modern-day pharmaceutical industry born, and thus through the 1950s was the pharmacist's role in compounding medication transferred from the prescription counter to the laboratory bench. Application of the scientific expertise assembled in the industrial laboratories to drug product development led to the discovery of ways to stabilize drugs and drug delivery systems to meet mass marketing needs and to development of standards for product uniformity and quality control far beyond the standards even the most skilled practitioner could meet. From both industrial and academic research laboratories came the further discoveries that the dosage form and the specific ingredients in the formulation could significantly modify drug availability for absorption by the body and that the absorption of a drug, its distribution throughout the body, and its elimination could be described very precisely by applying the principles of chemical kinetics.

Such a profound change in how and where medications were made was bound to affect the practice of pharmacy. And it did. The pharmacist of the 1950s grappled with a role change from compounder to purveyor of medications. Stifled by a code of ethics that specifically forbade "counter-prescribing" and discussing the therapeutic effects or composition of a prescription with a patient (American Pharmaceutical Association, 1952), the pharmacist turned to the product dispensed and to the development of high technology in the mechanical functions surrounding the dispensing function.

At the same time, pharmaceutical education was embroiled in its own turmoil. The Pharmaceutical Survey of 1946–1949 (American Council on Education, 1950), a comprehensive study of pharmaceutical education, led to a recommendation that initial steps be taken to develop and establish a six-year program of education and training leading to the professional degree, doctor of pharmacy. Concurrently with the Pharmaceutical Survey, the American Association of Colleges of Pharmacy (AACP) was deliberating the merits of a five-year curriculum. In time, but not without heated debate, a five-year program was supported by the National Association of Boards of Pharmacy (NABP) in 1953 and by the AACP in 1954. Action was finally assured in 1959 when the American Council on Pharmaceutical Education (ACPE) adopted a revision of its accreditation standards, to be effective July 1, 1960, that required a five-year undergraduate program leading to a baccalaureate degree. The standards also offered as an option a four-year program based upon two years of preprofessional instruction for which the doctor of pharmacy degree was authorized (American Council on Pharmaceutical Education, 1960).

In the face of disagreement over the duration of the curriculum, general accord on the nature of the curriculum content was reached. As a reflection of the discovery of new drugs in rapid succession during the 1950s and the growing recognition of the scientific base upon which drug products were formulated, curriculum content revisions put increasing emphasis on the pharmaceutical sciences. The product-oriented, purveyor role of the pharmacist was reflected by the addition of a new discipline, pharmacy administration, to the curriculum.

## Benchmarks Auguring Change: Federal Initiatives

Any effort to track the evolution of pharmaceutical education must be set in the context of the times. The aroused social consciousness of Americans in the 1960s precipitated many changes in the structure and behavior of our society. Government action to produce changes seen as in the national interest became commonplace and touched virtually every segment of our society, including the practice of pharmacy. Several such actions had such direct impact on pharmacy and pharmaceutical education that they must be cited.

*Kefauver-Harris Amendments to the Food and Drug Laws.* This legislation resulted from an investigation of the pharmaceutical industry by Senator Estes Kefauver. Provisions of the legislation that had particular impact on pharmacy were a requirement that a drug not be allowed on the market unless evidence was submitted to the Food and Drug Administration (FDA) to show that it was effective as well as safe, and a requirement that advertising and labeling of a drug include its generic name as well as adequate warnings of contraindications, potential side effects, and other hazards (Silverman and Lee, 1974). These provisions led to rapid expansion in clinical studies of new drugs and to increased consumer awareness of potential harm resulting from the use of drugs.

Task Force on Prescription Drugs. The Task Force on Prescription Drugs was established in 1967 by the Department of Health, Education, and Welfare and charged to study the costs of prescription drugs under the Medicare program (Silverman and Lee, 1974). The issue of clinical equivalency between brand-name and generic drug products was also assigned to the task force for resolution. The latter problem was resolved by accepting biological equivalency, or relative physiological availability, as a proxy for clinical equivalency, under the rationale that two preparations that provide the same blood concentration of drug will yield the same therapeutic effect. As the result of a recommendation of this task force, the Food and Drug Administration adopted a requirement that generic-name products not be allowed on the market unless they meet all compendial standards, and when required, adequate test data be supplied to demonstrate essentially equivalent biological availability.

Through the 1970s, consumer awareness of generic drug products, drug costs, and potential problems grew. By 1981, all but one state had passed legislation allowing or requiring the pharmacist to dispense a generic drug product if available, less expensive than the prescribed brand, authorized by the consumer, and not expressly prohibited by the prescriber. The pharmaceutical sciences, particularly pharmaceutics, biopharmaceutics, and pharmacokinetics have taken on new significance in both the pharmaceutical industrial laboratories and the academic research centers.

Health Professions Education Assistance Act. In 1968, in an effort to spur enrollments in the health professions, Congress extended the Health Professions Educational Assistance Program to include pharmacy and further expanded support to that field in 1971 (Hugill and Watzman, 1973). As part of the eligibility requirements for pharmacy schools, assurance had to be given that each student would undergo a training program in clinical pharmacy. This requirement, in effect, set educational policy, for it led directly to a change in accreditation standards to encompass a similar requirement.

## Developments Within Pharmacy

The first breakthrough in transforming pharmacy practice from a product-oriented mode to a patient-oriented mode can be traced to Eugene V. White (1978). In 1960, armed with a new tool he devised and named the Family Prescription Record System, White transformed his practice environment from a commercial pharmacy to a professional office setting. The record system introduced by White provided a continuing medication history for each member of the family. With it he monitored drug utilization and advised the patient and prescriber accordingly. The significance of this innovation did not escape the imagination of the profession's leadership. The attention of practitioners in all practice environments was drawn to the potential for direct involvement of the pharmacist in patient care.

Development of patient-centered pharmacy practice in the hospital setting is less easily traced. The seed of opportunity was planted in 1962 with the report that one medication error was committed for every six to seven doses administered by nurses under traditional intrahospital drug distribution systems. In response to these findings, the unit-dose system for medication handling was developed. This, in turn, led to other innovations in the delivery of pharmacy services in hospitals, such as providing a direct copy of the physician's order to the pharmacy and having the pharmacy assume responsibility for intravenous additive preparations, patient profiling, medication histories, patient education, and drug information services (Oddis, 1974). Implementation of these clinical pharmacy functions in the hospital setting occurred far more broadly than in community practice and with surprising rapidity.

The evolution of patient-oriented practice of pharmacy in the 1960s and the widespread support for the pursuit of this practice concept by the profession provided the impetus for a number of activities of major significance in shaping educational policy.

*Task Force on the Pharmacist's Clinical Role.* Following a multidisciplinary conference on pharmacy manpower in September 1970 (Graber and Brodie, 1970) and in response to one of the mandates from the conference, the National Center for Health Services Research convened an interdisciplinary task force to draft a set of criteria for definition of the clinical role to be played by the pharmacist in health care. The Task Force on the Pharmacist's Clinical Role (1971) decided that the criteria should be based on functions. Functions to be performed by the pharmacist in a clinical role were categorized as relating to prescribing drugs, dispensing and administering drugs, documenting professional activities, direct patient involvement, reviewing drug utilization, education, and consultation.

This report, emanating from a unit of the Department of Health, Education, and Welfare, coupled with the 1971 Comprehensive Health Manpower Training Act, which mandated clinical pharmacy education and training, could not be and was not ignored by pharmaceutical education. From an educational viewpoint the task force report was significant, not so much for the functions delineated, per se, but for the fact that the report gave credibility to the concept of a clinical role for the pharmacist. The path to curricular change through revision of accreditation standards was opened.

*Board of Specialties in Pharmacy.* In January 1973, the American Pharmaceutical Association (APhA) created a Task Force on Specialties in Pharmacy to consider the issue and to recommend a mechanism for recognition of specialties and the certification of specialists. Following more than a year of study and deliberation, the task force recommended that an official, independent board with decision-making authority be established and charged with recognizing specialties in pharmacy (American Pharmaceutical Association, 1974). The Board of Pharmaceutical Specialties was established in January 1976 and thus far has recognized one specialty, nuclear pharmacy.

In establishing criteria for specialty recognition, the task force emphasized that a specialized practice must be based on a specialized knowledge of the pharmaceutical sciences, that the special knowledge and skills be acquired by education and training and/or experience beyond the basic pharmaceutical education and training, and that the area of specialization be one in which schools of pharmacy and/or other organizations offer recognized education and training programs. This action has had a significant influence on the establishment of educational policy for the academic program requirements in pharmacy, particularly the doctor of pharmacy degree. The action has also provided a stimulus for the development of residency and other professional graduate degree programs.

*Study Commission on Pharmacy.* Another activity that contributed directly to the information base upon which policy decisions are made was the study of pharmacy and pharmaceutical education commissioned by the AACP. The study commission presented its report in 1975 after two years of examination, both of the *practice* of pharmacy as an integral part of the health service system and of the *process* of pharmacy education (American Association of Colleges of Pharmacy, 1975b). The basic thrust of the findings and recommendations of the study commission is summarized in the observations that pharmacists are health professionals who could make an important contribution to health care by providing information about drugs to consumers and health professionals, and pharmacy should be conceived as a knowledge system that renders a health service by concerning itself with understanding drugs and their effects on people and animals.

*Continuing Competence of Pharmacists.* Concerned about the reliance on registration and licensure as a means of assuring competence to practice, the AACP and APhA jointly created a Task Force on Continuing Competence in Pharmacy. The principal recommendation of the task force was the formation of a Pharmacy Practice Standards Commission with a primary responsibility for identifying and recommending national standards of competency that individual pharmacists would be required to meet (American Association of Colleges of Pharmacy, 1975a).

In response to this recommendation, the sponsoring organizations commissioned a national study designed to provide a model for developing standards of practice and to show how job analysis and practice standards could be used to develop instruments for assessing competence (Rosenfeld, Thornton, and Glazer, 1978). The findings reported in this study were then used to develop standards of practice for the profession of pharmacy (Kalman and Schlegel, 1979). At each step of this continuing project, starting with the report of the Task Force on Continuing Competence in Pharmacy, an assignment of responsibility was made to pharmaceutical education both in entry-level and continuing education programs.

### Interdisciplinary Influences on Practice and Education

The scenario describing factors at large that influenced the evolution of pharmacy education would not be complete if several interdisciplinary activities of national scope were not included. In 1967, the University of Michigan Schools of Pharmacy, Medicine, and Nursing sponsored a conference on health education for these three professions (Deno, 1967). The conference had as its objectives the exploration of new roles for pharmacy and pharmacists in the future and identification of ways to enable the pharmacist to meet the new service roles and to bring closer relations among medical, nursing, and pharmaceutical education. A conference with similar objectives, reflecting again the initiative taken by pharmacy in seeking interdisciplinary input into the definition of new roles for the pharmacists in patient care, was held in 1970 (Graber and Brodie, 1970). An outcome common to both conferences was agreement among the attendees that new roles for the pharmacist were desirable and would contribute to improved patient care. Less clear were outcomes defining what those new roles would be and how their implementation would be achieved.

In 1972, the Institute of Medicine of the National Academy of Sciences held a conference focusing on interrelationships of educational programs for health professionals (Institute of Medicine, 1972). This conference provided the first opportunity for leaders from the major health professions to meet on a national scale to define the issues in interdisciplinary education. An indirect conclusion of the conference for pharmacy resulted from the planning assumption that pharmacy, by virtue of a clinical role, must be part of interdisciplinary education and part of the model for health care teams that must be developed.

### Curriculum Evolution

The accreditation standards adopted by the ACPE on July 1, 1960, serve as a touchstone for tracing evolution of curricula in pharmacy. According to these standards, curricula were to include instruction in three natural divisions defined as nonscientific courses in general education (humanities, social studies, and economics), mathematics and the basic physical and biological sciences (algebra, trigonometry, qualitative and quantitative analysis, organic and biological chemistry, microbiology, and physiology), and courses in areas of professional instruction (pharmaceutical chemistry, pharmacognosy, pharmacology, pharmacy, and pharmacy administration). The curriculum as a whole was to "show logical balance among the three divisions . . . and among the five areas of professional instruction" (American Council on Pharmaceutical Education, 1960, pp. 19–20). The undergraduate program in pharmacy was to require not less than 150 weeks to complete, exclusive of holidays and vacation (five academic years), and was to be recognized with the award of a baccalaureate degree.

*Structure.* Curriculum surveys in 1959 (Adams, 1960) and in 1962 (Paul and Sperandio, 1962) of schools of pharmacy produced essentially identical data. Both surveys showed an average requirement of 165 semester credits for the baccalaureate degree. Although minor variations in the classification of courses existed, both surveys showed the distribution of credits among the three natural divisions to be approximately 20 percent general education, 35 percent mathematics and basic physical and biological sciences, and 45 percent professional instruction. It is of interest that even at the onset of the five-year curriculum, approximately one-third of the schools reported that the new curriculum would not provide adequate time to achieve the educational objectives proposed by the Pharmaceutical Survey (American Council on Education, 1950).

By 1968, concern that curriculum changes reflecting the expanding knowledge base of pharmacy were occurring at the expense of general education led to a charge to the AACP Committee on Curriculum to study general education and elective opportunities available to pharmacy students. A comprehensive survey of curricula of member schools was conducted in 1968-69 (Lemberger, 1968). The survey found that the median number of semester credits required for the baccalaureate degree was 162, the median number of required credits in general education was 15, the median number of directed elective credits was 8, and the median number of open elective credits was 12. While on the surface the accreditation guideline that 20 percent of the curriculum be devoted to general education was met, responses to the survey indicated that the average student devoted a significant portion of the available elective credit opportunity to elective courses in professional disciplines rather than general education. The survey also revealed that the percentage of the curriculum devoted to mathematics and basic physical and biological sciences remained at approximately 35 percent. Less clear was the distribution between general education and professional instruction. The data did indicate, however, that general education had declined to about 15 percent of the curriculum, and professional instruction had increased accordingly.

In the early 1970s, the erosion of general education requirements and opportunities was further exacerbated as clinical pharmacy education was added to curricula to meet the accreditation standards revised and adopted in 1974 (American Council on Pharmaceutical Education, 1975). The tide of erosion was stemmed in June 1976 when the ACPE reaffirmed its guideline that approximately 20 percent of the baccalaureate curriculum was to be devoted to general education and then adopted a rigorous stance in its enforcement.

The most recent attempt to review curricular change was reported by the AACP Academic Affairs Committee (formerly Committee on Curriculum) as part of its 1980-81 charge (Zelnio, 1981). Bulletins from twenty schools of pharmacy for 1970-71 and 1980-81 were used to analyze curricular changes that had occurred at each institution in the ten-year period covered. Within the sample chosen, there was evidence that the number of credits devoted to basic sciences and electives and the number of laboratory courses offered had been reduced to accommodate both clinical and general education. Particularly vulnerable were medicinal chemistry/pharmacognosy, chemistry, and physics. Reductions in pharmacy administration, drug assay, and pharmaceutics were also observed. Pharmaceutical sciences prerequisite to clinical courses such as biological sciences and pharmacology were slightly increased. The major change observed was the addition of pharmacy clerkships and externships as part of the professional instruction in pharmacy practice. Extrapolation of the data presented to curriculum structure is hazardous because only the basic science, elective, and professional instruction components were reported. However, among the schools comprising this sample there was no apparent increase in the overall credit requirement nor any significant shift in percentage distribution of the curriculum among the three natural divisions identified in the 1960 accreditation standards.

The twenty-year period covered in this review reveals no significant evolutionary trend with regard to the structure of the curriculum in pharmacy. The movement toward reduction of general education requirements to accommodate clinical education and the expanded knowledge base in the pharmaceutical sciences observed in the early 1970s was effectively reversed by the ACPE and has not been challenged by schools of pharmacy acting in concert. What innovations have occurred, then, must be found in curriculum content.

*Content.* From the time of adoption of the four-year baccalaureate program as a requirement for licensure to the implementation of the five-year curriculum requirement in 1960, pharmaceutical education had striven to achieve parity of academic recognition with baccalaureate programs in the arts and sciences. In the 1930s and 1940s, parity was sought through adoption of requirements in science and language commonly found in other baccalaureate programs. As the pharmaceutical sciences matured in the late 1940s and 1950s, curricula in pharmacy abandoned foreign language requirements and added mathematics, more rigorous chemistry, and additional biological science requirements. Professional courses, traditionally labeled pharmacy, became more commonly identified as pharmaceutics to reflect the added emphasis on the scientific approach to understanding dosage forms. The direction of this evolutionary movement warranted the pride of pharmaceutical educators because it signaled success to decades of effort.

The change in professional practice from a product to patient orientation, therefore, produced a need for profound change in the direction of evolution of pharmaceutical education. That a change of this magnitude should produce strain within the system is no surprise. Whereas pharmaceutical education had taken a position of professional leadership in elevating the qualification of practitioners for the product-oriented mode of practice, it found itself in a reactive posture as it attempted to adapt to the newly discovered educational needs of the profession.

*Emergence of the Clinical Component.* Evidence of the dilemma faced by pharmaceutical educators is found in the proceedings of the 1961 Teachers' Seminar on pharmacy (Lemberger, 1961). The theme of this seminar was "The Technical Pharmacy Courses." By and large, the formal presentations envisioned the pharmacy courses as being developed from the background of the physical sciences. However, a presentation made by Dr. John Autian (1961), calling for the terminal course in pharmacy to embrace topic areas perceived (remarkably accurately as seen retrospectively) as necessary to equip the pharmacist for an expanded role in health care proved to be controversial and provocative. The name "clinical pharmacy" was suggested as a title, and the course content proposed included communication, clinical evaluation of new drugs, evaluation of drug products, drug information, and application of drugs in the treatment of disease. To add further to the controversy, Autian suggested that techniques of compounding and dispensing, traditionally presented in the terminal course, could be minimized at this level and covered adequately in prerequisite courses. The syllabus proposed by Autian received the action to be expected; the group agreed with the spirit but did not accept it as the syllabus for any one course.

Another insight into the then widely accepted content of the entry-level curriculum in pharmacy was provided by the AACP Committee on Curriculum in 1967 (Gibson, 1967). Upon examination of what was purported to be "core" curriculum content, it is seen that consensus was achieved by inclusion of the full body of knowledge of each of the disciplines of pharmacy and that the topics proposed in the syllabus of each discipline reflected very traditional content. To be sure, the evolutional ferment in clinical education, then in its initial phase, could be seen by careful reading of the report—pharmacology's suggestion that selected students participate in clinical rounds, pharmacy's inclusion of biopharmaceutics, dosage form design, and professional services such as medication records are examples—but the value of the report stemmed from the curricular taxonomy it contained.

At about the same time (Biles, 1974; Beste and Herfindal, 1975), the University of Southern California and the University of California at San Francisco, which had adopted six-year doctor of pharmacy degree programs in the 1950s, began to experiment with placing pharmacy students in clinical clerkships. The experiment was an immediate success. To be sure, modification and adjustments needed to be made, and experience with this format of education so novel to pharmacy had to be gained, but the fancy of pharmaceutical education had been captured.

The nature, scope, content, and character of the terminal course in pharmacy came under intensive scrutiny (Gerraughty, 1967; Susina, 1967; Simonelli, 1967; Golod, 1968, 1969; Guess, 1968). By 1968, the use of the term *clinical pharmacy* had become commonplace. In an effort to avoid confusion and disagreement over the academic nature of clinical pharmacy, the AACP Committee on Curriculum offered a definition of this new instructional area in its 1968 report (Lemberger, 1968). The definition adopted stated, "Clinical pharmacy is that area within the pharmacy curriculum which deals with patient care with emphasis on drug therapy. Clinical pharmacy seeks to develop a patient-oriented attitude. The acquisition of new knowledge is secondary to the attainment of skills in interprofessional and patient communications" (p. 435). No attempt to delineate subject matter was made, but the objectives for instruction in clinical pharmacy were presented.

The committee further recommended that clinical pharmacy become an area of instruction in every curriculum in pharmacy. Additional observations and recommendations bearing directly on educational policy were:

• Clinical pharmacy should stand alone and on its own merits as an instructional area and not be considered a modification of existing courses.
• Full effect of this instructional area could not be achieved unless it was based on a breadth of prerequisite knowledge in pharmacology, dispensing, pathology, diagnostic techniques, medical terminology, and an orientation to the disease state.
• Ideal locus for clinical instruction is a health science center or teaching hospital. Any facility used should offer comprehensive health care.
• New types of faculty would be required, faculty who are practice oriented and involved in patient care. The academic environment of pharmacy would have to be modified to accommodate such faculty.
• Instruction in clinical pharmacy should not be introduced by the simple expedient of adding to the curriculum or displacing general elective credits.

A final observation, of such fundamental importance that it is quoted here, touched on the relationship between clinical pharmacy and internship. The report stated that "the relationship between clinical pharmacy and internship may, at first glance, seem to be one of conflict. Further examination of the objectives of instruction in clinical pharmacy reveals, however, that this subject area is intended to orient the pharmacist toward his expanding roles in health care, while internship training has as its primary objective the preparation of the student for current practice and the specific needs of the various practice environments" (p. 435). Educational policy issues and evolution of internship education are presented later in this chapter.

Student enthusiasm and support of the profession for clinical pharmacy instruction helped create an environment for change. However, the likely cause of its rapid adoption was the Health Professions Education Assistance Act of 1971, which required that instruction in clinical pharmacy be included in the curriculum for capitation grant eligibility. Significant for its impact on implementation of clinical education and in steering a common course nationally was the invitational workshop on clinical pharmaceutical practice and education sponsored jointly by the American Society of Hospital Pharmacists (ASHP) and the American Association of Colleges of Pharmacy (1971). More than sixty schools of pharmacy were represented at the conference to learn from each other about programs of clinical pharmacy instruction being implemented.

In this almost euphoric professional atmosphere of the early 1970s, full support for a major revision of accreditation standards was obtained with relative ease. The new standards, effective July 1, 1974, embodied two major changes (American Council on Pharmaceutical Education, 1975). Under the new standards, the ACPE began to accredit programs rather than institutions. This change was warranted by the fact that a number of schools of pharmacy had implemented two professional degree programs, the baccalaureate and the doctor of pharmacy. The second major change, reflecting the move to program accreditation, was the adoption of more detailed, explicit curriculum requirements and expansion of these requirements to include both degree programs recognized by the ACPE.

Under the 1974 standards, the three areas of the curriculum were identified as general education, preclinical sciences, and professional studies and training. Although made more explicit in the language of the standards, no major changes in instructional content were made under general education and preclinical sciences (formerly labeled nonscientific courses in general education, and mathematics and the basic physical and biological sciences, respectively). Major changes in professional instruction, however, were introduced. The traditional disciplines of professional instruction found in the 1960 standards were now included as a subdivision of professional studies and training and identified as pharmaceutical sciences. New inclusions to curricular requirements constituting further subdivisions of professional studies and training were biomedical sciences, social and behavioral sciences, management of pharmaceutical services, and clinical sciences and practice.

A particularly significant change in the standards was the inclusion of the statement: "The ACPE believes that the experiences students gain in the clinical courses (including clerkships and externships) should be of such caliber so as to serve in lieu of the internship requirement for licensure. The ACPE expects, therefore, that a curriculum be designed to include an externship and other clinical components that will lead to the degree of professional competence in students required for admission to the licensure examination" (American Council on Pharmaceutical Education, 1975, Section II-B, p. 5). This standard transferred responsibility for internship education from the profession, usually administered by the licensure board in each state, to pharmaceutical education. An appreciation of the enormity of this step as well as better perception of its ramifications can be developed by reviewing internship education in pharmacy.

*Internship Education and Licensure Requirements.* Historically, preparation for the practice of pharmacy was rooted in the apprenticeship system. As formal educational programs evolved, the amount of apprenticeship training required before a candidate could take the licensure examination was reduced to those who had completed such a program of study. Upon adoption of the four-year baccalaureate program as the academic requirement for licensure, most states reduced the apprenticeship time requirement to one year. Since this aspect of training could be completed in other than full-time and continuous employment, one year became defined as fifty-two weeks at forty hours per week. In the early 1950s, the profession acted to relabel the practical experience education requirement as internship, a term more in keeping with professional education and training. However, the substance of this training was not changed.

In spite of continuous efforts to upgrade the quality and to develop greater uniformity of internship training, little progress was made. While much of the failure to show progress was attributed to the fact that state pharmacy practice acts did not specifically authorize boards of pharmacy to regulate this training, the reality in many instances was that the resources of personnel, time, and money were lacking. One exception to this generalization was the state of Wisconsin, which amended its Pharmacy Practice Act in 1965 to create the Wisconsin Pharmacy Internship Board, an autonomous state agency specifically authorized to regulate internship education in pharmacy. In several other states, boards of pharmacy, by adopting additional regulations, were successful in upgrading the quality and uniformity of the internship. In the main, however, internship education remained more a function of the time of employment than of the experience gained in pharmacy practice activities.

On the national level, the National Association of Boards of Pharmacy (NABP) was deeply concerned about internship training, for the lack of uniformity in requirements from state to state seriously threatened reciprocity. The AACP was also concerned because of the growing disparity between the academic preparation and the practical preparation for the licensure examination and for practice. One concept of enduring value developed jointly by these organizations was that of establishing tripartite arrangements among the board of pharmacy, the state pharmaceutical association, and the school(s) of pharmacy in each state to deal with internship education. This concept was carried into the 1974 revision of the accreditation standards for relating externship education to the internship requirement for licensure (American Council on Pharmaceutical Education, 1975).

*The Pharmaceutical Sciences.* Driven partly by the change in educational objectives associated with preparing graduates for patient-oriented practice and partly by the time pressures within the curriculum created by the inclusion of a clinical component of education, instruction in the pharmaceutical sciences has moved to an emphasis on subject matter relevant to the functions proposed for the pharmacist in a clinical practice role. While all disciplines have undergone evolutionary changes, none has changed as dramatically as pharmaceutics. Galenical pharmacy has given way to scientific pharmacy. The compounding of capsules, ointments, and solutions is no longer the end point of instruction; these dosage forms are now viewed as drug delivery systems that can be formulated to modify and control the rate at which a drug becomes available for absorption. A new term, biopharmaceutics, has been coined to identify the aspects of pharmaceutics that interrelate drug absorption, distribution, metabolism, and elimination with the physiochemical properties of body tissues, the drug, and the dosage form. Instruction in dispensing pharmacy has been deemphasized; development of manual skills in extemporaneous compounding of dosage forms is no longer a major objective. Role playing and simulations involving problems in therapy are the modes through which problem-solving skills are developed. Theoretical courses emphasize the application of physical chemical principles to understanding drugs as chemical entities, as well as the behavior of dosage forms as complex systems designed to carry and deliver a precise dose of drug.

Biopharmaceutics and, more recently, pharmacokinetics provide a link between pharmaceutics and pharmacology that did not exist even a decade ago. This bridge permits the pharmacy student to gain unique insight into the mechanisms of drug action. Modern pharmacology instruction exploits the student's physical science background by emphasizing pharmacodynamics. The basic importance of pharmacology to clinical use of drugs is recognized by the greater prominence of this discipline in the pharmacy curriculum than in the curriculum of any other health profession. The needs of clinical pharmacy education and practice have also spawned expansion of instruction in toxicology, as evidenced by the emphasis in the curriculum on adverse drug reactions, drug interactions, and drug abuse. Other biological sciences recently introduced into the pharmacy curriculum are anatomy, pathology, and therapeutics.

In the discipline of pharmacognosy, the taxonomic approach to natural products has given way to a chemical approach. In current pharmacy practice, the graduate utilizes knowledge of antibiotics, blood, and blood products including immunizing biologicals, enzymes, and hormones on a daily basis; traditional classes of natural products such as volatile oils, resins, and gums are no longer emphasized. With the advent of medicinal chemistry as a discipline in its own right, the distinction between synthetic drugs and naturally occurring drugs has disappeared; thus, alkaloids, glycosides, and other naturally occurring chemicals with pharmacological effects are commonly taught as part of this instructional area. Stereochemistry is emphasized in order to develop a better understanding of mechanisms by which drugs exert their effects. The relationship between chemical structure and physiological activity is an important concept for the correlation of therapeutic applications. Synthesis of drug entities is taught mainly for its value in developing the ability to identify chemically reactive moieties. More recently, concepts of drug design, biotransformation, and genetic engineering have been introduced.

Administrative sciences, introduced into the curriculum with the expansion of the baccalaureate program to five years, have also undergone marked evolution. Originally this instructional area was identified closely with the business aspects of pharmacy, reflective of the then virtually exclusive curricular emphasis on the distributive functions of professional practice. Accounting, marketing, and management were the common elements of instruction and focused narrowly on drugstore operations. Expansion of the role of the pharmacist into patient-oriented activities, the growth of health programs—both governmental and private—that include medications in the benefit package, and the flood of legislation regulating the drug industry have markedly influenced educational policy decisions to broaden the scope of this area of the curriculum. In the modern curriculum, required course work has been redirected to include social and behavioral sciences so that the student gains perspective on pharmacy as a health profession within a complex social and professional milieu. For the most part, basic business courses such as accounting and marketing have been deleted from curricular requirements and, where available, are offered to pharmacy students as electives. Pharmacy law and management remain as discrete course offerings in most curricula.

## Programmatic Innovation

*Doctor of Pharmacy (Pharm.D.) Programs.* Earlier reference has been made to the adoption in the mid-1950s by the University of Southern California and the University of California at San Francisco of six-year programs of study leading to a doctor of pharmacy degree and to the recognition of such programs in the revised accreditation standards that became effective July 1, 1960. By the mid-1960s, both of these schools had introduced extensive clinical pharmacy into their curricula and the doctor of pharmacy degree began to acquire identity as a program for producing graduates who possessed a special level of skill in the clinical practice of pharmacy. In the decade from 1965 to 1975, doctor of pharmacy degree programs designed as postbaccalaureate programs ranging from one to three years in duration proliferated, further reinforcing the image of the Pharm.D. degree as a specialized, clinical practice certification. In 1966, only three schools, including the two California schools, offered a doctor of pharmacy degree program (Sprowls, 1967). The number of such schools had increased to eleven by 1970 (Orr, 1971), to twenty by 1975 (Schlegel and Rodowskas. 1976), and to twenty-seven by 1980 (Speedie, 1981). Additional schools have received or are actively seeking approval of doctor of pharmacy degree programs within their own universities.

The situation described above, in which more than one-third of the accredited schools of pharmacy offer programs of study ranging from six to nine years in length, designed both as first degree and as postbaccalaureate degree programs and culminating in the award of the same degree, is bound to result in confusion and divergence of opinion. Pharmaceutical educators have been attempting to deal with this conundrum in a systematic manner since the accreditation standards effective July 1, 1974, were issued. As these standards encompassed program accreditation, both baccalaureate and doctoral curricula were included. Concerned that the standards and guidelines for doctor of pharmacy programs adopted by the ACPE were inadequate to ensure uniform quality among doctoral programs, the AACP convened a special conference to develop specific guidelines for Pharm.D. program evaluation (American Association of Colleges of Pharmacy, 1975d). The formal report from this conference was accepted by the ACPE as a supplement to its proposed guidelines, but the basic issue of accreditation measures applicable to both first-degree and postbaccalaureate doctor of pharmacy programs remained largely unresolved.

In another attempt to settle this issue, the AACP began in 1975 a three-year cycle of study of the topic "Types of Pharmacy Personnel Required to Meet Society's Future Needs." Although broadly conceived, the study quickly narrowed to a debate on whether the doctor of pharmacy degree should be the sole professional degree recognized or whether the existing system of baccalaureate and doctoral curricula, both leading to licensure eligibility, should be continued (Walton and Doluisio, 1975; Haskell and Benedict, 1975). Also considered were societal needs for pharmaceutical services, professional aspirations for an expanded role, educational alternatives for the development of general clinical practice competencies and of specialized or differentiated practice competencies, and educational costs (Lee, 1976; Francke, 1976; Swintosky, 1976; Swintosky, Hopkins, and Vogt, 1975; Wolf, 1977; Lemberger, 1976; Beste and others, 1976; Institute of Medicine, 1974; Schwartz, 1976; Swintosky, Baumgartner, and Vogt, 1976; Rodowskas, Solandar, and Fischman, 1977). At the conclusion of the cycle of consideration of this issue, extended to a fourth year, a decision to maintain the bachelor's degree program as the minimum entry-level degree program was reached. While this action represented a policy action of the AACP, it remained only advisory to member schools. This policy decision has not been a deterrent to continuing development of doctor of pharmacy degree programs. In fact, the trend has been toward the development of such programs as an entry-level degree option.

Following the study and action on this policy issue, AACP continued with efforts to resolve concern of member institutions over the guidelines and standards used by the ACPE in evaluating doctor of pharmacy programs. A Task Force on Guidelines for Pharm.D. Accreditation was appointed in 1977 and reported its findings and recommendations in 1978 (Devenport, 1978). Evidence of the urgency attached to this matter was the recommendation that the AACP provide financial support to the ACPE to implement the recommendations of the task force. Subsequent dialogue with the ACPE led the AACP itself to pursue the matter of drafting specific minimum standards and guidelines for doctor of pharmacy degree programs through the appointment of a second Task Force on Pharm.D. Accreditation Standards. The report of this task force (Miller, 1981), presented in a format encompassing both standards and guidelines for baccalaureate as well as doctor of pharmacy programs, was approved as a policy statement by the AACP house of delegates in 1981 and transmitted to the ACPE for consideration and action.

*Specialty Education.* The first type of educational program intended to prepare graduates for a particular practice role was designed as a master's degree program and had as a particular objective the preparation of graduates for positions as directors of hospital pharmacies; thus, administrative sciences applied to the hospital setting were emphasized. Additional components usually found in the required course work were pharmaceutics related to sterile and special product formulation, pharmacotherapeutics, and research. With the advent of doctor of pharmacy degree programs, the relative merits of the master's and doctoral programs as a foundation for hospital pharmacy practice were debated (Zopf, 1968; Rowe, 1968). Preference for the doctoral program is evidenced by the fact that in September 1967, there were 270 students nationwide enrolled in master's degree programs in hospital pharmacy, and all thirty-five schools offering such a program reported enrollees (Nobles, 1968), while in 1980, there were only 155 students in such programs and only twelve of the thirty-two schools offering the program reported enrollees (Speedie, 1981).

An alternative route to a career in hospital pharmacy, particularly in community service–oriented hospitals, has been residency training. Since 1962, the American Society of Hospital Pharmacists (ASHP) has accredited residency programs designed to produce generalists for organized health care settings (Beste and others, 1976). With growth both in size and diversity of function, a need for breadth in residency training programs was identified, and the ASHP residency accreditation program has been expanded to recognize, in addition to programs leading to training of generalists, programs to train clinical practitioners, specialized practitioners and managers/administrators (American Society of Hospital Pharmacists, 1980a, 1980b). This accreditation program is voluntary and operated exclusively by the ASHP. In practice, residency programs are often combined with or are extensions of other professional education programs, and thus support for the involvement of the ACPE in the accreditation of residency programs is growing. The fact that specializations are now formally recognized by the profession through the Board of Pharmaceutical Specialties and that many people completing residency training programs are employed in other than hospital settings adds impetus to the perception of a need to broaden the accreditation of residency programs.

*Continuing Education.* The continued competence of health care providers has long been both a public and professional concern. The common approach to dealing with the issue of continuing competence in the health professions has been the imposition of a requirement to complete a stated number of hours of continuing education (CE) as a condition for relicensure, under the assumption that such participation would serve as quasi-assurance of competence. At the present time, twenty-six states require pharmacists licensed by that state to participate in CE for relicensure eligibility. Unique to pharmacy has been the development of a national program for the accreditation of providers of CE. The accrediting body for academic degree programs in pharmacy, the ACPE, also accredits providers of CE. All but three of the twenty-six states with mandatory CE requirements for pharmacy recognize ACPE–approved providers. Dissatisfaction with mandatory CE as a proxy for continued competence resulted in the joint APhA–AACP study of continuing competency in pharmacy reported earlier. Standards of practice have been promulgated and assessment instruments are under development. Success of this voluntary, profession-sponsored program of self-assessment and improvement is critically dependent upon CE as the major mechanism through which pharmacists can maintain their competence to practice. CE is also expected to serve a vital function in providing pharmacists with career mobility. Organized, sequential programs of study leading to certifiable skills necessary, for example, for specialty recognition and external doctor of pharmacy degree programs (Lowenthal, 1981; Mergener and Weinswig, 1977; Hanson, 1981a, 1981b) are forms of CE that differ in nature from those presently available. Such programs, however, are seen as necessary by the profession.

## Educational Research and Development

*Faculty Development.* A rather unique strategy for fostering educational development was the implementation of annual teachers' seminars by the AACP. The first such seminar, held in 1949 at the University of Wisconsin, focused on the emergence of pharmacy as a scientific discipline rooted in mathematics and physical chemistry. The Teachers' Seminars provided a forum for the exchange of ideas between teachers within a given discipline as well as across disciplines. The seminars also provided a mechanism for the continuing education of pharmacy educators during the period in which the pharmaceutical sciences flowered. The successful transition of pharmaceutical education from art to science accomplished nationwide in the 1950s was largely the result of these seminars.

By 1960, most schools of pharmacy had added an adequate number of young faculty members well educated in the sciences to their staffs, and therefore the need for the Teachers' Seminar to provide continuing education diminished. Relieved of this function, the Teachers' Seminar became exclusively the forum for exchange of educational philosophy, discussion of curriculum change, and presentations on new teaching technologies. In the period from 1960 to 1975, educational development was fostered by propagation of the wave of clinical education, by bringing visibility and credibility to continuing education, and by drawing attention to the concepts of competency-based education. The value of the Teachers' Seminar as a mechanism to advance educational innovation is evidenced by its reappearance in 1982, after a three-year moratorium, as a one-day program scheduled with the annual meeting of the AACP.

*Competency-Based Education.* Competency-based education in pharmacy has had a brief and varied history. Its genesis was in clinical education, in particular the experiential components. Awarding academic credit for educational experiences was a completely new concept to pharmacy faculties. Quality control and student evaluation were seen as necessary to assure that the desired learning had occurred. Defining outcomes in terms of measurable behavioral traits provided the solution to this problem. The ACPE, in its guidelines to the accreditation standards and its self-study guide, refers to the use of competency statements as part of curriculum design and management (American Council on Pharmaceutical Education, 1975). That competency-based instruction became an issue of great interest and discussion in the mid-1970s is reflected by the fact that the 1975 Teachers' Seminar was devoted to this topic (American Association of Colleges of Pharmacy, 1975c). However, consensus on this issue in the form of a policy decision has not been achieved, and the literature in pharmaceutical education has been relatively silent on this matter in the last several years.

*Independent Study.* Concurrent with active interest in competency-based education, the techniques of self-study and computer-assisted instruction were investigated for applicability to pharmaceutical education. Numerous attempts to develop individual courses in a self-study format and to create computer-assisted instruction modules have been reported. Such developments have been found to be successful in the hands of the instructor responsible for the work, but relatively little transfer of usage between schools has occurred. Most of the interschool sharing of computer-assisted instruction has been limited to computer-based games in administrative sciences and computer simulations in clinical sciences and practice.

Particularly noteworthy for its creativity and scope was the University of Illinois College of Pharmacy investigational program for self-directed study, known as the IPSDS (Purohit, Kulieke, and Manasse, 1980). The faculty of this school agreed to a curriculum-wide experiment in which the entire core curriculum was made available in a self-directed study format. The philosophy underlying the project held that, ideally, education should have as its goal the expected level of student achievement and allow time to be a variable, whereas traditional instructional formats fix time (semester, quarter) and allow achievement to be the variable. Several significant observations were made during the course of this study, but the chief conclusion reached was that neither students nor teachers were prepared for such a dramatic change in instructional delivery. Students who successfully completed the program were characterized by above-average academic achievement, a high degree of self-confidence, self-motivation, and independence, but it was not established whether these characteristics resulted from the IPSDS experience or whether such students were, in effect, self-selected because of the nature of the program.

Another school-wide experiment with self-directed study was conducted by the School of Pharmacy at Creighton University (Tindall and Koziol, 1976). The curriculum of the second professional year at that school was divided into modules, further subdivided into learning packages. As in the IPSDS, students advanced through the program by demonstrating attainment of a predetermined proficiency level for each module. Unlike the Illinois experiment, which was voluntary, all students at Creighton were required to complete the program, and a two- or three-semester time limit was imposed to assure student eligibility to enter the third professional year. Subjective observations similar to those made at Illinois confirm that students develop a sense of self-awareness and confidence in their ability to become self-teachers as well as learners.

### Unresolved and Continuing Policy Issues

In a careful review and analysis, an accurate perspective requires awareness that factors that shape destiny include actions that did not occur, as well as those that did. Tracing the impact of nonevents is difficult if not impossible; only examples and speculations can be provided. For pharmacy and pharmaceutical education, one such example would be the unfulfilled expectation of the 1950s that the pharmacist would become the "scientist on the street corner." Failure of this aspiration to materialize helped create an environment in which patient-oriented, health care-directed activities were readily embraced. Inaction in the updating of state pharmacy practice acts has also affected educational innovation and policy. Outdated laws constrain and in some states even limit the role of pharmacist to distribution of drug products, a limitation reflected in the setting of reimbursement fees for pharmaceutical services by federal, state, and private agencies. The economic barrier to establishing clinical pharmacy services in an ambulatory care setting is the primary deterrent to the routine implementation of such services. Failure to implement service, in turn, creates conflict within pharmacy when educational policy decisions on curriculum and degrees are approached.

Another observation arising from this review of educational development is that a systematic approach to the setting of policy is lacking. While at first glance this seems strange and almost irresponsible, further consideration reveals that forces external to pharmacy and pharmaceutical education have had an irresistible impact on policy decisions.

*Public Involvement.* The entitlement for public involvement in the setting of educational policy in the health professions is the monopoly granted each profession through licensure. This monopoly must be exercised in the public interest; thus, any change in educational policy must be consistent with the needs of the public. Governmental interest in health manpower supply and distribution follows as an expression of this control. However, the role of education need not be passive; in fact, education bears a responsibility to be active in assuring that any ultimate policy decision is, indeed, in the best interest of society. In the case of manpower, for example, care must be exercised that educational institutions are not viewed as factories whose sole mission is to produce health care providers efficiently trained for contemporary needs. Warping the educational system away from intellectual growth and in the direction of vocational training, albeit at a high-quality level, would be particularly harmful for baccalaureate programs in the health professions.

*Interprofessional Issues.* Interprofessional issues are also factors that help shape educational policy. Common to all health professions is a focus on serving the patient. Thus, as the capability for service of a given profession expands through educational advancement and as new areas for the provision of service are found, relationships between the professions as providers of service change. Interprofessional friction is often the result. In many instances, education is looked to for resolution of such problems. For example, education has been expected to bring the concept of a "health care team" to reality. The notion that this expectation can be achieved by the educational enterprise independently of actual practice behavior is erroneous, and the apparent lack of progress to date must be evaluated from this perspective.

An analysis of the progress made in achieving interprofessional education is also dependent on the definition chosen for the health care team. The common analogy of the health care team to a football team conjures up an image of all players being on the field simultaneously and a quarterback calling signals. A more apt analogy is to a medley relay team, where each member makes an individual and unique contribution to the team performance. The success of the team still depends on a combined effort, and the most important factor in success is the smooth passing of the baton.

Given the latter "team" as a concept, health professions education has been more successful than generally credited. Students today gain much better insight into the roles and capabilities of their health professions colleagues than ever before. Remaining shortcomings, to be overcome through joint study and policy decisions, are in the selection of clinical sites for education and in coordinating the educational activities of health professions students who share a common site for clinical work. Particularly detrimental to progress in this area is the current practice in the selection of clinical education sites. Schools select such sites independently rather than cooperatively and with virtual disregard for the quality of care provided by health professions other than their own at the sites selected. Thus, students educated at these sites may not be exposed to state-of-the-art quality of care in the other health professions with whom they share responsibility for patient care.

*Intraprofessional Issues.* Unresolved issues within pharmacy itself stem from the addition of clinical functions to the role of the pharmacist. As previously noted in this chapter, pharmaceutical education has responded rapidly through the introduction of clinical sciences and practice as a curricular requirement and through the adoption of clerkships and externships as instructional techniques. The second-generation policy issue that must now be addressed is that of establishing a healthy balance between pharmaceutical education as an intellectual pursuit and as a training program in preparation for professional practice. One ramification of this issue is the constraint on opportunity to prepare for specific career choices as a result of the intensive focus of the curriculum on preparation

for licensure. Closely related is the issue of the educational preparation of pharmacists for facets of pharmacy practice other than direct patient service. Another
need of the educational enterprise, generated by present accreditation requirements, is for the assignment of appropriate authority to determine the nature and
extent of practical training required for licensure.

Pharmacy must also address itself to the issue of types of personnel to be
utilized in the delivery of pharmaceutical services. Educational policy decisions
on future educational requirements for licensure, on professional graduate education (such as residencies and fellowships), on continuing education offerings
leading to both lateral and vertical career mobility, and on supportive personnel
training are closely woven into the fabric of this issue.

*Issues Within Pharmaceutical Education.* A number of issues within
pharmaceutical education remain unresolved. The expansion of knowledge
within the pharmaceutical sciences combined with a need for an expanded knowledge base to undergird additional functional roles has produced a glut for curricular content. This situation must not be resolved by adding to the student's factual
base of knowledge at the expense of effort devoted to developing problem-solving
skills, nor should it be resolved by the expedient of adding to the curricular
requirements. Alternatives that should be explored are competency-based education and subdivision of educational requirements according to identifiable functional roles. The latter alternative, in turn, implies the imposition of practice
limitations on a lateral as opposed to a hierarchical basis.

The overabundance of curricular content has already resulted in a significant loss of flexibility in curriculum design. Opportunity for students to individu-
alize their education has been seriously compromised. Erosion of opportunity for
educational innovation has also occurred, because new program thrusts normally
arise from elective, experimental programs of study. Policy decisions that will
foster high-quality educational research including curricular experimentation are
needed. One example of an area of need is the examination of clinical pharmacy as
an academic discipline in an attempt to elucidate that body of knowledge unique
to pharmacy and to identify the types of health care problems solvable with this
unique background. Another area for exploration is that of the relationship between basic pharmaceutical sciences and pharmacy practice. Discontinuity between basic science and clinical education must be avoided. Educational pathways
assuring the movement of pharmacy students into graduate education and research in the pharmaceutical sciences must be developed.

*Accreditation as an Issue.* The role of accreditation in providing firm policy directions and in creating a climate for change in educational programs leads
to another set of issues for continued study. The profound changes in pharmaceutical education since 1974 would not have transpired as rapidly and at such a
uniform level of quality in the absence of accreditation standards. As a process,
accreditation serves the public interest by assuring that all accredited programs
meet minimum acceptable standards, and it serves institutional interests by helping all schools improve through the process of internal and external review. This
latter function, carried to extreme, can be viewed as self-serving. Study of accreditation is timely in view of the current reduction in resources, the anticipated
falloff in enrollments, and the proliferation of accrediting and certifying bodies
in the fields of health care and health science education.

Another facet of the study of accreditation is the role of accrediting bodies in the professions. Particular scrutiny should be given to the use of accreditation as a mechanism to induce change. It is a given that accreditation must require change where necessary to meet stated norms, but the proper balance among the public interest, a profession, its educational arm, and the accrediting body in setting these norms must be maintained.

An accreditation-related study needed in pharmacy would explore the ramifications of program accreditation adopted in 1974 as compared to school accreditation as it existed before 1974. Since there are presently two different degree programs in pharmacy, each of which may be offered as a first-degree program and, as such, qualify a graduate for licensure, program accreditation seems necessary. However, the experience to date should be reviewed to determine whether the criteria used for evaluation preserve balance among the components of quality. Objective measures such as student/faculty ratios, required credits and credit distribution among curricular areas, budget figures, and assignable square feet must be employed; however, they cannot substitute for subjective measures of creativity, scholarship, and student performance in practice. Another aspect of program accreditation to be part of such a study is the potential role of the ACPE in the accreditation of graduate professional education programs, such as residencies and fellowships.

## Mission of Professional Education

This chapter reveals that much progress has been made in pharmaceutical education in the last two decades. Educational policy decisions, often made through an imperfect process, nonetheless have been sound. One overall concern needs to be raised as a concluding message. Any endeavor as fundamental as education attracts much interest and may easily become viewed as the focal point for change. It is of vital importance that any decisions on educational policy that are made are consistent with maintaining the primary mission of education as the preparation of young people for professional service to society. Other objectives not incompatible with this mission may also be adopted, if subordinate. Thus, using the educational enterprise to address such social problems as assuring availability and quality of health care within geographic or economic boundaries is a disastrous course to follow if the primary educational mission is compromised. Similarly, the use of education to fulfill professional aspirations for new roles or changes related to self-interest, no matter how well intentioned, is a pitfall that must be avoided in future policy decisions.

## References

Adams, J. G. "Report of the Committee on Curriculum, 1959." *American Journal of Pharmaceutical Education*, 1960, *24*, 353–355.

American Association of Colleges of Pharmacy. "The Continuing Competence of Pharmacists." *Journal of the American Pharmaceutical Association*, 1975a, *15*, 432–437, 457.

American Association of Colleges of Pharmacy. *Pharmacists for the Future: The Report of the Study Commission on Pharmacy.* Ann Arbor: Health Administration Press, 1975b.

American Association of Colleges of Pharmacy. "Proceedings of the 1975 Teacher's Seminar." *American Journal of Pharmaceutical Education*, 1975c, *39*, 555–574.

American Association of Colleges of Pharmacy. *Report of the AACP Conference on Guidelines for Doctor of Pharmacy Programs, October 26–28, 1975, Kansas City, Mo.* Bethesda, Md.: American Association of Colleges of Pharmacy, 1975d.

American Council on Education. *Findings and Recommendations of the Pharmaceutical Survey, 1948.* Washington, D.C.: American Council on Education, 1950.

American Council on Pharmaceutical Education. *Accreditation Manual.* (6th ed.) Chicago: American Council on Pharmaceutical Education, 1960.

American Council on Pharmaceutical Education. *Accreditation Manual.* (7th ed.) Chicago: American Council on Pharmaceutical Education, 1975.

American Pharmaceutical Association. *APhA Code of Ethics.* Washington, D.C.: American Pharmaceutical Association, 1952.

American Pharmaceutical Association. "Final Report, APhA Task Force on Specialties in Pharmacy." *Journal of the American Pharmaceutical Association*, 1974, *14*, 618–621.

American Society of Hospital Pharmacists/American Association of Colleges of Pharmacy. "Proceedings of the ASHP-AACP Invitational Workshop on Clinical Pharmaceutical Practice and Education." *American Journal of Hospital Pharmacy*, 1971, *28*, 842–843.

American Society of Hospital Pharmacists. "ASHP Long-Range Position Statement on Pharmacy Manpower Needs and Residency Training." *American Journal of Hospital Pharmacy*, 1980a, *37*, 1220.

American Society of Hospital Pharmacists. "ASHP Statement on Accreditation of Pharmacy Residencies." *American Journal of Hospital Pharmacy*, 1980b, *37*, 1221–1223.

Autian, J. "Fourth or Terminal Course in Pharmacy." In A. P. Lemberger (Ed.), *Proceedings of the American Association of Colleges of Pharmacy Teachers' Seminar*, Vol. 13. Bethesda, Md.: American Association of Colleges of Pharmacy, 1961.

Autian, J., and Berman, A. "Concepts of Drug Evaluations in the Dispensing Course of the Future." *American Journal of Pharmaceutical Education*, 1960, *24*, 299–308.

Beste, D. F., Jr., and Herfindal, E. T. "An Integrated Program of Clinical Pharmacy." *Hospital Formulary Management*, 1975, *10*, 172–182.

Beste, D. F., and others. "Final Report of the Special Committee on Accreditation of Residency Programs in Pharmacy." *American Journal of Pharmaceutical Education*, 1976, *40*, 494–495.

Biles, J. "Innovations in Clinical Pharmacy Education Program." *Wisconsin Pharmacist*, 1974, *43*, 273–275.

Deno, R. A. (Ed.). *Proceedings of Pharmacy/Medicine/Nursing Conference on Health Education.* Ann Arbor: University of Michigan, 1967.

Devenport, J. K. "Chair Report for the Task Force on Guidelines for Pharm.D. Accreditation." *American Journal of Pharmaceutical Education*, 1978, *42*, 490–493.

Francke, D. E. "Significant Issues Raised by the Study Commission on Pharmacy Report: A View from the Profession." *American Journal of Pharmaceutical Education*, 1976, *40*, 448–452.

Gerraughty, R. J. "Philosophy of the Terminal Pharmacy Course." *American Journal of Pharmaceutical Education*, 1967, *31*, 228–230.

Gibson, M. R. (Ed.). *Studies of a Core Curriculum*. Bethesda, Md.: American Association of Colleges of Pharmacy, 1967.

Golod, W. H. "Clinical Pharmacy: The Terminal Course: Part I." *American Journal of Pharmaceutical Education*, 1968, *32*, 65–69; "Part II." *American Journal of Pharmaceutical Education*, 1969, *33*, 226–228.

Graber, J. B., and Brodie, D. C. (Eds.). *Proceedings of an Invitational Conference on Pharmacy Manpower: Challenge to Pharmacy in the '70s*. U.S. Department of Health, Education, and Welfare Publication no. (HSM) 72-3000. Washington, D.C.: U.S. Government Printing Office, 1970.

Guess, W. L. "The Terminal Course in Pharmacy Today: Philosophy, Scope, and Syllabus." *American Journal of Pharmaceutical Education*, 1968, *32*, 876–884.

Hanson, A. L. "External Degree: Mechanism for B.S. Practitioners to Earn a Pharm.D." *American Journal of Pharmaceutical Education*, 1981a, *45*, 284–290.

Hanson, A. L. "External Doctor of Pharmacy Degree." *Möbius*, 1981b, *1* (2), 35–45.

Haskell, A. R., and Benedict, L. K. "The Universal Doctor of Pharmacy Degree." *American Journal of Pharmaceutical Education*, 1975, *39*, 425–427.

Hugill, P. R., and Watzman, N. "Comprehensive Health Manpower Training Act of 1971: An Update of Federal Support of Pharmacy Education." *American Journal of Pharmaceutical Education*, 1973, *37*, 237–241.

Institute of Medicine. *Education for the Health Team: Report of a Conference*. Washington, D.C.: National Academy of Sciences, Institute of Medicine, 1972.

Institute of Medicine. *Costs of Education in the Health Professions: Parts I, II, and III*. Washington, D.C.: National Academy of Sciences, Institute of Medicine, 1974.

Kalman, S. H., and Schlegel, J. F. "Standards of Practice for the Profession of Pharmacy." *American Pharmacy*, 1979, *19* (3), 133–145.

Lee, P. R. "The Family Pharmacist." *Journal of the American Pharmaceutical Association*, 1976, *16*, 396–397.

Lemberger, A. P. (Ed.). "*Proceedings of the American Association of Colleges of Pharmacy Teachers' Seminar*. Vol. 13. Bethesda, Md.: American Association of Colleges of Pharmacy, 1961.

Lemberger, A. P. "Report of the Committee on Curriculum." *American Journal of Pharmaceutical Education*, 1968, *32*, 435–437.

Lemberger, A. P. "Report of the Committee on Curriculum." *American Journal of Pharmaceutical Education*, 1969, *33*, 563–564.

Lemberger, A. P. "Specialty Recognition—Academic and Professional Alternatives." *American Journal of Pharmaceutical Education*, 1976, *40*, 453–456.

Lowenthal, W. "Obtaining Advanced Degrees in Pharmacy by Nontraditional Means." *American Journal of Pharmaceutical Education*, 1981, *45*, 77.

Mergener, M. A., and Weinswig, M. W. "A Case for a Professional Development Degree in Pharmacy." *Wisconsin Pharmacist*, 1977, *46*, 401–408, 442–447.

Miller, W. A. "Chair Report for the Task Force on Pharm.D. Accreditation Standards." *American Journal of Pharmaceutical Education,* 1981, *45,* 377–384.

Nobles, L. "Graduate Enrollment Data, September 1967, and Graduate Study in Member Colleges, 1968–1969." *American Journal of Pharmaceutical Education,* 1968, *32,* 117–119.

Oddis, J. A. "Patterns of Hospital Pharmacy Practice." *Wisconsin Pharmacist,* 1974, *43,* 309–312.

Orr, J. E. "Report on Enrollment in Schools and Colleges of Pharmacy, First Semester, Term, or Quarter, 1970–1971." *American Journal of Pharmaceutical Education,* 1971, *35,* 95–102.

Paul, D. B., and Sperandio, G. J. "A Survey of the Five-Year Curricula of Member Colleges." *American Journal of Pharmaceutical Education,* 1962, *26,* 461–467.

Purohit, A. A., Kulieke, M. J., and Manasse, H. R. *The IPSDS: Evaluation Results of a Five-Year Experiment in Pharmaceutical Education, University of Illinois College of Pharmacy.* Washington, D.C.: U.S. Department of Health, Education, and Welfare, 1980.

Rodowskas, C. A., Solandar, L., and Fischman, M. "B.S. to Pharm.D. Transition Costs: Some Early Speculations." *American Journal of Pharmaceutical Education,* 1977, *41,* 453–459.

Rosenfeld, M., Thornton, R. F., and Glazer, R. *A National Study of the Practice of Pharmacy.* Washington, D.C.: American Pharmaceutical Association, 1978.

Rowe, T. D. "The Pharm.D. Degree: A Possible Solution." *American Journal of Pharmaceutical Education,* 1968, *32,* 848–852.

Schlegel, J. F., and Rodowskas, C. A. "Enrollment Report on Professional Degree Programs in Pharmacy, Fall 1975." *American Journal of Pharmaceutical Education,* 1976, *40,* 279–293.

Schwartz, M. A. "An Analysis of the IOM Cost Study." *American Journal of Pharmaceutical Education,* 1976, *40,* 456–458.

Silverman, M., and Lee, P. *Pills, Profits, and Politics.* Berkeley: University of California Press, 1974.

Simonelli, A. P. "The Terminal Course in Pharmacy: Content." *American Journal of Pharmaceutical Education,* 1967, *31,* 237–241.

Speedie, S. M. "Enrollment Report on Professional Degree Programs in Pharmacy, Fall 1980." *American Journal of Pharmaceutical Education,* 1981, *45,* 399–414.

Sprowls, J. B. "Report on Enrollment in Schools and Colleges of Pharmacy: First Semester, Term, or Quarter 1966–1967." *American Journal of Pharmaceutical Education,* 1967, *31,* 41–47.

Susina, S. V. "The Scope of the Terminal Course in Pharmacy." *American Journal of Pharmaceutical Education,* 1967, *31,* 231–236.

Swintosky, J. V. "Maturing of Pharmaceutical Education." *Drug Intelligence and Clinical Pharmacy,* 1976, *10,* 153–160.

Swintosky, J. V., Baumgartner, R. P., and Vogt, D. D. "Institutional Resource Requirements and Cost per Student for Contemporary Pharmaceutical Education." *American Journal of Pharmaceutical Education,* 1976, *40,* 459–467.

Swintosky, J. V., Hopkins, H., and Vogt, D. D. "The Professional Degree in Pharmacy Reexamined." *Journal of American Pharmaceutical Association,* 1975, *15,* 683, 707.

Task Force on the Pharmacist's Clinical Role. "Report of the Task Force." *Journal of the American Pharmaceutical Association*, 1971, *11*, 482–485.

Tindall, W. N., and Koziol, R. J. "Development of a Pharmacy Curriculum Using Teaching Modules." *American Journal of Pharmaceutical Education*, 1976, *40*, 157–158.

Walton, C. A., and Doluisio, J. T. "Commitments for Tomorrow in Pharmacy Education: Two Professional Degree Programs." *American Journal of Pharmaceutical Education*, 1975, *39*, 418–424.

White, E. V. *The Office-Based Family Pharmacist.* Berryville: Va.: E. V. White, 1978.

Wolf, H. H. "A Matter of Degree." *American Journal of Pharmaceutical Education*, 1977, *41*, 520.

Zelnio, R. N. "Chair Report for the Committee on Academic Affairs." *American Journal of Pharmaceutical Education*, 1981, *45*, 361–364.

Zopf, L. C. "The Educational Needs of the Hospital Pharmacist Can Best Be Met by a Graduate Program." *American Journal of Pharmaceutical Education*, 1968, *32*, 844–847.

# 5

*Helen K. Grace*

# Nursing

Nursing education has engaged in a long and arduous struggle in moving from apprenticeship training, physician dominated and controlled by hospitals, into the mainstream of higher education. This struggle has been primarily political. Throughout this political process little attention has been given to building a research base to validate the gains or losses that have been achieved in the educational innovations attempted. For example, there are currently four types of educational programs preparing nursing students to take licensure examinations: (1) associate degree programs located in two-year community colleges; (2) certificate programs of hospital-based diploma schools of nursing; (3) baccalaureate degree programs offered by senior colleges and universities; and (4) the doctor of nursing degree program, a postbaccalaureate program preparing students for entrance into nursing and offered by Case Western Reserve University. These four types of programs prepare nurses for the same licensure examination. Although there are heated debates, both within nursing and without, over the type of educational preparation needed by nurses, little systematic research speaks to the differences among graduates of these very different educational systems. Rhetorical and philosophical arguments predominate, with little attention given to systematic research into broad-scope issues in nursing education. The reasons for this lack of attention to research are inherent in the types of political struggles that have surrounded the field. If nursing is to be controlled by other professions or to be held as a chattel by hospitals, there is little opportunity for investigation into educational innovation that might serve to challenge these controls. As nursing has moved out of the control of hospitals and

*Note:* This chapter has been prepared with special assistance from Olga Church, assistant professor of psychiatric nursing, College of Nursing, University of Illinois.

into the educational mainstream, extensive efforts have been mounted to meet the requirements of the "academy," that is, to prepare nurses at the doctoral level and to build a cadre of researchers. Nursing is only now at the point of beginning to investigate systematically its educational system.

## Social Forces Affecting Nursing Education

The development of nursing as a profession, in contrast to an occupation, has been hampered by a variety of social forces related to the status of women in the broader society. Ironically, as opportunities have expanded for women to engage in careers outside the boundaries of the traditional family, nursing, as a predominantly women's field, has not advanced accordingly.

Following World War II, it was anticipated that the nursing shortages experienced by hospitals during the war would be relieved by nurses returning from military service. However, only a small percentage of the military nurses returned to hospital nursing practice. The very considerable responsibility nurses had enjoyed in the Army and Navy led them to prefer more flexible and autonomous roles than were available in general duty hospital positions (Kalisch and Kalisch, 1978). Reasons given for the continuing shortage of nurses in the mid-forties were poor pay, long hours, increase in retirement and marriage of nurses, and opportunities for advanced education under the GI Bill (Kalisch and Kalisch, 1978). These same issues, in a somewhat altered form, are evidenced in the summary of public hearings conducted by the National Commission on Nursing under the auspices of the American Hospital Association in 1981: "Lack of recognition and understanding of the nurse's role in health care delivery by the public, other health care professionals, and nurses themselves was considered to be a key contributor to current nursing related problems . . . Nurses described themselves as overworked, underpaid, and lacking the respect of physician members of the health care team" (p. 9).

In the forties, as now, advanced education was viewed as a culprit in contributing to the nursing shortage. As the Kalisches (1978) report, "Edith W. Bailey, administrator of the Canonsburg General Hospital in Canonsburg, Pennsylvania commented: The nurses attending universities and colleges insist only on supervising—and strangely enough a sick person doesn't give a hang whether his nurse possesses a B.A. or B.S. The root question is, 'Can she make him comfortable?' Another comment along this line came from A. M. Frank, M.D., chairman of the staff at Lutheran Hospital, St. Louis. He predicted that practical nurses would be in greater demand than those with degrees and added that 'one definitely does not need a Ph.D. degree to carry a bedpan. The patients are only interested in whether it is hot or cold. Student nurses are spending too much time in the lecture halls and too little time on the floor so that we are getting too many desk models and insufficient floor models'" (p. 10).

Ironically, a consistent concern surrounds the overeducation of nurses. Historically, each nursing shortage that has occurred has resulted in some form of downgrading of the educational system. In the post–World War II years, it was the introduction and expansion of practical nurse education. Subsequently, the rapid evolvement of associate degree programs had the unplanned effect of shortening the educational preparation for nurses.

In the current national debate, one of the frequent discussions centers about the "bedside nurse." At the heart of this discussion is an assumption that nurses prepared at the baccalaureate level are not "bedside nurses" and that to fill this void we should recruit people off the street, provide them with short in-service education courses, and put them on acute hospital wards to provide bedside care. When one considers the acuity of illness experienced by the hospitalized patient, the complexity of medical terminology, and the advancement of knowledge in the health science fields, the argument that the "bedside nurse" does not need a knowledge base for practice is, on the face of it, an absurdity. But this argument bespeaks a much deeper conflict. The uneducated "bedside nurse" of the past was totally subservient to the hospital bureaucracy, on the one hand, and to physician authority, on the other. The educated nurse poses a threat to this control. As one of the witnesses at the hearings of the National Commission on Nursing (1981) commented, "As a result of a more liberal education, today's nurse is articulate, assertive and demanding of a professional practice environment that includes participative management techniques and recognition that nurses are colleagues of physicians and other health care providers. These nurses expect professional autonomy in determining the scope of nursing practice. Although committed to patient care, nurses express concerns over conditions of employment and expect appropriate financial compensation" (p. 10). Another witness, the president of a medical center, noted, "What happens when one of these young women, now an educated professional nurse . . . is presented with rotation of shifts, changing days off, two out of three weekends, and an inability to control her own leisure time and social life? . . . Today's nursing graduates have had a lot of assertiveness training, and they are willing to take on physicians and insist that 'nursing decisions' should be made by nurses . . . They were value programmed in what Tom Wolfe called 'the ME decade.' As a result, young nursing graduates are not going to accept the status quo and working conditions they see as unsuitable. They are going to look for alternatives to make their nursing careers meaningful, or they are simply going to quit" (p. 10).

Advanced educational preparation for nurses is viewed by many as a threat, with nursing education viewed as in a conflictual position with nursing practice. How this conflict is resolved today will perhaps be the determining factor in whether nursing moves forward in attaining professional stature or is pulled back into a continuation of its subservient occupational status of the past. A careful review of the past and the history of the role of women in society may provide insights into ways of more positively resolving the basic underlying conflicts.

### Modern Nursing Education

*Historical Antecedents.* Since the beginning of history, some form of "nursing" has existed, either as part of the mother's function in the family in caring for sick family members or, more recently, as a function of societal specialists trained to provide "nursing" in institutional settings outside the home. Indeed, one of the difficulties in defining nursing as a profession is that of distinguishing what nurses know and do from what the lay public knows and does. Hughes (1963) describes the problem of attaining professional status as, "Professionals profess. They profess to know better than others the nature of certain matters, and to know better than their clients what ails them or their affairs. This is the essence of the professional idea and the professional claim" (p. 656). In early history, care of the sick was provided within the family. If one had no family, then institutional care was provided, with the "nurses" as well as the patients being defined as societal outcasts. The role of women was carefully circumscribed and confined to the family. Nursing within an institutional context was considered a deviant societal role. The main contribution of Florence Nightingale was to identify nursing, outside of the family context, as an acceptable social role for women and thus make the first step in differentiating the nursing profession.

Inherent in this process was the establishment of an educational system to prepare nurses. As Hughes (1963) describes the process of attaining professional status, "Changes sought are more independence, more recognition, a higher place, a clearer distinction between those in the profession and those outside and a larger measure of autonomy in seeking colleagues and succcessors. One necessary validation of such change in status in our society is introduction of study for the profession in question into the universities" (pp. 661–662). The development of an educational system in nursing, as distinct from training, has been particularly complicated primarily because of the conflict over control of the process.

Early efforts to establish nursing education in this country were disorganized and isolated experiments until the importation and establishment of the Nightingale plan for three training schools in 1873. These first three schools, organized according to explicit principles of the plan as developed in England, are worth mentioning because they clearly provided a system with a certain amount of autonomy for the schools and their nursing superintendents. These early schools held to Nightingale's tenets that control of all aspects of the educational program should be administratively separated from hospital control (Dock, 1920, p. 155). Over the years, those aspects that related to the "control" placed in the hands of the matron (trained nurse) were de-emphasized, as compliance to medical authorities and institutional regulations emerged as predominant.

The inclusion of nursing education in the educational system of the country was a desired goal of the early nursing educators. The movement out of hospitals and away from the apprenticeship type of training, toward professional preparation in educational institutions, had begun at the turn of the century. However, during each national emergency, the concerns for expediency in producing needed numbers of nurses in hospital-controlled nursing schools took precedence. Student nurses constituted a stable work force for hospitals. However, fact-finding studies and surveys on nursing and nursing education repeatedly pointed to the general inadequacy of the average hospital training programs. The Goldmark report (Goldmark, 1923) concluded, "the average hospital training school is not organized on such a basis as to conform to the standards accepted in other educational fields; . . . the instruction in such schools is frequently casual and uncorrelated; . . . the educational needs and health and strength of students are frequently sacrificed to practical hospital exigencies" (p. 21).

The Goldmark report was surprisingly ineffectual in inspiring reforms in nursing education in contrast to those that followed the famous Flexner report on medical education in 1910. The timing of the report may have been one of the factors contributing to the lack of response. In 1923, the nation had come through a decade filled with critical social events. The initiation of the income tax in 1913, the First World War in 1918, and the feminist surge for suffrage had left the nation in a conservative mood, one not supportive of large-scale reforms for such progressive causes as women's education. The differing responses to the Goldmark report on nursing and the Flexner report on medicine may also have been partially due to the predominant sexist orientation of the society generally. Men were entitled to education for the medical profession, while women were destined to be trained to be their handmaidens.

Although the movement for women's rights in the first few decades of the twentieth century had culminated in the passage of the Nineteenth Amendment in 1920, the anti-feminist stance toward women who would aspire to become professional lingered on. This was especially apparent in such male-dominated professions as medicine (Means, 1963). The cost of educating women was considered to be a factor mitigating against women entering medical education; however, nursing was often viewed as a good preparation for marriage and in keeping with woman's innate nature. If women were to work, nursing and teaching were the socially accepted fields. Psychologically, it was considered desirable to have mutually reinforcing overlap between work and family roles (Bailyn, 1964). By staying within the confines of the authoritarian male-dominated health care system and playing out an extended maternal role, nurses were able to carve out a niche in the world outside the home. The nurse training system with its strong emphasis upon obedience to authority and the learning of caring skills was considered to be good preparation both for nursing and for marriage. There was not strong societal pressure to change the system. Certainly those in control of hospital-based training schools were not motivated to make changes during this period. The national economic collapse of the thirties and an accompanying oversupply of nurses further delayed the move of nursing into the educational mainstream. By 1935, only seven collegiate schools of nursing had been established.

*Impact of World War II.* Teachers College, Columbia University had offered programs for graduate nurses in such fields as economics and administration since 1899, and the first university-based nursing program had been established at the University of Minnesota in 1909. A standard curriculum was prepared by the Education Committee of the National League of Nursing Education in 1917. Recommendations for moving nursing education into baccalaureate-level preparation had been made in the Goldmark report of 1923, which advocated that university schools of nursing develop five-year programs that would include both professional studies and liberal arts. This was followed by the work of the Committee on the Grading of Nursing Schools directed by Mary Ayres Burgess (1928), which was to study the supply and demand for nurses and the status of nursing schools. Despite these concerns for and actual study of nursing education, the system of nurse training established in the United States in the late 1800s remained virtually unchanged. At the beginning of World War II, the major portion of nurse training was still occurring in hospital settings. Student nurses learned by doing. Their mentors were head nurses employed in the hospitals. The substantive content consisted of instruction given by physicians on particular disease entities and content in nursing ethics taught by nursing faculty. Students were expected to attend classes after having worked a full week (forty to forty-eight hours on duty). Changes were just beginning to occur as World War II broke out.

With the beginning of the war, attention shifted away from improvement in the quality of nursing education to a primary concern for quantity. At the onset of the war, nursing was faced with a depleted and changing nursing staff, a scarcity of students, and the need to sacrifice long-term goals to immediate and necessary demands (Whitehouse, 1941).

As outlined by the president of the National League of Nursing Education in 1943, significant among the liabilities of the wartime effort were the problems relating to the "depletion of the ranks of faculties of the schools of nursing and of the nursing staff of the hospital," along with the exploitation of students serving as substitutes for graduate nurses. The "dual responsibility of rendering . . . essential service and at the same time . . . maintaining sound educational practices in the preparation of young women for nursing . . . led to the development of the accelerated programs." Leaders of the nursing associations admitted that "it means unceasing vigilance in season and out of season to try to salvage a sound educational program" (Goostray, 1943, p. 50).

Turnover of staff within the hospitals was seen as a priority problem, and the shortage of staff nurses continued long after the war ended. Factors related to the shortages were listed as poor pay, poor working conditions (split shifts and longer hours than other occupations), and, as part of the generalized effect of the postwar conditions, the revival of the "cult of domesticity"—that is, earlier marriages, more babies, larger family responsibilities, and the fashionable quest for family togetherness.

By 1948, nursing was considered as a social necessity and public responsibility, yet advances toward more professional preparation in the educational foundation for such responsibilities had apparently faltered. An important document released at this time was the report of the findings by a noted social anthropologist, Dr. Esther Lucille Brown. This report, *Nursing for the Future* (Brown, 1948), is cited as having provided the final impetus for the movement of nursing education from its dependence on the hospital training programs and into the educational mainstream. Mincing no words, Dr. Brown clearly states her expert opinion: "By no conceivable stretch of the imagination can the education provided in the vast majority of the some 1,250 schools be conceived of as professional education. In spite of improvements that have been made in most schools over the years, it remains apprenticeship training" (p. 48). That nursing education in the United States could still be labeled as an apprenticeship system in 1948 by this respected social anthropologist was cause for considerable reaction and grave concern. The tradition of apprenticeship had been seen as appropriate by its proponents as it was a system that provided, as Ashley (1975) states, a "method of education most suitable for instilling a strong faith in superiors, a desire to cooperate, and a tendency to think less of oneself and one's own needs" (p. 50).

Although the war impeded the direct progression of nursing education into the academic mainstream, it had a profound impact upon the nursing profession. First, nurses who joined the armed forces found themselves in vastly expanded nursing roles. Secondly, when these nurses returned to civilian life, the GI Bill opened educational opportunities to them; nurses returning from the war enrolled in programs of study leading to advanced degrees in a variety of academic fields. Experience in expanded nursing roles in the armed services coupled with advanced educational preparation equipped this cadre of nurses to make marked changes within the nursing profession. Development of associate degree programs, establishment of collegiate programs leading to the baccalaureate degree, encouragement of doctoral preparation for nurse faculty, building of nursing research, preparation of clinical specialists at the master's level, and the development of doctoral programs in nursing are some of the tangible evidences of these changes.

*Post–World War II Associate Degree Nursing Programs.* The baccalaureate nursing programs initiated in the 1920s were still in existence post–World War II, and although they were located in universities, they retained many characteristics of the training school. The development of associate degree nursing programs provided an option of a shorter educational program offered in the community college system. While some may argue that the development of associate degree nursing programs impeded the move of nursing education into the university, others will counter that it was only through opening up a new and shorter route into nursing that the quantity of nurses could be produced. It was clear at the start that associate degree programs were designed to prepare technical nurses; it was only later recognized that a second level of nurses, prepared at the baccalaureate level, was necessary for the health care delivery system.

While collegiate baccalaureate education had been advocated by the Goldmark report in 1923 and two levels of nursing education had been advocated by Esther Lucille Brown in 1948 and again by Eli Ginsberg in that same year, it was not until 1952 that experimentation with an alternate model was initiated. Louise McManus, Director of the Division of Nursing Education at Teachers College, Columbia University, "explained that the purpose of the experiment was to determine if a two-year program, which would prepare bedside nurses for beginning general duty positions was feasible. Such an approach would reduce the critical shortage of nurses throughout the nation by producing more nurses faster; it would also help move nursing education into the overall system of American Higher Education" (Kalisch and Kalisch, 1978, p. 594). Mildred Montag became the project director for this experimental project. With funding from the W. K. Kellogg Foundation, seven community junior colleges from all over the country were selected for the five-year research project to test this model. These programs were designed so that one-third of the curriculum was reserved for general education with the balance available for nursing courses; 75 percent of the latter were courses in clinical practice. The results of the five-year study showed that the two-year program could prepare a registered nurse and that this type of educational program could be financed as any other.

Associate degree programs were not a welcome addition to the nurse "training" scene from the perspective of the hospital-based diploma programs. Although graduates were able to compete successfully on state board examinations, they did not have the same type of apprenticeship training as the nursing students who had spent long hours in repetitive practice as part of their training. Despite the lack of popularity of associate degree programs in the minds of diploma nurse educators and hospital administrators, the associate degree program has gained wide popular appeal for students entering nursing. This low-cost degree as an entry step in the nursing education process has made the associate degree route exceedingly popular with prospective nursing students.

Despite its popularity with nursing students, leaders in the profession argue that the two-year program prepares a technical nurse. These leaders assert that two types of nurses are needed in health care delivery: the technical nurse, prepared at the associate degree level, and the professional nurse, prepared at the baccalaureate level. However, to date, there has been great difficulty in differentiating these levels of practice.

*Baccalaureate Nursing Education.* Nurse training schools organized under the auspices of university-owned hospitals, like those in other hospitals, bore little resemblance to collegiate educational programs. In 1909, Richard Olding Beard was influential in seeing that the training school at the University of Minnesota was organized as an integral part of the institution. By 1916, sixteen colleges and universities had some form of nursing education. It was only a matter of time until opportunities to complete baccalaureate degrees within these college and university settings would be available. In this mode the nurse completed the "training" program preparing her to become a nurse, and then enrolled in a general education program within the university to complete baccalaureate degree requirements. No nursing content was offered in the baccalaureate completion portion of the program. The Kalisches (1978) report that although by 1926, some twenty-four universities offered this type of an option, there were only 368 students enrolled.

Though only seven baccalaureate nursing programs had been established by 1935, the opposition to this development was formidable. As the Kalisches (1978) describe the situation, "Opposition came from many private physicians who argued that nurses were overtrained, that the service they gave was too costly, and that brief training in hospital routines would be just as satisfactory. A number of hospital training schools maintained that nursing education meant acquisition of technical skills and manual dexterity only. They believed that intelligence and sound knowledge of theory were unnecessary and might handicap the prospective nurses" (p. 340).

In the mid-thirties, student nurses were the primary source of staffing for hospitals. Graduate nurses were used only as head nurses and in supervisory positions; student nurses provided the bulk of direct patient care. Once graduated, these nurses either provided care within homes or served as private duty nurses to patients who were hospitalized. Graduate nurses began to be employed in hospitals as a result of the Depression. With the Depression, there was suddenly a surplus of nurses; patients could no longer afford to pay for the private duty nurse either at home or in the hospital. Graduate nurses did bedside nursing in exchange for room, board, and laundry. The graduate nurse thus became an employee of the hospital rather than an employee of the patient or the family—a change that has had marked impact on the development of the nursing profession to this day. With the coming of World War II, the graduate nurses went off to war, once more leaving the student nurse as the backbone of hospital nursing services. The diploma schools of nursing were given new life. Attention was directed away from the development of baccalaureate programs to the war effort; graduate nurses were needed in large numbers, and student nurses in the diploma schools of nursing were needed to man the hospitals. Baccalaureate nursing education was to gain momentum only after the war; return of nurses with a more independent view of nursing and opportunities for higher education under the GI Bill, to-

gether with the development of associate degree nursing programs, served to accelerate this trend.

Though the argument about how nurses were to be prepared had persisted
since the early 1900s, virtually no research is evident to support or refute any of the
rhetoric. Research during this period consisted of a number of studies related to
the pattern of nursing education per se. As part of the utilization studies, activity
analysis became a popular area of investigation. For example, Johns and Pfefferkorn (1954) reported that out of 251 activities identified, 130 were nonnursing or
household tasks. This served to reinforce the notion that professional education
was unnecessary. Sister Frank (1959), Dean of the Catholic University School of
Nursing, described the nurse of the past: "The nurse was strictly a 'do-it-yourself'
girl. Everything from housecleaning, personal hygienic measures, preparation
and serving of diets, to some genuinely therapeutic procedures, were performed by
the nurse. She was a hospital housewife in the true sense of the word, with little
nursing on the side" (p. 19). No wonder that the resistance to change, both inside
and outside of the profession, was so great. As Partridge (1981, p. 42) cogently
poses the issue, "Why should any service-oriented institution operate on a basic
educational program (in any field)? The answer is to benefit the institution, not to
benefit the student and not the patient." She further notes, "The move toward
academically based education, the baccalaureate in particular, is an overt effort to
change nursing into an autonomous independent, devoid of wifelike, handmaid-
en's role."

Movement of nurse training out of the control of hospitals and physicians
and into the academic mainstream required that nursing faculty be prepared as
faculty in other academic disciplines. "Making it" in the academic mainstream
became the primary agenda of a whole generation of nursing leaders. The first
step in this process was that of seeing that at least the leadership—dean, directors,
and department heads—were doctorally prepared. Secondly, doctoral preparation
for faculty teaching in graduate programs was deemed necessary. At initial stages
the doctoral degree became an end in and of itself; only recently has the research
productivity of the cadre of doctorally prepared faculty become of concern. While
becoming part of the academic mainstream was of importance in making the
transformation from training for a trade to education for a profession, the clinical
component of nursing education was de-emphasized. The initial focus of graduate
education was upon the preparation of teachers and managers of nursing. In the
late sixties and seventies, the development of clinical specialty programs at the
master's level was an indication of renewed interest and concern for the clinical
aspects of the nursing profession. The late seventies and early eighties carry this
concern for the dichotomization between nursing and practice further with
numerous experiments in development of unified or collaborative models between
educational program and service delivery.

*Doctoral Education.* The first doctoral program designed specifically for
nurses was developed at Teachers College, Columbia University, about 1920. The
degree offered was the Ed.D., and the focus of this program was on the preparation
of teachers and administrators for nursing. The first phase of doctoral education
for nurses is considered to have occurred in the period from 1926 to 1959. During
this time span, 132 nurses earned doctorates. Eighty of this number earned their
doctorates in the field of education (Matarazzo, 1971, p. 67). This is a reflection of

the history of nursing education in which it was assumed that the knowledge base for nursing was borrowed from other disciplines. As we have seen, early nursing school curricula consisted of a combination of medical lectures on various disease entities and lectures by nursing faculty about the ethical behavior of the nurse. Doctoral preparation in education was focused on the administration of educational content and the transmission of knowledge, rather than on the generation of a knowledge base through research. This emphasis continued through World War II.

That war, with large numbers of soldiers identified as having psychiatric problems, created a burgeoning interest in the need for trained psychiatric personnel to treat the psychiatrically disabled. Because of the key role of nurses in providing treatment, nurses became identified as members of the psychiatric treatment team. Federal provision of monies to support the training of psychiatric professionals was of key importance in stimulating graduate education in psychiatric nursing. The development of graduate psychiatric programs necessitated that there be faculty with some specialized knowledge in this field. Nurses in increasing numbers began to enter doctoral study in behavioral science fields relevant to psychiatric nursing, such as psychology, sociology, anthropology, and education. Doctoral education in these related fields was supported by National Institute of Mental Health traineeships. It is significant that the first cadre of nurses prepared at the doctoral level were predominantly from psychiatric nursing and that these nurses moved progressively into key leadership positions within the profession. The prominent role of psychiatric nurses accounts, in part, for the emphasis on psychosocial content in general nursing education. The emphasis is further evidenced by the development, in 1960 at Boston University, of the D.N.Sc., the first professional doctoral program in nursing with an emphasis on psychiatric nursing. Although psychiatric nursing had taken the lead, other areas of nursing were not far behind. Establishment of graduate programs in other fields followed on the heels of psychiatric nursing and was supported in later years by federal monies allocated for the support of nursing and nursing education.

The federal government has played a key role, via its funding mechanisms, in influencing the course of doctoral development in nursing. Perhaps most significantly, through predoctoral research fellowships and then through the nurse scientist programs, nurses were provided support and encouragement to enter doctoral study in scientific fields of relevance to nursing. Between 1953 and 1960, the U.S. Public Health Service supported 156 students directly for doctoral study through Division of Nursing fellowships. The second source of funding, the nurse scientist programs, provided grants awarded directly to schools of nursing to finance Ph.D.–level education in disciplines related to nursing. The intent underlying the nurse scientist program was that of building a critical mass of faculty for the development of doctoral programs in nursing. Cleland (1976) explains that, "When programs like this were first established and federally funded in 1963, they were provided in the related discipline. This was necessary at that time because of the prejudicial treatment of women, including nurses in those disciplines" (p. 631). In a sense, the nurse scientist programs were a means of "buying a way in" to basic science programs that previously had been closed to nurses. Cleland further spoke to a change in these attitudinal sets: "Women are considerably more welcome to academia today. . . . In fact, with the current uneasiness about too many people with doctorates, the qualified nurse application is especially attractive, because job placement in nursing is not a problem. In addition, nurses have proven themselves as able students who also possess easy access to the health care system for research purposes" (p. 632).

Nurses prepared in basic sciences related to nursing have brought substantive knowledge and the research methodologies of these scientific fields into nursing. The introduction of this scientific content and research methods has done much to broaden the knowledge base for all of nursing education and practice. From 1960 to 1969, 449 nurses earned doctorates. Of this number, 215 earned Ph.D. degrees. During this same period, 191 nurses earned Ed.Ds (American Nurses' Foundation, 1973).

With this cadre of doctorally prepared faculty, the focus of the 1970s was upon establishment of doctoral programs in nursing; sixteen such programs were established during the seventies. As these programs developed, considerable attention was focused upon the content of the research doctorate in nursing. These programs have been shaped by a faculty whose own doctoral preparation is in a variety of scientific disciplines; these diverse scientific backgrounds have been joined in a focus upon research into nursing problems. A typical depiction of the argument for doctoral education and a proposal for how these diverse scientific fields are joined in nursing is that presented by Grace at a national conference in doctoral education in 1978: "While nursing is not, in one sense, a new field, in relation to building a scientific knowledge base, it might be so considered. The emergence of scientific fields has traditionally occurred out of a merger of recognized discrete bodies of knowledge. Biochemistry, bioengineering, and social psychology are familiar examples. These new fields of knowledge have emerged from a recognition of gaps among prior existing bodies of knowledge. Likewise, doctoral programs in nursing have developed based on a recognition of such gaps in the scientific knowledge base."

As evidenced by the wide array of investigators studying problems related to health or illness care, it becomes obvious that each is viewing one aspect of the person's problem and no one is looking at the totality. The physician is interested in the disease problem itself: its etiology, symptomatology, and treatment. Physiologists, while not frequently found in the clinical arena, most logically are interested in physiological changes under disease conditions. Psychologists investigate the person's responses to the illness or certain psychological patterns associated with disease states, while a sociologist looks at such things as the incidence of particular diseases in varying cultural groups and under certain socioeconomic conditions. As all these scientists pursue their research interests, valuable knowledge is generated, but frequently this knowledge is never integrated in a way that has impact on the patient.

A nurse researcher, in contrast, is apt to focus on the patient as a whole in the context of his or her living environment. Taking the research findings from related scientific fields as to the nature of the disease process, its psychological effects upon the patient, psychological traits, and sociological contingencies, the nurse researcher investigates ways of altering the conditions surrounding the patient and tests out the effects of these alterations. The nurse's approach to research on patient care problems is a holistic approach that considers the person within a broader social and environmental context. Thus, emerging from other

**Table 1. Distribution by Field of Preparation of Doctorally Prepared Nurses.**

| Percent | 1927–1949 N = 24 | 1950–1959 N = 75 | 1960–1964 N = 142 | 1965–1969 N = 289 | 1970–1973 N = 124 | 1974–1979 N = 994 |
|---|---|---|---|---|---|---|
| 100 | | | | | | |
| 90 | | | | | | |
| 80 | | | | | | |
| 70 | Education 75% | Education 80% | Education 70% | Education 57% | Education 61% | Education 59% |
| 60 | | | | | | |
| 50 | | | | | | |
| 40 | | | | | | |
| 30 | | | | 25% Social Science | 21% Social Science | |
| 20 | 12.5% Social Science | | 16% Social Science | | | 18% Social Science |
| 10 | 12.5% Natural Science | 8% Social Science | 7% Nursing | 8% Nursing | 10% Nursing | 16% Nursing |
| 0 | | 7% Nursing Administration | 5% Related Fields | 6% Public Health | 5% Natural Science | 3% Natural Science |
| | | 4% Natural Science | 3% Natural Science | 3% Natural Science | 3% Public Health | 4% Public Health |

*Source:* American Nurses' Foundation, 1973 and American Nurses' Association, 1980, ANA Publication No. G-143 6 M 8/80.

bodies of knowledge, the nurse builds a body of knowledge that is uniquely nursing. By 1980, there were 2,348 doctorally prepared nurses (American Nurses' Foundation, 1980). Table 1 shows the diversity of educational preparation of the cadre of nurses over the time span from 1927 to 1979.

## Research

*Nursing Care.* While the struggle to achieve doctoral preparation for faculty has been a matter of prime concern in making the transition from training to education, the more important question facing nursing at this time relates to the research productivity of this faculty cadre in generating a knowledge base for the profession. In 1952, the National Committee for the Improvement of Nursing Service proposed that studies in nursing for the previous decade, 1942–1952, be surveyed. Later the scope of this survey was extended to include studies reported from 1870 to the 1960s (Simmons and Henderson, 1964).

A review of nursing research prior to 1900 indicates no reported studies by nurses other than Florence Nightingale and little or no research on nursing before the turn of the century. As Henderson (1964, p. 12) points out, "Young women with research potentialities who entered these early schools were caught up in the rush of service, and as they increasingly demonstrated their value to the patient, to the doctor, and to the hospital, they had less and less time for anything but service . . . This was a woman's occupation and the nurse of the period epitomized the Victorian female who left intellectual and most creative endeavors outside the home to the male." Following in this tradition, methods of patient care were designed by doctors and implemented by nurses. In contrast to medicine, the greatest monetary rewards were given nurses who became administrators and teachers; clinical nursing practice was low on the prestige and reward hierarchy. It is understandable then that the earliest reported studies were related to administration and teaching.

The rapid expansion of nursing schools in the early 1900s stimulated studies pertinent to the quality of educational programs and upgrading of patient care. While most studies focused upon the nurse rather than on nursing care, a few studies of nursing techniques were reported. Experimentation in temperature taking, cleaning thermometers, and hand washing are examples of these early studies.

The Depression of the late 1920s and early 1930s and the accompanying unemployment precipitated a number of fact-finding studies. As an outgrowth, it was recommended that graduate nurses be employed to provide direct patient care. Up to this point, graduate nurses had primarily served as teachers and administrators, with care of patients the domain of student nurses. This signaled the beginning of nurses' involvement in clinical studies through participation with physicians conducting such research.

Throughout the 1940s the most conspicuous investigations are surveys of nurse manpower, while in the early 1950s studies related to functions of the nurse and allied nursing personnel predominate. In most of these studies nurses collaborated with social scientists. As increasing numbers of nurses with preparation in a variety of basic science fields reentered nursing, the influence of their basic science training is evident in the research produced. Investigation into psychological factors influencing patient response to medical procedures, physiological reactions to stressful events and cultural influences on health-seeking behavior are examples of this influence.

*Nursing Education.* Nurses with doctoral preparation in education similarly accelerated the investigation into issues specific to nursing education. Although most doctorally prepared nurses have earned their degrees in the educational field, research into educational problems can, at best, be described as scanty. This can most probably be attributed to the administrative leadership role this cadre of nurses has been called upon to assume in making the transition from nurse training to nurse education. In recent years, as research has accelerated generally, the investigation of educational problems in nursing has gradually increased.

In the late 1960s, with funding from the W. K. Kellogg Foundation, a commission was appointed to conduct a major study, sponsored by the American Nurses' Association and the National League for Nursing, of the system of nursing education (Lysaught, 1970). Known as the Lysaught report, three basic priorities were identified: (1) the need for increased research into nursing practice and nursing education, (2) the development of enhanced educational systems and curricula based upon the findings, and (3) increased financial support for nursing and nursing education to increase career opportunity.

The Commission on Nursing Research in 1975 identified the following priorities in educational research: (1) studies of manpower, (2) criterion measures for education, (3) the history and philosophy of nursing, (4) cost effectiveness of nursing utilization and preparation in relation to various levels of care, and (5) studies of nursing curricula (American Nurses' Association, Commission on Nursing Research, 1975). In summarizing educational research in nursing, Hill and others (1980) have categorized studies in five major categories: (1) program structure, (2) curriculum, (3) faculty, (4) learners, and (5) educational outcomes.

Because over 80 percent of the practicing nurses hold either a diploma certificate or an associate degree and lack baccalaureate preparation, the issue of educational mobility is an area of considerable concern. As a result, competency evaluation and program articulation have received some study. The National League for Nursing, for example, was influential in its sponsorship of study of an open curriculum approach (Johnson, 1971).

Curriculum development or modification was the primary focus of over one-third of the federally funded special project grants between 1968 and 1975. Of special concern was the move away from a disease-oriented curriculum to one focused upon health. This is indicative of the move toward professionalization and the differentiation of nursing from medicine. Despite the interest in curricular reform, there is little evidence regarding the long-range impact of these forms of curricular change on the graduate nurse. In keeping with the concerns of educational mobility, several studies reporting the use of alternative instructional methodologies are reported. These include studies related to use of videotapes, learning modules, programmed instruction, simulation, and computer-assisted instruction (Hill and others, 1980). While investigations of alternate instructional methodologies are described, little research is reported that compares methodologies and their effectiveness. An exception is the well-designed study of Huckaby (1981) in which she compares the effects of modularized instruction and traditional teaching techniques on cognitive learning and affective behavior of student nurses. She reports that a combination of independent study and lecture-discussion is more effective than either methodology used separately.

Research on faculty has been concerned primarily with the faculty member as a role model for nursing students. Research on students has centered around studies of student characteristics. These are commonly reported to include altruism, preference for helping people, social, ethical, and religious values, femininity, and personal satisfaction (Muhlenkamp and Parsons, 1972). However, this topic of research has recently dropped out of vogue and since the studies do not extend beyond 1970, it may be assumed that, given the impact of the women's movement, characteristics of nursing students may be somewhat altered.

As for educational outcomes, considerable current research centers around attempting to differentiate characteristics of graduates from varying types of educational programs. In summarizing studies in this area, Sikes (1982) notes, "Nursing today as an organized entity is struggling in an attempt to settle the controversy over what educational preparation constitutes entry into professional practice. Many assertions are made in the nursing literature that differences exist in the preparation of the ADN, BSN, and diploma graduate. However, research findings, to date, have failed to provide valid evidence of significant differences in cognitive performance of nurses from different educational programs. The research that does exist is either limited in geographical scope, has low or unknown validity, has small samples, is published in dissertation abstracts only or offers conflicting evidence.''

Research on educational issues in nursing is similar to other areas of nursing research; though many studies are reported, there is little evidence that systematic areas of research have developed within the field. Rather the approach has been a scattered one, despite the many areas of theoretical interest that have implications far beyond the field of nursing. To date, changes in nursing education have been based primarily upon philosophical argument, with little documentation of the impact of these changes on programs, students, or the health care delivery system. This constitutes a major handicap in that the arguments for change ultimately become political, rather than scientific ones buttressed by a sound base of knowledge.

### Realignments Between Nursing Education and Practice

In its efforts to move from training to education, nursing has engaged in a valiant struggle to secure for itself a place in institutions of higher education. In so doing, primary concerns have been for obtaining control over the education of nursing students, for achieving—through doctoral preparation of nursing faculty—recognition within the university as legitimate, and for developing a conceptual approach to the definition of the discipline of nursing that provides structure for educational programs. In many ways, these concerns relate to the form of nursing education rather than to its substance. But without the achievement of its place within the educational system, nursing would never have gained the degree of autonomy necessary to address the substantive issues related to the generation of knowledge on which the teaching and practice of nursing ultimately rests.

The primary issue facing nursing today is that of developing a rapprochement between nursing education and practice. Nursing education is viewed by the practitioners of nursing as being in an ivory tower, far removed from the day-to-day demands of nursing practice. Conversely, nursing practice is viewed by nursing educators as outmoded, controlled by physicians, and falling short of professional standards. While much attention within this chapter has been focused upon conflicts between nursing and those outside of the field, perhaps the most pervasive element in this whole historical saga is that of divisions within nursing itself, and between those who would view nursing as a profession and those who see it in the position of physician handmaiden. Like the current women's movement in which some argue for equal rights while others prefer a more dependent and therefore less responsible role, the nursing profession disagrees on a wide range of basic issues. With the nursing educators being on the side of greater independence and autonomy and many in the practice setting not wishing to be disturbed, the strains between factions often surface.

Given this situation, a major current theme concerns the ways in which the service-education gap in nursing might be bridged. Unification between nursing education and nursing practice is a topic of national concern, as evidenced by recent nursing publications. Some argue that nursing education and nursing practice should be organized under one leadership, with the dean of nursing also being the director of nursing service within university-affiliated hospitals. In these models, it is argued, that nursing faculty become the practitioners of nursing, and the student no longer needs to isolate the educational experience from the world of practice. However, such a unified model carries the implicit risks that faculty who also have practice responsibilities will be overloaded, that the educational needs of students will take second place to the patient care demands, that the educational model will be focused on acute care settings and disease rather than on a broader view of nursing as related to health and health promotion, and that organizational charts indicating a unified structure will not work out that way in reality. Further, in such a system, nursing administrators see themselves as being taken over and controlled by nursing educators.

Others propose the development of collaborative, or semiunified models. Case Western Reserve is the oldest example of such a model. There the merger occurs where department heads are responsible both for nursing services within their clinical area and for the educational program within the academic structure. A director of nursing has overall responsibility for the nursing service activities of the hospital, while the dean of the College of Nursing has responsibility for academic programs. Joined through a complex committee structure, linkages are built throughout between practice system and educational system.

At the University of Illinois, work has been focused upon the development of a collaborative model that will develop an interface between the department of nursing in University Hospital and the College of Nursing (Grace, 1981). Using a process approach, projects of mutual interest have been stimulated. As these projects are developed, the structural and governance issues are identified and addressed. For example, continuing education in the college, staff development for nurses in the hospital, patient education, and professional development for faculty were identified as a cluster of activities of common interest. A consolidated structure in the form of an Office of Continuing Learning and Professional Development has been established, which brings resources of the hospital and the college together into a common structural unit. As cohesiveness has developed between the members of the Nursing Council (that is, the representatives of nursing education and nursing practice), attention has been turned to the creation of joint education-practice roles, the participation of clinical specialists in the teaching programs of the college, and the initiation of jointly sponsored clinical research projects. Established as an experimental unit, the development of this unit and its productivity are being carefully researched.

While most of the current "unification" models are specific to settings in which there is a university hospital, most clinical practicum experience of nursing students takes place outside the university structure. The clinical instructor who accompanies students as they go to a wide range of affiliated hospitals for their clinical experiences is commonly assigned the role of "guest in the house." To deal with this situation, the University of Illinois is building a collaborative model with the Evanston Hospital Corporation. In this model the Evanston Hospital Corporation has agreed to close its diploma school of nursing in exchange for becoming a clinical teaching site for the nursing programs at the University of Illinois. Under terms of this agreement, a significant number of nursing students, generic baccalaureate, R.N. completion, and graduate students will be placed in this quality clinical facility for their clinical practicum experience. Nurses of the Evanston Hospital Corporation who meet criteria for faculty appointment at the University of Illinois will be given joint appointments of varying percentages of time, based upon their responsibilities. In their faculty capacity, they will function as clinical specialists within the hospital system but will also share in the teaching of nursing students. The open-curricular methodology developed at the Evanston Hospital Corporation is a national model and will be applied to the baccalaureate curriculum of the University of Illinois College of Nursing. A Learning Resource Laboratory at the Evanston site will be used to make mediated instruction available to students. Students who have chosen Evanston as their primary clinical site will have the opportunity of self-pacing through portions of the baccalaureate curriculum while participating with other students of the College of Nursing in specifically designed learning activities. This combination of resources makes possible a more flexible approach to nursing education. Extensive research comparing outcomes of this experimental program with the more traditional programs of the College of Nursing should provide data that will lead to further program innovation. It is hoped that as more flexible approaches to delivery of instruction are achieved, these models may be used to enrich regional approaches in addressing issues of maldistribution and to provide valuable insights into new ways of linking the educational system to practice settings.

## Challenges of the Future

*Nursing Research.* For nursing to become a profession in its own right, it must develop a data base to underpin both nursing education and practice. Unlike medicine, which has incorporated basic scientists into the structure of medical research and education, nursing is instead developing its own cadre of nurse researchers. This is necessary to achieve a focus upon nursing and its distinct domain of concern. Medicine's focus in research has been primarily upon disease and its treatment; basic scientists and their focal areas can readily be incorporated into this domain of investigation. In contrast, nursing has as its focus the promotion and maintenance of health and the patient's (individual and social network) response to disease. The nursing role is that of influencing this process. Knowledge needed for the practice of nursing is an amalgam drawn from biological and behavioral scientists, applied and tested in the nursing care of patients.

The development of doctoral programs in nursing has been critical in preparing a cadre of nurse investigators who are progressively mapping out the domain of nursing knowledge. The focus of nursing research has changed dramatically as evidenced by the areas of investigation of doctoral research over the last ten years (Table 2). The challenge to nursing research is to organize and build the domains of nursing knowledge that will constitute a solid base for education and practice.

*Nursing Education.* In the early stages of nursing education, content was limited primarily to the communication (usually by physicians) of basic knowledge of diseases and their treatment, plus a code of proper behavior. More recently, emphasis has been placed on the scientific base, both biological and behavioral, for the practice of nursing. The assumption has been that the nurse must have a

**Table 2. Research Conducted by Doctoral Students in Nursing Doctoral Programs, 1972–1982.**

| Research Study Category | Number | Percentage |
|---|---|---|
| Clinical Research on Problems Related to Nursing Care | 413 | 65 |
| Model and Theory Development (Instrument Development) | 30 | 5 |
| Organization of Patient Care | 18 | 3 |
| Studies of Nurses | 55 | 9 |
| Health Economics | 2 | .03 |
| Health Manpower and Educational Studies | 94 | 13 |
| Ethical Studies | 9 | 1 |
| Historical Studies | 18 | 3 |
| | 639 | 99.03 |

scientific knowledge base, but little attention has been given to the question of how this knowledge is applied in the nursing care of patients. For example, it is extremely important that the nurse have an understanding of the biochemical base for fluid and electrolyte balance in adjusting the flow of intravenous fluids into patients. At a different stage of the health/illness process, it is of equal importance that nurses be able to incorporate this knowledge in patient teaching, so that patients may ultimately assume some responsibility for their own self-care. In short, the challenge of nursing education is that of incorporating the scientific knowledge base into programs of patient care directed toward patient understanding and responsibility for participation in the care process. To achieve this end, the rigorous scientific base of nursing education must be maintained but balanced with equal attention to the application of this knowledge in the clinical practice of nursing.

*Nursing Practice.* Practice and education cannot stand as separate entities; nursing research and education must be solidly rooted in clinical practice settings. Traditionally, nursing practice in hospital settings has been structured on a bureaucratic model. Hierarchical decision making and extensive rules and regulations (as evidenced in policy and procedure manuals) are indices of this bureaucratic model. Movement to a professional model of participatory decision making, with responsibility and authority vested in the professional nurse, presents a challenge and, in many instances, a threat to nurse administrators, particularly those who are firmly entrenched as a part of hospital administration. Clearly, the professionalization of nurses poses a threat to the traditional forms of control, as outlined in the tortuous history of nursing. However, this professionalization is essential if the full potential of nursing in health care delivery is to be realized.

## Summary

Nursing education has struggled for the past 100 years to move from nurse "training" to nurse "education" as part of the process of becoming a profession. Entangled with broader issues of women in society, each time advances have been made or proposed for the educational system, diverse societal forces have intervened to make advance difficult, if not impossible. Fears of overeducation of women, as well as women's ambivalence about professional and family role obligations, have held back progress. Nurse shortages throughout the history of nursing have always occurred when nursing is just on the brink of making a significant breakthrough. World War II and the need for nurses for the war intervened, just as nursing was moving toward baccalaureate nursing education. When the wartime nurses returned, they did not return to practice in hospitals but rather went into the universities to attain a higher level of education. Others, caught up with the predominant societal value system of the family and traditional women's roles, withdrew from nursing. As nursing was once more on the brink of achieving agreement on educational preparation and levels of practice, nurse shortage became a predominant national concern.

To secure a place within the academic mainstream, nurses have had to place emphasis upon attaining the credential required of university faculty—the doctoral degree. As large numbers of nurses have become doctorally prepared, they have been diverted in many instances from the clinical settings in which nursing is practiced. Additionally, since the emphasis has been first upon doctoral preparation of administrators for both education and practice, the research productivity of the small numbers of doctorally prepared faculty has not been as great as might be desired. As greater numbers of nursing faculty are now doctorally prepared, it is anticipated that research productivity will increase.

While educational innovation has been a consistent theme throughout nursing history, little research documenting the impact of educational changes has been reported. Building a data base to validate the impact of change is a crucial challenge facing the profession. Additionally, achieving renewed linkage between nursing education and practice is essential, if long-range changes within the system are to occur. If nursing is to upgrade the educational system so that the baccalaureate degree is required for entrance into professional nursing practice, nursing educators, nursing administrators, nursing faculty, and nurses in practice must develop a united view of the profession and of its future direction. If this is not attained, nurse shortage, and the political pressures that are adjunctive, will once more pull the educational system downward and history will once more repeat itself.

## References

American Nurses' Association, Commission on Nursing Research. *Position Paper: Statement on Nursing Research*. Kansas City, Mo.: American Nurses' Association, 1975.

American Nurses' Foundation. *International Directory of Nurses with Doctoral Degrees*. Kansas City, Mo.: American Nurses' Foundation, 1973.

American Nurses' Foundation. *Directory of Nurses with Doctoral Degrees*. Kansas City, Mo.: American Nurses' Foundation, 1980.

Ashley, J. *Hospitals, Paternalism, and the Role of the Nurse*. New York: Teachers College Press, 1975.

Bailyn, L. "Notes on the Role of Choice in the Psychology of Professional Women." *Daedalus*, 1964, *93* (2), 708.

Brown, E. L. *Nursing for the Future*. New York: Russell Sage Foundation, 1948.

Burgess, M. A. *Nurses, Patients, and Pocketbooks.* New York: National League for Nurses Committee on the Grading of Nursing Schools, 1928.

Cleland, V. "Developing a Doctoral Program." *Nursing Outlook,* 1976, *24* (19), 631–632.

Dock, L. L. *A Short History of Nursing: From the Earliest Time to the Present Day.* New York: Putnam's, 1920.

Frank, C. M. "The Professional Nurse—Yesterday, Today, and Tomorrow." *Nursing World,* 1959, *133* (3), 26–32.

Goldmark, J. *Nursing and Nursing Education in the United States: Report of the Commission for the Study of Nursing Education.* New York: Macmillan, 1923.

Goostray, S. *Address of the President: Forty-Ninth Annual Report.* New York: National League of Nursing Education, 1943.

Grace, H. "The Research Doctorate in Nursing." Paper presented at Second National Conference on Doctoral Education in Nursing, Rush University, 1978.

Grace, H. "Unification, Reunification, Reconciliation, or Collaboration: Bridging the Education-Service Gap." In J. McClosky and H. Grace (Eds.), *Current Issues in Nursing.* Boston: Blackwell Scientific Publications, 1981.

Henderson, V. "Development of Research in Nursing." In L. Simmons and V. Henderson, *Nursing Research: A Survey and Assessment.* New York: Appleton-Century-Crofts, 1964.

Hill, M. S., and others. "Educational Research in Nursing." *International Nursing Review,* 1980, *27* (1), 10.

Huckaby, L. "The Effects of Modularized Instruction on Cognitive Learning and Affective Behavior of Student Nurse." *Advances in Nursing Science,* 1981, *3* (3), 67–83.

Hughes, E. A. "Professions." *Daedalus,* 1963, *92* (4), 656–662.

Johns, E., and Pfefferkorn, B. *The Hopkins School of Nursing, 1889–1949.* Baltimore, Md.: Johns Hopkins University Press, 1954.

Johnson, W. L. "Status of the Open Curriculum in Nursing." *Nursing Outlook,* 1971, *29* (10), 656–664.

Kalisch, P. A., and Kalisch, B. J. *The Advance of American Nursing.* Boston: Little, Brown, 1978.

Lysaught, J. *Abstract for Action: National Commission for the Study of Nursing and Nursing Education.* New York: McGraw-Hill, 1970.

Matarazzo, J. *Perspective in Future Directions for Doctoral Education.* Report of conference held at Bethesda, Md., Jan. 20, 1971. U.S. Department of Health, Education, and Welfare Publication no. (NIH) 72–82. Washington, D.C.: U.S. Government Printing Office, 1971.

Means, J. H. "Homo Medicaus Americanus." *Daedalus,* 1963, *92* (4), 720–721.

Muhlenkamp, A., and Parsons, J. D. "Characteristics of Nurses: An Overview of Recent Research Published in a Nursing Research Periodical." *Journal of Vocational Behavior,* 1972, *2,* 261–273.

National Commission on Nursing. *Summary of the Public Hearings.* Chicago: American Hospital Association, 1981.

Partridge, R. "Education for Entry into Professional Nursing Practice." *Journal of Nursing Education,* 1981, *20* (4), 42.

Sikes, M. "Effects of Formal Education on Cognitive Skills of Nurses." Unpublished doctoral dissertation, University of Chicago, Department of Education, 1982.

Simmons, L., and Henderson, V. *Nursing Research: A Survey and Assessment.* New York: Appleton-Century-Crofts, 1964.

Whitehouse, W. N. "A Challenge to Nursing." *American Journal of Nursing,* 1941, *41,* 800.

*Charles W. Ford*　　　　　　　　　　　　　　6

# Allied Health

Allied health is both a concept and a term that reflects more diversity than singularity. For some, the term connotes an alliance of persons and professions joining together to support patients and professionals. For others, the term is an anathema, cloaking the identity of practitioners in a set too encompassing to have any significance.

Allied health personnel presently number between two and three million. The precise figure depends on which occupations are included. Does the term *allied health* apply to some 200 health occupations listed in the occupational index, or does it apply only to persons who have access to practice through certification, licensure, or registry? The answer is, of course, in qualifiers such as allied health occupations. An early definition found in federal legislation (Title VII, Section 795 of the Public Service Act) has been used in the past decade: "The term *allied health personnel* means individuals with training and responsibilities for (a) supporting, complementing, or supplementing the professional functions of physicians, dentists, and other health professionals in the delivery of health care to patients, or (b) assisting environmental health control and preventive medicine activities."

This definition has been annoying to those in allied health for two reasons: It uses the term *personnel* rather than *professional*, and it suggests that allied health practitioners always work under the supervision of another person. An attempt to overcome these objections is found in Senate Bill 2375, which proposed to amend Section 795 as follows: "The term *allied health personnel* means individuals trained at the associate, baccalaureate, master's, or doctoral degree level in a health care related science, with responsibility for the delivery of health care or health care related services (including services related to the identification, evaluation and prevention of diseases and disorders, dietary and nutrition services,

113

health promotion, rehabilitation, and health systems management), but who, for the purposes of this title, are not graduates of schools of medicine, osteopathy, dentistry, veterinary medicine, optometry, podiatry, pharmacy, or nursing."

The National Commission on Allied Health Education (1980, p. 14) endorsed the following definition of *allied health personnel*: "All health personnel working toward the common goal of providing the best possible services in patient care and health promotion." In this chapter *allied health* is used as a generic synonym for other terms readers may find more acceptable, such as health sciences or associated medical/dental sciences.

## Manpower Training

For the public at large, care in a health institution is often portrayed as being delivered by the doctor and the nurse. Present estimates are that there are fifteen allied health personnel for every physician, a marked change since the turn of the century when the ratio was three to one. Though the dramatic increase has come to an end, the ratio will continue to change. Regardless of the status of physician manpower, ongoing technological development will demand new or expanded allied health professions—both in medicine and dentistry.

Specialization of service requires specialized manpower. For the array of persons under the rubric of allied health, the needs were first evident in health care settings. Thus, as in most professions, educational needs were first established at the site of the delivery services, in this case health care institutions; training was on the job. Training requirements were dictated by the service needs of local facilities, not by established standards. These on-the-job training programs eventually became formalized, leading to the establishment of occupations and professions with national standards and organizations, including licensure, certification, and/or registration requirements.

The transition from on-the-job training to training in formal institutions of higher education has been a phenomenon of the last two decades. The rapid growth in both programs and graduates has resulted from the establishment of certificate, associate degree, and baccalaureate degree programs in educational settings. Despite the increased number of such programs, health care institutions continue to be a major training site. Over half of the nearly 3,000 programs listed in the 1980 *Allied Health Education Directory* were in health care institutions (American Medical Association, 1980). From this, one might incorrectly assume that health care institutions are responsible for the majority of programs. However, based on a combination of survey results and conjectures, the National Commission on Allied Health Education (1980) determined that there are approximately 14,000 allied health programs with 52-56 percent of the programs housed in collegiate settings, 33-35 percent in health care institutions, and the remainder in other settings.

On-the-job training programs in health care institutions were started to meet local needs. The size of the average hospital is presently less than 100 beds. Hospitals of this size are not in large metropolitan centers where a variety of options is available, so local needs continue to be a factor in the site of programs. In contrast, the majority of university health sciences centers are in metropolitan areas. For many leaders addressing manpower needs in the sixties and the seventies, the health sciences center appeared to be the ideal location for housing the majority of allied health programs. In fact, most of the early programs were established in medical schools; by 1940, 60 percent of medical schools had established allied health programs.

The ideal of learning together and working together was promulgated by a number of persons. Perry (1968), an early leader in allied health education, addresses the issue in numerous publications: "Through coordination and communication among these allied health professions there will be maximum benefits in curriculum development, faculty enrichment, combined research efforts, and student recognition of mutual respect for all other health professions" (p. 1116). Various models of organizations were developed ranging from separate colleges of allied health to divisions within colleges of medicine. Rosenfeld (1972) provides one of the first comprehensive views of the variety of organizational designs for allied health education, and King and Dietrich (1980) examine the bureaucratic, collegial, and political models in the context of allied health structures. They relate these models to organizational maturation in accord with predictions from contemporary management theory. They also relate the past to some projected needs of the eighties.

As manpower needs increased, some health sciences centers incorporated programs varying from certificate to graduate degrees. Others concentrated on upper-division programs. Four-year institutions that were not part of health sciences centers also initiated programs. While clinical facilities were a necessary part of the centers, four-year institutions had to look to the community for clinical instruction. Similarly, two-year community colleges responded to changing societal needs; currently the largest segment of allied health students resides in these institutions.

The great expansion in the number of programs and of graduates that occurred in the seventies has placed a heavy burden on clinical facilities. The competition for space is acute in some geographic areas. Need forced educators to examine alternative ways of providing instruction, such as simulation laboratories and coordination of clinical sites. Problems in the delivery of educational programs were also associated with problems in the integration of education and practice that required the development of new models.

As a result of a two-year study of clinical education, Ford (1978) focused on the major generic issues as they unfolded and developed. At about the same time, others conducted a study examining both the general issues of clinical instruction and their specific application in physical therapy (Moore and Perry, 1976). Supported by a grant from the Robert Wood Johnson Foundation to the American Association of Community and Junior Colleges, Hawthorne and Perry (1974) examined community colleges and primary health care. Extant efforts in other areas of clinical education include limited research on costs (Moore, Perry, and Clark, 1976). Blayney (1977, p. 1115) laments that "it seems ironic that in the past decade so much effort and money have been expended on increasing the quality of on-campus education, while very little attention has been paid to comparable improvements of clinical education."

Manpower training faces a dilemma in the eighties caused by the unprecedented expansion in the seventies. What are the new priorities as fiscal constraints become a way of life in both health care and academic institutions?

Indications are that allied health programs in health sciences centers are the most expensive to operate and often subject to the political pressures that exist within the hierarchy of the health professions. Indeed, the first closings of schools and divisions of allied health have been in health sciences centers. Allied health programs in four-year institutions have become main-line programs, particularly in four-year institutions that have comprehensive offerings. Prestige of the allied health programs is generally high in such institutions; thus these programs are less vulnerable to reduction or elimination. Though a few two-year colleges, both public and private, are suffering retrenchments in programs, including those in allied health, the number of programs in two-year colleges is still increasing nationwide.

Programs in all types of institutions were started with a sense of urgency and in response to perceived needs; now that the immediate needs have been met and jobs are less available than they once were, new problems are emerging. Addleman (1981), recent president of the American Society of Allied Health Professions, addresses the changing nature of federal largess in his remarks to the Association of Academic Health Centers:

> Allied health schools in two-year and four-year institutions seem, generally, to be faring very well in these hard times. The great majority of these institutions have not hitched their wagons to the star of federal generosity and now, as the glitter of that star fades, they are less anxious than others of us in the higher education community about the lean years ahead.
>
> I wish I could say the same for those of our schools in academic health centers. I can't. Schools of Allied Health for some years now have accustomed themselves to surviving without federal capitation funding. Other schools in academic health centers, on the other hand, have been the fortunate beneficiaries of capitation funding. Now that that's changing, what we're beginning to see develop in a number of academic health centers is the situation where Schools of Allied Health are being looked to as the principal locus of funding reductions made necessary by the loss, in other schools, of capitation funding.

Nonetheless, other sites for programs continue to develop. For example, in the private sector, short-term vocational training in the health occupations has continued to expand. Similarly, the armed services have enlarged their offerings and have established more formalized programs. While generalizations are risky, one is safe: The period of rapid growth is over. Growth will continue, but in a slow, undulating way and with a careful delineation and determination of needs, in contrast to the seventies in which programs were often started without extensive long-term planning. One dean expressed it candidly, "I thought it would be a good program to have—particularly before State started one." The growth mentality did not just happen; it was a creature of need coupled with the strong input of national policy as evidenced by federal legislation.

### Development of Allied Health Education

*Impact of National Legislation.* Though the origin of the term *allied health* is not clear, its widespread use is a direct result of the definition arising from federal legislation. St. Louis University first added an X-ray technician program to the School of Nursing in 1929. A School of Allied Medical Professions at the University of Pennsylvania, now closed, was established in 1950. A College of Health Related Professions was established at the University of Florida in 1957 (McTernan, 1972).'Nevertheless, credit for first using the term *allied health* for a freestanding unit should be given to Indiana University, which in the fifties established a Division of Allied Health Science as a part of the School of Medicine (National Commission on Allied Health Education, 1980).

In 1966, the Allied Health Personnel Training Act (P.L. 89–751) was passed by Congress. This legislation was a result of several federal studies and conferences. For example, in 1966 the National Conference on Health Manpower identified four issues with legislative implications: "(1) The unemployed and underdeveloped constitute a potential source of manpower for entry jobs in the health service industry; (2) training programs for health and related service workers must be expanded; (3) research and demonstration programs in the health occupations are needed; and (4) federal resources for training and related manpower programs need to be utilized more extensively for programs in the health fields" (Hatch and Kress, 1972, p. 121).

The 1966 report of the Allied Health Professions Education Subcommittee of the National Advisory Health Council was published approximately six months after the enactment of the 1966 legislation, but it serves to indicate the thinking of the time: "Needs in medicine, dentistry, and nursing have received major attention for a number of years, and fairly well-defined goals for educational progress and expansion had been established. But with a few exceptions relatively little attention has been given to the needs and the education potential for the many allied health occupations which are essential to modern health services. There are now major unmet needs for health manpower. Indeed, the lack of adequate health manpower is a most serious problem as we aspire to bring the full potential of modern medicine to all members of our society" (Hatch and Kress, 1972, pp. 121–122).

The Bureau of Health Manpower was created within the Public Health Service in 1966. Its prime activities were directed toward increasing health manpower. As a result of several organizational changes occurring in the latter sixties, the Division of Allied Health Manpower was established within the bureau to implement legislation.

In order to improve the educational opportunities available in programs preparing allied health personnel, Congress approved funds in five major areas. In the first area, funds were authorized for the construction of teaching facilities, the purchase of equipment, and the payment of salaries. A second area of funding was for the improvement of allied health programs that existed in a setting along with other programs. The third and fourth areas of funding were for specific projects, such as curriculum studies encompassing self-paced instruction, laddered program design, minority enrollment, core curriculum, competency-based education, and clinical education. The last category of monies appropriated by Congress was to support trainees in allied health education. Both administrators and faculty in allied health education were eligible for traineeships to offset tuition. Stipends were provided for graduate students and certain upper division students. The ability of institutions to furnish stipends during this period assured a pool of qualified students (Burnett, 1972; Task Force on Allied Health Clinical Education, 1974; U.S. Department of Health, Education, and Welfare, 1975). Although the funding for this legislation never exceeded $36,000,000 in any single year (*Health Planning and Manpower Report,* 1981), its impact at the time was significant. Yet, in retrospect, follow-up research has been sporadic and inconclusive. The use of allied health personnel in an interdisciplinary health care team has been attempted in a variety of settings. Yet Ducanis and Golin (1979, p. i) report that the team approach "has generated more rhetoric than research and an adequate theory of team has yet to be formulated." In many instances federal monies were supplemented by grants from private foundations, most notably the W. K. Kellogg Foundation. Kellogg encouraged a variety of experimental projects, especially in the area of institutional development of instructional personnel (Kellogg Foundation, 1977). Kellogg has continued support of allied health education through the American Society of Allied Health Professions. In the seventies, it funded the National Commission on Allied Health Education and the National Conference on Continuing Education in Allied Health. In 1981, it funded a three-year project to establish a National Center for Allied Health Leadership to disseminate and implement recommendations of the National Commission on Allied Health Education.

Some allied health leaders now support selective funding if new legislation is forthcoming. These leaders believe that it will be better to support allied health programs in institutions that have stability and proven track records in contrast with the "something for everyone" policy. Study of previous efforts could provide a basis for this decision, an area of research that has been largely untapped. This is not to say that no data are available or no examination of efforts has occurred. In the Health Manpower Act of 1968, the legislation included a requirement that the secretary of Health, Education, and Welfare submit a report to the president and Congress. The report, submitted by Secretary Harris in April 1969, summarizes the effects of the earlier legislation. Statistical information together with observations concerning the development of allied health educational programs was provided. The report concludes with nineteen recommendations, directed to support of the national policy for major health objectives and strategies in the following areas (U.S. Department of Health, Education, and Welfare, 1969):

- Health care cost containment
- Patient safety and effectiveness of health care through assurance of the competency of personnel
- Better capabilities for health planning
- Improved opportunities for minorities
- Equality of access to health services
- Career opportunities for veterans
- Efficient use of educational resources

These recommendations were for the seventies; while the first three are likely to be reemphasized in the eighties, it is uncertain whether the last four will continue to receive federal attention. However, one thing is certain: The legislation of the sixties was successful in stimulating a rapid growth in the number of allied health education programs from 2,500 in 1966 to more than 8,000 in 1980 (American Society of Allied Health Professions, 1980a).

*American Society of Allied Health Professions.* The American Society of Allied Health Professions (ASAHP) was founded in 1967 to create a "national voice for the allied health professions." This society, originally named the Association of Schools of Allied Health Professions, was formed as a result of thirteen representatives joining together to sponsor an interdisciplinary and interagency approach to allied health education. Although ASAHP projects do change with time, early in its history nine areas needing attention were identified (Gertz, 1972):

- determination of needs and priorities
- development and continuance of quality programs
- recruitment and retention of qualified students
- recruitment and retention of qualified faculty
- programs of continuing education
- career mobility and testing
- career mobility for those with military experience
- physician assistant programs
- research

While the list has changed somewhat since 1967, most of the areas are still relevant.

As an organization committed to interdisciplinary education, ASAHP has attempted to serve as an umbrella agency for the many allied health professions. Although the society was founded in the belief that those who practice together should both plan and be educated together, its success has been jeopardized by the reality of "professional turf." Practitioners' allegiances and efforts are normally directed first to their practice and secondarily to their profession, leaving little motivation or time to devote to interdisciplinary efforts, even when interest exists. As a result of these and other factors, the society has not been totally successful in attracting all the major associations that speak for the various allied health professions or their rank-and-file practitioners.

ASAHP has, however, been successful as a marketplace for exchange of ideas among certain types of institutions involved in educational programs. Specifically, most of the major colleges and universities offering allied health programs have been active in the society, but two-year colleges and hospitals—institutions that were noted earlier as accounting for the largest number of programs—have been noticeably absent. This may not be surprising, since it was deans who organized the society and after a decade of searching for a constituency, it still remains, in effect, a "dean's club." Curtailment of travel, rising membership costs to institutions, and competition with other organizations for membership hinder the umbrella function that the organization had hoped to realize. In response to these concerns, the society modified its organizational structure in 1981. These changes, along with those in membership standards, may make ASAHP more appealing to a larger segment of allied health professions personnel.

Despite its limited membership, the society does function as a national voice on issues affecting interdisciplinary efforts in allied health. It serves as a focal point for discussion of educational issues, funding concerns, and leadership issues. One of its first acts was to establish the *Journal of Allied Health,* dedicated to multidisciplinary efforts. The *Journal* has become the national forum for reporting on curriculum and research projects that are multidisciplinary or interdisciplinary in nature and on experimental curricula tested in colleges and health care settings. Areas such as continuing education, accreditation, and core curriculum are other prominent *Journal* themes, while research on clinical practice is usually reported in specialty journals that cater to their own individual constituencies.

ASAHP's national conferences have also provided a forum for consideration of issues that cut across many professions such as continuing education (American Society of Allied Health Professions, 1980b) and accreditation (American Society of Allied Health Professions, 1980c). These conferences have been successful in bringing together persons concerned with multidisciplinary efforts as well as those representing single disciplines. Specialized projects launched by the society or other groups can be traced to these national forums. For example, the efforts to establish a center for continuing education in allied health arose from one of these conferences.

Training workshops, a major activity of ASAHP provide a mechanism to reach instructors, administrators, and practitioners. Workshops in teacher preparation, administrative skills, leadership training, publishing, and faculty development are examples of programs the society has sponsored, largely through federal support. Most of the training efforts relate to educational programs. In the view of the society, programs in specialized disciplines are within the purview of specific associations or single educational or health care institutions, whereas issues that address practice and educational preparation in multidisciplinary settings are within the scope of training activities appropriate for the society. Regional training workshops dealing with the handicapped are illustrative of the latter.

Research projects, such as sponsored studies in accreditation, clinical facilities, and program offerings, are a major part of ASAHP's activities. These studies have generated useful planning data to assist institutions in launching new programs based on actual need rather than sentiment (Anderson, Nunn, and Sedlacek, 1976; American Society of Allied Health Professions, 1975). A major project sponsored jointly with ASAHP was an accreditation study known as SASHEP, for Study of Accreditation of Selected Health Education Programs. This study has become the benchmark for improving the process of accrediting programs. Due to the political realities of vested interests, such a study would have been difficult for any discipline to sponsor separately (Selden, 1972).

In summary, ASAHP has been a visible and viable force, bringing together an array of diverse groups and helping to meet the very real need for continued research in areas such as accreditation, continuing education, and clinical education that encompass many professions. As a relatively young organization in an arena as amorphous as allied health, ASAHP must continue to define and redefine its purpose and constituency, particularly in a world in which competition for time and energy is unparalleled.

### Present and Future Concerns

In any look at the future, a combination of insight and luck are at play. The eighties leave open many possibilities, ranging from continuing geometric increase in the technology of health care to the effects of reduced numbers of high school graduates.

*Funding.* During the seventies, most outside funding for allied health programs originated with federal legislation. One may easily conclude therefore that the Reagan administration is responsible for the reduction in federal largess. However, many of the reductions in health manpower programs were begun under the Carter administration. The Carter administration concluded that increased manpower did *not* lower medical costs. Rather, as more health manpower became available and as specialty areas developed and grew, costs increased. Although inflation has been a factor in increasing costs, the rise in medical costs has exceeded that caused by inflation. Thus the Carter administration, while trying to put a ceiling on hospital reimbursement, began simultaneously to dismantle the legislation that had pumped money into manpower. As Kelty (1981, p. 153), a futurist, stated in the keynote address at a recent ASAHP national meeting, "In the immediate future, it is unlikely that Congress will appropriate increased funds for any health programs."

The 1981 *Health Planning and Manpower Report* (1981, p. 3) quoted Hoover, acting director of the Bureau of Health Professions, Division of Associated Health Professions, as saying that the rationale for cutting allied health entirely in the recent budget measure is that "there is no national shortage and therefore we don't need any money." In an address at a health care productivity conference in Arlington, Virginia, on July 1, 1981, Richard S. Schweicker, secretary of Health and Human Services, put it simply: "The further the government has gotten into health care, the higher prices have climbed."

These decisions have had an impact on allied health programming. With the reduction in federal support, growth in new programs in academic health sciences centers and in four-year colleges has been curtailed. Programs largely funded on "soft" federal dollars have been cut back and, in several instances, entirely eliminated. In addition, several schools of allied health housed in academic health sciences centers have chosen to discontinue as separate entities. During the past decade, programs in academic health centers were in a strong financial position. Funds in the form of research and project grants, student traineeships, and particularly capitation funds supported expensive programs. Although capitation funds were never directed to allied health, the money, nonetheless, supported the entire academic health sciences center. With these funds reduced, the scramble for state and local funds has become severe. Today, Richard Dowling, executive director of ASAHP, voices particular concern about some sixty allied health schools that are part of health sciences centers. "Health science centers in search of money to balance their books (may look) to schools of allied health to do that" (*Health Planning and Manpower Report*, 1981, p. 3).

In contrast, four-year colleges have developed programs that are relatively low in per capita costs. The competition for funds is with programs that are facing sagging enrollments, such as liberal arts and teacher education. Health program growth and enrollment compares favorably with business and engineering in these colleges. Although the reduction in federal money may affect future growth and development somewhat and may limit special projects, the impact will be felt less than in the academic health sciences centers. This is particularly true for comprehensive regional universities that have established themselves in the past fifteen years as regional centers for allied health and that have institutionalized budgets for these programs. Two-year colleges, never large recipients of federal health dollars, have programs that are less expensive to operate and they continue to draw students. They will continue to show steady growth, particularly as health care institutions leave the education business.

As educational costs increase, health care institutions are examining their role in education. As a result, it is probably inevitable that small and medium-sized hospitals in which education has been an "add-on" will discontinue all educational programs. Meanwhile, in large health care institutions, where teaching is a major function, the model will become one of regional centers of education that combine separate discipline programs and clinical education. These regional institutions will not be limited to allied health education but will encompass all of the health professions.

As noted previously, the federal government has not been the sole source of financial support; state and local funds have been a sustaining force, as have grants from private foundations. However, since projections are that foundation funding will also be reduced, it is likely that the bulk of funding will have to come from local and state resources. Those institutions that have not nurtured these sources may face the greatest hardships in the next decade.

*Alliances.* One positive outcome of the struggle for survival is the development of new forms of alliances. In the eighties, private alliances will emerge as a result of the difficulties posed by limited resources. While the seventies witnessed the development of programs without regard to need or their geographical proximity to each other, the fiscal situation of the eighties will demand joint planning and decisions. Institutions interested in functioning independently will find that combined pressure from the state and from competing institutions will make it difficult if not impossible to make programmatic decisions in isolation. Alliances to share educational and clinical resources will become a necessity and joint program development and sharing of resources will become the norm. Although contracts may develop, the emphasis will probably be on informal alliances based on mutual trust. While, theoretically, formal alliances do work and can break down the barriers of institutional protectionism, it is unlikely that they will occur, since they rarely reduce overall costs, and institutions are wary of giving up their autonomy in the absence of some obvious gain.

*Accreditation.* As noted previously, monographs have been written and conferences held on accreditation in allied health. In some disciplines accrediting bodies are independent, while others work jointly with the Committee on Allied Health Education and Accreditation of the American Medical Association (AMA). Millions of dollars are spent every year to develop self-studies, conduct site surveys, and determine accreditation status in committees. The array of professionals has led to a parallel array of "essentials" and/or "standards" for each profession. Duplication of efforts between regional accrediting bodies and separate allied health programs is evident and much of the same material is required in multiple formats. The move toward an independent umbrella accrediting agency that incorporates standard formats and coordinated site visits is perhaps more wishful thinking than reality for the eighties. Although the Committee on Allied Health Education and Accreditation (CAHEA) has played a major leadership role in these areas, many allied health professionals do not support that effort due to the committee's involvement with the AMA. However, issues about who will bear the cost preclude any sudden and rapid development of an independent body. Program accreditation changes will occur more by evolution than revolution, and alliances based on cost-effective considerations will provide the impetus for this evolution.

*Planning.* Allied health in the seventies was characterizd by activity short on planning but long on growth; the reverse will be true in the eighties. Planning will encompass the areas already mentioned and will specifically address educational growth and development, especially within alliances.

Perhaps more importantly, planning will be required for retrenchment. Applicant pools are already producing shortfalls in some programs; others have decided to modify or close. During retrenchment the protection of students and faculty must be foremost in the planning process. For example, faculty will continue to be required as programs are phased out and as student enrollment declines. How should the decline be brought about: by reducing annual intake or by placing a one-year moratorium on admission? What is the current situation with respect to need for allied health professionals? Shall institutions retain marginal programs or reduce the number in order to elevate their quality? Ideally, research will accompany the planning needed to address these questions.

⟍ *Research.* Research has not been a high priority for allied health education. Practitioners have not sufficiently documented various treatment modalities, nor have educators adequately documented educational outcomes. Many areas are targets for research. In *The Future of Allied Health Education,* the National Commission on Allied Health Education (1980, pp. 159–160) lists fifteen recommendations that reflect six basic themes:

- Allied health personnel provide essential health care.
- Allied health education is essential for provision of a competent and sufficient work force.
- The primary purpose of allied health education is to prepare students for health service.
- Flexibility in the educational processes for preparing students to meet performance objectives is essential.
- Interests of the student or the public should be served above any special interest of educational institutions and professional groups.
- Coordination of resources and collaborative problem solving are essential.

These themes are expanded and explained in fifteen recommendations and sixty-three corollaries. While any suggestions risk important omissions, the following high-priority areas for research may be noted:

- Clinical practice education: What are the various modalities of treatment and how effective are they? How do they compare in cost and outcome with alternatives, including nonintervention? What are the most effective means of organizing clinical education? How effective is simulation in teaching the integration of cognitive and psychomotor skills? What are entry-level competencies?
- Accreditation: How effective is it in assuring minimal standards? Are there alternatives that would obtain the same results with less effort? Can unit

accreditation replace program accreditation? Does survey coordination save time and money?

- Curriculum design: What are the outcomes of existing educational programs and what are the programmatic alternatives? Does the curriculum include too many specifics unrelated to practice? Can multicompetent professionals serve multiple roles?

- Cost containment: Will the reduction in federal funds provide for stability or retrenchment? Will a competitive model of health care result in an increased use of allied health professionals? How can programs in allied health examine practice from an economic standpoint?

- Health promotion: How can health promotion be made a way of life and an attitude that permeates society? How can public attitudes be modified in the five areas that most influence health: smoking, drinking, eating, sleeping, and exercising? How can allied health professionals become advocates for better health through better habits?

## Summary

The allied health professions are young as compared with the other health disciplines and their futures are fraught with uncertainties about care and levels of practice. Goals and objectives are not solidified nor will they be in the near future. This suggests a time for self-examination in the cycle of need analysis, implementation, synthesis, and evaluation. Allied health education is just finishing the third phase, synthesis, in which organizational structure and experimentation are being resolved. We need now to get on with evaluation, both retrospective and prospective, to examine where we have been and to provide guidance for the future. Over a decade ago Mase (1968) proposed "three c's for allied health education: communication, collaboration, and cooperation," processes that are as valid for the eighties as they were for the seventies. To these we must add two more: contribution and conviction. We must posssess the conviction that allied health education can make a contribution to close the distance between the rhetoric and the reality.

## References

Addleman, A. D. "Critical Issues Facing Allied Health." In *Proceedings: Meeting of the Committee of Presidents of the Health Professions Educational Associations.* Washington, D.C.: Association of Academic Health Centers, 1981.

American Medical Association. *Allied Health Education Directory.* (9th ed.) Chicago: American Medical Association, 1980.

American Society of Allied Health Professions. *Survey of Clinical Facilities, Allied Health Education Programs in Junior and Senior Colleges, 1973–1974: Guidance Edition, NIH.* Bethesda, Md.: Bureau of Health Manpower, Health Resources Administration, 1975.

American Society of Allied Health Professions. *Collegiate Program Survey.* Washington, D.C.: American Society of Allied Health Professions, 1980a.

American Society of Allied Health Professions. *Proceedings: National Conference on Continuing Education in Allied Health.* Washington, D.C.: American Society of Allied Health Professions, 1980b.

American Society of Allied Health Professions. *Proceedings: National Forum on Accreditation of Allied Health Education.* Washington, D.C.: American Society of Allied Health Professions, 1980c.

Anderson, P. W., Nunn, R. S., and Sedlacek, W. E. *Collegiate Programs in Allied Health Occupations.* Washington, D.C.: American Society of Allied Health Professions, 1976.

Blayney, K. D. "A Review of Clinical Education in Allied Health." In J. Hamburg (Ed.), *Review of Allied Health Education.* Vol. II. Lexington: University of Kentucky, 1977.

Burnett, E. *Report on Core Curriculum in Health Professions.* Washington, D.C.: U.S. Department of Health, Education, and Welfare, 1972.

Ducanis, A. J., and Golin, A. K. *The Interdisciplinary Health Care Team.* Germantown, Md.: Aspen Systems Corporation, 1979.

Ford, C. W. (Ed.). *Clinical Education for the Allied Health Professions.* St. Louis, Mo.: Mosby, 1978.

Gertz, R. M. "The Association of Schools of Allied Health Professions." In E. J. McTernan and R. O. Hawkins (Eds.), *Educating Personnel for the Allied Health Professions and Services.* St. Louis, Mo.: Mosby, 1972.

Graduate Medical Education National Advisory Committee. *Summary Report.* Vol. I. Washington, D.C.: U.S. Government Printing Office, 1980.

Hatch, T. D., and Kress, L. M. "Government Support for Allied Health Professions Education." In E. J. McTernan and R. O. Hawkins (Eds.), *Educating Personnel for the Allied Health Professions and Services.* St. Louis, Mo.: Mosby, 1972.

Hawthorne, M. E., and Perry, J. W. *Community Colleges and Primary Health Care: Study of Allied Health Education Report.* Washington, D.C.: American Association of Community and Junior Colleges, 1974.

*Health Planning and Manpower Report.* Arlington, Va.: Capitol Publications, 1981.

Kellogg Foundation. *Action Programs for Developing Allied Health Education.* Battle Creek, Mich.: Kellogg Foundation, 1977.

Kelty, E. J. "Half-Past Tomorrow." *Journal of Allied Health,* 1981, *10,* 149–153.

King, E. C., and Dietrich, M. C. "The School of Allied Health—a Political Model of University Government." *Journal of Allied Health,* 1980, *9,* 242–252.

McTernan, E. J. "Introduction: The Philosophy of Allied Health." In E. J. McTernan and R. O. Hawkins (Eds.), *Educating Personnel for the Allied Health Professions and Services.* St. Louis, Mo.: Mosby, 1972.

Mase, D. J. "Whither Now." Paper presented at first annual meeting of Association of Schools of Allied Health Professions, Miami Beach, Fla., 1968.

Moore, M. L., and Perry, J. F. *Clinical Education in Physical Therapy: Present Status/Future Needs.* Washington, D.C.: American Physical Therapy Association, 1976.

Moore, M. L., Perry, J. F., and Clark, A. W. *Clinical Education in the Health Professions: An Annotated Bibliography.* Washington, D.C.: American Physical Therapy Association, 1976.

National Commission on Allied Health Education. *The Future of Allied Health Education: New Alliances for the 1980s.* San Francisco: Jossey-Bass, 1980.

Perry, J. W. "The Allied Health Professions: Change Is the Name of the Game." *Journal of the American Physical Therapy Association*, 1968, *48*, 1115-1121.

Rosenfeld, M. H. "Organizing for Allied Health Education in Educational Institutions." In E. J. McTernan and R. O. Hawkins (Eds.), *Educating Personnel for the Allied Health Professions and Services*. St. Louis, Mo.: Mosby, 1972.

Selden, W. K. (Ed.). *Study of Accreditation of Selected Health Education Programs (SASHEP)*. Washington, D.C.: American Society of Allied Health Professions, 1972.

Task Force on Allied Health Clinical Education. *National Assessment of Clinical Education of Allied Health Manpower*. Vols I, II, III. Washington, D.C.: Booz, Allen, and Hamilton, 1974.

U.S. Department of Health, Education, and Welfare. *A Report on Allied Health Personnel*. Washington, D.C.: U.S. Government Printing Office, 1969.

U.S. Department of Health, Education, and Welfare. *Allied Health Education Programs in Junior and Senior Colleges*. Vols. I and II. Washington, D.C.: U.S. Government Printing Office, 1975.

*Cecil G. Sheps*

# 7

# Public Health

Specialized education for public health had its beginnings in the United States with the establishment of a school of public health at Johns Hopkins University in 1916. By 1960, twelve such schools existed, six at private universities and six at public universities. Since 1960, the number of schools of public health has almost doubled, with twenty-three schools now admitting students and others being planned. Starting in the 1930s, special programs in other graduate schools as well as a few baccalaureate programs were also established. There are now numerous programs, both graduate and undergraduate, in specialized fields provided in many different academic settings. This growth is a reflection of the changing meaning and scope of public health in the United States.

## Scope of Public Health

Initially, public health consisted primarily of governmental regulations and services to control epidemics of infectious diseases by quarantine and later by immunization measures. This was accompanied by controls governing the protection and purification of water supplies and the safe disposal of sewage and other wastes, as the vital role of such measures in preventing disease became clear. Appreciation of the widespread need for these protective measures led to the establishment of state and local—city and county—health departments. In the twentieth century, these activities became firmly established and widespread. As the role of nutrition, sanitation, and medical care in preventing infant and maternal mortality became clear, public health departments took on the responsibility of educating the general public regarding the importance of these measures and also, in many instances, of providing these services to those who would otherwise not receive them. The great achievements that resulted from public health programs are well known. Communicable diseases are largely under control in the United States, and it is now generally recognized that public health measures have been primarily responsible for the great increase in life expectancy in the twentieth century. Government efforts aimed at prevention have formed the basic foundation of public health.

Since World War II, the conceptual base and scope of public health has been significantly broadened. Though the emphasis on prevention continues to be the central concern of public health, its meaning has been expanded to include a much wider range of health and related social problems that now encompasses not only the prevention of the onset of a disease but also includes limiting its progression, preventing disability, and rehabilitating the disabled. Simultaneously, there has developed in the United States, as in all industrialized nations, the acceptance of a new national standard: the expectation that all persons should be able to obtain medical care services, regardless of their ability to pay. Thus the delivery of diagnostic and treatment services, under both private and public auspices, has become a public concern and, increasingly, a public responsibility. The scope of public health has also been enlarged as a result of the greater understanding, particularly in the past few decades, of the effects of the physical and social environment on the health of the public. However, eliminating from the physical environment the hazards of toxic substances that result from industrial production is much more complex than immunizing children; eliminating pathological elements in the social environment is at least equally difficult. For this reason, the development of policies and procedures in this field reaches into the interstices of our economy and touches the roots and currents of our life-style.

For the purpose of this discussion, the definition of public health which seems most appropriate is that developed by the Milbank Memorial Fund Commission (1976) in *Higher Education for Public Health*: "Public health is the effort organized by society to protect, promote, and restore the people's health. The programs, services, and institutions involved emphasize the prevention of disease and the health needs of the population as a whole. Public health activities change with changing technology and social values, but the goals remain the same: to reduce the amount of disease, premature death, and disease-produced discomfort and disability" (p. 3).

The leading health problems of our nation today are inequities in health status, the chronic diseases, and environmental hazards. The network of activities that we have developed to protect the health of our citizens and to prevent and treat disease consists of three major elements: personal medical care, environmental controls, and health promotion and education. The concern and activities of public health today range from the planning, financing, and management of health services to the identification and control of substance abuse and of hazardous substances in the workplace. The major public health responsibilities are prevention of disease; promotion of the health and well-being of the population; efficient and effective use of health resources by the entire population; and monitoring of the health status of the population, health-related problems, and health resources throughout the community, the state, and the nation. These responsibilities encompass both private and public institutions and activities. They are of key public concern and interest and typify the field of public health in modern times.

In response to the increased scope of public health in recent decades, there has been a concomitant growth in the number and types of professional personnel needed and employed. These individuals play increasingly specialized roles and, hence, need to be adequately prepared for their respective tasks. If the aims of public health are to be carried out fully in the public interest, an adequate supply of appropriately trained professional personnel is needed. The effectiveness of science, technology, and managerial skills will, however, depend on the manner in which decisions on health policy issues are made and on the nature of those decisions. There is also a need, therefore, for a cadre of leaders trained to address broad issues of social policy as they affect the health of the public. To do this, they need to be qualified to assess community health problems effectively, establish priorities, identify the forces that affect health, establish feasible health goals, assemble resources, and then organize programs to achieve these goals and evaluate existing programs.

### Knowledge Base for Public Health

As the scope of public health has broadened, the knowledge base from which its activities are drawn has expanded far beyond its beginnings in medicine and engineering to include a widening range of biological and physical sciences, the social sciences, law, and ethics. This has clear implications for, and presents a serious challenge to, the educational programs aimed at preparing professionals to work effectively in this increasingly complex field of public service. Given the breadth that modern public health now encompasses, it is evident that it does not represent a single scientific field organized and applied in a uniform manner. Rather, its knowledge base is multidisciplinary and its modes of application are pluralistic.

Despite the involvement of many distinct, established fields of expertise in public health, there is a knowledge base for public health that can be codified into two categories. The first consists of three elements that are fundamental to public health and that flourish best in public health settings: the measurement and analytic sciences of biostatistics and epidemiology, social policy and the history and philosophy of public health, and the principles and practice of organization and management for public health. The second group consists of fields developed outside of public health that are cognate to it and includes the clinical sciences of medicine, dentistry, nursing, and some aspects of social work. Though these sciences are directed primarily to individual patients, it is important that some of their insights and methods be adapted to community health programs aimed at communities and populations. Other fields cognate to public health are the biomedical sciences, which provide information regarding disease that may suggest methods of control; the environmental sciences, which relate human health to the physical environment; and the social sciences, which shed light on social issues, on group and individual behavior, and on the distribution and costs of health services. Law and ethics are also increasingly pertinent.

Except with some aspects of the public health measurement sciences of biostatistics and epidemiology, maximally effective public health activity requires the application and interaction of some of the cognate as well as the generic elements in the knowledge base. Not only is public health work done by different types of personnel, but it calls for different levels of responsibility. Therefore, there is a need for different mixes and levels of professional education and training. The clustering of needed elements and the depth of attention given to each should be determined by the particular type of public health activity for which persons are being prepared. Virtually all elements in the knowledge base are relevant, in some degree, to any special field of public health. The elements of the knowledge base generic to public health are fundamental to all.

### Personnel for Public Health

Early in this century, the central figure in public health was the health officer who was usually a physician, often assisted by a sanitarian or, in larger areas, by an engineer. Today the physician is no longer numerically dominant. In some fields, such as the environment, there are subspecialized professionals, such as environmental engineers, environmental technologists, and industrial hygienists. What brings these diverse professionals together was best expressed by a statement in the report to the Rockefeller Foundation by Welch and Rose (1916) that led to the founding of the first school of public health in this country: "Unity is to be found rather in the ends to be accomplished—the preservation and improvement of health—than in the means essential to that end" (p. 415).

To meet the special educational needs of the members of the different professions who apply their knowledge and skills to public health programs, the distinction must be made between two kinds of professional functions. One is the use of people from many different professions, such as medicine, dentistry, nursing, or social work, who apply the knowledge and skills of their profession directly or with some slight adaptation within an already designed public health program. This type of function does not require anything more than a general orientation to the program. The second type of function is quite different. It uses professionals such as epidemiologists, biostatisticians, administrators of health programs, nutritionists, health educators, and environmental specialists, whose knowledge and skills are centered primarily on public health problems and programs. Higher education for public health is essential in preparing such persons for this type of work.

There is yet another type of professional in public health. These are people with varied earlier professional training and experience who are given major management responsibilities as executives, policy makers, and planners, all of whom should have broad expertise in the field of public health generally. These are the persons who actually develop priorities, assemble resources, plan, implement, and evaluate programs. Clearly, when this is done in public health, substantive knowledge of the issues generic to public health is fundamental to success.

The American Public Health Association has recently identified at least forty different professional-level specialties in public health (American Public Health Association, 1981). Though many more are employed in public health in various capacities, it has been estimated by the Division of Associated Health Professions of the Department of Health and Human Services that in 1979 there were approximately 150,000 professional persons wholly engaged in such work

(U.S. Department of Health and Human Services, 1980). In developing their estimate of the number of core public health workers, the Division of Associated Health Professionals grouped them as follows: (1) health services administrators and planners, employed by hospitals, health departments, other governmental agencies, nursing homes, voluntary health agencies, and medical group practices; (2) health statisticians; (3) epidemiologists, about half of whom are M.D.s; (4) public and community health educators; (5) environmental health personnel, including sanitarians, industrial hygienists, and environmental health engineers and scientists; (6) public health nutritionists; and (7) public health physicians, dentists, nurses, veterinarians, and related personnel. These personnel are employed by health departments and other governmental agencies at federal, state, and local levels; by hospitals and other medical care institutions both private and public; by voluntary health agencies, some of which have quasi-governmental responsibilities; by health professions schools and other educational institutions; and by corporations, unions, and others.

## Educational Programs

Specialized education for public health in the United States began with the establishment of schools of public health. Today, the curriculum of these schools differs sharply and uniquely from that of the schools of all other professions. Unlike other professional schools that admit all students to the same curriculum, schools of public health admit almost all students to distinctly specialized tracks and do not graduate a single type of professional. In sharp contrast with the situation in schools of law, architecture, or medicine, admission to schools of public health or to programs offering public health training in other parts of the university is the responsibility of the individual department or program. Since students are admitted to a particular field of public health, such as health administration, the curriculum consists predominantly of courses given within a specific department or program, with few courses of a "core" nature given by other departments. Often, even "core" courses, such as research methods, are given within the particular department and while this gives the faculty of the department greater control over the development of their students, it carries the risk of differential standards and is likely to be more costly.

Unlike other professional schools, schools of public health differ greatly among themselves. Although all offer programs in the generic public health disciplines, they vary widely in their emphasis on different cognate disciplines and fields of application, as well as in their internal departmental organization and in the nature of faculty interest, skills, and fields of competence. All offer a master of public health degree (M.P.H.), and most offer a master of science (M.S.); both are generally of two years' duration. The latter degree is offered in hygiene, hospital administration, environment, maternal and child health, epidemiology, biostatistics, industrial hygiene, and other specialized fields. In 1977–78, 95 percent of the students in public health schools were enrolled in sixteen different areas of specialization (American Public Health Association, 1981). Doctoral programs in special fields are also offered in all except the most recently established schools. The degrees of Ph.D., doctor of public health (Dr.P.H.), and doctor of science (D.Sc.) are given in specialized fields of science basic to public health or in fields of application.

The growth in the number of schools has been accompanied by an even greater growth in the number of students. In 1974, the total number of graduate degrees awarded by schools of public health was 2,510, twice the number granted in 1968. In 1960, 5 percent of the degrees were at the doctoral level (Milbank Memorial Fund Commission, 1976); in 1977-78, 19.6 percent of the student body in schools of public health were registered in doctoral programs, and another 0.8 percent were registered in postdoctoral programs (American Public Health Association, 1981).

As the need was recognized for a widening range of professional backgrounds and disciplines to be applied to public health, dentists, social workers, teachers, administrators, and laboratory scientists as well as physicians and engineers were admitted to schools of public health. By the 1960s, these schools were enrolling from over twenty disparate, specific professional groups. At approximately the same time, another change occurred in the nature of the student body. Until the early sixties, the great majority of students enrolled after having already obtained their basic professional preparation in fields such as medicine, dentistry, nursing, and engineering, and many of these already had some field experience in public health work. They enrolled to obtain special graduate education in order to learn to apply their professions more effectively in public health work. This is still to some extent the case today, with a few schools even concentrating on attracting such students; however, in recent decades, schools have begun to admit more students without a professional or graduate degree or any prior experience in health work. These younger students are being admitted not only to programs in biostatistics, epidemiology, or environmental sciences but also to applied fields, such as health services administration and health education. This approach draws a much larger pool of potential candidates for public health work; however, it constitutes a substantial change in policy and creates a new problem of developing educational programs suitable for students with widely varied levels of educational background and experience.

Another significant development over the past forty years is that growing numbers of core public health professionals have been educated at graduate schools other than schools of public health, especially in health services and hospital administration, public health nutrition, public health nursing, public or community health education, and environmental health. The number of graduates in the last three categories has, in recent years, exceeded those from schools of public health. The location of these programs reflects the developing interest and capacity of the sponsoring school or department since they are offered in such diverse settings as schools of engineering, business, public administration, medicine, education, allied health sciences, and home economics. Though comprehensive national data on these programs are not available, it appears that graduate degree programs are now being offered by at least 50 institutions in health services and hospital administration, 36 in environmental health, approximately 100 in public and community health education, and 8 in public health nutrition (American Public Health Association, 1981). In addition, some students are enrolled in graduate programs in biostatistics and epidemiology outside schools of public health.

In the past decade, in particular, college programs at the baccalaureate level have also developed and grown rapidly, mainly in health education, environmental health, and nutrition. It has been estimated that there are now well over 200 such programs in operation (Milbank Memorial Fund Commission, 1976). In response to perceived manpower needs, a few schools of public health have recently initiated baccalaureate degrees that are designed to prepare the graduate for entry-level positions in such fields as health services administration, biostatistics, nutrition, and health education. Though graduates of these programs are prepared to function in only a limited manner, they appear to provide a useful service, and they can, of course, subsequently pursue further graduate study in their areas of interest.

## New Directions in Educational Programs

*Part-Time Students.* As was noted earlier, the majority of personnel now employed full time in core professional work in public health have not had graduate-level education. Most cannot take the time needed from work to enroll in a full-time academic program, though many are eager to further their professional education in public health. Consequently, in contradistinction to most other professional programs, those in public health have developed special opportunities for part-time students, a significant proportion of whom already work in public health or health agencies of one type or another. For example, most schools of public health, as well as programs in other institutions, register a few part-time students for their standard programs; a few of the latter offer night courses for such students. In the past decade, a few innovative programs have been developed to meet the need; four of these are described below.

Since the early 1970s, the School of Public Health of the University of North Carolina has offered a master's degree program in health administration at four off-campus sites at varying times for students engaged in health work of some type. Faculty from the school teach two courses each semester, one day per week. A degree can be earned in three years, and of the approximately 150 students so far enrolled, 100 have already earned their degrees. A concentration in public health nursing has recently been added to this program.

In 1972, the School of Public Health of the University of Michigan initiated an on-the-job/on-the-campus M.P.H. program in medical care administration, designed for persons with current administrative responsibilities related to the delivery of personal health services. Although people without a degree but with a record of considerable achievement and experience are considered, most candidates are required to have a bachelor's degree. Students attend class four days per month for twenty-five months and, between the classroom sessions, prepare for class and do work-related projects at the site of their employment. Approximately 200 students will have completed the program when the sixth class is graduated in June 1982. Recently, this program was expanded to include a dental public health concentration.

In the late 1970s, Boston University established a school of public health offering courses in the late afternoon and evening, to meet the professional education needs of persons who could not become full-time students. Most of the students are employed in health agencies and take, on the average, three years to complete the requirements for a master's degree. Despite this radical departure, this school obtained accreditation from the Council on Education for Public Health, the national accrediting body for schools of public health. Since its inception, the school has admitted a small number of full-time students; however, by retaining its primary objective, it continues to enjoy an enrollment of adequate size.

In 1980, the School of Public Health of the University of North Carolina instituted an experimental regional program in health administration combining on-campus and independent study. Its purpose is to promote access to a master's degree program of study for candidates working in health activities who live out of state. Current candidates, located in eight states, are required to spend one week in January and a summer session of six weeks on the Chapel Hill campus for two years. They also obtain a maximum of 30 percent of the required credits at another, presumably nearby, university. Specially designed modules for independent study have been developed. It is expected that the average time to complete the degree will be three years, with five as the maximum. Twenty-two students were enrolled in the first class, with the expectation that forty will be admitted to the second.

*Field Experience for Faculty and Students.* An unsettled question in public health programs is the role of field exposure and experience for faculty as well as students. Since the great majority of public health professionals practice in the field, one might expect that work in actual field situations would be the context for much of the teaching. One also might expect that the faculty charged with preparing students to function effectively in the field would have had, and would continue to maintain, significant direct and responsible involvement in field-related problems. However, this is the exception rather than the rule, both in schools of public health and in outside programs. Where faculty have had such experience, it is often uneven and fragmentary. Since the validity of the theoretical approaches to public health practice and the conceptual framework for the role models that are identified by the faculty for the graduates are usually influenced by the nature and degree of field experience of the faculty, many directors of field agencies are critical of the new graduates as being inadequately prepared for the realistic tasks they face in the field. They raise concerns as to the degree to which faculty, given their background and activities, can fully understand field-related problems and practice. Nonetheless, some institutions and departments regard responsible field experience, past or current, as of little relevance, if not actually dysfunctional, in upgrading the qualifications of the faculty in applied fields.

In contrast, the Milbank Memorial Fund Commission (1976) recommended that "educational institutions should develop reciprocal relationships with health agencies and community organizations to bring greater realism to the classroom and academic expertise to the field. They should also solicit, and be responsive to, evaluations of their educational programs provided by these agencies." The commission also recommended that "supervised programs of field experience in connection with academic activity must be an integral and significant part of education for public health," and that "faculty members in schools of public health should undertake periodic, if not continuous, formal responsibilities in the operation of community health services which are relevant to, and will be supportive of, their respective fields of academic responsibility" (pp. 131–132).

This latter recommendation was particularly controversial in view of the persistent attitude among many public health faculty that a strong and consistent linkage between professional education and professional practice is irrelevant unnecessary, and does not contribute to academic "excellence." However, in the past ten years, at least two schools have taken action along work-teach and work-study lines as a matter of school-wide policy. The School of Public Health of the University of North Carolina established a special Division of Community Health Service for the express purpose of making its faculty expertise available to meet the needs of communities, where these matched "to the mutual benefit of the school and the community" (University of North Carolina School of Public Health, 1979). The Division's activities now include continuous collaboration with relevant state health agencies by such departments as environmental sciences and engineering, biostatistics, epidemiology, maternal and child health, and others. Following another model of interaction, the School of Public Health and Community Medicine of the University of Washington at Seattle carries out analytic studies for both the state legislature and the executive branch, through a Health Policy Analysis Program, arranged through the Graduate School of Public Affairs and Institute of Governmental Research.

Recently, a new and unique program has been developed by the Johns Hopkins School of Hygiene and Public Health. In 1977, it established a Health Program Alliance as an expression of its new policy. The alliance is charged with establishing mutually beneficial programs and relationships between the school and health institutions, organizations, and agencies in the four neighboring states of Maryland, Virginia, West Virginia, and Delaware and the District of Columbia. The stated objectives of this development include: improving curriculum relevance and relevance of research undertaken by the faculty and better "coupling (of) classroom work to a period of involvement with an operational program so that the student becomes sensitive to the gap between theory and practice." This synergistic relationship is also expected to assist the school in evaluating: "(1) the utility and applicability of its various training programs, courses, educational modalities, and educational objectives, and (2) the relevance of its applied research, the development of research strategies, and research priorities" (Johns Hopkins University, 1977).

Hopkins expects to achieve these goals in the context of providing consultation and technical assistance to field agencies using the range of disciplines and capacities represented on its faculty. The alliance has an impressive set of field activities under way involving faculty, physician residents in preventive medicine, and other selected students. Three full-time professional personnel are occupied in the program's overall direction and operation, in addition to other faculty who provide consultation and technical assistance. This recognition of the ineluctable value of the interaction between theory and practice is most encouraging and represents a point of view that was unfashionable in programs of higher education, especially during the past fifteen years or so. Experiments, research, and evaluation are badly needed to determine the optimum role of field experience and professional practice of public health field work in producing faculty and educational programs of highest quality. Evaluation of the Hopkins experience and that of other institutions that may perhaps adopt the same approach can be expected to be crucial to understanding the effectiveness of various approaches to professional education for public health.

   *Continuing Education.* Like other professional schools, programs in public health are responsible for continuing education activities. In fact, they were involved in this area earlier than most other professional institutions. Growth in these programs has been fostered by the recent trend to make participation in continuing education a required component for relicensure or recertification and a prerequisite for continued membership in professional societies. The 1980 federal report on public and community health personnel concluded that "approximately 50 percent of the 'core' work force (150,000 persons) need short-term training in specialized subject matter, or to obtain a clear view of the economic, social, political, or technological context in which they work" (American Public Health Association, 1981, p. 210).

   Though there are many courses and programs of continuing education in public health conducted by academic institutions, they can generally be characterized as consisting "of a series of miscellaneous efforts, haphazardly conceived" (Milbank Memorial Fund Commission, 1976, p. 149). While some are sponsored by professional groups or field agencies, it is expected that in public health, as in other professions, academic institutions will play the predominant role. The essentially random nature of most continuing education activities is mainly due to the fact that academic institutions have not accepted the responsibility for this type of education, in the form of comprehensive programs organized and directed toward target groups of professionals to fill the identified knowledge gaps generated by new policies, scientific or technologic developments, or needs in the fields of operation. Greater awareness of the importance of this role for academic institutions and more realistic assessment of the fiscal restraints they currently face lend support to the hope that continuing education will occupy a distinct and prominent role in their overall program planning. In the field of continuing education, the research issues are the same as in other professions. They include such questions as how to determine needs, how best to meet them in terms of form and content, and how to measure the effects of programs in terms of altered professional behavior. Special attention, of course, must be paid to the context of changes in public health knowledge, policy, and opportunities for the full exercise of professional competence.

   *Research.* Research is fundamental to the effectiveness of public health activity. In addition to its substantive value, the conduct of research by faculty contributes, as in any other field, to the quality of educational programs in unique and essential ways. The substantial amount of research now being done is diversified, reflecting largely the competence and interests of faculty. Federal support has made most of this research possible and has influenced the selection of subjects to be studied. While federal priorities may, and often do, realistically reflect the needs and interests of the nation, they may also be determined by political pressures and may not reflect scientists' views of areas promising immediate or long-term gains. The immediate and long-term social purpose of public health makes it somewhat easier to establish priorities in terms of both basic and applied research at the institutional, as well as the national, level.

## Agenda for Change

*Manpower Planning.* Information about manpower requirements for public health is fragmentary, uneven, and entirely inadequate for planning at the national, state, or institutional levels. While not unique to public health, this deficiency is especially significant here because of the high cost of educational programs in this field, because government bears a goodly share of the cost in the form of financial support both of students and of programs, and because the great majority of public health professionals are employed in the public sector. This is not the case in professions such as law, pharmacy, architecture, or accounting. Though several studies in recent decades have attempted to describe the public health professional work force and to quantify the production of personnel (Milbank Memorial Fund Commission, 1976; U.S. Department of Health and Human Services, 1980; White and others, 1976; Goldston and Padilla, 1975; U.S. Department of Health, Education, and Welfare, 1967; Hall and others, 1982; Moore and others, 1982; Association of Schools of Public Health, 1980; Hall, Jackson, and Parsons, 1980), we have yet to see any significant efforts to estimate and project personnel requirements or to identify and study the problems that may exist with regard to validated qualifications for various types of responsibilities.

The most recent listing of relevant studies is found in the bibliography prepared by Hall, Jackson, and Parsons (1980). On the basis of their review, they concluded that "most studies of public health personnel tend to be quite limited in the scope, data base, or setting, and are more apt to be descriptive than analytical. The most obvious gaps concerning public health personnel include: operational definitions and categorization of the specialty; studies of the determinants of supply and demand; estimates of career stability in the various public health jobs; estimates and characterization of the production of public health; rigorous evaluations of the major alternative modalities of public health training" (p. 57).

In the first of a series of biennial federal reports on public and community health personnel mandated by legislation passed in 1978, the report asserts that "the inability to document a shortage or surplus of public health manpower is due primarily to lack of uniform and fixed qualifications for employment, and secondarily to inexact demand" (U.S. Department of Health and Human Services, 1980, p. 209). As suggested earlier, these problems are especially difficult because the field encompasses a broad range of specialties and includes both persons who do not have any formal training in public health and those who enter the field in mid-career. The same federal report concludes that there are about 550,000 persons, or one out of every ten health workers, who have some responsibilities or functions in the public health area. Of those, a core group of about 150,000 are wholly engaged in public health work. Of this group, it is estimated that about 25 percent have had graduate-level preparation in public health (p. 209).

It is clear, therefore, that a basic need in this field is the establishment and implementation of a national public health manpower data base and monitoring system. In making this recommendation, the Milbank Memorial Fund Commission (1976) pointed to the need for "a continuing program for the systematic collection and monitoring of data in the current and projected balance between the supply of, and need for, public health manpower. This monitoring is (now) done in many other fields. Such a system would provide information on the nature of the pool of applicants, training categories, and educational programs. It could provide a basis for discussion on the best location of centers for advanced training, sites of new educational programs, and curriculum emphasis based in service needs and employment opportunities. The responsibility for generating and overseeing such a surveillance system should be assumed by the federal government and shared with universities and relevant professional organizations" (p. 49). In a current report, Hall and others (1982) set forth the objectives of such an information system in greater detail under such headings as defining health manpower, monitoring manpower production, and supply and demand.

A reliable data base is essential if we are to develop a national and optimally effective public policy for public health manpower. This not only presents a complex research task in itself, but data from such a system are crucial to tackling other research issues regarding the education of public health professionals. A contract in late 1981, awarded to the American Public Health Association by the Health Resources Administration of the Department of Health and Human Services, gives promise that perhaps some headway is being made in this direction. The objectives of this eighteen-month project are: (1) to develop working and functional definitions for those major areas of specialization in public health that form at least four-fifths of the public health personnel category; (2) to define the data elements necessary for a system capable of determining work force supply and requirements and to identify the principal or desired sources of such data; (3) to design a cost-effective system of collection and analysis of the above data (American Public Health Association, 1981).

Without a basic data and surveillance system to monitor the need, demand, and production of professional manpower for public health, effective planning of educational programs at any level is impossible. However, this should be only the beginning; there are many issues needing scientific investigation. As noted, a distinctive feature of professional education in this field is that, while schools of public health were first in this field, a major and growing portion of public health education is carried out in graduate programs located elsewhere in the community. Yet, schools of public health have been established and continue to behave almost as though they were the only source of appropriately trained personnel; at the same time, graduate programs in single fields in various other parts of the university have developed without regard to the total framework of higher education for public health. The issue is the optimum role of university programs of a different focus: separate schools versus individual programs lodged in other schools or departments. As this author has recently written, "A rational approach to the future of higher education for public health calls for answers to a series of questions." These include: "Do these diverse auspices (for the conduct of programs) represent important differences in the nature and quality of educational programs? Do they differ in cost? In effectiveness? Is the competition among these programs real? Is it helpful? Is more or less diversity needed?" (Sheps, 1980, p. 9). Though implementation might be difficult, a series of research projects to answer these questions could readily be designed.

Finally, in the past decade or so, much attention has been given to the special and severe health problems of minority groups in the United States. The 1980 federal report on manpower presents and discusses data dealing with the issues affecting personnel who deal with these problems. It concludes that "educational programs frequently are deficient in preparing students to appreciate and deal with the public health problems of minority groups" (U.S. Department of Health and Human Services, 1980, p. 211). More demonstrations, experiments, research, and evaluation in this field are also needed.

*Optimum Use of Faculty Resources.* The multidisciplinary character of the knowledge base for public health raises important challenges in the organization of faculty resources to conduct educational programs. The disciplines and professions cognate to public health are usually represented in universities by separate existing departments and schools. Graduate programs in special fields of public health organized outside schools of public health usually make arrangements to associate with their program existing faculty in fields cognate to its focus. On the other hand, schools of public health rarely do so; instead, they usually recruit members from the cognate disciplines directly to their faculty. This practice raises issues both of quality and of possible duplication in educational offerings. To avoid these problems and despite the generic difficulties involved, a number of universities have arranged joint activities and interchange among different schools and departments. The Harvard School of Public Health has developed two M.S. curricula that use faculty resources in other schools of the university and at its neighbor, the Massachusetts Institute of Technology. Clearly, research and evaluation in this area of the optimum use of faculty resources and the effects of different arrangements on the quality of the education program is timely and potentially significant.

Objective analysis and evaluation is also needed to determine the effectiveness of diverse educational programs as measured, inter alia, by the performance of graduates in the field and by a follow-up of their perceptions of the relevance and adequacy of their academic preparation. Two such studies have recently been reported (Clemmer and Bertrand, 1980; Monroe, Tuttle, and Lorimer, 1980); many more are needed. Here too, from the national point of view, an overall research strategy can be developed.

Finally, significant contributions to the achievement of public health objectives can be made by members of other professions. This is true not only of the human service professions, such as medicine, dentistry, social work, and nursing, but also of law, engineering, education, and communication. Experiments and demonstrations should be conducted to determine the most effective means of providing students in each of these professions with appropriate knowledge and understanding of public health perspectives and programs.

## Conclusion

In the past two decades, professional education for public health has been characterized by exponential growth, great diversity, and very little planned experimentation or research into the process of education. The few recent studies completed and those now under way may be viewed as early harbingers of the additional work that must be done. Policy in the field of education is being made daily by interested and sincere parties with deeply held and varied views, commitments, and biases. Perhaps the research agenda set forth in this chapter would provide a sounder basis for such decisions.

## References

American Public Health Association. *Survey of Public Health/Community Health Personnel: A Proposal by the American Public Health Association.* Washington, D.C.: American Public Health Association, 1981.

Association of Schools of Public Health. *Educational Data Project, 1974–1979.* U.S. Department of Health and Human Services Publication no. (HRA) 80–43. Washington, D.C.: U.S. Department of Health and Human Services, May 1980.

Clemmer, D. I., and Bertrand, W. E. "A Model for the Incorporation of Alumni-Faculty Feedback into Curriculum Planning." *American Journal of Public Health,* 1980, *70,* 67–69.

Goldston, S. E., and Padilla, E. "The Professional Public Health Worker: Educational and Demographic Profiles." *American Journal of Public Health,* 1975, *65,* 831–836.

Hall, T. L., Jackson, R. S., and Parsons, W. B. *Schools of Public Health: Trends in Graduate Education.* U.S. Department of Health and Human Services Publication no. (HRA) 80–46. Washington, D.C.: U.S. Department of Health and Human Services, May 1980.

Hall, T. L., and others. *The Job Market for Graduates of Schools of Public Health: Experiences of the Classes of 1978 and 1979.* U.S. Department of Health and Human Services Publication no. HRP–090–4360. Springfield, Va.: National Technical Information Services, 1982.

Johns Hopkins University. "The Development of a Johns Hopkins University Health Program Alliance." Personal communication, 1977.

Milbank Memorial Fund Commission. *Higher Education for Public Health.* New York: Prodist, 1976.

Monroe, L. B., Tuttle, D. M., and Lorimer, R. J. "Job-Related Activities, Academic Preparation, and Continuing Education Needs of Graduates of Schools of Public Health." *American Journal of Public Health,* 1980, *70,* 70–73.

Moore, F. I., and others. "Anthology of Studies of Public Health Graduates." Paper presented at a conference cosponsored by the Bureau of Health Professions, U.S. Department of Health and Human Services, and the American Public Health Association, Washington, D.C., March 30–April 2, 1982.

Sheps, C. G. "Identifying the Relationship Between Higher Education for Public Health and the Field of Practice." *American Journal of Public Health,* 1980, *70,* 7–9.

U.S. Department of Health and Human Services. *Report of Public and Community Health Personnel.* U.S. Department of Health and Human Services Publication no. (HRA) 80–43. Washington, D.C.: U.S. Department of Health and Human Services, April 1980.

U.S. Department of Health, Education, and Welfare. *Report of the National Commission on Health Manpower.* Vols. I and II. Washington, D.C.: U.S. Department of Health, Education, and Welfare, 1967.

University of North Carolina School of Public Health. "To Serve the State: Division and School Work Together." *The Body Politic,* 1979, *7,* (1).

Welch, W., and Rose, W. *Annual Report to Trustees of the Rockefeller Foundation in the Institute of Hygiene.* New York: Rockefeller Foundation, 1916.

White, P. E., and others. *Graduates of American Schools of Public Health: A Survey of Graduates, 1956–1972.* Washington, D.C.: Association of Schools of Public Health, 1976.

*Howard G. Sachs*
*W. Ann Reynolds*

8

# Graduate Programs in Health Sciences

Graduate education in the health sciences center is a distinct and unique educational entity. To the health professional educator, the way in which graduate education is carried out, the governance of graduate programs, the processes of graduate degree curricular design, and the relative insulation from the intrusion of accrediting agencies, all are anomalies within the academic affairs of the health sciences center. To those familiar with graduate education in the arts and sciences, the unique relationship between the graduate dean and the professional school dean, as well as the interdigitation of graduate faculty and professional school faculty, is viewed with a mixture of curiosity and distrust.

Few educators and administrators in the health sciences are familiar with the roots of graduate education in the United States. Because graduate education has changed remarkably little over the past half century, particularly at the doctoral level, it is important to study its history in order to develop an appreciation of the parallels in evolution of graduate and professional education. While the recent history of medical, dental, and other health sciences curricula has been marked by cyclical trends, experimentation, and a great deal of introspection, such has typically not been the case in the graduate school. The influences of educational philosophy, research in educational methodology, and models of alternative methods of instructional delivery have been felt in the health sciences center but not generally within the graduate programs offered in that arena.

The graduate school in the health sciences center is often ill understood, ill cared for, and in general cast in the role of the stepchild to a family of importance and lineage. The responsibility for graduate programs in the health sciences lies with both parents, the professional school as well as the graduate school. To many, the way in which graduate programs in the health sciences are conceived, delivered, and cared for will seem haphazard, and perhaps even capricious and arbitrary. This chapter seeks to convey an understanding of the forces at work in the health sciences center that shape the destiny of graduate degree programs. A more facilitative attitude on the part of those whose primary responsibilities lie in the professional schools is crucially needed, particularly at a time when fiscal reality and financial exigency come dangerously close. While this chapter does not provide proscriptive advice, suggestions for improvement of the health of the stepchild are advanced.

## Laying the Foundation

In comparison with medical education, graduate education in the United States as we know it today is a relatively recent phenomenon. Prior to the establishment of Johns Hopkins University in 1876, there had been attempts to establish graduate programs at several major American institutions, including Harvard, Michigan, Yale, Columbia, Western Reserve, and Virginia, but for the most part these efforts failed. For those students who had progressed through the typical undergraduate curriculum of Greek, Latin, mathematics, and moral philosophy, with an occasional seasoning of natural science, Europe—France or Germany—was virtually the only direction to travel in search of a research-based graduate education.

The emergence of graduate programs of significance in American institutions can be traced to the founding not only of Johns Hopkins University but also of Clark University in Massachusetts in 1889 and the University of Chicago in 1892. Clark began as a "purer" version of the German model established at Johns Hopkins (Veysey, 1965) and is regarded as the first all-graduate institution in the United States, emphasizing the pure sciences. Of the three most important founding members of the German school in the United States, only Clark soon found itself without any associated program of instruction in medical sciences, although all three institutions had undergraduate programs within a few short years. Medical education meanwhile was evolving along two paths, the freestanding school of medicine and the university-associated school or department of medical instruction. The University of Pennsylvania is credited with establishing the first medical school in the United States, founded in 1765. Harvard College began the instruction of physicians in 1782, and by the mid-nineteenth century there were nearly a dozen university-associated programs of medical instruction. Johns Hopkins was in existence as a graduate, and later undergraduate, institution for only thirteen years before building a hospital; it started medical instruction four years later, thus probably establishing the first academic "health sciences center." From the beginning of the graduate program at the University of Chicago, President Harper had the vision of a major university including a medical school, for he wrote to major benefactor John D. Rockefeller in 1905 that he had not completed his "work," wanting to see the establishment of schools of music, technology, and medicine (Veysey, 1965). However, it was not until 1927 that the University of Chicago could boast of having fulfilled the dream of Harper and established a school of medicine.

The relationship of the medical school to the university is a critical determinant of the success of graduate education in the health sciences. It is worth a small time investment to examine the evolution of the relationship in order to appreciate more fully the present position of the graduate school today.

Few American universities established a faculty of medicine in their original plans. Generally, at the turn of the twentieth century, most would-be physicians were trained at proprietary, nonaffiliated schools. The numbers of such establishments had swelled in the years prior to the Flexner report of 1910, but many were already beginning to suffer financial problems. Stevenson (1967) noted that by 1926, half the schools that had been functioning twenty years earlier were no longer in existence.

Many influences led to the evolution of health sciences centers as parts of universities. William Welch, the great physician who led Johns Hopkins to preeminence, noted in 1907 that "The historical and proper home of the medical school is the university, of which it should be an integral part coordinate with the other faculties" (Stevenson, 1967, p. 22). Welch early recognized the relationship of the health sciences faculty to the graduate faculty and the faculty of the arts and sciences. The Flexner report is most often cited as the landmark that influenced the joining of the medical school and the university, although clearly financial considerations were of at least equal if not paramount importance. Flexner did write that "It is precisely the advantage of university status that while, to accomplish a professional purpose, a professor is a member of a professional faculty, nonetheless, as scientist, he is a member of a university with freedom and incentive to pursue truth in any direction whatsoever" (Eisenhower, 1967, p. 18).

In the early post-Flexner years, proprietary schools closed their doors or merged with each other or with universities. Sufficient income then, as today, could not be derived from student fees to pay for facilities and faculty salaries, much less research undertakings. Further, indigent patients who had no choice but to submit their care to physicians in training quickly became a fiscal burden for proprietary medical schools. New medical schools were not established until 1925. Of the twenty-one medical schools established between 1925 and 1962, all but one began as university-affiliated institutions; the lone independent began as a two-year school and was absorbed into the state system at the time of expansion of the curriculum to four years (Smythe, 1967). From 1964 until 1971, sixteen more medical schools were founded, and in each case the medical school was university affiliated from its inception, which, according to Smythe, "affirms the conviction and is a reflection of the pressures promoting the decision that American medical education is best conducted in a university setting" (p. 995).

### Administration of Graduate Degree Programs

"The presidents and graduate deans of the AAU universities held a symposium on 'The Ambiguous Position of the Graduate School Dean.' Most observers, I think, consider it just as ambiguous after that discussion as before, mainly because ambiguity is inherent in the situation as universities are now organized. Administrative and organizational problems have characterized graduate work so long that most people have become used to them" (Berelson, 1960, p. 119).

As is clear from the preceding brief history of the development of American medical and graduate education, some institutions began with a clear sense of purpose—there was to be a place in the university for graduate work as there was to be a niche for health education. Milton Eisenhower points out that often each was built on a firm foundation and cites a speech by Daniel Gilman, the first president of both Johns Hopkins University and the Johns Hopkins Hospital, who observed that "the advancement of learning and the relief of suffering—the foundations—are set apart . . . There is still a great want to be supplied, an arch to rest upon these pillars" (Eisenhower, 1967, p. 21). The degree to which that arch has been constructed and indeed the manner of its construction vary considerably across the spectrum of academic health sciences centers.

Just under two-thirds (73 of 112) of the academic health sciences centers that offer graduate instruction are located on the campus of a university or are freestanding educational institutions. Within this category, 77 percent of the institutions are true universities, with undergraduate, graduate, and professional programs on the same campus, while 12 percent (nine institutions) are publicly supported health sciences centers, and 10 percent (seven institutions) are private health sciences centers. The manner in which the graduate school interacts with the academic health sciences schools varies considerably. Only in part does the relationship depend on the relative sizes of the units. For example, in the academic health sciences center that consists essentially of a medical school, a hospital, and some associated academic units, such as the graduate school and a nursing program, the dean of graduate studies often also serves as the associate dean of the school of medicine. In the larger academic health sciences centers, those within a university structure, the dean of the graduate school has line responsibilities and does not serve in a staff capacity within any of the health professional units.

Certainly the relationships within the university are not static; there have been numerous changes within the past twenty years or so. At one time, both the dean of the medical school and the dean of the graduate school served in those capacities on a part-time basis. The responsibilities assigned to the respective offices were simpler, and the organizational tree of the university had far fewer limbs. But times change, and within the complex university with a health sciences center, the changes occurring over the past twenty years or so have been profound. Between 1965 and 1975, a new position, that of vice-president for health affairs, has emerged in academic health sciences centers. In 1965, just over half the institutions had such vice-presidencies, and one-third of the vice-presidents also served as dean of the medical school. By 1975, 80 percent of the health sciences centers had a vice-president for health affairs, and essentially only the newest institutions had the same person serving as dean of the medical school (Hogness and Akin, 1977). Similarly, the dean of the graduate school began to take on additional responsibilities, so that today almost all graduate deans serve as dean and chief research officer. The result of these changes has been to make the relationship between dean of graduate studies and the graduate faculty in the health sciences more encompassing and more complicated than it was some ten or twenty years ago.

The administration of graduate programs in a significant number of institutions can be described either as subordinate to the graduate school on the main university campus or as separately administered. Why have some gone to one extreme, while others remain an integral part of the graduate administration on the main (but remote) campus? Analysis of the enrollment data for graduate programs in academic health sciences settings does not reveal a simple answer. Using the data provided by the institutions and published in the *Graduate Programs and Admissions Manual* (Graduate Record Examinations Board and Council of Graduate Schools in the United States, 1981-1983) and the *Education Directory of the National Center for Education Statistics* (1980-1981), several interesting points emerge. Many graduate schools at health sciences centers function as separate schools from the main campus graduate school and yet have enrollments in health sciences of less than 100 graduate students, a number often far less than 10 percent of the number of students in the main campus graduate programs. Conversely, there are many health sciences campuses with hundreds of graduate students where the local administration of graduate programs is by an associate dean or director of graduate studies who is subordinate to the dean of the graduate school on the main university campus. In most cases of the subordinate mode of administration, the health sciences campus is located close to the main campus, and there are only a few where the distance is over twenty miles. Public and private institutions do not differ in this respect; nine public and ten private institutions administer graduate programs in the subordinate mode.

How, then, do we arrive at the diversity of administrative structures? In part the variations are explained by differences in individual institutional history, but certainly the increased responsibilities of the office of graduate dean in the area of research administration have played a role. What once was a part-time position now requires a full-time dean and staff, often including several full-time assistant and associate deans. To a large extent, the burgeoning research enterprise in the academic health sciences center as well as the markedly increased demands for compliance with federal regulations has created the demand for this level of organization in the graduate school. At one time in the history of most academic health sciences centers, there was but one professional school, medicine. The graduate programs associated with the medical school were relatively few in number, being mainly restricted to the basic sciences—such as anatomy, biochemistry, physiology, and microbiology—and the numbers of graduate students in those programs remained small. Growth of the graduate enterprise paralleled the growth of the health sciences professional schools. Dental schools, schools of pharmacy, schools of nursing, allied health, and public health have sprung up, clustered in the health sciences center. This cadre of faculty lobbied for expansion of the graduate programs into their areas of interest, and both the number of programs and the number of students increased. No longer was the graduate deanship a part-time position for a faculty member in the medical school in those institutions where the health sciences center was geographically separated from the main campus or where the health sciences center was on the university campus. These same pressures have been brought to bear on the administration of graduate programs on the "unified" campus, and the health sciences faculty has become a force to be dealt with.

Furthermore, it is not only the faculty of the health sciences nor the graduate dean who have been the strong influences on the development of the graduate school–health sciences relationship. The external accrediting bodies for the health sciences have also had an impact on the graduate programs. For example, the Liaison Committee on Medical Education (LCME), the official accrediting agency in medicine, has stated that "The graduate school of the university may provide assurance that graduate programs conducted by the faculty of the school of medicine will be of a high quality" (Crispell and Vogel, 1980, p. 41). Such influence by vigorous accrediting bodies is also clear in the development of graduate programs in nursing and certain of the allied health fields.

## Relationships Between Professional Schools and Graduate Schools

Within the university there are few more highly charged issues than the manner in which a graduate school selects its faculty and conducts the graduate degree programs for which it was formed. No structural diagram can convey the emotion contained in a colleague's remark: "My salary may be paid by the College of Medicine, but my soul belongs to the Graduate College." David Saxon, president of the University of California, described the problem in his statement that "The arrogance of medical faculties is a bar to genuine interdisciplinary activities, and so is the arrogance of some in the academic world who view their fields as the only truly academic ones and view medical and other professional schools as trade schools" (Saxon, 1976, p. 994). Within the academic health sciences center, it is clear that tensions exist not only vertically between the various health profession faculties, with a resultant "pecking order," but also horizontally between the professional schools and the graduate school.

Does tension between the graduate and professional schools facilitate or impair achievement of the overall educational mission of the health sciences center? Two studies that relate to this issue are that of Charns, Lawrence, and Weisbord (1977), who analyzed the multiple functions of health sciences faculty, and more recently the Kellogg Foundation–supported study of the organization and governance of academic health sciences centers (Crispell and Vogel, 1980), published in three volumes by the Association of Academic Health Centers. In the first study, the authors analyzed the perceptions of medical faculty regarding five functions: undergraduate medical education, graduate degree education, research, house staff education, and patient care. They found considerable blurring in the perception of these functions and substantial differences in the degree of uncertainty surrounding them. Patient care followed by research were the most clearly defined functions, and functions related to graduate education more defined than those related to undergraduate education. The authors concluded that an appropriate organizational model was a matrix in which individuals are responsible both to a department chairman and to different directors for each function they perform. Unfortunately, the study was limited to clinical departments in the school of medicine, and so the perception of the roles of graduate faculty and clinical faculty in other health sciences was not investigated. The study for the Association of Academic Health Centers was more far ranging, encompassing responses from university presidents as well as professional school deans and including several questions about the probability and desirability of certain changes in the academic health center over the next decade. For example, university presidents approved, by a wide margin, the proposal that all Ph.D. degrees be awarded by the graduate school of the university, though they were less confident that this would occur. Deans of medicine regarded such a development as both less desirable and less likely. Here we have evidence of the tension between the academic and professional administration, which probably reflects faculty bias as well. However, not all health sciences deans shared the evaluation made by deans of medicine. Deans of pharmacy schools were more conservative in their responses than either deans of medical schools or university presidents; 97 percent felt that it was most desirable that the Ph.D. be the exclusive province of the graduate school, compared to 62 percent of the deans of medicine. Despite the expectation of most health sciences deans that the number of graduate students in the basic medical sciences would decline within the next decade, these responses reveal the distinct rivalry between the graduate dean and the professional school dean, generally the dean of the medical school, for administration of graduate programs.

This issue of control of graduate programs in the health sciences becomes acute when the subject turns to such programs as the doctorate in nursing or the professional degrees in public health. However, the problem is not restricted to doctoral programs but also has an impact on the training of health personnel at the master's level. Essentially, the debate is one involving the faculty role in program development and operation—and the real question is *which* faculty, the graduate or the professional school faculty.

In the vast majority of graduate institutions, particularly those granting the doctorate, the graduate faculty has been a distinct set of individuals who also share to some extent the responsibilities for professional education. Virtually all faculty in basic science departments within medical schools are members of the graduate faculty, while few in the clinical areas hold graduate appointments. In terms of the analogy of President Gilman of Johns Hopkins, the pillars of professional education and graduate education are set as far apart as the difference between the professional and graduate faculties. The bridge that must be constructed to rest upon those pillars will have different dimensions, depending on the nature of the program to be offered. If we look at the pillars erected on the foundations of biological chemistry in the university and in the medical or dental school, they will be close together, while the engineering problems in spanning the gap between the pillars of clinical nursing education and the graduate school can be formidable. This holds true for the bridges being built between professional education in allied health and the graduate school. For many faculties and many institutions, the solution is to ignore the presence of the latter, not to try to bridge the gap, but rather to stand yet another structure atop a single crowded pillar.

## Graduate Faculty

Two major considerations must be addressed in any graduate program: Who is responsible for its administration, including monitoring of quality, and who is responsible for the delivery of the instruction, be it didactic, seminar, or laboratory in nature? We have already discussed the issue of administration to some extent; however, we will shortly investigate the distinctions between program types and discuss their implications for housing the administration of a program. What concerns us now is the nature of the faculty whose responsibility it is to develop the program of study, deliver the instruction, supervise the apprenticeship of the graduate student, and, finally, certify that the student has passed the minimum standards appropriate to the degree and the field. The graduate faculty is indeed a peculiar beast. While for the most part, the graduate faculty represents a subset of the total teaching faculty of an institution, it often functions in a manner appropriate to a second, distinct collection of individuals. The dichotomy of perceived faculty roles has been studied by Charns, Lawrence, and Weisbord (1977), but these investigators never asked the question in evolutionary terms: How did the two faculties develop?

In the great experiment of the Clark and Johns Hopkins models for higher education, there was no separation of responsibilities, for in fact there was no undergraduate faculty per se. As institutions grafted on the responsibilities for undergraduate education and later yet the responsibility for medical education, it was the graduate faculty that came to be regarded as "the" faculty. Today in many institutions there is a scholarly core identified as the "graduate faculty of arts and sciences," and membership in the graduate faculty of an institution has become an elected position. In the health sciences, one finds considerable variation in the extent to which the graduate faculty coincides with the professional faculty. In some institutions, particularly those in which the graduate programs are exclusively in the basic medical sciences, the graduate faculty is the same as the academic faculty; all faculty in departments that offer graduate programs are able to serve on graduate committees and act as advisers to graduate students. Included in this group of health sciences institutions are a few of the larger health sciences centers as well as many of the centers that arose about an existing medical school.

The predominant model for graduate governance is that based on the university model. Appointment to the graduate faculty is not automatic upon hiring; rather the candidate is required to demonstrate to some constituent group that he or she has the qualifications necessary to carry out the tasks of graduate teaching and advising. A typical example is Ohio State University, where all regular faculty are eligible for appointment to the graduate faculty at one of three levels of appointments, representing different degrees of involvement in graduate program activities. Category I–graduate faculty can teach graduate-level courses, serve on master's committees, and be readers on doctoral dissertation committees. Such faculty must have a terminal degree appropriate to the field and college teaching or professional experience. Category II–faculty can further serve as advisers to master's students and direct master's theses; candidates for this level of appointment must also demonstrate scholarly and research attainments. The highest level, Category III–faculty, can direct doctoral dissertations and must have demonstrated "mature, sustained, independent work in scholarly, research or creative activities" (Graduate School Handbook, Ohio State University, 1981). Another variation on this model is found at the University of Illinois at Chicago Health Sciences Center. Graduate programs at this center are administered by a Graduate College separate and distinct from that on the other campuses of the university. This Graduate College has the reputation of offering what is probably the broadest spectrum of degrees and programs of any health sciences center. Faculty who wish to participate in graduate degree–related activities must be members of the graduate faculty. Two levels of appointment are made: full, with all privileges associated with supervision of doctoral programs, and associate, which allows full participation and supervision of students in master's programs and limited participation in doctoral activities.

In our experience, the multiple levels of appointment to the graduate faculty can serve an important role in the development of faculty, particularly in fields where there is concomitant development of graduate programs. In an area where an institution has not previously offered a master's-level program, a cadre of faculty will have to demonstrate sufficient research productivity to satisfy the appropriate graduate faculty committee that the applicant can adequately serve the new program in a variety of tasks, including course development, student advising, and supervision of theses if there is a thesis requirement. Often this stimulates the professional teaching faculty, individually and collectively, to begin to organize research activities appropriate to the field and, perhaps for the first time in their careers, to publish. In the case of the development of a doctoral program in an area such as nursing, a second factor comes into play: In order to qualify for graduate faculty status for supervision of doctoral students, the faculty must be doctorally prepared. In such areas where there were few doctoral-level programs nationally, faculty are stimulated to enter or complete graduate training in an ancillary area, such as the basic medical sciences, the social sciences, or education. Thus an institution can build a graduate faculty from the existing professional base, and the diverse graduate training of the faculty is often a real asset to the program development process, serving to broaden the base of the new program.

### Graduate Programs: Practice-Oriented and Research-Oriented

It is appropriate at this point to note that there is diversity in the governance of graduate programs not only in terms of the faculty allowed to participate in teaching and supervision but also in terms of the precise administrative unit that is responsible for the program. The particular arrangement depends to a large extent on the nature of the program and the ecological niche its graduates are expected to occupy. Some postbaccalaureate programs are designed to train professional practitioners, while others are established to train teacher-researchers to "push back the frontiers of knowledge."

One group of educators representing both the graduate schools and the accrediting agencies has defined these two graduate program thrusts as follows: "Practice-oriented graduate degree programs, where the primary objective is to train graduate students through the master's or doctor's level as preparation for professional practice directed mainly toward the application or transmission of existing knowledge," and "Research-oriented graduate degree programs, where the primary objective is to train graduate students through the master's and doctor's level as preparation for scholarly or research activity directed mainly toward the acquisition of new knowledge" (*The Joint Statement on Accreditation of Graduate Work* of the Council of Graduate Schools, the Federation of Regional Accrediting Commissions of Higher Education, and the National Commission on Accrediting, n.d., p. 3; quoted in Ohio Board of Regents, 1977, p. 50). To some extent, the difference of emphasis in the two types of programs is reflected in the naming of the degrees, where the research-oriented degree is usually denoted as the master of science, while the practice-oriented degree is often in a named practice area, such as the master of business administration.

In the health sciences, some programs clearly fall into one or the other category, and some bridge the gap. For example, the Ph.D. has been awarded for more than a century in this country in such areas as anatomy and physiology. More recently, Ph.D. programs have evolved in such hybrid fields as biophysics, toxicology, "medical sciences," and bioengineering. Most of the practice-oriented programs in the health sciences are at the master's level, with the master of nursing science as a representative program. Some of the degree programs that have emerged over the past few decades are designed to produce more highly trained health professionals, yet require research activity and serve to encourage future contributions to the "acquisition of knowledge" by their recipients. In this category are doctorates in public health and nursing science. The degree to which research and scholarly creativity are required in any of these programs is largely a function of the faculty who have designed the program and the unit responsible for its administration. Graduate faculties often resist the inclusion of new areas of the health sciences into the traditional portfolio of graduate degree programs administered by the graduate school, even when such new programs require thorough grounding in experimental design and a thesis based on an original contribution to the literature. In some cases such resistance by the entrenched interests has resulted in the assignment of new titles to the degrees, making them resemble practice-oriented programs, or in the reversion of administrative control for the graduate degree program to the professional school or college. Examples can be found in such degrees as the master of associated medical sciences (allied health) and the master of health professions education, both degrees administered by the Graduate College at the University of Illinois at Chicago Health Sciences Center and requiring completion of requirements equal to those for the master of science degree at that institution. In both of these cases, graduate faculty committees agreed that if the early experience with the new degrees proved satisfactory, then a name change to the master of science would be acceptable.

This caution reflects in part the graduate faculty perception that the newly developed degree programs lacked the quality of the master of science degree, despite the fact that a research thesis was required and that special pains were taken to demarcate the boundary between the "high ground" and the new territory. Interestingly, in Berelson's 1960 study, 63 percent of the graduate deans felt that graduate schools had wrongly allowed the master's degree (master of arts and master of science) to deteriorate in quality, and 64 percent of the deans agreed with the statement that the standards of the master's should be restored. Of the graduate faculty surveyed, 41 percent felt the quality had deteriorated, and 52 percent were in favor of restoration of the standards.

In some institutions, all graduate-level degrees are administered by the graduate school, including the master of business administration and the master of social work. However, in the health sciences the assignment of responsibility for administration of a graduate program is often made consistent with the prevailing policy in a field. Such is the case with the professional degree of doctor of public health, often administered by the school of public health. Generally, however, the faculty that supervise the Dr.P.H. students in their studies also act as advisers and dissertation mentors to Ph.D. students in public health. It is questionable whether this division of responsibility is made in the best interests of the education of the student.

## Developing Graduate Programs in New Areas

The preceding section has touched on the problems confronting an academic unit seeking to develop a new graduate program. We can examine the situation in greater detail by referring to several cases: graduate programs in the basic sciences at developing medical schools, the development of doctoral programs in nursing, and the emergence of graduate programs in a variety of allied health specialties.

*Basic Sciences.* As new medical schools were founded in the past few decades, the faculty teaching the basic sciences to the medical students were also expected to develop research programs as part of their responsibilities. In fact not only did their own promotion and tenure depend to a significant extent on the mounting of aggressive research programs, but also the accreditation status of the college became dependent on the success of those research endeavors. Furthermore, in some of the teaching areas, as the number of medical students grew above a token level, the load placed on faculty in terms of student contact and contact hours became an argument for hiring nontenure track assistants. What better, inexpensive labor than the graduate teaching assistant? Even in those states or regions where there were more graduates in the basic sciences than could be accommodated by the job market, pressure has been brought to bear on the administration of the institution, as well as on state agencies responsible for overseeing higher education, to approve new graduate programs in the basic medical sciences. In the *Higher Education in Ohio Master Plan: 1976*, the Ohio Board of Regents (1977) states that "Considering existing factors, the Board of Regents believes that Ohio's current graduate programs are largely adequate to produce the needed graduate-trained personnel at the Ph.D. level over the next several years," and yet also wrote that "The Ph.D. programs being developed for the new medical schools . . . are perceived as falling within the category of those which can be approved" (p. 62). Often the basic science departments are too small to justify individual Ph.D. programs in anatomy, physiology, and the other disciplines, and so there has been the formation of programs leading to a Ph.D. in basic medical sciences, with a combined faculty adequate to qualify as a critical mass.

*Nursing.* The development of the doctorate in nursing is largely a story of the last two decades. In *A Guide to Graduate Study* (Ness, 1960) prepared for the American Council on Education, there is only one entry under nursing—the University of Pittsburgh. Between 1955 and 1959, only two Ph.D. degrees were awarded in that program. Over the intervening twenty years, there has been a slow but steady increase in the number of programs and graduates, so that in 1979, 101 doctorates were awarded by a total of twenty-five programs in nursing or nursing education (Vaughn, 1980). Comparing the periods of 1975–1977 and 1978–1980, there was an overall increase of over 50 percent in doctorates awarded, and every program showed an equal or increased number of graduates in the second period (graduate programs reporting data to the Educational Testing Service, and reported in the *Graduate Programs and Admissions Manuals*, 1979–1981 and 1981–1983). One-third of the programs award a professional degree, usually the doctor of nursing science, while the rest lead to the Ph.D. The number of programs is clearly increasing, and nursing is one of few areas in the health sciences where there is currently a demonstrated critical need for doctorally prepared graduates. There has been an almost explosive increase in the demand for nurses trained beyond the master's level to serve as faculty, not only in the almost 400 baccalaureate programs in nursing but also in the 127 master's programs, and to act in a broader range of capacities within the health care delivery system. The increase in demand has not been met by the slow but steady increase in both the number of programs and graduates at the doctoral level. Thus, a number of institutions that for years had trained nursing graduates only to the master's level are now in the process of developing doctoral programs, presenting university administrators with critical resource allocation and faculty development problems.

Graduate degree programs are costly enterprises. The very nature of doctoral work, with its heavy emphasis on small seminar classes and the intense expenditure of time on the adviser-student relationship means that doctoral instruction on a per-student basis is many times more expensive than baccalaureate instruction. An institution needs to assess carefully not only the cost of delivery of instruction but also the costs entailed in supporting thesis and dissertation research. There are probably few, if any, examples of institutions that have mounted doctoral programs with adequate resources. This is certainly particularly true of nursing. Morris (1980), in one of the position papers on academic health center governance commented that "Nursing in the academic health center demonstrates, in a collective sense, many of the characteristics of a developing nation" (p. 158). Development of doctoral programs in nursing clearly requires reallocation of resources, not only with the budget of the nursing educational unit, be it school or college, but also significant largess on the part of the university or health sciences center. The graduate school must also play a supportive role and back that position with available funds for graduate student research support.

While not playing down the magnitude of the financial resources needed to support a new doctoral program, even when built upon an existing master's program, perhaps the most crucial problem facing units embarking on a doctoral program in nursing is that of sufficient faculty resources. Doctoral programs need doctoral faculty and in a field such as nursing, where for many years the master's was the terminal degree, there are simply too few nurses with the necessary credentials. Some of the existing faculty obtained those degrees in nursing, but the majority received their doctoral training in the social sciences and education. The nurse-scientist training program of the sixties and early seventies added doctorally trained nursing faculty in the biomedical sciences. However, the number of faculty fall far short of that required. At Ohio State, for example, official school records indicate that only 26 percent of the regular faculty in the School of Nursing have doctorates.

Nor will adding doctorally trained nurses to the teaching faculty alone solve the problem. As indicated earlier, attainment of graduate faculty status commensurate with that required to direct doctoral dissertations generally requires that a candidate present evidence of research and scholarly productivity. A recently completed study on nurse faculty development in the Midwest by McElmurry (1982) reveals the extent of this problem. Few nursing faculty have full-time research positions (3 percent) and while 73 percent indicated that they had some research involvement, less than half of those spent as much as 40 percent of their time on this endeavor. The data on research productivity are even more startling:

only 25 percent of the respondents in the survey indicated that they had been an author or coauthor of a research publication (McElmurry, 1982). In contrast, 77 percent of those with a doctorate in biological sciences in 1947–48 published one or more titles other than the dissertation within the next eight years, and 51 percent of those who had received their degrees in education had published papers (Berelson, 1960). The most distressing observation by McElmurry is that "Our bias is that the Midwest nurses may actually be quite productive scholars when their publication rates over time are compared to other regions" (p. 3).

Despite the strains created by restricting the number of faculty, maintenance of requirements for admission to the ranks of the graduate faculty can serve a positive function in faculty development. For example, at the University of Illinois productivity of the nursing faculty in terms of publications increased dramatically within a few years, when the graduate faculty as a whole elected to maintain classes of faculty membership. In the long run, such selective pressures will cause many of the doctorally trained faculty who have never published to venture forth and submit manuscripts. This is critical if the faculty in these emerging programs are to serve as successful role models in performing and publishing their research.

*Allied Health Specialties.* The situation with programs in allied health is somewhat different. (Fields of study administered under allied health vary considerably from one institution to another. The definition used here is restricted to such areas as physical therapy, occupational therapy, medical records administration, medical illustration, and similar programs; it does not include such areas as medical care administration, which could be included in allied health in one institution and in public health in another.) The major problems in establishing graduate programs in this area are the omnipresent limited resources and the reorientation of the faculty to the differing conceptual bases of undergraduate and graduate education. While it is difficult to say exactly how much more it will cost to operate a program with both graduate and undergraduate thrusts, the total and true costs are generally underestimated by the faculty and administration. Rarely does one find such a thorough analysis of instructional costs as was done at the University of Pennsylvania in examining the future of the School of Allied Medical Professions. Langfitt (1980) wrote of the process that led to the closing of the school: "Everyone had agreed that master's programs were necessary in order for the school to continue its position of eminence in allied health. The establishment of master's programs plus other improvements would result in a 50 percent increase in the direct expenses of the school. Since long-term federal or state funding of the programs was unlikely, and there was little chance that the school could raise significant sums of money from private philanthropy, it was clear the university would need to reallocate unrestricted funds to the School of Allied Medical Professions from other units" (p. 227). The cost of developing graduate programs in allied health is clearly a major factor in limiting their numbers. In 1969, there were only eighteen schools with graduate programs in the area of occupational therapy or physical therapy; of these, seven offered occupational therapy only, and six gave degrees only in physical therapy. Eleven years later, in 1980, the number had reached a modest twenty-eight, with an increase of six schools in physical therapy only and four with programs in both physical and occupational therapy.

Few programs have developed in recent years with the ambitious goal of simultaneous emergence of graduate tracks in occupational and physical therapy, medical illustration, medical laboratory technology, and human nutrition. This was the case several years ago at the University of Illinois at Chicago Health Sciences Center, and the lessons learned are useful for anyone interested in the problems of faculty development—one of the important "hidden costs" in developing graduate programs in allied health. In all the areas just mentioned, the School of Allied Health (later renamed the College of Associated Health Professions) had strong existing undergraduate programs. All the allied health tracks in this new degree program sprang from a core of course work that all graduate students were to take. The necessary approval of the courses by the Graduate College came after approximately nine months of close cooperation between the core teaching faculty from allied health and a committee of the Graduate College, with representatives from both the basic sciences and other graduate programs in the professional health sciences. Only a few faculty had earned doctorates but, as the terminal degree in the field had been the master's, some of the existing faculty could qualify for admission to the graduate faculty if they could provide evidence of scholarly activity and previous involvement with graduate students. However, developing a critical mass of qualified graduate faculty to direct thesis research in the research-based master's of associated medical sciences proved to be a major hurdle. As students began enrolling and taking core courses in health team theory and other areas preparatory to choosing advisers and initiating the thesis portion of the degree program, three related concerns arose almost simultaneously: What topics would be appropriate for graduate thesis work, who was to advise the students, and how would the research be paid for?

There was nothing unique in these problems—they face all developing graduate programs; nor were any unique solutions developed. What did happen was that the administrations of the allied health school and of the graduate school united in a commitment to help support the research programs in allied health from limited Graduate College discretionary funds, and in a concerted effort to develop an awareness in the primarily baccalaureate-level teaching faculty that they *could* do research, that they *could* publish in peer-reviewed journals, and that there were ample opportunities within the health sciences center to develop collaborative research programs capable of generating outside funding. The dean of the allied health unit also made it clear to his faculty that promotion and tenure decisions in that unit would be determined in large part by the ability of the faculty to rise to the new challenges. And rise they did! Within two years following the initiation of the degree program, the faculty were holding research forums and publishing with considerably increased frequency. Further, a significant percentage were being appointed to the graduate faculty, including election to membership on the executive committee of the Graduate College. The message here is that such an effort could only be successful when the graduate school, the school of allied health, and faculty from all over the health sciences center worked to raise the level of a primarily baccalaureate-oriented teaching faculty to that expected by the research-oriented, and largely doctorally trained, graduate school faculty. There would have been little faculty development, and ultimately slippage in the reputation of the allied health programs at all levels, if the graduate school had capitulated to those who sought "grandfathering" of the existing teaching faculty into the graduate faculty.

## Physician-Researchers and Graduate School

Within the past decade, there has been heightened awareness of a problem in our medical school faculties: fewer physicians are interested in the practice of academic medicine in the context of traditional forms of promotion and tenure. The problem has reached crisis proportions in some schools and departments. As faculty come up for tenure action, there is an increasing tendency to evade or erode the criteria for performance in one or more of the areas of teaching, clinical service, and, most importantly, research. Several medical schools are now exploring alternative staffing models that would allow for maintenance of the professional ranks but in a clinical track that might not be a tenure-accruing one.

The involvement of the graduate school, until recently, has been circumspect. As indicated earlier, the study by the Association of Academic Health Centers (1980) revealed that many medical school deans think it highly desirable that house staff have the "status" of graduate students, and from time to time the suggestion has been made that all residents be registered through the graduate school within the university or the health sciences center. This recommendation is heavily influenced by the widespread belief that graduate student status will obviate employee status and head off the specter of unionization. For the most part, such suggestions have fallen on deaf ears at the graduate school. However, it is clear that within the next decade the graduate school will need to become involved in the problems of clinical departments in medical and dental schools and to devote significant energy, and possibly resources, to the training of physicians in the art and science of research. This will have to come about through efforts on at least three fronts: reconsideration of the M.D.–Ph.D. programs nominally available at the majority of medical schools, involvement in postdoctoral research training for some residents and faculty members, and review of the existing programs in the clinical medical specialties. Bickel and others (1981) have taken the position that federal intervention is required to solve the problem. From 1968 to 1980, there was a slow and steady decrease in the number of National Institutes of Health postdoctoral traineeships, and concomitantly the number of physicians in this program declined from just over 4,000 to under 1,750, with new trainees accounting for approximately half the total each year. However, there is little information regarding the retention of those trainees in research after conclusion of the training period. The authors felt that a more productive program was the federally supported medical scientist training program, which assists medical students to complete a Ph.D. program in concert with the medical degree. However, there is no evidence to support the contention that this program serves to increase the pool of medical researchers five or more years after completion of the degree programs, a time when the retention of medical faculty with demonstrated promise as researchers begins to have an impact on the medical school. Wyngaarden (1979) has advocated an increase in the number of federally funded postdoctoral fellowships for M.D. and M.D.–Ph.D. graduates as a means of increasing the number of clinical investigators. All the evidence he presents shows that there is little difference in the grant-getting powers of the M.D.–Ph.D. or the M.D. when compared to the Ph.D.-only recipient. Furthermore, it is only in the attainment of research career development awards that the M.D. appears to be at a disadvantage in terms of number of grants awarded, while other categories, such as the Young Investigator Awards, are made in approximately equal numbers to the Ph.D., the M.D., the D.D.S., and the applicants holding a professional degree plus the Ph.D.

In short, there is little to suggest that the entire problem lies with federal funding; the medical profession must also be regarded as an accomplice to the problem. Singled out for criticism by Wyngaarden is the American Board of Internal Medicine. It is the board's policy, requiring consecutive years of clinical practice during postgraduate training, that has constrained the young physician from seeking intensive research experience. Certainly the diplomate boards must address themselves to the problem of the quality of the research faculty in clinical medicine, but it is also a responsibility of the medical and dental school and the graduate school, acting in concert. New programs should be developed that are appropriate to the discipline, as well as the institution. Faculty who want to embark on research careers, as well as engage in clinical practice, should be encouraged to do so by the departments, and financial incentives must be in place so that the clinical researcher is not at a hopeless competitive disadvantage in salary considerations. It is mainly the opportunity to do research that keeps specialists in remunerative fields such as cardiovascular surgery, neurosurgery, plastic surgery, and gynecologic oncology in the fold of academic medicine. Thus, adequate funding in support of research from *any* source is probably the most critical issue in encouraging the young physician to choose academic medicine.

We are convinced that funding sources are available for the academic clinician-to-be that have not yet adequately been tapped. These include private donors, often interested in major disease entities such as diabetes and cancer, and the pharmaceutical industry, for whom research in the clinical setting is of paramount importance. We have found that residents in surgical specialties were willing and outstanding laboratory instructors in gross anatomy, where experienced teachers are in short supply. Salary supplements for such teaching are legitimate in most universities, and since the time required is predictable, such teaching is compatible with research.

Flexible approaches to research training must be developed by graduate schools. The incubation period of the researcher is a long one and must continue under a succession of mentors. A one-year experience in the laboratory is good initial exposure for fostering germination of the clinical researcher but must be followed by subsequent supervised and collaborative experiences in the research arena.

Many universities and health sciences centers have in place graduate programs in such fields as surgery, medical sciences, radiology, and other medical or dental specialties. Many of these programs are moribund, and should be. For the most part, a one-year program of research and course work cannot accomplish much beyond a superficial view of the research laboratory. There is little time for the development of a research topic independent of an ongoing program, and almost certainly no time for the productive education that comes from the analysis of research failures or for the output of the published paper. Graduate schools that still have such degree programs on the roster would best initiate program review in the hope that a viable alternative would emerge that would better serve the needs of the medical community. We desperately need fresh, creative approaches to developing research expertise in clinical faculty, both through formal course work on experimental design and via laboratory experience in planning and performing a research project. This is a subject that the American graduate school has studied and refined over the past hundred years, and this proven experience should be brought to bear on the problem at hand.

## Program Review

For most health professions educators, program review experience has been associated exclusively with the accreditation of the professional degree programs, as for example, conducted by the Liaison Committee on Medical Education in reviewing the programs leading to the M.D. degree. Programs of study leading to the master's or to the doctorate have also been reviewed as part of the accrediting process for professional baccalaureate programs, and leaders in the field of nursing are very much aware of this aspect of program review. The same situation is true in the review of allied health programs, and in one area, biomedical illustration, the accrediting body has indicated to the institutions that offer both baccaluareate and master's-level instruction that after 1983, the accrediting process will only be carried out for programs leading to a master's degree. However, most graduate faculty have been relatively isolated from the review processes and immune from the effects of review except as it directly influences their instruction of professional degree candidates. Nevertheless, program review of graduate programs is upon the horizon for most programs and has already begun to affect some institutions. Pressure for program review activity has come from within the institution and also from the state regulatory agencies for higher education. While the history of informal program review dates back to the early formalization of the university, it is only within the past ten to twenty years that most institutions have formalized their review processes, sometimes of their own volition, and not occasionally, under threat of state-mandated and -conducted review of programs receiving state support.

In the late 1970s, for example, the Illinois Board of Higher Education began to consider seriously program review in selected areas of higher education, including nursing programs. And in Ohio, the Board of Regents noted in their 1976 Master Plan (1977): "In the state system of higher education, the Board of Regents helps assure quality through the process of program review . . . Over the past few years, the board has become more active in weighing questions concerning the need and possible duplication of programs at the graduate . . . level(s) . . . The board therefore recommends that each state institution of higher education begin a review of its programs on a five-year cycle and report its findings to the board" (p. 35). In the cases cited here, the state regulatory agencies did not establish a prescriptive formula for the review process. The issue of a state-mandated process has, however, raised the sensitivities of at least one well-respected group of educators, the Carnegie Commission, who spoke to the issue in their 1980 report (Carnegie Council on Policy Studies in Higher Education, 1980). Said the members of the panel: "We are doubtful about state-mandated review of academic programs. We believe such review is better conducted by the institutions themselves . . . we question the wisdom of this great intrusion into academic affairs" (p. 124). Whether institutions of higher education are in favor of review or not, for the state-supported schools it is a fact of life in the eighties and beyond.

Financial considerations weigh heavily in this reality, and the same reality faces the private institutions. We have already cited the case of the review of the School of Allied Medical Professions at the University of Pennsylvania (Langfitt, 1980), and others are sure to exist.

The review processes employed by departments within medical schools have been examined in a comprehensive survey by Smythe and others (1979), who report that 60 percent of the medical school deans responding indicated that there was a departmental review procedure in place, and 70 percent of these used such a process on a regular cycle rather than on an ad hoc basis. It is interesting that only 6 percent of the deans regarded the primary purpose of departmental review as a university-based evaluation of the work of the medical school. The most prevalent purpose indicated was to serve in the evaluation of the status or performance of the department, while approximately equal numbers of respondents felt the primary purpose was to evaluate the performance of the incumbent department chair or to review objectives and goals. A further important point emerged in follow-up interviews, in that many of the faculty and chairmen felt that departmental review was an intervention initiated to investigate perceived weaknesses in the quality of faculty work.

Universities that have initiated program review structured on too narrow a basis usually soon discover that the self-imposed restrictive review is less than satisfactory. This was the case with the review process formerly employed at Ohio State (Poland and Arns, 1978), when the emphasis was exclusively on graduate programs. In the revised set of processes, the entire spectrum of functions of the educational unit is considered. For example, in the Ohio State model, almost fifty reviews are either in process or completed, and the units reviewed include departments, schools, colleges, research institutes, and even one scholarly journal.

The basic questions posed in program review vary somewhat from institution to institution. For example, the essential issues in the Ohio State reviews are (Poland and Arns, 1978, p. 2):

- Who are we?
- What do we do?
- How much does it cost?
- Why do we do it, and what do we seek to accomplish?
- How does what we do relate to why we do it?
- What difference does it make whether we do it or not?
- How well do we do it?
- What is needed to make what we do more valuable, or to help us do it better?

While at Stanford, the basic issues are reduced to four (Miller, 1980, pp. 206-207):

- Is the program academically important?
- Is there now, and will there continue to be, student interest?
- Can we, as an institution, be outstanding at this program?
- Can the program be securely funded?

Each institution, or for that matter, each review, may need to establish a list of relevant questions to serve as a framework on which to build the review process.

Experience with program review in the health sciences suggests that one cannot effectively evaluate a graduate program in isolation from the other activities of the unit responsible for the administration of the program. For example, in a department of pathology, there is an interaction between the service and educational programs; not only does the department serve in training medical students and house staff, but it may also have post–M.D. and postbaccalaureate students in a Ph.D. program. Furthermore, a department of pathology is a clinical service unit, with anatomic and microscopic pathology service functions and, often, responsibility for the hospital clinical laboratory operation. There is mixing of faculty responsibilities, sharing of resources, and, often, resource reallocation within such a department. Thus, it is worth the effort for any effective program review process in health sciences departments to be as comprehensive as possible.

Graduate education in the health sciences is changing, and institutions should actively employ some form of program review to adapt to present conditions and to prepare for the next decade. The curriculum in medical education has shifted away from a reliance on laboratory experiences in the preclinical years, so that in most schools only anatomy has a full complement of teaching laboratories (anatomists have always been masochists!). This has meant a decrease in the number of graduate teaching assistantships available to the basic science departments to use in attracting graduate students. More and more, funded researchers are being asked to put graduate student stipends on grant monies. In addition, the infamous federal circular A–21 from the Office of Management and Budget has placed tuition waivers in the category of direct cost rather than the indirect cost pool. In short, graduate programs are in a more critical condition than ever, and program review processes that lead to a concrete set of resolutions and actions can be helpful. In the Ohio State model, for example, a Memorandum of Understanding is signed by all relevant parties to assure that some action will eventuate. These could take the form of a proposed merger of small, duplicative units or reorganization within a department. Other programs, such as those in allied health, public health, or nursing, might be capable of sustaining an expansion, and a plan of action could be formulated under program review that would serve to assure the allocation of necessary resources.

Program review might establish that there are needs for graduate-level programming offered in a format different from the traditional master's or doctoral program of study. For example, many health professionals want access to the courses offered in a graduate program but may not want to take them for degree credit. Program review undertaken jointly by the Office of Continuing Education and the Graduate College at the University of Illinois at Chicago Health Sciences Center in 1979–80 led to the establishment of a mechanism to allow students to enroll in graduate-level courses in one of three ways: for credit to be applied to a degree program, for graduate credit on a nondegree basis, or for continuing education credit. The program was established in 1980, and during fiscal year 1981 almost 100 students had registered. For fall 1982, registrations reached well over 100 for that quarter alone. Clearly, here was an unfilled need that was effectively dealt with following program review.

We earlier discussed the crisis in clinical research and mentioned the ill health of the master's programs in specialties such as surgery. Institutions with such lingering programs would be well-advised to undertake a comprehensive review of their offerings. The situation at Ohio State, which has master's programs in anesthesiology, medicine, obstetrics and gynecology, ophthalmology, pediatrics, physical medicine, psychiatry, radiology, and surgery is illustrative: Only six students in all were enrolled in these programs in 1981. One high-quality program designed to train clinical researchers would surely serve the interests of both the professions and the institution far more effectively.

## Summary and Conclusions

The graduate school is a unique entity within the health sciences center, for it is the only unit that has degree-granting responsibilities and no paid faculty. The emergence of the American graduate school and the evolution of the relationships between the graduate school and the health professional schools have been described as a basis for understanding the status of the graduate school today. We have attempted to present a picture of the diversity of graduate administration models in place at universities and health sciences centers and to develop an appreciation of the roles played by the graduate dean and the graduate faculty. Despite the rich history and fertile territory for educational research, little evidence of critical studies is found in the literature. Some scholars have studied the organization of responsibilities and the governance of graduate programs as part of the overall health center environment, but there is little in the way of research into curricular design or program development. Perhaps one reason this is so is that graduate schools and graduate faculties appear to resist change to a greater degree than almost any other educational unit. The ritual for obtaining the doctorate today differs little from that of a century ago, and yet the areas of specialization have indeed changed with the times.

Increasingly, graduate deans and faculty are faced with mandated review of programs. The next decades will bring changes in the composition of student populations and the economics of higher education. Program review that takes the long view and that studies the graduate programs as integral functions of units in the health professions can help to revitalize graduate work. New program formats may well emerge in the next few years. The graduate school acting in concert with the health professional schools has the potential for reinvigorating clinical research. The stepchild on the health center campus may yet lead the way to the promised land.

## References

Association of Academic Health Centers. *The Organization and Governance of Academic Health Centers: Presentation of Findings*. Washington, D.C.: Association of Academic Health Centers, 1980.

Berelson, B. *Graduate Education in the United States*. New York: McGraw-Hill, 1960.

Bickel, J. W., and others. "The Role of the M.D.-Ph.D. Training in Increasing the Supply of Physician-Scientists." *New England Journal of Medicine*, 1981, *304*, 1265–1268.

Carnegie Council on Policy Studies in Higher Education. *Three Thousand Futures: The Next Twenty Years for Higher Education*. San Francisco: Jossey-Bass, 1980.

Charns, M. P., Lawrence, P. R., and Weisbord, M. R. "Organizing Multiple-Function Professionals in Academic Medical Centers." In P. C. Nystrom and W. H. Starbuck (Eds.), *Prescriptive Models of Organization*. Amsterdam: North Holland Publishing, 1977.

Crispell, K. R., and Vogel, L. L. "University–Health Center Relationships: A Reappraisal." In K. R. Crispell and T. W. Langfitt (Eds.), *The Organization and Governance of Academic Health Centers: Position Papers*. 3 vols. Washington, D.C.: Association of Academic Health Centers, 1980.

Eisenhower, M. S. "An Arch upon These Pillars." *Journal of Medical Education*, 1967, *42*, Part II, 11–21.

Hogness, J. R., and Akin, G. C. "Administration of Education Programs in Academic Health Centers." *New England Journal of Medicine*, 1977, *296*, 656–663.

Langfitt, T. W. "Management of Change: Closing a School." In K. R. Crispell and T. W. Langfitt (Eds.), *The Management of Change in Academic Health Centers*. Washington, D.C.: Association of Academic Health Centers, 1980.

McElmurry, B. J. Unpublished abbreviated final report, Division of Nursing, Public Health Service–supported, Grant no. NU 25030, 1982. (Mimeographed.)

Miller, W. F. "Institutional Policy Setting: A Dynamic View." In W. K. Frankena (Ed.), *The Philosophy and Future of Graduate Education*. Ann Arbor: University of Michigan Press, 1980.

Morris, A. L. "Interschool Relationships in Academic Health Centers." In K. R. Crispell and T. W. Langfitt (Eds.), *The Organization and Governance of Academic Health Centers: Position Papers*. 3 vols. Washington, D.C.: Association of Academic Health Centers, 1980.

Ness, F. W. *A Guide to Graduate Study: Programs Leading to the Ph.D. Degree*. Washington, D.C.: American Council on Education, 1960.

Ohio Board of Regents. *Higher Education in Ohio Master Plan: 1976*. Columbus: Ohio Board of Regents, 1977.

Poland, W., and Arns, R. G. "Characteristics of Successful Planning Activities." *Planning for Higher Education*, 1978, *7*, 1–6.

Saxon, D. "Is the Medical School a Proper Part of the University?" *Journal of Medical Education*, 1976, *51*, 991–995.

Smythe, C. M. "Developing Medical Schools: An Interim Report." *Journal of Medical Education*, 1967, *42*, 991–1004.

Smythe, C. M., and others. "Departmental Review in Medical Schools." *Journal of Medical Education*, 1979, *54*, 284–293.

Stevenson, L. G. "The University and the Medical School." *Journal of Medical Education*, 1967, *42*, Part II, 22–32.

Vaughn, J. C. "Educational Preparation of Nursing—1979." *Nursing and Health Care*, Sept. 1980, pp. 80–86.

Veysey, L. R. *The Emergence of the American University*. Chicago: University of Chicago Press, 1965.

Wyngaarden, J. B. "The Clinical Investigator as an Endangered Species." *New England Journal of Medicine*, 1979, *301*, 1254–1259.

# 9

*Edwin F. Rosinski*

# Curricular Trends

## Critical Review and Analysis

Reviewing curriculum developments in the health professions of medicine, nursing, pharmacy, and dentistry, and some of the research associated with these developments from the late 1950s to the 1980s is a formidable task. Screening the findings from the literature and organizing them into a logical sequence is even more demanding and difficult. Nevertheless, a pattern of events that shaped curriculum development and research over time does evolve. It begins with the ferment of the early 1960s, when the die was cast for curricular modification. This was followed by the emergence of governmental, student, faculty, philanthropic foundation, and other interest groups whose roles and influence on the educational goals of the health professions became increasingly significant. The third period reflects a confluence of forces exerting pressure for curricular modification. Finally, the period of the mid-1970s can probably best be described as a period of cumulative additions of specific courses and activities. In this chapter, the curricular changes in health professions at each of these periods are described, their implications are examined, and the future course of action in curriculum development and research is considered.

### Period of Ferment

By the end of the 1950s, ferment in health professions education had almost become a way of life. In nursing, the move to collegiate programs had begun. In pharmacy, the transition from four- to five-year programs was accelerating. In medicine, organization of subject matter by body (organ) systems was gaining popularity. In dentistry, the use of chairside assistants and the emerging influence of preventive dentistry was prompting a critical review of educational objectives. To those involved in health professions education at that time, it appeared as if every institution was engaged in some curricular modification, either requiring a major revision or some minor adjustment in course sequence or content.

*Medicine.* Probably because medicine was perceived by many to be the most traditional in its educational outlook, it received considerable attention when changes in its educational programs began to occur. During the 1950s and early 1960s, several major medical schools initiated a curriculum that encompassed both preprofessional and undergraduate professional education; other medical schools experimented with teaching comprehensive care. Case Western Reserve introduced the concept of organizing the curriculum according to body (organ) systems, while the State University of New York at Buffalo (the University of Buffalo) focused its attention on improving the quality of teaching through its Project in Medical Education (Miller, 1980). Many of these revisions in medical education and accompanying educational research are succinctly described in a monograph published by the Association of American Medical Colleges (Lee, 1962).

A number of medical schools subjected curricular revisions to considerable study. For example, Boston University in 1961 selected a group of students and allowed them to combine their undergraduate education with medical education in a six-year sequence. Fifteen years later, a report (Lanzoni and Kayne, 1976) revealed that, except for differences in scores on the Medical College Admissions Test and National Board of Medical Examiners Test, students following the two tracks were no different. Because so much attention was focused on these six-year programs, many of them were closely monitored. A recent literature review (Daubney, Wagner, and Rogers, 1981) of many of the articles and research on these programs concluded that there were few significantly distinctive characteristics of the students in these programs; the programs could be called "successful."

The fervor of curriculum reform in the United States slowly spread to Europe. While integration of the basic and clinical sciences was also taking place, many European medical educators focused on improving the quality of teaching while at the same time developing curricula that offered both the M.D. and Ph.D. degrees. In reviewing some of the European trends, Tysarowski (1968) points out that, unlike the United States, in some European medical schools changes in curriculum were mandated by national law, while other schools did not have the flexibility or authority to innovate. Also, he notes that there was less emphasis placed on the role of research related to curriculum revisions.

Through the early 1960s, the trend accelerated. Existing medical schools continued to change their curricula and the new medical schools being created, such as at the University of Connecticut, the University of Arizona, and the University of New Mexico, to name only a few, began to develop eclectic curricula that embodied not only significant changes in the format of the curriculum but also in the content and in the organization of the faculty to teach that content. It got to the point in the early 1960s that it was almost impossible to keep up with the changes being instituted in medical education. Although most of the literature at the time dealt with descriptions of those changes, there was a paucity of data justifying them or documenting their effects. There were probably as many ideas on how to reform medical education as there were faculty, and as the ranks of medical school faculties were being supplemented with social and behavioral scientists, those disciplines were gaining a foothold in medical education and playing a role in curriculum development. The influence of those disciplines had major effects on the curricula of the medical schools at the Universities of Kentucky, Florida, and Oregon. By the end of the sixties, the social and behavioral sciences had exerted significant influence in medical education; yet, data on the results were in short supply. When in 1969 an international seminar ("The Social Sciences in Medical Education," 1970) was held on the social sciences in medical education, there was little hard evidence to back up the argument that medicine could be enhanced if the following courses were introduced into the curriculum: social sciences as a unifying concept of behavior, human development, human response to illness, communication, organization of medical care, and problems of society and man. A review of any contemporary medical curriculum will reveal the presence of all or some of these courses, with little justification given for their presence other than that they appeared appropriate.

Curriculum reform, however, did not sail on a smooth sea. In some schools, reform and modification were initiated by decree, and faculty involvement was minimal. Many of these changes met stiff resistance and, in some cases, quickly reverted once there was an administrative change. Other medical schools had to contend with faculty who were satisfied to rest on past laurels and continued to espouse conventional attitudes on medical education. The lack of leadership often stymied efforts, and as noted by Rosinski (1971), this was more common in new medical schools where curriculum had a lower priority than many other activities. Still other schools failed to define their institutional goals so that curriculum reform became a piecemeal operation, often leading to educational discontinuity and dissatisfaction among students and faculty. Furthermore, curriculum revision was an expensive undertaking, and until the middle and late 1960s, the federal government did not have the authority to support medical schools in their quest for improving the quality of medical education. Fortunately, the vision of such philanthropic foundations as the Commonwealth Fund, the Rockefeller Foundation, the John and Mary R. Markle Foundation, and the National Fund for Medical Education, to mention a few, made it possible for several schools to progress with their curricular revision and research. Many schools, on the other hand, did not have the benefit of extramural funds to undertake such changes. Finally, some schools encountered difficulty because they tended to equate the improvement of the teaching/learning environment with curricular modification. In many cases, the high expectations of change in the curriculum did not produce an appreciable change in student and faculty attitudes. Perhaps the one medical school that continued during the first five years of the 1960s the legacy established at the State University of New York at Buffalo with its emphasis on pedagogy, rather than curricular change, was the University of Illinois.

The question will always remain in medical education: If more research had been conducted on the teaching/learning process, would as many schools have embarked on the option of major curricular revisions?

*Nursing.* During the late 1950s, curricular developments in nursing education were not as radical as in medicine. Nursing's primary concern was the upgrading of the quality of nursing education, especially through a dramatic development of baccalaureate and associate degree programs. In 1960, there were 69 associate degree programs; only four years later there were 174 ("Educational Preparation for Nursing," 1966). But perhaps the real change in nursing education can be seen in another set of data, which revealed that, in 1957, there were only two accredited associate degree programs in the country ("A Report on Progress in Nursing Education," 1958). The quest for upgrading nursing education continued to be a major goal of nursing educators throughout the 1960s. This desire occurred for many reasons, but it was evident that the ranks of nursing would have to be bolstered by more baccalaureate nurses if the upgrading was to occur. A startling report in 1956 (Division of Nursing, 1957) estimated that of approximately 430,000 nurses, 91.7 percent held *no* degree. Faced with such shocking information, it is no wonder that nursing educators were more concerned about the quality and respectability of their educational offerings than with innovations in existing curricula.

The transition to baccalaureate and associate degree programs, however, met considerable opposition from many nursing educators and administrators who defended the status quo. The literature published at that time brought to the forefront many of the arguments for and against change. Erne (1966) pleaded to reduce the vehemence of the arguments and suggested that an orderly transition of nursing education into institutions of higher education take place. As Erne states, it appears that every twenty-five years or so an idea comes to nursing that, because of its importance, either draws together or divides the profession. In spite of professional conflict, changes in nursing curricula were taking place, and research was being done on those programs. Research on students, faculty, cost of education, and the like (Davis, 1975) reveals the concerns of nursing educators as the transitions were being made.

Perhaps the most significant changes were being made in the baccalaureate curricula. A review of the literature during the early and middle 1960s clearly indicates that some of the changes paralleled those in medical education. Among them was the increased emphasis on the psychosocial aspects of nursing and organizing the curriculum according to the body (organ) system approach. Similarly, additional science courses were being introduced, not only to keep pace with developments in medicine but to enhance further the academic background of nurses who planned to pursue higher degrees.

Two other factors played an important role in curriculum development in nursing at that time. One was the academic background of many of the nurses in leadership positions. Because many nursing educators had advanced degrees from schools of education, educational courses were common, not only in graduate nursing education but also in the baccalaureate programs. The popular argument for this was that since many graduates of the baccalaureate programs would themselves be assuming positions of leadership in nursing education, they should have a strong background in education. Critics of this trend countered with the need for a "discipline of nursing" based on science and technology with a strong psychosocial orientation toward patient care. An interesting by-product of the leadership being educated in graduate schools of education was that most of the research produced by schools of nursing was a reflection of what was being done in schools of education. A corollary to this was that schools of nursing were especially sensitive to the development of educational or learning objectives that enabled some of them to evaluate their curricular changes.

Another important factor that played a role in curriculum development was the emergence of physician assistants being trained in medical schools or under other auspices. Initially, nursing looked on this new type of health worker with suspicion, but eventually it became evident that the role of the nurse could be modified to assume many of the responsibilities assigned to physician assistants. This, in turn, required some curricular modification that will be described later in this chapter when the issue of conflicts among the health professions is considered.

*Pharmacy.* The history of pharmaceutical education is long and troubled, but by the late 1950s, a pattern of education began to emerge that, while it still stirred controversy, reduced its vehemence. In one of the most informative and erudite studies on the history of pharmacy, Mrtek (1976) sheds light on many previously obscure issues and brings into focus an appreciation for the conflicts and turmoil that accompanied the development of pharmacy education. Mrtek makes it quite evident that pharmacy, like all the other health professions, did little research related to curricular reform, and that what was produced was spotty and inconclusive.

Perhaps the greatest change in pharmacy education was the increased emphasis on the basic sciences in therapeutic counseling. In addition, by the early 1960s, there was a strong move toward the pharmacist's greater participation in health care as a member of the health team. At that time, a number of pharmacy educators (Apple, 1961) were concerned that public health was not receiving attention in the pharmacy schools, while others (Parks, 1967) cited the need for innovations that included courses in pathology, greater emphasis on clinical pharmacology, and courses on professional practice. Some of these were, indeed, incorporated in many curricula, but the conflict between schools of pharmacy graduating dispensing pharmacists and those graduating pharmacists concerned with total care continued. At a meeting of the American Association of Colleges of Pharmacy, the deans of pharmacy were encouraged (Rosinski, 1968) to redefine their educational goals, develop a curriculum to meet those goals, improve the quality of pharmacy education by being more sensitive to the learner, provide varied career opportunities, and develop a new type of pharmacist known as the clinical therapy consultant. What finally began to emerge in pharmacy education was a curriculum that prepared the graduate pharmacist to be the manager of all drug-related resources, to be a professional responsible for drug counseling, to be a drug consultant to other health professionals, and to be responsible for the chronically ill who depend on proper medication. All of this was accompanied by a move to lengthen the curriculum and to include more basic and medical sciences, as well as social and behavioral sciences.

Even these more recent curricular developments were not all met with enthusiasm. There were some medical educators who thought that the clinical pharmacist was intruding into professional areas that were the concern of the physician. There were pharmacy educators who continued to support the dispensing pharmacist as the only legitimate role. The issues surrounding clinical pharmaceutical education and practice were frequently on the agenda of professional meetings to the point where they were the subject of an invitational workshop

("Proceedings of the 1971 Invitational Meeting," 1971) at which deans of pharmacy, physicians, nurses, and pharmaceutical and hospital administrators tried to resolve some of the issues.

In a personal communication in 1981, Warren Weaver, dean of the School of Pharmacy at the Medical College of Virginia in Richmond, said: "The last four-year graduates finished in 1963. Enrollments in the mid-sixties were down . . . some pharmacy educators lost sight of the mandate of the five-year program, which was to put more liberal arts, social sciences, and humanities in the programs . . . Along came the 'clinical' concept, plus the need to incorporate the experiential into the five-year program. With all of this there were people saying that the five-year programs never were fairly evaluated and the six-year programs still need to prove themselves." Once more, in another health profession, curricular reform took place and continued with little, if any, evaluative or research data.

*Dentistry.* Curricular reform in dental education was neither as extensive nor as intensive as in the other health professions. This may have been attributable to the educational goals of dentistry that were more oriented to psychomotor skills or to the attitudes of dental educators, many of whom in the late 1950s were still only part-time clinicians devoting a considerable portion of their time to private practice. While there were some attempts at curricular modification, they consisted mostly of adding or rearranging courses. However, by the end of the 1960s, some significant changes began to occur, many motivated by developments abroad. In England (Allred and Slack, 1968), dental education was altered by such influences as epidemiological studies, the teaching of advanced skills, and patient attitudes. The London Hospital Medical College Dental School embarked on a major curricular reform and did what was unheard of in dental education by creating an educational research unit that provided evaluation and research data on what future modifications should be. Also in Europe, a major conference ("Undergraduate Dental Education in Europe," 1970) reviewed most of the issues facing dental education. These included the organization of dental schools, admission of students, use of auxiliary personnel, and the importance of public health, including epidemiology, biostatistics, behavioral sciences, and the organization of public health services.

Slowly the pattern of dental education began to change. Perhaps the initial motivating factor was the emergence and widespread use of chairside assistants. These included not only dental assistants, who were viewed as "another pair of hands," but also dental hygienists who provided limited direct patient care under supervision. In the case of some experimental programs, such as the one at the U.S. Public Health Service Dental Manpower Training facility, Louisville, Kentucky, they were the dental equivalent of the physician assistant and provided limited primary dental care (Lotzkar, Johnson, and Thompson, 1971). The use of these new types of personnel modified the role of the dentist, and, consequently, required the curriculum to change to satisfy this new role.

But other curricular changes were also beginning to occur. At Harvard, dental and medical students attended the same basic science courses, with faculty unaware of who were the dental and who were the medical students. At the new dental school at the University of Connecticut, the same approach as at Harvard was initiated but extended to include other conjoint educational experiences. At the Universities of Kentucky and Oregon, which had influential groups of social scientists engaged in the health professions, the social and behavioral sciences were introduced. At Howard University, some fifteen major components of the curriculum were revised (Henry and Sinkford, 1974), with special attention placed on improving the teaching skills of the teachers. Still other schools attempted to copy some medical curricula by reorganizing according to the body (organ) system approach. The importance of preventive dentistry became so paramount that dental educators were forced into critically reviewing their educational programs. The role of preventive dentistry and patient attitudes and the varied background of dental students prompted one dental educator (Oaks, 1970) to make a strong appeal for even greater reform in dental education. Finally, a study (Brown, 1976) on dental education in the United States was sponsored by the Council on Dental Education of the American Dental Association.

In 1981, William Feagans, dean of the School of Dentistry at the State University of New York at Buffalo, an individual with a distinguished career in medical and dental education and administration, offered an excellent summary of key dental curriculum developments in a personal communication to the author. He listed these as preventive dentistry, introduction to patient care earlier in the curriculum, the trend toward providing total patient care, increased awareness of the total health of patients, increased productivity through the use of assistants, integrated basic sciences, trend to full-time faculty, greater flexibility in course offerings, and the influence of the social and behavioral sciences. Unfortunately, even to a lesser degree than medicine, nursing, and pharmacy, dental educators did little to support their curricular reforms and modification through evaluative or research studies.

 *Reaching a Plateau.* By the beginning of the 1970s, the fervor for curricular reform and modification began to subside. An editorial in *Science* magazine (Stetten, 1968) at that time cautioned against new names for old courses and emphasized that what was important was not curricular revision but the dedication of teachers and the enthusiasm of students. Nevertheless, changes continued but, in general, at a more moderate pace. This more cautious approach resulted from the fact that in the late 1960s, a number of problems, directly and indirectly related to curricular reform, began to emerge.

One of these was the increased frequency of "town-gown" conflicts. As more full-time faculty were hired, part-time teachers saw themselves threatened and viewed many of the programs under which they were educated as being "corrupted." At the Medical College of Virginia, where major reform was taking place in the medical school, the conflict between the medical educators and private practitioners became so public and vehement that it almost prompted an investigation of the curriculum changes by the state legislature (Rosinski, 1976). Practicing nurses complained that the baccalaureate programs were losing sight of the ideals of nursing, while dental practitioners and dispensing pharmacists complained that dental and pharmacy educators were moving too fast with reform and modification. In the presence of such hostile attitudes, many deans decelerated their curricular efforts.

Still another reason for not initiating major changes in some schools was the absence of faculty commitment to the endeavor. Without a doubt, getting involved in the curriculum was a time-consuming activity, an activity that would require a reordering of faculty priorities, a reordering that many were unwilling to make. Then, too, curriculum revision inevitably altered the status quo, and there were always some individuals who felt insecure with impending change. Without faculty commitment to change, even minor curricular revisions were most difficult to achieve. A corollary to the lack of faculty commitment was the lack of dynamic leadership. Even a cursory review of the schools that were involved in a searching analysis of their programs revealed that there was always one individual present who provided the leadership and was able to get the faculty committed to the undertaking. Such a person was the spark that ignited others and was able to fill in when others began to falter. Many schools, unfortunately, lacked individuals with this kind of commitment and dedication.

Then, too, faculty were not always in complete agreement about what was transpiring. Most of the efforts to integrate the basic and clinical sciences failed because of continued vested interest in how a subject should be taught or even whether it should be integrated at all. Basic scientists often saw the earlier introduction of patient care as merely another intrusion into their teaching time. Many clinical faculty saw electives as a poor use of time that could more profitably be devoted to core courses. As new disciplines were added to the faculties, competition for time in the curriculum grew. With conflicts among faculty arising with greater frequency, agreement on curricular change became more difficult. Furthermore, faculty and administration were occasionally at odds about the goals of curricular change. Some deans saw themselves as not being "tuned in" to the times unless their schools were engaged in curricular change. Frequently, however, faculty did not share such deans' enthusiasm for change, and both subtle and obvious stumbling blocks to change were placed in the way. Conversely, faculty were often eager to get involved, while the dean saw the ferment in curricular reform as a fad. As a result, some schools reached a standoff between the dean and faculty, with only minor, cosmetic changes in the curriculum.

Nor were legislators always enthusiastic about the reforms taking place, especially in state-supported institutions. Vested interests were heard to complain that no longer were generalists in medicine and dentistry being graduated, there was too much emphasis on the specialties, university-educated nurses were not interested in taking care of patients, and neighborhood pharmacists would disappear. When politicians spoke and threatened budgets, it was natural that caution would prevail in educational reform.

There were other reasons for not initiating major changes after the first decade of frenzied activity. After several schools embarked on their new curricula and others tried to copy them, it became obvious that it was an expensive enterprise, especially if evaluation and research were to be part of the modification. Most schools did not have the funds to support such an activity, and it was not until the middle to late 1960s that the federal government made grants available to improve the quality of education in the health professions. Furthermore, the few philanthropic foundations that supported curriculum changes and studies had fully committed themselves to the pioneering efforts that had already demonstrated their value. Clearly, a lack of funds prohibited many schools from engaging in curricular change, with its accompanying evaluation and research.

But without a doubt, the major reason for not initiating major changes was the lack of data, including data from other schools on the effects of the change, to support the argument that a change was needed. Especially damning was the absence of any pre- and postevaluation of a major curricular revision. The pioneering effort of Case Western Reserve in changing its medical school curriculum was copied by numerous other schools, but there was no objective evidence that the "new" curriculum was any better than the "old" one. The only medical school known to design and carry out a major pre- and postevaluation (Rosinski, 1976) did not have data available until the early 1970s because of the way the study was designed. Considering that faculty in the health professions are immersed in the scientific approach, it is no wonder that many were reluctant to change their educational programs in the absence of data to support that change. Change for the sake of change was not a convincing argument.

During the early 1970s, another educational phenomenon occurred that had a stifling effect on curricular change, and it is probably best described as a growing conflict about institutional objectives within academic health centers. This phenomenon could be seen, for example, in the conflict between training physician assistants and nurse practitioners. In an international symposium (Pitcairn and Flahault, 1973) dedicated to the training of physician assistants, arguments were repeatedly made that physician assistant training programs were not necessary because nurses could fill those roles as well if given additional training. The same arguments could be heard on many campuses, and it was the rare institution (Fowkes, O'Hara-Devereaux, and Andrus, 1979) that trained both groups of practitioners in a combined program. Nursing educators were cautioned (Schlotfeldt, 1976) not to become involved in such institutional arguments but to assume leadership for stimulating learning and research in nursing education. Nevertheless, conflicts persisted in many institutions, and these in turn had an adverse effect on curriculum change. Not only were there intrainstitutional arguments about the role of the physician assistant and the nurse practitioner, but arguments were heard on the conflicts that can arise between the role of the physician assistant and the physician. In the first descriptive book (Rosinski and Spencer, 1965) on the international use of physician assistants, considerable attention was given to the potential conflicts that can arise in the training of physician assistants. This was further substantiated (Sadler, Sadler, and Bliss, 1972) after several programs got under way in the United States. However, whenever studies (McCally, Sorem, and Silverman, 1977) were undertaken to examine the roles of the physician assistant, the nurse practitioner, and the physician, clear distinctions were evident. Nonetheless, intrainstitutional arguments continued that directly and indirectly had an effect on curricula.

Although not as vehement, similar arguments were being made regarding the education of clinical pharmacists (pharmacy) and clinical pharmacologists (medicine) and dental assistants and dentists. As the question of the role of each health professional was argued, it had its fallout on the educational programs, including specific courses and content of courses. In summary, the conflict in institutional goals about who should be educated and what should comprise that education had an effect that precluded many significant developments in curriculum revision and reform.

## Emergence of New Interest Groupings

The doldrums in educational activity in the health professions were broken in the middle and late sixties by the emerging influence of governmental, student, faculty, foundation, and other interest groups. Among these, the role of the federal government was, without a doubt, the greatest since it assumed primary responsibility for increasing the supply of health manpower, and no school in the health professions was untouched by its influence.

*Federal Government Influence.* One of the most significant developments at that time was the availability of federal funds to develop three-year curricula in medicine and dentistry. Schools were given financial incentives to develop these three-year programs, and many immediately became engaged in necessary curricular modification. Other schools combined undergraduate education with professional education (Pritchard, 1976; Campbell and DeMuth, 1976), while others (Green, 1970) embarked on converting their previous two-year schools of basic sciences to full-fledged medical schools. Tufts, one of the first dental schools to convert to a three-year program ("Tufts Dental School to Initiate Three-Year Degree Program in 1972 by Operating on a Twelve-Month Curriculum," 1971) did so with strong faculty support and planned to evaluate the results of the new program. However, a great opportunity to evaluate and compare two dental schools in close geographic proximity, one—the University of the Pacific—taking the option to develop a three-year curriculum (Redig, 1976), the other—the University of California at San Francisco—taking the option to remain a four-year program (Pavone, 1976), was missed. The deans of both schools gave convincing arguments as to why they selected a particular option but offered no data to support the programs and, even more unfortunate, had no plans to evaluate or compare results.

The federal role in the health professions was evident in other areas at the time. Funds were made available not only to train physician assistants but nurse practitioners as well. As many of these programs got started, some educators with vision saw the opportunity to study these programs and the roles the practitioners played. One such study (Andrus and others, 1977) demonstrated the effectiveness of nurse practitioners as teachers in a family medicine program, while another (Stillman and others, 1978) described the use of nurse practitioners in teaching physical examination skills. Because of the availability of federal funds not only to initiate new programs but also to evaluate them, research findings and evaluative studies were reported with increasing frequency.

Another significant development brought about through federal initiative was the creation of new medical schools. These new medical schools were located in a variety of settings, ranging from the traditional university to community-based schools capitalizing on local human and physical resources. Curricula in these schools took various forms with the proponents (Evans, 1973) of the community-oriented schools arguing that their programs contributed to better health care and were more responsive to the needs of society. Some of the new schools designed elaborate evaluation schemes, but data from these evaluation efforts are yet to be made generally available.

Not only was the federal government involved in the expansion of health manpower but also in developing ways to make more efficient use of that manpower. Specifically, for the first time, funds were made available for research in health professions education. For example, in nursing, comparisons between types of programs and types of curricula were made (Kaiser, 1975; Farley, 1978). In dental education, studies on how to educate dentists were not uncommon (Rose and Escovitz, 1974). In addition, the health team was garnering attention, and studies were directed toward improving interdisciplinary teamwork (Mazur, Beeston, and Yerxa, 1979).

Still another significant development during those years was the federal government's commitment to primary care, that is, the education of the family practitioner and non–family medicine internist. Vast sums of money were made available for the education of these types of practitioners, with curricula and residency programs developed or modified accordingly. So much attention was being focused on primary care that a supplement to one of the issues of the *Journal of Medical Education* was dedicated to primary care and medical education (Hudson and Nourse, 1975). One spin-off from this interest in primary care was a series of studies that examined rural settings for medical education and contrasted them with university-based experiences (Johnson and Haughton, 1975; Garrard and Verby, 1977).

Still one other federal intervention had an impact on curricula in the health professions, and that was the emphasis on recruiting students from varied social and economic backgrounds. With greater cultural diversity in the student body, curricula in many schools were modified to benefit from this expanded and diverse student population. In nursing, deTornyay (1976) emphasized the need for curricula to be responsive to cultural diversity, and the journal in which deTornyay's editorial appeared was devoted to describing curricular models to implement the cultural diversity. Similarly, medicine examined some of the ethnic and social-cultural issues in medical education ("Medical Education and Minorities," 1978), and numerous programs were initiated that were geared to the diverse student body now attending medical schools.

*Other Influences.* In addition to the federal government, there were other forces that also had an impact on health professions education at that time. One of these was the steady state in the physical expansion of university medical centers. In both private and state-supported institutions, funds were becoming limited for physical growth and "off-site" clinical facilities were sought for the education of students. Pharmacy began to make use of community hospitals (Whitmore, 1970), nursing began to develop a whole series of outreach programs (Love, 1978), and medicine began to evaluate the educational activities in which medical students engaged at multisite clinical clerkships (Kettel and Vanselow, 1978). With the expansion of health maintenance organizations (HMOs) at university medical centers, the educational function of the HMOs had to be examined (Kalinowski and Ackerman, 1973).

Further conspiring to influence curricula in the health professions was the decreasing number of patients seeking medical care at university medical centers, while at the same time there was a corresponding increase in student enrollment. With fewer patients available, other learning resources had to be sought out or developed. Consequently, such things as simulators, patient management problems, skills laboratories, and the like were being utilized with increasing frequency. Perhaps one of the greatest values of the use of these new techniques was that they permitted more objective evaluation of students' clinical judgment and performance in a course (Sherman and others, 1979; Ruffman, Tobias, and Speedie, 1980).

This was also a time marked by greater student and faculty concern for "relevance" in the curriculum, as manifested in many different ways in each profession. Dentistry had finally become so aware of the importance of preventive dentistry that guidelines for inclusion of it in the dental curriculum were established (American Association of Dental Schools, 1980). Problem solving received so much emphasis that in some schools the entire curriculum was problem based (Bandaranayake, 1980). Because the composition of the student body was shifting and because student career goals were being established earlier, curricula were being developed that offered students options or tracks. In nursing, many of the schools that formerly had a student body of middle-class, white female students now had a population of some males, married older women, ethnic minorities, and low-income individuals. With such diversity, curricula had to be developed that permitted students to select a particular option or track (Stevens, 1971). Several medical schools developed second tracks that permitted greater use of patient problems and integrated the basic concepts of the biomedical, behavioral, and social sciences (Echt and Chan, 1977).

Faculty and students were also influential in increasing the amount of free time students had in the curriculum and increasing the availability of electives, partly in response to the diverse career goals of the students. One curricular development that had a great deal of promise but was never fully implemented was the concept of a core curriculum in which students from *all* the health professions in a university medical center would participate. While it was attempted in several universities, it apparently has taken hold in only one—King Abdulaziz University, Saudi Arabia (Basalamah, Rosinski, and Schumacher, 1979).

Still another area in which faculty and students, with governmental encouragement, had some influence on the curriculum was in the use of community resources. While some students and faculty saw this move as motivated by greater curricular relevance, it was also necessitated by a shortage of facilities and patients. As already indicated, the proponents gave convincing arguments for the value of these settings (Evans, 1973), but perhaps some of the research findings did more than anything else to encourage the further use of these external sites (Gordon, Hadac, and Smith, 1977; Johnson and Haughton, 1975; Garrard and Verby, 1977). Not only was the use of rural sites and community orientation indigenous to the United States, but in many developed countries, dentistry was placing strong emphasis on community dentistry, health planning, and preventive dentistry (Nasir and Woo, 1980).

Accompanying the use of community resources was the early exposure of students to patients. While some of the comprehensive health clinics established in the mid-1950s did permit students, especially medical students, to obtain this experience, greatest strides in this direction were made during the late 1960s. As pharmacy students were becoming more patient-oriented, some schools developed courses in patient communication (West, 1975), while in dentistry, the suggestion was made that students work as dental assistants in the first year of the curriculum, with greater opportunities to work in the basic sciences throughout the entire curriculum (White, 1971). The desire to develop curricula that provided earlier patient contact was so infectious that even in France, not noted for its curricular reform, schools were giving students early exposure to patients (Mensh, 1967).

One of the more idealistic goals of curriculum reform in the 1950s and 1960s was the integration of the basic and clinical sciences. In fact, integration of the basic and clinical sciences had been a long-held goal (Sanger and Hurd, 1946), but there was little evidence of how it was to be accomplished or what were the consequences of that integration when it did occur. As recently as 1980, the American Association of Colleges of Pharmacy devoted a significant portion of its annual meeting to a series of presentations on how the gap between the basic and clinical sciences could be bridged ("Proceedings of the 1980 Annual Meeting," 1980). Though the dichotomy between the basic and clinical sciences was not as great in nursing, curricular efforts were also being made there to "integrate" the entire curriculum. As often has been the case in the health sciences, curriculum change and reform progressed more by enthusiasm than by documentation. In the case of nursing, Levine (1979) suggested caution in jumping on the bandwagon of the integrated nursing curriculum, and she warned that "during this time of accountability it is hard to believe that a curricular plan could be so widely accepted and implemented and so scantily documented" (p. 46). She further lamented the general lack of curricular evaluations.

*Foundation Support.* Even though the federal government was playing an increasing role in the health professions, there were certain educational areas that were not receiving financial support. There was still a need for support to develop even more efficient curricula, better and more thorough evaluation of existing programs, and health services research, including the role of health policy decisions in medical education. Fortunately, as they had done in the past, a number of philanthropic foundations entered the scene and began to provide funds for a number of these activities. The appeal of foundation support was that fewer restrictions were placed on how the funds were to be used; therefore, health professions educators had greater leeway in what they could do to further improve the quality of the education programs. With foundation support, some schools focused on the organization of the curriculum, others introduced new courses like health economics, while still others developed such things as family practice sites that could be used for patient care and teaching. Often the foundations' efforts were so successful that subsequent federal legislation permitted federal support of similar activities.

Perhaps the one single activity at that time that drew the greatest attention and held out the greatest promise for health professions education was health services research. The ultimate goal of health services research was to bring down the cost of health care by conducting research related to every aspect of health care, including education. In a comprehensive review of health services research (Flook and Sanazaro, 1973), its importance to health professions education was considered and recommendations were made as to how its role could be widened. The importance of health services research to medical education was further noted when the *Journal of Medical Education* devoted a full issue to the subject, with several authors suggesting its importance to the curricula of the health professions ("Teaching Quality Assurance," 1976). By the late 1970s, there were so many activities related to health services research that a special work group (Magraw,

Fox, and Weston, 1978) on health professions education and health policy was formed to suggest more productive approaches for future studies.

*Influence of Major Curricular Modifications.* With the federal government exerting its influence, with students and faculty becoming more involved, with the physical expansion of health sciences centers in a steady state, with student enrollment and composition of the student body changing, with philanthropic foundations supporting unexplored areas, and with numerous other forces exerting their influence, it is interesting that most of the curricular changes in the health professions were minor; only occasional exceptions are worthy of special note.

In medicine, perhaps the most significant curriculum development took place at McMaster University in Canada in 1969. This new school instituted a tutorial program that was completely oriented toward problem solving, encouraged independent learning, and made extensive use of teaching/learning resources. Hamilton (1976) cites the advantages as being the following: Learning is active, students learn to deal with problems, it allows for individual learning differences, and integration of the basic and clinical sciences is accomplished. He lists the problems as being: Free time is limited, faculty at times tend to dominate the teaching/learning sessions, and occasionally faculty "slip back" to traditional approaches. Campbell (1970) attributed the program's success to the diversity of the student body and continuous revision in teaching. Still another review (Neufeld and Barrows, 1974), written after the program had been in operation for five years, attributed its success to the continuous evaluation by students, integrated learning, and comprehensive educational planning. It is a program that has probably been examined by more educators than was Case Western Reserve some fifteen years earlier, and it had the advantage of planning considerable research on the curriculum before the program began, as well as while it was in operation.

Halfway around the world, a similar novel approach to medical education was taking place at the medical school in Newcastle, New South Wales, Australia. In planning the curriculum, the dean (Maddison, 1978) cited some deficiencies current in medical education; interestingly, Maddison's criticisms were almost identical to those voiced thirty years earlier by Sanger and Hurd (1946). These included, among others, lack of provision for individual differences, being too vocationally oriented, and incorporating too much detail in the curriculum. As one medical student saw it, the program embodied the scientific approach to medical problems, teamwork, self-learning, development of professional characteristics, and early patient contact (Colditz, 1980). As a member of the faculty saw it, its success could be attributed to faculty and student cooperation (Clarke, 1978). While several other medical schools, notably the new ones, were introducing innovative curricula, the ones at McMaster and Newcastle stand out because their design was such a radical departure from conventional thinking. They drew considerable attention and, of course, criticism. To their credit, both schools early on developed a strong research and evaluation program to monitor their programs continuously and to make appropriate changes.

In nursing, several major reforms were also taking place. Many schools had already developed programs for career mobility, allowing registered nurses to obtain baccalaureate degrees. Perhaps the more significant curricular innovation since the development of the baccalaureate degree, and the one that received the greatest attention, was the program leading to a combined baccalaureate and master's degree that offered a university course of study to graduates of associate degree programs. The graduate degree was especially appealing, since it permitted many students to pursue specialty training in such fields as nurse practitioner, surgical nursing, and the like. Furthermore, the extended program provided a broader-based education emphasizing the basic, clinical, and social/behavioral sciences.

Pharmacy continued its conversion to a professional doctorate degree, with heavy emphasis on the pharmacist as a therapy consultant on the use of drugs. Because student enrollment in all the health professions was increasing, many schools of pharmacy developed community affiliations and evaluated them in detail. In one elaborate study, a surprisingly large number of students—81 percent—thought their rotation through a community hospital was the best learning experience they had encountered (Campbell, 1975).

Despite these examples of major curricular change, most modifications were minor; others were merely cosmetic. Throughout, however, there were those who were averse to any change. For example, Nicholls (1980) warned London's medical schools against change and suggested that they remain small, give a solid basic science education keeping the basic and clinical sciences separate, and be cautious of integration "for it creates more problems than it solves" (p. 429). In a more moderate vein, Sheldrake and others (1978), in a comprehensive study of medical education in Australia, recommended no radical changes but suggested that slow, rational change, change responsive to the health needs of the people should determine the organization of the curriculum, its content, and how medical education is administered.

## Confluence of Forces—Change by Accretion

By the middle and late 1970s, there appeared to be a confluence of forces exerting pressure for curricular modification, albeit minor, while at the same time urging reappraisal. Perhaps the era can best be described as marked by the involvement of pressure groups, each with a vested interest in a portion of the curriculum, and each claiming that its particular interest, specialty, discipline, or course would enhance the entire curriculum. Curricula in many of the health professions became a series of cumulative amplifications, characterized by the addition of specific courses and activities. At times, the additions had a compelling logic to them; in other cases, it was difficult to see why a particular addition was made to the course of study. With some humor, but obvious seriousness, Abrahamson (1978) saw the inherent problems in curricular change and noted quite accurately that the term *curriculum* is often equated with courses, hours, and the like.

Be that as it may, the number of changes in curricula brought about by the addition of new courses was impressive, and some were evaluated with remarkable thoroughness. Perhaps the earliest of these changes was bioethics. Although it was first introduced into medical school curricula, it spread rapidly to all of the professions and often was treated and taught as an interdisciplinary subject. What made bioethics an especially appealing subject to students was that it often used case studies extensively, avoided didactic lectures, and introduced a relevance that students often found missing in many required courses (Fromer, 1980). Where bioethics began as an elective, it quickly gained a niche as a required course with a strong clinical orientation.

At about the same time that bioethics was emerging, so was sex education, or human sexuality as it soon became designated. The pioneering programs at the University of Pennsylvania and the University of California at San Francisco had strong evaluation components. As other schools began to develop their own unique courses, evaluation and research related to them became even more important (Lamberti and Chapel, 1977). Again, in many university medical centers human sexuality was offered as an interdisciplinary course and received enthusiastic support. It appears that one of the reasons that bioethics and human sexuality were so thoroughly evaluated was that many of the programs initially received extramural financial support, and the agencies and foundations supporting the programs required that they be evaluated. Often a full-time evaluator was hired to design and carry out the studies.

Another development, although one that did not have an immediate impact on health professions education, was the emerging role of health policy groups in a number of medical centers. These groups were amalgams of medical economists, anthropologists, sociologists, health planners, lawyers, bioethicists, and the like who, working with physicians, nurses, dentists, pharmacists, and public health individuals, began to address some of the critical issues in the delivery of health care. As noted earlier, a national group was formed that made recommendations that, hopefully, would result in more productive future research on which more rational policy decisions could be made (Magraw, Fox, and Weston, 1978). As health policy groups began to develop on some of the major campuses, their influence began to be felt in many of the curricula in the health professions. Indeed, as health needs began to be projected into the future and recommendations made on how those needs could be met, health professions educators began to respond to those projections.

In the 1970s, a significant portion of our society became quite conscious and concerned about good nutrition. This carried over to students in the health professions, many of whom became actively involved in making nutrition a specific course in the curriculum. While many health professions educators argued that nutrition was adequately taught in other existing courses, such as biochemistry, students and indeed some faculty insisted that it be included in the curriculum as a separate course. The most persistent arguments were made by medical and dental students since nursing had apparently long recognized the importance of nutrition, including the cultural, economic, and religious factors that influence nutrition, as part of the nursing curriculum (Newton, 1960). Adding to the argument was a study that determined that nutritional knowledge of medical students was, at best, modest (Podell, Gary, and Keller, 1975). Within several years, as the subject of nutrition either became an elective or was expanded into an existing course, it was often offered or presented as an interdisciplinary course.

In the 1970s, others in our society were concerned about alcohol and drug abuse, later expanded and classified under the rubric of substance abuse. While alcohol abuse was a concern of some health professions educators as early as the 1960s, it was not until the decade of the seventies that most health professions schools felt a social responsibility to deal with the issues. In some programs, it was offered as an elective, while in others it was taught by the department of pharmacology or the school of pharmacy as part of an existing course. Unlike nutrition, it tended not to be taught as an interdisciplinary course but rather as a subject geared to the needs of a specific health profession. Pokorny, Putnam, and Fryer (1978) found in a survey of U.S. medical and osteopathic schools that the number of hours devoted to teaching about drug abuse and alcoholism ranged from 0 to 126.

Although some new medical schools, Pennsylvania State University at Hershey an excellent case in point, established humanities departments, it was not until the 1970s that more schools saw the need for expanding the humanistic base of the health professions. However, no distinct pattern emerged as to how the humanities were included in the curriculum or were taught. For example, in one department the consideration of some human issues was designed around extracts from classic literary works (Moore, 1976). Here it was not intended as a literature course but to help students appreciate human behavior as relevant to the study of medicine. That the humanities in the health professions did not evolve in a single characteristic pattern, as did so many other courses, is perhaps attributable to the fact that there was no body of knowledge that could be identified as the humanities. Furthermore, faculty involved in the humanities included historians, philosophers, theologians, and many others who, working with their health professions counterparts, molded the humanities in the curriculum according to their own particular disciplines. The differing roles that the humanities play in medical education, for example, are well described by Self (1978), who argues convincingly that the background and orientation of the individual responsible for teaching largely determines what comprises that content. There are no data on how many schools of the health professions include the humanities in their curricula, probably because the way the "subject" is taught makes it impossible in many cases to identify it as the humanities. Its influence, however, is felt in many schools.

Occupational and environmental health was still another addition to the curricula of the health professions, largely motivated by public attitudes of the seventies. Although dentistry had earlier recognized the importance of prevention and the impact of the environment on dental health, the other health professions did not as immediately respond to the need to include the topic in the curriculum. Medical schools had been teaching toxicology for many years, but the contemporary issues related to occupational health and the environment required new approaches to defining the content of the subject and how it was taught. Once more, in many schools it was included as an expansion of an existing course or as a totally new one. The one characteristic that appeared to unify the teaching of the subject was that it placed heavy emphasis on prevention, and in some cases that was the major theme (Wegman and others, 1978).

Death and dying, a common occurrence at university medical centers, was often viewed as a taboo subject in medical school curricula, with the nurse often delegated to deal with the terminally ill patient and his or her family. The role of the nurse in dealing with death has been reported from different perspectives, including that of a psychiatrist (Renshaw, 1979). Perhaps because of the strong psychosocial and bedside teaching orientation of nursing, nursing curricula had a long history of dealing with the subject. Medical education, on the other hand, began to face the issue in the 1970s, and a review of the literature on the subject reveals that it was not until that time that it began to be included in the curriculum. A survey in 1976 revealed that forty-four medical schools offered minicourses on death and dying, while forty-two reported offering a lecture or two (Schachter, 1979). Characteristic of so many other courses added to curricula at that time, the nature of the presentation of courses or lectures on death and dying varied considerably. A survey done in 1975 and again in 1980 indicated that most often a team approach was used, with some theologian or clergy present. Most of the courses on the subject were offered during the clinical years, although one medical school taught it during the first year, in connection with a course in anatomy (Marks and Bertman, 1980). Though long established in the curricula of nursing schools, it was not until the 1980s that death and dying finally became part of the curriculum in a majority of medical schools.

Including medical economics as a subject in many curricula was an outgrowth of the development of health policy programs previously described. Many of the early efforts to include a medical economics course were unsuccessful, but when cost containment became a national concern, including it in medical and dental curricula spread. By 1979, approximately 34 percent of all the medical schools in the United States had programs under way or planned, and most of these had been initiated since 1977 (Hudson and Braslow, 1979).

Perhaps because the federal government has a high health priority on aging, the topic attracted individuals from various disciplines. At first, most educators and practitioners were reluctant to classify aging as a distinct and separate entity that could be studied, but as more social and behavioral scientists became involved in research and teaching on aging, the educators and practitioners began to take notice and give attention to this dynamic and critical issue. Again, nursing educators led the field, though the topic was handled in many different ways— among others, by integrating gerontological content in a course on adult health in the nursing curriculum (Strumph and Mezey, 1980). Though as early as 1961, pharmacy was being criticized by its leadership for failing to respond to the welfare of senior citizens (Apple, 1961), it was not until the late 1970s that the subject began to receive serious attention. Its importance to pharmacy became so evident that a major part of the report of a special study commission was devoted to pharmacy and the elderly (Study Commission on Pharmacy, 1975), where a strong plea was made for pharmacy curricula to reflect the needs of the elderly through learning about them in different settings and working with other health professionals (Schlegel, 1980).

In medical education, concern about the elderly was also growing, and some research on the subject was being conducted. In a study on student attitudes toward aging, data revealed that after a seminar on the subject, three things were necessary to develop positive attitudes: availability of factual information on aging, contact with the sick and well elderly, and positive role models in physicians (Wilson and Hafferty, 1980). In another study, Goodson and others (1981) described the demographic, residential, and health characteristics of patients over seventy and how students develop skills to deal with that group of patients. In a description of a humanistic approach to geriatric care in a public subsidized housing unit, evaluation of the program revealed that it was highly acclaimed by tenants, physicians, and students (Rose and Osterud, 1980). It is apparent that for at least the next two decades, the issue of aging will receive considerable attention in the curricula of the health sciences, and it is likely that more social and behavioral scientists will join the teaching and practice teams.

Two other curricular developments occurred during this time that should be noted. In pharmacy, it was the teaching of pharmacokinetics and in nursing, the move toward "areas of concentration." Pharmacokinetics—the study of the absorption, disposition, metabolism, and excretion of drugs—was a natural development as pharmacy curricula became more patient consultant-oriented. By being familiar with the mechanism of pharmacokinetics, the pharmacist can adjust drug dosage for optimal effect. Consequently, as pharmacy curricula increased their emphasis on the role of the therapy consultant, more curricular time was provided to pharmacokinetics.

The introduction of areas of concentration in nursing curricula permitted nursing students to develop an expertise or specialization in, for example, gerontology or occupational health some time during the last year of study. Where previously there was little flexibility, nursing curricula were modified to accommodate student specialty interests.

During the time that all these additions were being made in the curricula, there were simultaneous pressures to expand existing courses and subjects, to give students greater free time, and to offer more electives. All this transpired when there was no visible evidence that other courses were being reduced or eliminated. As already noted, it became essential that education of the health professionals extend beyond the confines of university walls, so that a whole host of community resources could be utilized to implement the ever-changing and expanding curricula.

## A Time of Reappraisal

The middle and late 1970s were also characterized by some reversion, some accommodation, and some continued progress.

*Reversion.* There is little doubt that the most startling development was the abandonment of the three-year curriculum in medicine and dentistry that had previously been encouraged with such enthusiasm by the federal government. In the case of medicine, the height of the three-year program was 1973, when 27 percent of the schools moved to this option. Some other schools developed combined baccalaureate and medical degree sequences, but these did not generate the strong feelings that the three-year curricula did. Several reasons have been put forth as to why most of these three-year programs were abandoned. Beran (1979) attributed the failure to the "quality of life" for students and faculty alike; there was little, if any, free time and all courses were presented at a hectic pace. Even before Beran's article appeared, some students were citing the strains of a three-year program and were recommending that it be abandoned (Greenberg, 1976). Study of faculty attitudes toward the programs revealed the view that they lacked substance, students were pushed too hard, students were deficient in the basic sciences, and students were not good in developing problem-solving ability (Trzebiatowski and Peterson, 1979). Another school, the University of Arizona, initiated and abandoned the three-year curriculum because it was stressful, compacted the basic sciences, reduced student-faculty contact, forced a reduction in vacation time, and developed negative attitudes on the part of the faculty (Kettel and others, 1979). Others argued that a three-year curriculum increased the number of graduates by one class only, and thereafter the number would be indefinitely stable (Beliveau, 1976). In rebuttal, Garfunkel (1976) argued that not enough time had elapsed to make judgments on the merits or demerits of the three-year curricula. Nonetheless, in a matter of only a few years, they began to fade away. Almost all the arguments against the three-year medical program were voiced also by dentistry in three succinct statements: (1) rejection by the faculty, (2) lack of flexibility, and (3) negative attitudes of practicing dentists toward the quality of the graduates (Formicola, 1978).

When Harvard and Yale reverted to some "old" curricular practices, the move received considerable attention, probably because it occurred at Harvard and Yale. In describing the change at Harvard, Goldhaber (1973) reports that in part because of poor performance on National Board examinations, the core curriculum was abandoned, grades were reinstituted, and teaching was again organized by departments rather than body (organ) systems. Fairly similar changes occurred at Yale, and many schools that had developed a core curriculum in the 1960s were reducing the amount of time devoted to the basic sciences. There is, however, little evidence to show that students' performance had suffered.

As many new courses were added and few, if any, deleted, infringements were being made on elective and free time. Though there are no known studies of how free time was used by students, it was held sacrosanct when it was initially instituted; it was perhaps inevitable that slowly, almost imperceptibly, inroads into that time would be made.

While many medical schools were reverting to former curricular activities, it is interesting to note that one, the University of Illinois, developed an independent study program within an organized curriculum that permitted a small group of highly motivated students to do independent and creative work and allowed them to proceed through the curriculum at their own pace (Johns and Smith, 1973). Unfortunately, there is no indication as to whether the two groups of students will be studied as they move along their careers.

*Accommodation.* In pharmacy, the emphasis on clinical pharmacy continued through the seventies. As increasing numbers of graduates found positions where they could apply their clinical skills as drug therapy consultants, more schools began to make appropriate curricular modifications to accommodate students seeking such programs. Also, schools continued to affiliate with a greater number of hospitals and clinics beyond the confines of the university medical centers. In nursing, there was a continued increase in "second step" programs that enable graduates of associate degree programs to obtain baccalaureate degrees.

*Continued Progress.* Two of the more significant events that prompted additional curricular modification were the further expansion of primary care and the greater use of community resources. As already noted (Hudson and Nourse, 1975), the *Journal of Medical Education* devoted a special supplement to the implications of primary care for medical education. Fortunately, primary care programs were subjected to close scrutiny. Both the Robert Wood Johnson Foundation, which initially funded several programs, and the federal government insisted that programs with substantial funding be studied and evaluated. Trends in primary care education in U.S. medical schools and also in the general residency programs of the many teaching hospitals were examined (Giacalone and Hudson,

1977). In another study of two approaches to the teaching of primary care, Sarnacki (1979) concludes that the best approach to producing competent primary care practitioners is to modify the curriculum rather than to look for student characteristics that would likely motivate them to go into the field. In a national study, Rosinski and Dagenais (1980) compared the original nine programs funded by the Robert Wood Johnson Foundation with the first seven programs funded by the federal government. This study examined numerous questions, beginning with how the programs' objectives were developed to how (and if) the programs were supported by university funds. In examining many of the curricula of the primary care programs, it is evident that most embody the eight general objectives recommended by Vandervoort (Vandervoort and Ransom, 1973). By the late 1970s, almost every medical school provided or required a clerkship in primary care, dentistry was gearing up for primary care, and nursing schools were emphasizing it, often through nurse practitioner programs.

The greater use of community resources for teaching/learning was prompted by dramatic shortages of clinical facilities and patients in university medical centers and by the gradual awareness of some health professions educators that varied educational experiences could be most enriching when they took place in off-campus sites. Nursing probably took the leadership in utilizing urban and rural clinical settings for the education of nurses in baccalaureate programs. In a study of one such program that took place in a rural community hospital in a town of 800 people, Pakieser (1978) concluded that it provided experiences that could not be matched at the university medical center and, furthermore, that it motivated a large number of graduates to seek rural positions.

As already noted, other professions also continued to expand their programs to off-campus sites. If there was any single factor that prompted the health professions to move to off-campus sites, it was the federal legislation that authorized the creation of Area Health Education Centers (AHECs). The AHECs were an outgrowth of the report of the Carnegie Commission on Higher Education (1970) that recommended that universities develop and strengthen rural community resources related to education for the health professions, as well as improve patient care resources. The legislation authorizing AHECs was just the incentive that many university medical centers needed, and eleven such AHECs were originally funded. The programs that the university medical centers established in conjunction with their affiliated communities ran the entire gamut of the health professions. While there was strong sentiment for the development of AHECs, some individuals cautioned educators and administrators against moving too fast on them (Mike and Ross, 1975). Though each of the original eleven AHECs recruited an individual who was responsible for the evaluation of the program, much of the evaluation was for management or in-house purposes. The evaluation of one of the programs was based solely on evaluating each one of the component programs by first developing the objectives for each component part and then determining the extent to which the objectives were met (Rosinski, 1978). Attempts to evaluate the entire national AHEC program were initiated several times, but in some cases the evaluations were aborted as they got under way, and in others the results were so questionable that they were never published. In frustration, the directors of the AHEC programs themselves contracted to have the program evaluated, and a report was finally published (Odegaard, 1979).

It is worthy of note, if for no reason other than historical, that by the end of the 1970s, all the old two-year medical schools that offered only the basic sciences expanded by adding the clinical years of instruction to become four-year schools, with the curricula resembling those of most other schools. Also, Congress authorized and the president signed Public Law 92-541, the Veterans' Administration Medical School Assistance and Health Manpower Training Act, authorizing the creation of eight new medical schools affiliated with veterans' hospitals. To date, little has been written about the curricula of these new schools or whether any research and evaluation of their programs is taking place. In addition to the establishment of new or expansion of old schools, some curricular modification in medical education continued. In a symposium at the 1979 Conference on Research in Medical Education (Association of American Medical Colleges, 1979), seven schools reported on such modifications. While all the schools had different objectives, in essence they reported efforts to strengthen some of the subjects, such as the humanities and the social and behavioral sciences, and attempts to avoid needless repetition. A depressing conclusion of the symposium was that evaluation was considered difficult, but, in a more optimistic tone, it was felt that if the quality of life of the student was positively affected, the changes were worth it. It is not known whether the same sentiments are expressive of the other health professions, but it is evident that much of the curricular modification in all the health professions was based on a desire for change rather than on data obtained through research or evaluation that clearly indicated a change was necessary.

Finally, the 1970s marked the emergence of the competency-based curriculum, on which some research was conducted. For example, in the State of Illinois the Board of Higher Education decreed that as new medical schools were developed in the state, performance was to be constant and time the variable. Some descriptions of the programs developed in Illinois also report limited evaluations (Quinlan, 1975), and the volume of curricular behavioral objectives developed for the Southern Illinois University School of Medicine (Mast, 1980) is, without question one of the most impressive of its kind ever compiled. Other health professions, likewise, explored the appropriateness of competency-based curricula. In 1975, the American Association of Colleges of Pharmacy devoted a portion of its national meeting to a consideration of competency-based curricula ("Proceedings of the 1975 Annual Meeting," 1975). A number of nursing schools implemented such curricula (Peterson and others, 1980), but studies comparing a competency curriculum to a conventional one are rare in all professions.

## Implications of Curricular Reform and Changes

A review of the implications of the curricular efforts since the beginning of the 1960s appears in order. The first question must be: What were the reasons for instituting change? Certainly they were multiple, and there can be little doubt that health professions educators were attempting to develop a better learning environment and to make teaching/learning more efficient. But probably the most important reason is that educational objectives were in a constant state of flux. It has always been an axiom of the health professions that their educational objectives are derived from three sources: the needs of society, the needs of the profession, and scientific and technical developments. If that is, indeed, the case, then it is no wonder that curricula were being modified in an attempt to find the best way to satisfy the dynamic objectives of the health professions. For example, Walsh (1966) stated that the health needs of society should be the prime determinants of a dental curriculum and gave examples of what a comprehensive dental curriculum should look like. Hixon (1973) described, in a most erudite fashion, the philosophical and historical evolution of change and civilization and related those changes to changes in dentistry and dental education. There is ample evidence that one of the reasons that curricular modifications were initiated and continue to date is that health professions educators were often knowingly responding to the health needs of society, the needs of the professions, and to scientific and technical developments, although not necessarily in that order.

Curricular changes were also made because of genuine dissatisfaction on the part of students, faculty, and some segments of society. The first major reforms in medical education were brought about because there were faculty who recognized the need to apply some of the same scientific rigor exercised in their laboratories and clinics to an examination of the educational process. Instituting the body (organ) system approach to organizing a curriculum, for example, made obvious sense, since a physician does not examine a patient by "subjects" but by body systems. Nursing educators, who recognized the need for a nurse who could respond and adapt to evolving major developments in medicine and could deal more effectively with patients and colleagues, saw the need for the baccalaureate curriculum. Pharmacy educators, who saw that the need for the conventional dispensing pharmacist was diminishing, recognized the potential for a new type of pharmacist and moved toward developing curricula that would produce the clinical pharmacist. Dental educators, who saw beyond the manual or skill orientation of the profession, prompted dental curricula to become more scientifically based, with increased emphasis on the social and behavioral sciences as an adjunct to developing clinical skills. Many other educators were probably responding directly to the fundamental observation that there must be a better or more efficient way to organize the curriculum, and they then proceeded in an attempt to find that way.

Student dissatisfaction with the curriculum did not surface until the late 1960s, when there was widespread criticism by many university students of certain aspects of society. Students voiced concern that some curricula lacked relevance and that the health professions should be more directly involved in solving the health problems of society. It was partially through student action that community storefront clinics were opened, health care provided to migrant farm workers, interdisciplinary courses instituted, and many new, especially elective, courses added. Student involvement in curricular change was not limited to the United States; in certain European countries also students influenced curricular change, though not to the same degree as in the United States (Mensh, 1978).

Some segments of society voiced concern that health professions education was neglecting their needs. A case in point is the rapid rise of the family and nurse practitioner, whom many saw as the answer to the almost extinct general practitioner of old. Even though the memory of that type of practitioner was blurred by time, still there was a perceived need for a practitioner who would provide "total family care." Another case in point was the rise of geriatrics in the curricula of all the health professions. Once more a segment of society, feeling that its needs were not being met, lobbied and pressured for appropriate curricular changes. The physician assistant, primary care, and nurse midwife programs represent a few examples of the federal government's perception of ways of meeting these dissatisfactions.

Other dissatisfaction with the educational programs was voiced by faculty and students who did not see the relevance of the students' education to their ultimate career goals. As more students made career choices earlier in life, they wanted curricula that gave them an opportunity to begin preparing for that goal. Consequently, tracking was instituted in many medical schools, areas of concentration provided in some nursing schools, and greater freedom to select from a broader variety of electives given students in pharmacy and dentistry.

The litany of scientific and technical developments that had an impact on education is amazingly long: genetic counseling, DNA and RNA, neurophysiology, the noninvasive techniques used for eliciting physical findings, and countless others had to be added to the armamentarium of health professionals in order to enable them to provide state-of-the-art care. Curricular changes obviously had to be made to accommodate these and many other important scientific and technical developments.

As discussed earlier, there continued to be resistance to all these curricular modifications, whether minor or major, on the part of some educators and administrators. There were those who opposed organizing the curriculum by body (organ) system because it would blur the distinctions among the basic science disciplines. There were those who opposed the addition of the behavioral and social sciences because they would infringe on precious time that could be given to the established and entrenched disciplines. There were those who opposed strengthening the scientific base of nursing for it would detract from the nurses' humanistic orientation. There were those who opposed any change in dental education because they perceived any modification as a distraction from the well-established and accepted goals of a dental education. There were those who objected to the development of the clinical pharmacists because they detected them as being in competition with other existing health practitioners. Opposition to change is not unidirectional. Many of the schools that made radical curricular modifications also resisted any changes. Fraenkel (1978), who on several occasions visited McMaster University in Canada to examine the remarkable curriculum there, was surprised that during all those years the program resisted reversion to a more conventional/traditional one. While there is a tone of cynicism in Fraenkel's observation, there is also considerable admiration in his listing of the reasons some programs are able to resist change: faculty enthusiasm, student pride, international recognition, and the presence of an administrative system that makes changes difficult.

In the final analysis, however, it appears that the greatest obstacle to curricular modification has been the absence of data to document the need for change or the result of any change. Abrahamson (1977) notes that there is a greater willingness to change a curriculum now, but he laments that many faculty still do not apply the same scientific rigor to work related to curricular change as they do to their research. To some extent, this has been corrected by the creation in many schools of offices of research, staffed by trained educational researchers. But for these offices to be successful, it is necessary that they have the support and participation of the faculty who will be responsible for judging the need for change, instituting the change, and then assessing the results of that change. Unfortunately, that participation and support are often lacking or minimal.

## A Program for Action

What processes and procedures promote rational change? First of all, there is a need to define in detail institutional and teaching objectives. This has been stated so often by so many educators that one would think it was an accepted truism. Yet, it continues to be ignored by many individuals and many schools, though we all "know" that without objectives, curriculum reform is arbitrary and precludes a systematic evaluation of any program (Mast and Bellanti, 1976).

Secondly, we require objectives that are better related to needs of society and the profession and to scientific and technical developments. Furthermore, it is necessary to reexamine those needs and developments constantly so that appropriate adjustments can be made. Constant reappraisal of educational objectives is necessary if education is to be a dynamic process.

Thirdly, faculty involvement must be present in all aspects of curriculum activities. By being involved, faculty will have a stake in what is being done and will more readily support projected changes or modifications. Faculty who are not involved will have no vested interest and will often hinder change or disassociate themselves from the educational program.

Finally, it is imperative that we have more data, based on sound research and evaluation. As has been evident in this chapter, a considerable amount of curricular revision was generated by personal feelings, with objective data supporting the need for change or the effects of change in seriously short supply.

What lies ahead in research on curriculum development? Miller (1980) partially addressed this question in the final chapter of his book. However, he focused on research in medical education in general, not specifically on the effects of curricular modification so, to some extent, the question remains unanswered. Perhaps the question can best be answered by analyzing the reasons for modifying a curriculum.

First of all, changes in a curriculum are made so that learning is more efficient. That being the case, it should appear obvious that research on whether that learning is, indeed, more efficient should be conducted. There are some studies addressing this issue, but by and large they have been ex post facto and provided little comparative data. As future curricular modifications are made, pre- and poststudies on learning efficiency should be planned. Granted, these studies will be difficult to conduct, but to do less will provide little justification for curricular modification other than a subjective impression that a change was necessary.

Secondly, curricular changes are made to make learning more effective. All the requisite knowledge, skills, and attitudes should be acquired in a meaningful way. To determine whether effective learning has taken place will require considerably more evaluative research than has taken place to date. This, in turn, will necessitate the definition of behavioral objectives and the development and application of techniques to assess whether the objectives are being achieved. Health professions schools have done a remarkable job during the past twenty years in progressing toward defining curricular and teaching/learning objectives. Still, a great deal more must be done in this area so that sound evaluative research can be undertaken on the effectiveness of learning brought about by a curricular change.

Third, curricular modification occurs in order to introduce new knowledge and skills that enable the student to function as a capable contemporary professional. The problem, however, is that often the additions made to a curriculum are arbitrary, lacking any rational justification. Recent years have seen the introduction of the concept of "needs assessment," and it appears that this concept must be applied to a greater extent in curriculum research. For example, other than the work conducted at the University of Southern California little has been done to examine the role and function of the practicing health professional, and to relate those roles and functions to a curriculum (The Robert Wood Johnson Foundation, 1981; Mendenhall, Girard, and Abrahamson, 1978). Until now, additions of a wide range of courses and subjects to curricula have not been accompanied by even a modest subtraction of existing ones. By conducting needs assessments in relation to postgraduate education and to the practicing health professional, changes in a curriculum can be made that will reflect a positive relation between what is taught and learned in school and what is necessary to function skillfully as a practicing health professional.

In concluding this chapter, no attempt has been made to provide a litany of specific curricular research topics in which health professions educators might engage. The specific topics can only be determined by the particular curriculum of each school. If attention is given to examining and to evaluating whether a curriculum is efficient, effective, and relevant, the contributions to education for health professions will be considerable.

## References

Abrahamson, S. "Changing Curriculum in the Medical School." *Journal of Medical Education*, 1977, *52* (9), 778–779.

Abrahamson, S. "Diseases of the Curriculum." *Journal of Medical Education*, 1978, *53* (12), 951–957.

Allred, H., and Slack, G. L. "The Changing Pattern of Dental Education." *British Journal of Dentistry*, 1968, *125* (5), 187–193.

American Association of Dental Schools. "Curriculum Guidelines for Preventive Dentistry." *Journal of Dental Education*, 1980, *44* (9), 533–555.

Andrus, L. H., and others. "A New Teacher in Medical Education: The Family Nurse Practitioner." *Journal of Medical Education*, 1977, *52* (11), 896–900.

Apple, W. S. "Some Missing Links in Pharmaceutical Education." *American Journal of Pharmaceutical Education*, 1961, *25*, 222–226.

Association of American Medical Colleges. "New Experiments to Improve Premedical and Medical Education: A Symposium." In *Annual Conference Research in Medical Education*, No. 18, pp. 317–327. Washington, D.C.: Association of American Medical Colleges, 1979.

Bandaranayake, R. (Ed.). "Trends in Curricula II: The University of New South Wales." In *Review Paper No. 3*. Kensington, New South Wales, Australia:

Center for Medical Education, Research, and Development, University of New South Wales, 1980.

Basalamah, A., Rosinski, E., and Schumacher, H. "Developing the Medical Curriculum at King Abdulaziz University." *Journal of Medical Education*, 1979, *54*, 96–100.

Beliveau, R. R. "It Takes Four Years." *Journal of the American Medical Association*, 1976, *235* (14), 1424.

Beran, R. L. "The Rise and Fall of Three-Year Medical School Programs." *Journal of Medical Education*, 1979, *54* (3), 248–249.

Brown, W. R. "National Dental Curriculum Study." *Journal of Dental Education*, 1976, *40* (9), 592–594.

Campbell, C., and DeMuth, G. R. "The University of Michigan Integrated Premedical/Medical Program." *Journal of Medical Education*, 1976, *51* (4), 296–298.

Campbell, E. J. "The McMaster Medical School at Hamilton, Ontario." *Lancet*, 1970, *2* (676), 763–767.

Campbell, R. K. "Student Pre- and Post-Evaluation of an Off-Campus Clinical Clerkship." *American Journal of Pharmaceutical Education*, 1975, *39* (3), 238–244.

Carnegie Commission on Higher Education. *Higher Education and the Nation's Health: Policies for Medical and Dental Education*. New York: McGraw-Hill, 1970.

Clarke, R. "The New Medical School at Newcastle, New South Wales." *Medical Journal Australia*, 1978, *1* (15), 255–256.

Colditz, G. A. "The Students' View of an Innovative Undergraduate Medical Course: The First Year at the University of Newcastle, New South Wales." *Medical Education*, 1980, *14* (5), 320–325.

Davis, C. "Relation of University Preparation to Nursing Practice." *New York League Exchange*, 1975, *108*.

Daubney, J. H., Wagner, E. E., and Rogers, W. A. "Six-Year B.S./M.D. Programs: A Literature Review." *Journal of Medical Education*, 1981, *56* (6), 497–503.

deTornyay, R. "Cultural Diversity and Nursing Curricula." *Journal of Nursing Education*, 1976, *15* (2), 3–4.

Dickinson, G. E. "Death Education in U.S. Medical Schools, 1975–1980." *Journal of Medical Education*, 1981, *56* (2), 111.

Division of Nursing Resources. *A Report of the Public Health Service, Department of Health, Education, and Welfare*. Washington, D.C.: U.S. Public Health Service, 1957.

Dixon, A. D. "Dental Education in the U.S., 1976. Part II: Curriculum Study Findings." *Journal of Dental Education*, 1978, *42* (5), 237–243.

Echt, R., and Chan, S. W. "A New Problem-Oriented and Student-Centered Curriculum at Michigan State University." *Journal of Medical Education*, 1977, *52* (8), 681–683.

"Educational Preparation for Nursing." *Nursing Outlook*, 1966, *14* (9), 58–61.

Erne, M. J. "Implications of Trends in Nursing Education." *Nursing Outlook*, 1966, *14* (9), 36–39.

Evans, R. L. "Medical Education, Medical Care, and Our Public." *Journal of the American Medical Association*, 1973, *226* (13), 1563–1564.

Farley, V. "An Evaluative Study of an Open Curriculum/Career Ladder Nursing Program." *New York League Exchange*, 1978, *118*.

Flook, E. E., and Sanazaro, P. J. *Health Services Research and R and D in Perspective*. Ann Arbor: University of Michigan, Health Administration Press, 1973.

Formicola, A. J. "Reflections on the Three-Year Program." *Journal of Dental Education*, 1978, *42* (10), 572-575.

Fowkes, V., O'Hara-Devereaux, M., and Andrus, L. H. "A Cooperative Education Program for Nurse Practitioners/Physician's Assistants." *Journal of Medical Education*, 1979, *54* (10), 781-787.

Fraenkel, G. J. "Medical Education: McMaster Revisited." *British Medical Journal*, 1978, *2* (6144), 1072-1076.

Fromer, M. "Teaching Ethics by Case Analysis." *Nursing Outlook*, 1980, *28* (10), 604-609.

Garfunkel, J. M. "It Takes Four Years—A Rebuttal." *Journal of the American Medical Association*, 1976, *235* (16), 1701-1702.

Garrard, J., and Verby, J. E. "Comparisons of Medical Students' Experiences in Rural and University Settings." *Journal of Medical Education*, 1977, *52* (10), 802-810.

Giacalone, J. J., and Hudson, J. I. "Primary Care Education Trends in U.S. Medical Schools and Teaching Hospitals." *Journal of Medical Education*, 1977, *52* (12), 971-981.

Goldhaber, S. Z. "Medical Education: Harvard Reverts to Tradition." *Science*, 1973, *181* (104), 1027-1032.

Goodson, J. D., and others. "Characteristics of Older Patients in an Urban Teaching Practice." *Journal of Medical Education*, 1981, *56* (6), 459-466.

Gordon, M. J., Hadac, R. R., and Smith, C. K. "Evaluation of Clinical Training in the Community." *Journal of Medical Education*, 1977, *52* (11), 888-895.

Green, R. L., Jr. "Medical Education: A Summary of Revolutionary Changes." *West Virginia Medical Journal*, 1970, *66* (8), 251-256.

Greenberg, R. M. "It Takes Four Years." *Journal of the American Medical Association*, 1976, *235* (16), 1689.

Hamilton, J. D. "The McMaster Curriculum: A Critique." *British Medical Journal*, 1976, *1* (6019), 1191-1196.

Henry, J. L., and Sinkford, J. C. "Trends in Dental Education." *Journal of Dental Education*, 1974, *38* (8), 425-427.

Hixon, E. H. "A Future For Dentistry in New Zealand." *New Zealand Dental Journal*, 1973, *69* (315), 5-17.

Hudson, J. I., and Braslow, J. B. "Cost Containment Education Efforts in U.S. Medical Schools." *Journal of Medical Education*, 1979, *54* (11), 835-840.

Hudson, J. I., and Nourse, E. S. (Eds.). "Perspectives in Primary Care Education." *Journal of Medical Education*, 1975, *50* (12), Part II.

Johns, C. E., and Smith, R. D. "An Independent Study Program in Medical School." *Journal of Medical Education*, 1973, *48* (8), 732-738.

Johnson, K. G., and Haughton, P. B. T. "An Outreach Program for a Rural Medical School." *Journal of Medical Education*, 1975, *50* (1), 38-45.

Kaiser, J. "A Comparison of Students in Practical Nursing Programs and Students in Associate Degree Nursing Programs." *New York League Exchange,* 1975, *109.*

Kalinowski, R. H., and Ackerman, S. J. (Eds.). "HMO: Program Development in the Academic Medical Center." *Journal of Medical Education,* 1973, *48* (4), Part II.

Kettel, L. J., and Vanselow, N. A. "Experience with College of Medicine Department Reviews." *Journal of Medical Education,* 1978, *53* (7), 556–564.

Kettel, L. J., and others. "Arizona's Three-Year Medical Curriculum: A Postmortem." *Journal of Medical Education,* 1979, *54* (3), 210–216.

Lamberti, J. W., and Chapel, J. L. "Development and Evaluation of a Sex Education Program for Medical Students." *Journal of Medical Education,* 1977, *52* (7), 582–586.

Lanzoni, V., and Kayne, H. L. "A Report on Graduates of the Boston University Six-Year Combined Liberal Arts/Medical Program." *Journal of Medical Education,* 1976, *51* (4), 283–289.

Lee, P. V. *Medical Schools and the Changing Times: Nine Case Reports on Experimentation in Medical Education, 1950–1960.* Washington, D.C.: Association of American Medical Colleges, 1962.

Levine, L. "Through the Looking Glass at the Integrated Curriculum." *Journal of Nursing Education,* 1979, *18* (7), 43–46.

Lotzkar, S., Johnson, D., and Thompson, M. "Experimental Programs in Expanded Functions for Dental Assistants: Part I—Base Line and Part II—Training." *Journal of the American Dental Association,* 1971, *82,* 101–122.

Love, J. "Using the Community Hospital as a Learning Center for Community Nursing Students." *Journal of Nursing Education,* 1978, *17* (7), 5–12.

McCally, M., Sorem, K., and Silverman, M. "Interprofessional Education of the New Health Practitioner." *Journal of Medical Education,* 1977, *52* (3), 177–182.

Maddison, D. C. "What's Wrong with Medical Education." *Medical Education,* 1978, *12* (2), 95–96.

Magraw, R. M., Fox, D. M., and Weston, J. "Health Professions Education and Public Policy: A Research Agenda." *Journal of Medical Education,* 1978, *53* (7), 539–546.

Marks, S. C., and Bertman, S. L. "Experiences with Learning About Death and Dying in the Undergraduate Anatomy Curriculum." *Journal of Medical Education,* 1980, *55* (1), 48–52.

Mast, T. A. (Ed.). *Curricular Objectives, 1980.* Carbondale: School of Medicine, Southern Illinois University, 1980.

Mast, T. A., and Bellanti, N. D. "Expanding the Role of Behavioral Objectives in Dental Education." *Journal of American College of Dentists,* 1976, *43* (4), 249–256.

Mazur, H., Beeston, J. J., and Yerxa, E. J. "Clinical Interdisciplinary Health Team Care: An Educational Experiment." *Journal of Medical Education,* 1979, *54* (9), 703–713.

"Medical Education and Minorities." *Journal of Medical Education,* 1978, *53* (8), 627–666.

Mendenhall, R. C., Girard, R. A., and Abrahamson, S. "A National Study of Medical and Surgical Specialties: I—Background, Purpose, and Methodology." *Journal of the American Medical Association,* 1978, *240,* 848–852.

Mensh, I. N. "Changing Patterns of Medical Education." *Journal of Medical Education*, 1967, *42* (12), 1101–1110.

Mensh, I. N. "French Medical Education: Years of Change." *Journal of Medical Education*, 1978, *53* (9), 741–745.

Mike, L. H., and Ross, R. J. "Area Health Education Centers: What Are They and Where Are They Going?" *Journal of Medical Education*, 1975, *50* (3), 242–251.

Miller, G. E. *Educating Medical Teachers.* Cambridge, Mass.: Harvard University Press, 1980.

Moore, A. R. "Medical Humanities: A New Medical Adventure." *New England Journal of Medicine*, 1976, *295* (26), 1479–1480.

Mrtek, R. G. "Pharmaceutical Education in These United States: An Interpretative Historical Essay of the Twentieth Century." *American Journal of Pharmaceutical Education*, 1976, *40*, 339–365.

Nasir, V. M., and Woo, N. I. I. "Increasing Awareness in Community and Preventive Dentistry: Trends in Curricula II." *In Review Paper No. 3.* Kensington, New South Wales, Australia: Center for Medical Education, Research, and Development, University of New South Wales, 1980.

Neufeld, V. R., and Barrows, H. S. "McMaster Philosophy: An Approach to Medical Education." *Journal of Medical Education*, 1974, *49* (11), 1040–1050.

Newton, M. "What Every Nurse Needs to Know About Nutrition." *Nursing Outlook*, 1960, *8* (6), 316–317.

Nicholls, J. G. "American Lessons for London's Medical Schools." *Lancet*, 1980, *1* (8165), 429.

Oaks, J. H. "The Need for Curriculum Innovation in Dental Education." *Journal of the American Dental Association*, 1970, *80* (5), 1027–1029.

Odegaard, C. E. *Area Health Education Centers: The Pioneering Years, 1972–1978.* Berkeley, Calif.: Carnegie Council on Policy Studies in Higher Education, 1979.

Pakieser, R. "A Rural Hospital Practicum." *Nursing Outlook*, 1978, *26* (4), 249–251.

Parks, L. "Pharmaceutical Education for the Future." *American Journal of Pharmaceutical Education*, 1967, *31*, 22–28.

Pavone, B. W. "The New Four-Year Curriculum at University of California, San Francisco." *Journal of the California Dental Association*, 1976, *4* (2), 34–36.

Peterson, C., and others. "Competency-Based Curriculum and Instruction." *New York League Exchange*, 1980, *124*.

*Pharmacists for the Future: The Report of the Study Commission on Pharmacy.* Ann Arbor: University of Michigan, Health Administration Press, 1975.

Pitcairn, D. M., and Flahault, D. (Eds.). *The Medical Assistant: An Intermediate Level of Health Care Personnel.* World Health Organization Public Health Papers, No. 60. Geneva, Switzerland: World Health Organization, 1973.

Podell, R. N., Gary, L. R., and Keller, K. "A Profile of Clinical Nutrition Knowledge Among Physicians and Medical Students." *Journal of Medical Education*, 1975, *50* (9), 888.

Pokorny, A., Putnam, P., and Fryer, J. "Drug Abuse and Alcoholism Teaching in U.S. Medical and Osteopathic Schools." *Journal of Medical Education*, 1978, *53* (10), 816–824.

Pritchard, H. N. "The Lehigh Medical College of Pennsylvania Six-Year B.A./M.D. Program." *Journal of Medical Education,* 1976, *51* (4), 283–289.

"Proceedings of the 1975 Annual Meeting." *American Journal of Pharmaceutical Education,* 1975, *39* (5), 556–572.

"Proceedings of the 1980 Annual Meeting." *American Journal of Pharmaceutical Education,* 1980, *44* (4), 359–384.

"Proceedings of the 1971 Invitational Meeting." *American Journal of Hospital Pharmacy,* 1971, *28* (11), 842–888.

Quinlan, T. "The Rockford Experience: Competency-Based Medical Curriculum." *American Journal of Pharmaceutical Education,* 1975, *39* (4), 439–449.

Redig, D. F. "The Three Year Curriculum at the University of the Pacific." *Journal of the California Dental Association,* 1976, *4* (2), 38–42.

Renshaw, D. "The Nurse's Role with Parents of the Dying Child." *Journal of Nursing Education,* 1979, *18* (1), 17–21.

"A Report on Progress in Nursing Education." *Nursing Outlook,* 1958, *6* (6), 336.

The Robert Wood Johnson Foundation. *Medical Practice in The U.S.: Special Report.* Princeton, N.J.: The Robert Wood Johnson Foundation, 1981.

Rose, B. K., and Osterud, H. T. "Humanistic Geriatric Health Care: An Innovation in Medical Education." *Journal of Medical Education,* 1980, *55* (11), 928–932.

Rose, L. F., and Escovitz, G. H. "A Medical-Dental Interdisciplinary Teaching Program." *Journal of Medical Education,* 1974, *49* (8), 756–762.

Rosinski, E. F. "The Challenge to Pharmacy in Meeting the Health Needs of Society." *American Journal of Pharmaceutical Education,* 1968, *8*, 385–393.

Rosinski, E. F. "The New Medical Schools and Curriculum Innovation." *Journal of the American Medical Association,* 1971, *216* (2), 322.

Rosinski, E. F. "Curriculum Reform and Medical Education." Unpublished report of the evaluation of the Medical College of Virginia School of Medicine curriculum, 1976. Available from the University of California at San Francisco School of Medicine.

Rosinski, E. F. "The Central San Joaquin Valley Area Health Education Center." *Western Journal of Medicine,* 1978, *128* (4), 355.

Rosinski, E. F., and Dagenais, F. *Non–Family Medicine Resident Training for Primary Care: A Comparative Evaluation of Federally and Nonfederally Supported Primary Care-Oriented Medical Residency Programs.* Federal Contract HRA 232-78-0115. Washington, D.C.: U.S. Department of Health and Human Services, 1980.

Rosinski, E. F., and Spencer, F. J. *The Assistant Medical Officer: The Training of the Medical Auxiliary in Developing Countries.* Chapel Hill: University of North Carolina Press, 1965.

Ruffman, D., Tobias, D., and Speedie, S. "Validation of Written Simulations as Measures of Problem Solving for Pharmacy Students." *American Journal of Pharmaceutical Education,* 1980, *44* (1), 16–24.

Sadler, A. M., Jr., Sadler, B. L., and Bliss, A. A. *The Physician's Assistant—Today and Tomorrow.* New Haven, Conn.: Yale University Press, 1972.

Sanger, W. T., and Hurd, A. W. "What the Educator Thinks the Ideal Medical Curriculum Should Be." *Journal of the Association of American Medical Colleges,* January 1946, 2–12.

Sarnacki, R. E. "A Comparison of Two Approaches to Producing Competent Primary Care Physicians." *Journal of Medical Education*, 1979, *54* (3), 224–229.

Schachter, S. C. "Death and Dying Education in a Medical School Curriculum." *Journal of Medical Education*, 1979, *54* (8), 661–663.

Schlegel, J. F. "Pharmacy Education: Looking Ahead." *American Pharmacy*, 1980, *20* (5), 18.

Schlotfeldt, R. "Can We Bring Order Out of the Chaos of Nursing Education?" *American Journal of Nursing*, 1976, *76* (1), 105–107.

Self, D. J. (Ed.). *The Role of the Humanities in Medical Education*. Norfolk, Va.: Teagle and Little, 1978.

Sheldrake, P. F., and others. *Medical Education in Australia*. Educational Research and Development Committee Report no. 16. Canberra: Australian Government Publishing Service, 1978.

Sherman, J., and others. "A Simulated Patient Encounter for the Family Nurse Practitioner." *Journal of Nursing Education*, 1979, *18* (5), 5–16.

"The Social Sciences in Medical Education." *World Health Organization Chronicle*, 1970, *24* (10), 278–281.

Stetten, D. W., Jr. "Medical School Curricular Reform." *Science*, 1968, *160* (834), 1293.

Stevens, B. J. "Adapting Nursing Education to Today's Student Population." *Journal of Nursing Education*, 1971, *10* (1), 15–20.

Stillman, P. L., and others. "The Nurse Practitioner as a Teacher of Physical Examination Skills." *Journal of Medical Education*, 1978, *53* (2), 119–124.

Strumph, M., and Mezey, M. "A Developmental Approach to the Teaching of Aging." *Nursing Outlook*, 1980, *28* (12), 730–734.

Study Commission on Pharmacy. *Pharmacists for the Future: The Report of the Study Commission on Pharmacy*. Ann Arbor: University of Michigan, Health Administration Press, 1975.

"Teaching Quality Assurance." *Journal of Medical Education*, 1976, *51* (5), 363–394.

Trzebiatowski, G. L., and Peterson, S. "A Study of Faculty Attitudes Toward Ohio State's Three-Year Medical Program." *Journal of Medical Education*, 1979, *54* (3), 205–209.

"Tufts Dental School to Initiate Three-Year Degree Program in 1972 by Operating on a Twelve-Month Curriculum." *New York Journal of Dentistry*, 1971, *41* (5), 184–185.

Tysarowski, W. "Current Trends in European Medical Education." *Journal of Medical Education*, 1968, *43* (5), 521–525.

"Undergraduate Dental Education in Europe." *World Health Organization Chronicle*, 1970, *24* (11), 506–511.

Vandervoort, H. E., and Ransom, D. C. "Undergraduate Education in Family Medicine." *Journal of Medical Education*, 1973, *48* (2), 158–165.

Walsh, J. "New Trends in Dental Education." *International Dental Journal*, 1966, *16* (4), 480–489.

Wegman, D. H., and others. "Teaching Occupational Health to Physicians." *Journal of Medical Education*, 1978, *53* (9), 746–751.

West, D. "Understanding and Communicating with Patients: An Undergraduate

Course in Communication and Medical Sociology." *American Journal of Pharmaceutical Education,* 1975, *39* (6), 30–34.

White, E. "Revolutionary Curriculum Reform." *Journal of Dental Education,* 1971, *35* (8), 521–522.

Whitmore, J. "Developing an Undergraduate Clinical Pharmacy Course in the Community Teaching Hospital." *American Journal of Pharmaceutical Education,* 1970, *34* (2), 69–77.

Wilson, J. F., and Hafferty, F. W. "Changes in Attitudes Toward the Elderly— One Year After a Seminar on Aging and Health." *Journal of Medical Education,* 1980, *55* (12), 993–999.

# Part Two

---

## Research
## on Health Professions
## Education:
## Findings and Implications

# Introduction:

# Current Research Trends
# and Future Directions

## Richard P. Foley

The chapters comprising Part Two examine the past twenty years of research relating to the various rites of passage that a health professional must go through to become and remain a professional. Rezler first reviews the process of admission into health professions schools and colleges. Foley then follows with an examination of the instructional approaches used to educate students who have been admitted, and McGuire looks at how these students are evaluated and ultimately licensed to practice as professionals. Once credentialed, Caplan and Stritter deal with the professional in practice from the respective standpoints of remaining a competent practitioner and educator.

It is apparent from Part One of this book that curricular reform was abundant in virtually every health profession during the last thirty years. By the late 1970s, for example, the three-year curriculum in dentistry and medicine was being eliminated, and in the latter field, thought was being given to introducing a five-year course of study. As Rosinski notes, however, little substantive research and evaluation were undertaken in the midst of this curricular fervor, and he wonders if as much reform would have taken place had more been conducted. The research reviewed in Part Two was, in part, affected by these changes. For example, the training of new types of health personnel occurred in almost all professional schools, and this influenced admission policies, while curricula that included self-instruction, independent study, and problem-based learning demanded new instructional skills of faculty. Therefore, for the richest understanding of the developments in this part of this volume, some familiarity with the preceding chapters is suggested.

### Integrating Research Findings into Educational Practices

A retrospective review of the research conducted in any field, of course, allows an author the luxury of assessing what has been learned, bemoaning what was not discovered, criticizing the methodologies employed, and recommending how future investigations should be conducted. It is clear from each of the chapters that follow that much was learned during the past two decades that should be heeded by those interested in advancing our current knowledge of how to educate health professionals during the next twenty years. Benjamin Bloom* argues, in fact, that we can no longer remain innocent of the findings of educational researchers; there are things we know that should guide us when admitting, teaching, and evaluating health professionals. A few of the recommendations germane to most of the chapters in this section are discussed here.

*Criteria for Selecting, Evaluating, and Certifying Health Professionals.* These criteria have not been related to professional practice. Regarding admissions, Rezler found that personality, value, and attitudinal measures show the most promise for predicting an individual's career choice, income, and attitudes toward medical practice twenty years after graduation, but as yet such measures are not being employed in the selection process. To the contrary, she found that in all the health professions, there is an increasing emphasis in the selection of students on the basis of prior academic achievement and on test scores purporting to measure academic aptitudes and/or achievement. These academic predictions, however, fail to predict clinical performance in any of the professions studied.

McGuire observed that at least until the mid-sixties all types of examinations used to test students during their schooling and at the certification and licensure levels sampled behaviors that usually had little relevance to the professed goals of professional education or to what were thought to be the essential components of professional competence. And while considerable progress was made during the sixties and seventies toward introducing more reliable and more valid techniques of assessing professional competence, McGuire is concerned that the problem of relating standards to realistic requirements derived from health care delivery settings is far from resolved.

*Multiple Types of Learning Experiences.* Educational programs should provide a variety of ways for health professionals to learn. In his review of instructional methods and media, Foley found that despite the homage paid to the importance of differences among individuals, most researchers have proceeded as if students were a homogeneous group and have given scant regard to the fact that students have personal learning characteristics that are likely to affect achievement and satisfaction. Stritter argues that while improvement in faculty instruction is relative, it can occur; however, a variety of approaches must be employed to bring about improvement, and no single approach is effective with all instructors, at all times, and in all contexts. Caplan similarly concludes that

*Bloom, B.S. "Innocence in Education." *School Review*, May 1972, pp. 333–352.

continuing education programs must maximize individualization by providing multiple types of learning experiences.

*Limits of Short-Term Educational Experiences.* To expect behavioral changes as a result of short-term educational experiences is unrealistic. Foley cautions researchers about placing too much credence upon student achievement scores that are purported to be the result of receiving one brief instructional intervention versus another. He states that a particular technique may be most effective within very narrow aspects of the learning process and that it makes greater sense to investigate larger sequences of instruction in light of educationally sound principles of learning. Stritter points out that while brief faculty development programs can increase knowledge or heighten awareness of ways to improve teaching skills, they are not likely to produce any lasting change in performance unless skill practice and specific feedback continue after a program's conclusion. Similarly, Caplan is concerned with inappropriate expectations of the impact of short-term continuing educational experiences on the quality of practitioner performance and notes that audits of practice following an educational activity have fallen short of the promise they seemed to offer.

These are just a few of the broader conclusions made by the authors of Part Two, and more specific ones can be found in each chapter. The knowledge gained from the past twenty years of research in these educational areas should prove useful to both researchers and to those who implement educational practices. However, as Mawby states in Chapter Twenty-Three, "A great deal more is known about what good health care could be—and should be—than is generally put to use." The same can be said of health professions education.

## Recommendations for Future Research

Each author in this part has also taken a sharp look at the nature of the research conducted and, in many instances, the appropriateness of the methodologies employed. Again, very specific suggestions are given regarding the areas of research that should be examined and the types of investigations that, if conducted, would enhance our present knowledge of the processes of educating health professionals from admission to lifelong learning. A number of recommendations were made by some or all of the authors, and several are worth noting here.

*Less Descriptive Research.* Stritter laments that the reported research on faculty development and evaluation of teaching has not been conducted systematically, that it has been mainly descriptive, and that many of his conclusions must be, therefore, largely impressionistic. Foley writes that the majority of the articles published on instruction were merely descriptive and without adequate documentation, but that authors nonetheless have concluded that a new technique, course, or program was effective. While not as frequent in the evaluation of professional competence, McGuire similarly found that the preponderance of the literature she examined had little or no documentation, save subjective impressions.

*Eliminate Focus on Trivial or Obvious Issues.* Foley believes that the work on instructional methods has been misdirected for the most part; it continues to belabor the same weary issue of whether one instructional method is superior to another and has not drawn upon the findings from parallel studies in general education. McGuire reports that throughout the period she reviewed, investigators continued to report the obvious ad nauseum—an example being that the typical examination, be it objective, essay, or oral, evaluated essentially low-level cognitive information. McGuire further points out that despite the plethora of studies on individual evaluation, there is little evidence from twenty years of research to substantiate the effects of system-wide modifications.

*Need for Follow-Up Research.* Rezler is concerned with the lack of follow-up studies evaluating the validity of present-day admission practices. She questions, for example, what happens to students with mediocre or lower intellectual qualifications: Do they graduate? Do they remain in practice? Foley raises the issue that once a promising program appears in the literature it is seldom heard of again, while the lack of qualitative and quantitative research on the effects of faculty development activities is of concern to Stritter.

*Emphasize Learner Characteristics.* Research should relate learner characteristics to specific learning strategies and to practice. Foley found that much of the research on instructional methods was flawed by the lack of attention paid to student and faculty characteristics; he believes that if faculty preferences for certain teaching formats and student preferences for particular learning methods were studied in conjunction with instructional sequences, we would acquire important information capable of influencing our present understanding of the education of health professionals. Rezler suggests that a major effort of research should be directed toward the refinement and development of assessment methods in order to measure noncognitive characteristics of students and their possible relationship to clinical performance. Caplan and Stritter both emphasize the need for research that examines possible relationships between the characteristics of the health professional as practitioner and teacher and the effectiveness of alternative learning strategies for continuing education and faculty development activities.

*Educational Interventions and Behavioral Outcomes.* Research must be concerned with assessing the behavioral outcomes that result from an educational intervention. In varying ways, each author in Part Two is concerned with this issue. Caplan believes that too much emphasis is placed on the fact that continuing education has merit only if its usefulness can be proved. McGuire is concerned that after thirty years of research, we do not as yet have a satisfactory methodology for evaluating professional habits and attitudes. Rezler raises doubts about the wisdom of an exclusive reliance on grades to validate the selection of students because there is no proven relationship between grades and the quality of subsequent professional performance. Stritter and Foley both urge that methods be found to enable us to assess the behavioral outcomes, as well as changes in knowledge and attitudes, that result from a specific educational intervention.

*Educational Practices and Health Care Practices.* Research should relate educational practices to health care practices. Again, most of the authors address this concern in some manner. Caplan, unlike the others, does not feel that educators should be held responsible for the improvement of health care delivery, arguing that there are too many variables that influence health care outcomes. Conversely, Rezler believes that practitioners and consumers of health care should be involved in identifying the essential, noncognitive qualities in the practice of the various health professions and asks such basic questions as whether today's graduates are acceptable to the patients they serve. Foley notes that studies are rare that examine the cost of a particular instructional technique, and even rarer are those that relate instructional strategies to health care outcomes. McGuire asks what effect the shifting emphasis in the aspects of professional competence that are evaluated has had on the quality of health care delivered.

It will become clear in reading the ensuing chapters that there has been a serious discontinuity between the education of health professionals and actual practice. And it seems likely that there is an equally serious discontinuity between practice based upon this education and the health of our populace. Such discrepancies should clearly dictate the focus of our health professions research agenda for the next two decades.

# 10

*Agnes G. Rezler*

# Student Selection
# and Admission

The process by which applicants are admitted to programs preparing students for different health professions is being viewed with increasing sensitivity for legal and social implications. This is due in part to the current climate in which the validity of many traditional modes of operation is being challenged. In addition, the large applicant pools force admissions committees to refine and justify admission standards and processes. They see their task as one of finding an equitable and efficient means of identifying the most promising applicants who are most likely to succeed, not only in school but also in practice.

Between 1970 and 1980, the number of students increased in all health professions. This increase has been due in part to growth in college enrollment and to expanded employment opportunities in many health fields (Nassif, 1980). Presently, however, there are not enough applicants to fill four-year nursing programs and barely enough for available places in allied health. At the same time, medical schools attract three to five times as many applicants as can be admitted. The image of each health profession, economic and social considerations, and cultural stereotypes influence the number and types of students who apply.

Selection invariably starts with a pool of applicants exhibiting different kinds of characteristics. The first task of an admissions committee is to define and reach consensus on the characteristics thought to be essential or desirable in entering students. The second problem is to decide how to measure these characteristics. The third step is to relate these measures, usually referred to as predictors, to selected measures of performance, called criteria. The fourth step is to establish and study the relationship between the predictors and the criteria to decide if the selection process should be continued or modified.

This chapter reviews and discusses trends pertaining to the characteristics of applicant pools, the selection and measurement of predictors, the choice of criteria, and the relation between predictors and selected outcome measures in five health professions—allied health, dentistry, medicine, nursing, and pharmacy. (Only B.S. programs are discussed and, in keeping with the literature on selection, allied health is treated as one field, despite the fact that it embraces several distinct professions.) The results of prevailing admissions practices are summarized and their implications for professional performance, manpower distribution, and consumer satisfaction are discussed.

## Student Characteristics

What kinds of students are attracted to the health professions? How old are they at entrance? Which profession attracts males or females exclusively? How are minority groups represented? Do different health professions attract applicants with different personalities? What are the career orientations of entering students?

*Age.* Professional programs differ in the number of years of college required for admission. Accordingly, to the extent that age is taken as an indication of maturity, entering students in the several professions vary in level of maturity.

The figures for allied health and nursing shown in Table 1 apply only to college-based programs leading to a B.A. or B.S. degree. Older students are willingly accepted into these programs, and many R.N.s return to college to obtain a B.S. degree. Since applicants to nursing and pharmacy programs are the youngest, one would expect them to have less well-developed study skills and more frequent shifts in interest, both of which interfere with success and perseverance. This expectation was substantiated in a study of the rate of attrition among first-year students at the University of Illinois in 1978.

*Sex Distribution.* At one time, medicine and dentistry were considered primarily male occupations and nursing and allied health primarily female. During the last decade, the percentage of women students in dental, medical, and pharmacy schools has been growing steadily. The figures in Table 2 approximate current figures, except in pharmacy where entering classes may now contain 40 to 50 percent women. During the same period, there has been some growth in male admission to nursing schools. In B.S. programs, the increase ranged from 2 percent to 7 percent. Hence, nursing and most allied health professions are still predominantly female professions.

*Minority Status.* Favorable admissions policies and intense efforts to encourage minority students to apply have resulted in some increase in minority student enrollment, though participation fluctuates from program to program.

**Table 1. Ages of Entering Students in Five Professions.**

| Profession | Completed Years in College | Age at Entrance |
|---|---|---|
| Allied Health | 2 or 3 | 20 or 21 |
| Dentistry | 4 | 22 |
| Medicine | 4 | 22 |
| Nursing | 1 | 19 |
| Pharmacy | 1 | 19 |

Table 2. Percentage of Women in Entering Classes of Dental, Medical, and
Pharmacy Schools.

| Year | Dentistry | Medicine | Pharmacy |
|------|-----------|----------|----------|
| 1971–1972 | 3.1 | 13.7 | 24.9 |
| 1972–1973 | 4.2 | 16.8 | 26.5 |
| 1973–1974 | 7.2 | 19.7 | 28.3 |
| 1974–1975 | 11.2 | 22.2 | 30.4 |
| 1975–1976 | 12.3 | 23.8 | 33.2 |
| 1976–1977 | 13.5 | 24.7 | 36.8 |

Source: U.S. Department of Health, Education, and Welfare, Bureau of Health Manpower, 1978.

Since 1976, efforts to increase minority participation in the health professions
have persisted; nonetheless, two-year programs continue to attract more minority
students than do longer programs.

*Personality Profiles.* In addition to such demographic characteristics as
age, sex, and race, the personality profiles of applicants are also relevant. Though
each profession attracts students with varied personalities, studies show that professional prototypes do exist. McCaulley (1978) and Rezler (Rezler and French,
1975; Rezler and Buckley, 1977; Rezler, Manasse, and Buckley, 1977) found significant differences on the Myers-Briggs Type Indicator (MBTI) among students in
different health professions. While they found sizable numbers of both Extroverts
and Introverts in each profession, differences were more pronounced on the
Sensing-Intuition dimension. Only medical and occupational therapy students
are primarily Intuitive; all other professions attract a larger proportion of Sensing
individuals. Proportionately more women are Feeling types, irrespective of the
profession they have chosen; hence, fields where the majority of entering students
are females are also fields where the majority are Feeling types. Students in most
health professions appear to prefer to work in an organized, predictable environment; therefore, most health fields attract more Judging than Perceptive types
(Tables 4 and 5).

Table 3. Percentage of Minority Students in 1976 Entering Classes in
Nine Health Professions.

| Profession | Percent Admitted |
|------------|------------------|
| Dietetics | 13 |
| Medical Records | 19 |
| Medical Laboratory | 16 |
| Occupational Therapy | 7 |
| Physical Therapy | 8 |
| Dentistry | 11 |
| Medicine | 12 |
| Nursing | 14 |
| Pharmacy | 9 |

Source: U.S. Department of Health, Education, and Welfare, Bureau of Health Manpower, 1978.

**Table 4. Scales on the Myers-Briggs Type Indicator (MBTI).**

*Extrovert-Introvert (E-I)*
E people attend to the outer world of people and things in action, making confident use of trial and error.
I people focus on the inner world of ideas and like to reflect at great length before acting.

*Sensing-Intuitive (S-N)*
S people tend to be realistic, practical, observant, fun-loving, and good at remembering and working with facts.
N people tend to value imagination, inspiration, and possibilities and are good at new ideas, projects, and problem solving.

*Thinking-Feeling (T-F)*
T people tend to analyze, weigh facts, and think that impersonal logic is a surer guide than human likes and dislikes.
F people tend to sympathize, weigh the personal values, and feel that human likes and dislikes are more important than logic.

*Judging-Perceptive (J-P)*
J people live in a planned, decided, orderly way, aiming to regulate life and control it.
P people live in a flexible, spontaneous way, aiming to understand life and adapt to it.

*Note:* These scales are bipolar; thus, an individual is labeled either E or I, S or N, T or F, J or P.

**Table 5. Percentage of Students in Different Health Professions on
Contrasting MBTI Scales.**

*MBTI Scales**

| Profession | E | I | S | N | T | F | J | P |
|---|---|---|---|---|---|---|---|---|
| Dietetics | 66 | 34 | 56 | 44 | 24 | 76 | 69 | 31 |
| Medical Technology | 49 | 51 | 59 | 41 | 41 | 59 | 62 | 38 |
| Medical Records | 50 | 50 | 70 | 30 | 26 | 74 | 68 | 32 |
| Occupational Therapy | 61 | 39 | 40 | 60 | 23 | 77 | 49 | 51 |
| Physical Therapy | 55 | 45 | 56 | 44 | 28 | 72 | 56 | 44 |
| Dentistry | 53 | 47 | 59 | 41 | 50 | 50 | 69 | 31 |
| Medicine | 49 | 51 | 34 | 66 | 39 | 61 | 54 | 46 |
| Nursing (B.S.) | 60 | 40 | 61 | 39 | 26 | 74 | 62 | 38 |
| Pharmacy | 47 | 53 | 56 | 44 | 48 | 52 | 59 | 41 |

*E = extrovert, I = introvert, S = sensing, N = intuitive, T = thinking, F = feeling, J = judging, P = perceptive. See Table 4 for further explanation.
*Source:* McCaulley, 1978, Tables C-14, D-2, E-5, G-3, I-3, J-2, K-2, L-2, S-10.

Given these similarities and differences, it is clear that many health professions can accommodate a variety of personality types, but certain types will fit in better with the duties and demands of certain professions. Some professions—for example, medicine—offer considerably more room for multiple roles and settings than others. A future pathologist and a future practitioner of family medicine are likely to represent different personality types, although both are M.D.s. Other professions—for example, medical records—will satisfy mainly Sensing and Judging students.

*Career Choice.* In a large-scale survey of health career aspirants, Holstrom (1975) asked prospective medical technologists, occupational and physical therapists, nurses, and dentists to state their reasons for wanting to enter these professions. In general, they rarely spoke about the congruence between their personalities and their chosen profession; reasons given referred mainly to different characteristics of the profession. Medical technicians cited the availability of jobs, high earnings, chance for steady progress, and the prestige of the occupation; most of them expected to work in a hospital or clinic. Occupational and physical therapists, on the other hand, wanted to work with people and ideas and sought opportunities for originality. They hoped to do counseling with their patients, in addition to occupational or physical therapy. Only one in three wanted to work in a hospital, and one-third desired to work with children in schools. Nursing was chosen by aspirants because of patient contact, opportunity to help and to make a contribution to society, steady progress, chance for administrative responsibilities, and availability of jobs. Dental candidates cited high earnings as their primary reason for choosing dentistry. The prestige of the profession and the autonomy offered were other important factors in their career choice. Most dental students wanted to go into general practice when they entered; they did not know about dental specialties until they started to study dentistry. Most of them expected to go into solo practice.

Other studies have shown that prospective pharmacists are interested in combining the technical and scientific aspects of the field with organizing efficient delivery systems. Retail pharmacy was preferred by 50 percent of the males, while 34 percent of the females selected hospital pharmacy and only 26 percent wanted to work in retail. There was little fluctuation in career choices from the freshman to the senior year. The only downward trend was in manufacturing; fewer seniors than freshmen wished to go into industry (Rezler, Mrtek, and Manasse, 1976).

Medicine attracts students for a variety of reasons, including scientific interest, desire to help, autonomy, prestige, and high income. It offers a wide range of specialties to choose from, with varying degrees of patient contact. Though medical students are aware of specialties at the outset and consider a wide range of possibilities, numerous studies show that about 50 percent change their specialty preference between the freshman and the senior year. The shift in student interest from scientist to clinician-specialist to primary physician has been described in an interesting study by Funkenstein (1970).

This brief sketch of the personality patterns and career interests of entering students in different health professions is included to remind readers that vocational interest and personality are strong motivators. Their potential contribution, as compared with academic indicators, has not been fully exploited in selecting students for admission.

## Selection Methods

Student characteristics found to be important in selection may be divided into four categories. Measures that indicate what an individual is capable of doing intellectually belong in the first group. The grade point average (GPA), class rank, aptitude, and achievement test scores are good examples. Although an aptitude test is designed primarily to predict success in some future learning activity and an achievement test is customarily used to measure past learning, both have been employed to predict future performance. The second category includes such characteristics as interest, motivation, attitudes, values, personal adjustment, and social habits. A wide variety of procedures is available to assess these characteristics, but only interviews and letters of recommendation have been widely used. The third group contains biographical data, such as age, sex, race, family status, place of origin, volunteer activities, work experience, and specific career goals. A biographical inventory and written statements of goals are the usual methods for collecting these data. The last category consists of psychomotor skills, usually measured by some kind of test. Although psychomotor skills are important in several health professions (for example, in surgery, medical technology, nursing, occupational therapy, physical therapy), they are measured only in dentistry at the time of student selection.

Since applicants outnumber available places in some health professions programs and some unpromising candidates apply to all, admissions committees must establish priorities. In medical, dental, and pharmacy schools, past achievement and scores on entrance exams determine acceptance. In allied health schools, motivation and personality have counted more heavily than test scores in the past. Johnson, Arbes, and Thompson (1974) surveyed thirty-seven occupational therapy programs and found that the characteristics listed in Table 6 were preferred in applicants.

Nursing schools use many different methods to select students as is shown in Table 7, which is based on a survey of 1,439 schools (Nash, 1977). In a more recent article, Schwirian (1976) observes that admissions procedures are changing in nursing schools. There is increasing reliance on academic achievement and entrance test scores and less concern about motivation and personality. This change is related to nursing faculties' recent emphasis on problem solving, independent judgment, self-direction, and leadership in nursing education.

*Measures of Intellectual Ability.* Despite the variety of preferred applicant characteristics, most investigations have been limited to studies of the predictive

**Table 6. Preferred Characteristics of Applicants to Occupational Therapy Programs.**

| *Preferred Characteristics* | *Percent of Programs* |
| --- | --- |
| Motivation | 98 |
| Personality | 97 |
| Academic Achievement | 86 |
| Academic Ability | 46 |
| Experience in Health-Related Activities | 24 |
| Knowledge of OT | 19 |
| Health | 16 |
| Social Achievement | 14 |
| Minority Student | 5 |

*Source:* Johnson, Arbes, and Thompson, 1974, p. 599.

Table 7. Methods Used by Nursing Schools to Select Students.

| Selection Methods | Percent of Schools |
|---|---|
| Application Form | 85 |
| Health Form | 82 |
| High School Rank | 79 |
| Interview | 72 |
| Entrance Tests | 72 |
| Statement of Motivation | 62 |
| References | 54 |
| Biographical Inventory | 47 |
| Statement of Financial Ability | 23 |

Source: Nash, 1977, p. 12.

power of cognitive measures. In using these measures, selection committees generally consider the applicant's grades first, since it has been shown repeatedly that the grade point average (GPA) from preprofessional school is the best single predictor of achievement in a professional program. Maintaining high grades over a period of time reflects motivation and work habits, in addition to subject matter knowledge. To allow for variations in the standards of different colleges, many schools weight the GPA according to the applicant's college.

In addition to overall achievement represented by the GPA, standardized entrance tests have been employed in all professions. The American College Test (ACT) and the Scholastic Aptitude Test (SAT), once popular in allied health and pharmacy, were replaced in the 1970s by custom-made entrance test batteries, such as the Allied Health Professions Admissions Test (AHPAT) and the Pharmacy College Admissions Test (PCAT). Unique entrance test batteries have been available to schools of medicine and dentistry for a long time. The four major specialized entrance tests in current use and their respective subtests are shown in Table 8.

Scores from the entrance tests listed in Table 8 have been used to supplement grade point averages for a number of reasons. By rating applicants on a standardized instrument, the grade record can be verified. Variations in the quality of undergraduate institutions, grading standards, and the difficulty level of undergraduate courses can be counterbalanced. Finally, standardized entrance tests can provide estimates of overall ability of students whose early college performance was not distinguished but who showed substantial gains in the later years, the so-called late bloomers.

The Dental Aptitude Test (DAT) and the Medical College Admissions Test (MCAT) have been used since the 1950s and continue to play a major role in admission decisions. A recent survey of admissions procedures conducted by the Dental Aptitude Test Committee (Boyd, Teteruck, and Thompson, 1980) showed that the most heavily weighted factors in selecting applicants to dental school were preprofessional grades and DAT scores, including scores on the Perceptual Motor Ability subtest—a measure of manual dexterity.

In the 1960s, the MCAT came under heavy criticism from many medical educators. They argued that while it predicted academic performance in the basic sciences, it failed to predict clinical performance either during medical school or

**Table 8. Admissions Test Batteries.**

| *Allied Health Professions Admissions Test (AHPAT-1975)* | *Dental Aptitude Test (DAT-1950)* | *Medical College Admissions Test (New MCAT-1977)* | *Pharmacy College Admissions Test (PCAT-1973)* |
|---|---|---|---|
| Verbal Ability | Academic | Reading | Verbal Ability |
| Reading Compre- | Verbal | Quantitative | Reading |
| hension | Reasoning | Biology | Quantitative Ability |
| Quantitative | Reading | Chemistry | Biology |
| Ability | Comprehension | Physics | Chemistry |
| Biology | Quantitative | Science Problems | |
| Chemistry | Reasoning | | |
| | Biology | | |
| | Chemistry | | |
| | Manual | | |
| | Perceptual | | |
| | Motor Ability | | |

in subsequent practice. It was also argued that the MCAT overstressed recall of specific facts but failed to measure analytical skills or such personal qualities as empathy, responsibility, and flexibility desired in the practice of medicine. In response to these criticisms, the Association of American Medical Colleges mobilized a nationwide task force in 1972–73 to revise the MCAT and to consider the addition of noncognitive measures. The new MCAT differs from the old MCAT in several respects: It has six subtests, as shown in Table 8, while the old test had four—Verbal, Quantitative Ability, General Information, and Science. The number of test items requiring scientific application rather than simple recall was increased. Comparison of the old with the new MCAT indicates that both are two-factor tests (Molidor and Elstein, 1979). In the old MCAT, the Verbal and General Information subtests accounted for the greatest total amount of variance. In the new MCAT, the scientific and quantitative tests account for most of the variance. Hence, if a student wants to be admitted to medical school, achievement in biology, chemistry, and quantitative skills is more important than ever.

Both the AHPAT and the PCAT were developed in the 1970s. The major impetus was to provide a more accurate prediction of performance than was possible from using the ACT or SAT scores obtained in high school, since the longer the elapsed time from the predictor to the criterion, the greater the inaccuracy is likely to be (Katzell, 1977). Since allied health students customarily enter in the junior year of college, the AHPAT tests are based at the college sophomore level.

There is a great deal of similarity among these four entrance test batteries. Each contains achievement tests in two or more sciences, usually chemistry and biology, as well as measures of verbal and quantitative ability and reading comprehension. None contains tests in the humanities or the social sciences. Thus, students who major in a science should score higher than students who major in a social science. Further, all four batteries are limited to multiple-choice type questions that reward the convergent rather than the divergent thinker. Finally, none of these examinations includes a test of written communication skills although writing case studies, case summaries, interview notes, referral notes, and reports are pertinent tasks required in many health professions. The omission of writing tests suggests that admissions committees do not consider writing skills crucial in the health professions.

*Measures of Other Characteristics.* Many admissions committees are reluctant to base the selection of students solely on intellectual qualifications and test scores, despite the importance they attach to these credentials. Faculty insist that the task of selection should not be left entirely to a computer, for there is more to a person than is disclosed by an academic record and achievement test scores. Hence, applicants are often interviewed to determine whether they have the desired attitudes, values, interests, and personality. However, the interview as a selection device has been a source of controversy for a long time. Many committee members have felt and will continue to feel that the interview is the best way to appraise personal qualities. However, research has cast a good deal of doubt on the validity of this position (Wright, 1969).

Interviewers often disagree when they rate the same applicant (Morse, 1971; Mann, 1979; Litton-Hawes, MacLean, and Hines, 1976; Gordon and Lincoln, 1976). Social graces are often mistaken for empathy, motivation, and maturity. Focusing on the assessment of personal characteristics during the interview has proved to be counterproductive, but assessment of the candidate's knowledge about program demands appears to be productive (Weinstein, Brown, and Wahlstrom, 1979).

Perhaps the purpose of selection interviews needs to be reconsidered. For example, Reeves (1978) bemoans the lack of clear specifications for the sort of person that is needed in nursing. But even if everybody should agree that maturity and integrity are important, it is doubtful that the degree to which a candidate possesses these qualities could be accurately determined in a brief selection interview.

Some educators criticize negative research findings on the ground that interviews should not be expected to predict grades, and there is at least one study that demonstrates that selection interviews do predict the quality of the internship evaluation letter given to senior medical students (Murden and others, 1978). It might be fruitful to explore further the value of interviews in relation to nonacademic criteria. Other suggestions concerning selection interviews include using a highly structured format, training interviewers, employing group interviews, and using students and representatives from the profession, in addition to faculty members, as interviewers. Irrespective of research findings, the interview is likely to continue as a selection device because admissions committees have faith in it.

Letters of recommendation are usually requested for the assessment of personal characteristics. Unfortunately, these letters often fail to evaluate the applicant's strengths *and* weaknesses or the importance of his or her extracurricular activities. In addition, they may fail to indicate the applicant's standing in comparison with peers.

Personality and interest tests have been widely used in research but rarely in selection. For example, a survey of 117 medical schools shows that a wide variety of noncognitive tests was used to measure educational process, professional development, skills in patient care, and personal adjustment (D'Costa and

Schafer, 1972). Many studies have been reported in the literature where personality tests were employed to predict clinical performance, primarily in medicine and nursing (Schofield, 1972). Some of these studies are discussed more fully later in this chapter.

*Biographical Data.* Biographical data are routinely collected from all applicants and reviewed by admissions committees. Certain parts of the data are given special attention. At one time, *age* was considered to be an important factor in admission; upper age limits were set in many schools. In the 1970s, age limits have been extended upward; more older women have been admitted, particularly in nursing and allied health. *Race* now receives preferential treatment, in keeping with affirmative action. Special efforts are being made by most schools to attract minority students. The applicant's *place of origin* may be given special attention in some schools, since it has been found that students from rural areas are more likely to return to rural areas to practice than are those from cities and suburbia (Hutt, 1976). Health-related *work experience* is considered highly desirable in some programs, based on the assumption that those students who have assisted health professionals will have a more realistic picture of their intended profession.

In addition to age, race, place of origin, and work experience, some programs focus on other biographical details. For example, Gellhorn and Scheuer (1978) report equal weight given to academic and nonacademic qualifications in selecting students into a two-year biomedical program. Elstein and Teitelbaum (1974) developed a system for quantifying biographical data to reduce the cost and time of selecting a small number of students from a large applicant pool.

*Tests of Psychomotor Skills.* Dentistry is the only health profession where psychomotor ability is tested as part of the admissions process. Its weight in accepting or rejecting applicants has not been reported. Tasks performed by other health professionals (for example, occupational therapists and surgeons) also require manual dexterity, but students for these professions are not selected on that basis.

### Relation Between Selection and Outcome Measures

Admissions committees strive to select students who will perform well in school, graduate, and become competent professionals. Thus, the value of any selection method depends on its ability to predict a given outcome. These predicted outcomes may occur as early as the first year in a program, during the latter part of the program, or even after graduation. Table 9 shows predictors grouped along qualitative lines and outcomes by time of occurrence, immediate or delayed. Illustrative outcome measures are listed in each cell. Findings from representative studies of allied health, dentistry, medicine, nursing, and pharmacy are reviewed here.

*Allied Health.* Most studies since 1960 attempt to predict two kinds of outcomes—grade point averages and clinical ratings. For prediction of GPA, the following measures of intellectual ability were used: entry GPA, the American College Test (ACT), the Scholastic Aptitude Test (SAT), and the AHPAT (Schimpfhauser and Broski, 1976; Leiken and Cunningham, 1980; Blaisdell and Gordon, 1979). In all studies, entry GPA was the best predictor of academic performance in allied health; this held true for studies based on samples of physical

Table 9. Predictors and Outcome Measures.

| Predictors | Immediate Outcomes | Intermediate Outcomes | Long-Range Outcomes |
|---|---|---|---|
| Intellectual (verbal and quantitative ability, specific knowledge) | Success in first year of school; GPA, no attrition, progress to second year without delay | Success in later years in school; GPA, clinical grades, passing external professional examinations | Professional knowledge judged by peers; demonstration of professional growth via publications and leadership |
| Nonintellectual (values, attitudes, personality, interests) | Interaction with peer groups and faculty | Interviewing and patient teaching skills; clinical performance ratings; interpersonal relations with other health professionals; ability to cope with stress | Establishment of satisfactory professional and patient relations; achievement of patient cooperation; demonstration of professional commitment |
| Biographical (sex, age, socioeconomic background, work experience) | Choice of school and profession | Choice of specialty and work setting | Choice of specialty and of practice arena; supervision, teaching, or administration |
| Psychomotor | Dissection skills; laboratory skills; technical procedures | Laboratory, dental and minor surgical skills; art and crafts skills in occupational therapy; technical procedures in occupational therapy and physical therapy | Dental and surgical skills; laboratory skills |

Source: Hutchins, 1972.

therapy, occupational therapy, medical technology, and dietetics students. Both the ACT and the AHPAT improved prediction of GPA to varying degrees ($r = .10$ to .72), depending on the subtest and the program. Due to substantial overlap between the ACT and the AHPAT, one or the other is sufficient to select applicants who are most likely to succeed academically. Clinical performance is much less predictable than academic performance. Tidd and Conine (1974) studied physical therapy students over a twelve-year period and found that the entry GPA of each class was strongly related to grades in academic courses ($r = .88$) but much less to grades in clinical courses ($r = .29$). Interests, rather than intellectual predictors such as entry GPA and the Florida Placement Examination, appeared to predict clinical performance (Anderson and Jantzen, 1965; Bailey, Jantzen, and Dunteman, 1969). Graduation or withdrawal was also influenced by measured interests and values but was not affected by entry grades or Scholastic Aptitude Test (SAT) scores (Blaisdell and Gordon, 1979).

Since the number of studies that relate selection measures to outcome measures is limited in allied health, suggestions rather than generalizations are offered. Admissions committees can depend mainly on entry GPA and, to a lesser extent, on either ACT or AHPAT scores in selecting students who can be expected to earn satisfactory grades in academic subjects. Clinical performance may be slightly influenced by intellectual ability but depends more on measured interests and values. While interviews are widely used in allied health schools to screen applicants, studies could not be located where interview ratings were used to predict either academic or clinical performance. In view of the predictive potential of measured interests and values, the use of interest and value inventories, along with biographical data, may prove to be more productive than interviews for selection purposes.

*Dentistry.* Several dental educators claim that the predental GPA is the best single predictor of success in dental school (Hood, 1963; Chen and Podshadley, 1967; Kreit and McDonald, 1968; Rasmussen and Boozer, 1978). Ross (1967) believes that entering GPA is a good predictor of a student's ability to cope with the basic sciences but has little value in predicting overall success. The predictive power of both the academic and the manual scores from the Dental Aptitude Test (DAT) has been studied in relation to freshman as well as senior performance. Correlations between grades in theory courses and DAT academic scores range between .21 and .28, while the correlations between grades on theory courses and entering GPA range from .34 to .38. As recently as 1980, Boyd concluded that preprofessional grades are still the best predictors of success in dental school (Boyd, Teteruck, and Thompson, 1980).

The score on the Perceptual Motor Ability subtest of the DAT correlated positively with technique grades in twenty-one of thirty-three dental schools studied (American Dental Association, 1978).

Academic predictors have been supplemented by interviews and personality tests to obtain more accurate predictions of success at different levels. However, in the majority of the studies, little or no relationship was found between these measures and success. Gough and Kirk (1970) utilized the California Psychological Inventory (CPI) to predict grades. Scales that correlated with academic performance in dental school were Sense of Well-Being, Responsibility, Socialization, Tolerance, Communality, Achievement via Conformance, Intellectual Efficiency, and Flexibility. While these results are encouraging, it should be noted that they were obtained under conditions in which student responses to the CPI did *not* influence admission. The fact that applicants tend to select socially desirable answers to improve their chances when personality tests are used to screen for admission limits the practical implications of this study.

The attrition rate nationwide during four years of dental education has been about 7 percent, and withdrawals for personal reasons outnumber withdrawals for academic reasons (American Dental Association, 1979, p. 1). The most frequent reasons for withdrawal are change of career objective and general lack of interest. When withdrawal is due to academic causes, the problems arise in didactic courses.

*Medicine.* The large pool of qualified applicants, of whom only 39 percent are accepted nationwide, permits a high degree of selectivity (Gordon, 1979). Selection is based primarily on college grades and scores on the MCAT test—that is, measures of cognitive achievement. Hence, it is not surprising that 98 percent of those who enter finish medical school, and attrition occurs mainly for personal reasons.

The relationship between entry GPA, scores on the old Medical College Admissions Test (MCAT), and grades during the preclinical years has been repeatedly studied (Edwards, 1978; Friedman, 1979; Sanazaro and Hutchins, 1963; Erdmann and others, 1971; Gough, Hall, and Harris, 1963; Ingersoll and Graves, 1965). Results have been mixed, but in general, low correlations have been found between MCAT scores and performance in medical school during the first two years. This had led to justifications of the MCAT (Sanazaro and Hutchins, 1963; Erdmann and others, 1971), as well as criticisms and suggestions as to its appropriate use (Molidor and Elstein, 1979; Gough, Hall, and Harris, 1963; Bartlett, 1967). It has been repeatedly observed that one of the main purposes of the MCAT was to identify the marginal applicants, rather than the individuals likely to perform at the top level. Nevertheless, it appears that medical schools have utilized MCAT data in such a way that individuals with higher scores are more likely to be accepted for admission than individuals with lower scores (Funkenstein, 1966; Stefanu and Farmer, 1971; Williams and others, 1977; Hamberg, Swanson, and Dohner, 1971).

At this time, studies relating new MCAT scores only to first year GPA are available. Erdmann (1980) reports that in three out of five students, new MCAT scores are better predictors than GPAs. McGuire (1980), on the other hand, finds that maximum predictability is achieved by the joint use of entry GPA and the Science Problems subtest of the MCAT. Actually, it seems that only two subtests make a major contribution to predicting basic science grades: the Science Problems and the Science Knowledge subtests (Cullen and others, 1980; Friedman and Bakewell, 1980).

Although most prediction studies of preclinical performance are limited to cognitive predictors, a few researchers experimented with the addition of noncognitive measures. In one study, measures of a variety of personality traits were added to the usual cognitive predictors (Roessler and others, 1978). The addition of personality variables greatly enhanced the prediction of basic science grades and National Board of Medical Examiners (NBME) Part I scores. Multiple correlations increased from .25 to .55. Barratt and White (1969) found that students who were unusually high or low on both anxiety and impulsiveness performed less well than those in whom these traits were balanced.

Several writers have suggested the importance of distinguishing between performance in the earlier and later years of medical school. In a follow-up study on admissions, basic science grades were compared with those from clinical rotations (Rhoads and others, 1974). Only about half the students who excelled in the basic science portion of the curriculum did so in the clinical portion. Admission data predicted only performance in the basic sciences, not in the clinical years. Similar findings are provided by a study covering four years of medical education, where correlations of entering GPA and MCAT scores with grades were shown to range from a maximum of .28 in the first year to .00 in the senior year (Gough, Hall, and Harris, 1963).

If the MCAT is useless in predicting clinical performance, what other tools could be employed? The California Personality Inventory, the Adjective Checklist, the Personality Research Form, the Edwards Personal Preference Schedule, the Allport-Vernon Study of Values, the Strong Vocational Interest Blank, and the Minnesota Multiphasic Personality Inventory (MMPI) have all been studied as predictors of clinical performance (Johnson and Hutchins, 1966; Rothman, 1973; Jiske, Ort, and Ford, 1964; Korman, Stubblefield, and Martin, 1968; Gough and Hall, 1964). The criterion itself in clinical performance has also been studied and shown to embrace two major, independent performance dimensions: academic achievement and clinical potential. Clinical potential includes clinical effectiveness with patients and the utilization of knowledge and ability in the practice of medicine. This latter factor is moderately related to such personality characteristics as sense of well-being, responsibility, self-control, tolerance, achievement via conformance, nurturance, affiliation, and deference. Personality measures offer promise as forecasters of clinical competence, although results to date fall short of a satisfactory level of predictive accuracy for individuals. This state of affairs may be attributable to the questionable validity and/or reliability of faculty ratings, the most often used criterion of clinical performance.

In the studies just cited, the samples included only medical students. The clinical performance of residents has also been studied, using a combination of cognitive and noncognitive variables as predictors (Kegel-Flom, 1975; Keck and others, 1979). The latter study included twenty selection and evaluation measures divided into three categories: cognitive, noncognitive, and performance based on observations. The criterion, the Resident Evaluation Form, contained thirty-three scales covering cognitive abilities, professional responsibilities, clinical skills, and interpersonal relations. The results indicate that a combination of cognitive and noncognitive measures functions best in predicting the resident's clinical performance. Two personality tests, Holland's Self-Directed Search and the Omnibus Personality Inventory, enhanced prediction substantially by contributing information that is relatively independent of other predictors.

In the final analysis, selection procedures are meant to identify individuals who will turn out to be "good" practitioners of medicine. One could expect that the major criterion used to validate selection procedures, namely grades in medical school, would relate to measures of medical practice. This assumption has been challenged by a review of the literature, which indicates little or no correlation between grades in medical school and performance in professional practice (Wingard and Williamson, 1973). The authors explain that grades often reflect only the ability to memorize isolated facts, whereas career performance measures include observations of actual medical practice and review of clinical records (Peterson and others, 1956; Clute, 1963; Price and others, 1964). These studies challenge the exclusive use of grades as criterion measures during medical school and draw attention to the often inadequate tests upon which grades are based.

Although the Association of American Medical Colleges (AAMC) longitudinal study (1979) of medical school graduates does not focus on the *quality* of performance in practice, the findings are pertinent for selection in relating five types of predictors to five measures of career choice (Table 10). When overlap among predictors is taken into account and only unique, independent contributions are considered, achievement measures add nothing significant to the prediction of any of these five outcomes. Personal qualities and attitudes, however, predict all outcomes except the size of the community chosen for practice.

**Table 10. Summary of Hierarchical Regression Results, with Predictors Entered in the Order Listed.**

| Predictors | Outcomes | | | | |
| --- | --- | --- | --- | --- | --- |
| | Academician vs. Practitioner | Primary vs. Nonprimary Care | Size of Current Practice Community[a] | Physician Income[b] | Orientation Toward Government Involvement in Medical Care |
| Background | Δ | Δ | Δ | | |
| Personal qualities/ attitudes | ΔΔΔ | Δ | | Δ | ΔΔ |
| Achievement | | | | | |
| Type of premedical college | | | | | Δ |
| Type of medical college | ΔΔ[c] | | | | Δ |
| Personal constraints | | | | | |

Key:    Δ indicates significant increase in explained variance of between 1 and 5 percent.
ΔΔ indicates significant increase in explained variance between 5 and 10 percent.
ΔΔΔ indicates significant increase in explained variance of more than 10 percent.

[a] Analysis performed for specialty.
[b] Analysis performed controlling for specialty and hours worked.
[c] Interpretation modified by the presence of a significant interaction between type of medical school and personal qualities/attitudes.

*Source:* Association of American Medical Colleges, 1979, p. 8.

Studies pertaining to selection and admission to medical school could fill several volumes. In spite of some disagreements among investigators, there is more agreement than disagreement, and certain themes recur in the literature, summarized as follows:

- The best predictors of preclinical achievement are the preentry GPA and the Science Problems subtest of the new MCAT.
- There are two independent performance dimensions in medical school: academic achievement and clinical performance. The former includes mainly memorization of factual information; the latter includes application of knowledge and interpersonal effectiveness with patients.
- Clinical performance cannot be predicted from cognitive entrance tests or from preclinical grades. Different kinds of personality tests have enhanced the prediction of clinical performance substantially. A combination of cognitive and noncognitive variables best forecasts clinical performance.
- Personality and attitude measures are also related to career choice, income, and attitudes toward medical practice twenty years after graduation from medical school. Academic achievement in medical school is not related to these outcomes.
- Quality of medical practice is unrelated to grades in medical school.

Given the above findings, it is not surprising that many medical educators counsel changes in the selection process. For example, Keck and others (1979, p. 765) conclude: "These findings lend support to a widespread subjective dissatisfaction with the tendency to subordinate personal attributes to cognitive measures in selection and evaluation of medical students. The point of diminishing returns may have been reached in regard to the use of cognitive criteria. Given the cognitive homogeneity of most medical school applicants, it no longer suffices to select those intellectually capable of completing their medical education. Almost all are capable. The prime objective of medical education should be to select and train those who will perform best as physicians. Consideration of noncognitive criteria appears to be essential in order to further this objective." In spite of these sentiments, the tendency to focus on cognitive selectors continues with the new MCAT, and there is no organized effort to reorient the selection procedure.

*Nursing.* Prediction of success in nursing programs is complicated by multiple routes to becoming an R.N. One route is the two-year community college program leading to the A.A. degree, to which students are admitted after high school. Another route is the hospital-based diploma program, which is being phased out. The third, the one most favored program by nurse-educators, is the B.S. program, which requires one year of college prior to entry. While the A.A. program emphasizes technical skills, the B.S. program provides the scientific and theoretical foundations of nursing practice. Admission variables to these three kinds of programs have been related to four kinds of criteria: (1) academic achievement, (2) attrition, (3) performance on state board examinations, and (4) on-the-job performance. Although the goals and the curricular content differ among the three programs, many prediction studies are based on mixed samples. Hence, reported findings apply to more than one kind of program unless stated otherwise.

The most frequently used criterion measures of academic achievement are course grades and the GPA at different levels in the program. As in other health professions, the best predictor of academic achievement in nursing school is prior academic achievement. Test scores provided by the ACT, SAT, and other academic aptitude tests have only moderate predictive value (Chissom and Lanier, 1975; Lewis and Welch, 1975; Michael and others, 1971; Yess, 1980). In a large-scale study conducted in Toronto to identify the characteristics of successful generic nursing students, the best predictors of academic achievement were the number of science courses taken in high school and college, as well as grades in English courses (Weinstein, Brown, and Wahlstrom, 1980). Entry liberal arts GPA was the best predictor of exit liberal arts GPA for R.N.s who enrolled in a B.S. continuation program, irrespective of the time elapsed since the entry GPA was obtained. Age was not a factor in achievement (Rezler and Moore, 1978). Other factors associated with the successful completion of a B.S. program to obtain an R.N. were the National League for Nursing (NLN) medical-surgical test score and the SAT verbal score. Personal and family responsibilities did not interfere with completion of the degree program (Raderman and Allen, 1974).

Only a few studies chose to look at clinical performance, apart from performance in theory courses. Those that did agree that neither academic aptitude and achievement (Michael, Haney, and Jones, 1966; Johnson and Leonard, 1970) nor personality tests or interviews with students (Hagarty, 1976; Weinstein,

Brown, and Wahlstrom, 1979) predict clinical performance. Whether the observed lack of relationship is due to the predictors or to invalid and/or unreliable criterion measures cannot be ascertained from the studies, since nursing faculty feel less confident about clinical performance evaluation than about evaluating the knowledge of the students in the classroom.

Attrition from nursing programs has been consistently high over the years. Throughout all types of nursing programs, about 33 percent of all entrants fail to graduate (Sherman, 1978). Among this group, 80 percent drop out during the first year. A recent study based on a national sample found that 27 percent of the two-year students and 41 percent of the four-year students withdrew (Munro, 1980). Added to the high rate of attrition is the nationwide shrinkage in the supply of applicants to nursing programs (National League for Nursing, 1981). Under these circumstances, it is very important to identify causes of attrition in order to increase retention.

Attrition has been related to many different kinds of predictors, among them measures of academic aptitude and achievement (Raderman and Allen, 1974; Hutcheson, Garland, and Prather, 1973; Wittmeyer, Camiscioni, and Purdy, 1971; Backman and Steindler, 1971; Knopke, 1979). Although different tests were used as predictors in different studies, the findings agree that students who withdrew voluntarily did not differ in aptitude/achievement at entrance from those who continued in nursing school, and students who were dropped tended to have lower high school rank or GPA and tended to score lower on measures of scientific aptitude and achievement.

However, academic difficulties account for only about 40 percent of the students who leave nursing school. To identify the nonacademic components of attrition, measures of personality, interest, values, and attitudes were related to voluntary withdrawal (Levitt; Lubin, and DeWitt, 1971; Klahn, 1969; Smith, 1965; Baker, 1975; Jones, 1975; Warnecke, 1973; Knopke, 1979; Hutcheson, Garland, and Lowe, 1979). No clearly defined pattern of relationships emerged from these studies, partly because personality dimensions measured by different tests varied from study to study. In addition, a student with a given personality may continue in a program that fits his or her needs but may withdraw from a program whose goals are incongruent with that student's predispositions. For example, students with high need for dependence, order, and nurturance were found to be more likely to succeed in a traditional program (Thurston, Brunclik, and Feldhusen, 1965, 1968); on the other hand, a program that emphasized leadership skills was found to lose deferent, dependent students. Hence, attrition may be the outcome of incompatibility between the environment and the student's personality (Knopke, 1979). Since the image of the nurse is being reshaped nationwide, the personality attributes of entering students should be considered in relation to the particular program the student wishes to enter. In addition to personality tests, nonacademic causes of attrition have also been related to biographical data and to expressed interests. Only age and marital status helped to predict graduation; older and married students were more likely to graduate (Knopf, 1972; Baker, 1975). Other biographical variables did not affect attrition.

Reasons for attrition have also been studied using questionnaires. Rotenberg (1978) observes that reasons given by administrators or faculty often do not coincide with reasons given by students and that most data have been collected from administrators. An exception is Miller's (1974) follow-up of voluntary dropouts where a wide gap was found between reality and students' expectations from nursing education. In a study by Knopke (1979), students gave four types of reasons for leaving: change in career choice, difficulties with basic science courses, inability to work with sick people, and inability to adjust to the program. Loss of interest in nursing and becoming interested in another career are perhaps the two most frequent reasons for voluntary attrition (Munro, 1980; Warnecke, 1973). In Canada, a selection interview that focused on the applicant's knowledge of program demands helped to reduce attrition (Weinstein, Brown, and Wahlstrom, 1979). It seems that students who have a realistic view of nursing and of the program they wish to enter are more likely to persevere, provided they have the academic qualifications.

Since a license to practice cannot be obtained without passing state boards, prediction of performance on the state board examination has been the subject of several studies (Brandt, Hastie, and Schumann, 1966; Baldwin, Mowbray, and Taylor, 1968; Ledbetter, 1968; Muhlenkamp, 1971; Deardorff, Denner, and Miller, 1976; Bell and Martindill, 1976; Wolfle and Bryant, 1978). Those studies that included NLN Achievement Test scores clearly showed that these tests are the best predictors of State Board Test Performance Examination (SBTPE) scores. The NLN Nursing of Children Test is a particularly strong predictor. To a lesser extent, theory grades and GPA from nursing school were useful predictors, but clinical performance was not. The latter finding supports previous studies where no relationship was found between academic achievement and clinical performance.

The most important criterion in any profession is on-the-job performance. In most studies, nursing performance has been rated by supervisors and occasionally also by physicians and by students rating themselves. In these studies, clinical practice grades from nursing school were found to be the only predictors that related to on-the-job ratings; GPA, grades from theory courses, and scores from achievement tests were all unrelated to work performance (Bohan, 1966; Brandt and Metheny, 1968; Saffer and Saffer, 1972; Dubs, 1975; Seither, 1980). In a somewhat different kind of study, Kelly (1974) used promotion into leadership positions in agencies as the criterion and four personality tests as predictors. The qualities characterizing nursing leaders were independence, self-assurance, intelligence, capacity for status, and being distant, relaxed, and resistant to psychological pressure.

In conclusion, the studies reviewed relating to nursing reveal that both academic achievement and performance on the state board examination are predictable from prior academic achievement and, to some extent, from standardized aptitude and achievement tests. However, academic failure accounts for less than half the dropouts from nursing schools. Since 33 percent of all students who enter a nursing program leave prior to graduation, the reduction of attrition is a serious challenge. The present tendency to use more cognitive tests in selection may help to reduce academic attrition but will not affect that large group of students who quit for nonacademic reasons. Lack of realistic orientation to nursing and incompatibility between a student's personality and the learning environment have been the major causes of nonacademic attrition.

The lack of relationship between grades and on-the-job performance is cause for concern. It suggests that the qualities valued by supervisors are different from those that lead to high grades in school. Superior clinical performance depends on many factors that do not influence academic performance. This finding is not unique to the nursing profession.

*Pharmacy.* Concern with the prediction of the academic success of pharmacy school applicants has increased since the 1970s. One reason for this concern is growth in the student population in certain schools. Increase in the number of applicants has been accompanied by parallel growth in the number of highly qualified candidates. This situation has created the need to research selection procedures.

Most of the studies reported in the literature relate preadmission data to GPA at the end of the first year. This criterion is chosen, possibly because pharmacy educators observed that student failure occurs mainly during the first year. The best predictor is entry GPA; the second best predictor is usually the PCAT Reading subtest; the third best predictor is either the Chemistry, Biology, or Quantitative Ability subtest of the PCAT battery (Munson and Bourne, 1976; Lowenthal, Wersin, and Smith, 1977; Liao and Adams, 1977). One study using entry GPA and grades in different preprofessional subjects found that only entry GPA and grades in chemistry were useful predictors of first-year GPA (Waldman and Leavitt, 1974). In another study, entry GPA and the type of college attended were found to be most useful predictors, and none of the PCAT tests made significant contributions (Jacoby and others, 1978).

Considering that pharmacy education is undergoing an ideological change, from a dispensing to a patient-centered approach, it is surprising that only one study was found that focused on performance in clinical pharmacy (Torosian and others, 1978). Predictors included entry GPA, SAT, SCAT, and ACT scores, all of which measure academic aptitude and achievement. Only entry GPA and previous achievement in mathematics and science courses were found to be correlated with grades in the third year of pharmacy school.

In conclusion, first-year GPA can be predicted from entry GPA and the Reading, Chemistry, Biology, and Quantitative Ability subtests of the PCAT. Type of college attended has also been a valuable predictor in some schools. With limited exceptions, prediction of achievement beyond the first year has not been investigated. Predictors in all studies measure exclusively academic potential; nonacademic predictors have not been employed in any study.

### Summary of Major Findings

Widespread admission trends and practices in health professions in the United States can be summarized as follows:

- Competition for admission is most pronounced in medicine and, secondly, in dentistry. In allied health, nursing, and pharmacy, steady growth in the number of applicants during the 1970s has recently been reversed, to the extent that some schools find it necessary to engage in vigorous recruiting.
- The number of women admitted to traditionally male professions—that is, medicine and dentistry—has increased substantially. There has been no com-

parable increase, however, of male applicants in traditionally female occupations.

- Limited growth in the proportion of minority student applicants has occurred in all health professional programs and has been facilitated by concentrated recruiting efforts.
- Selection in all health professions depends increasingly on prior academic achievement and test scores measuring academic aptitudes and/or achievement. In dentistry, medicine, and pharmacy, this practice is of long standing. At one time, admissions decisions in allied health and nursing were heavily weighted by personal interviews, written references, and qualitative judgments; the recent shift to academic criteria is particularly pronounced in nursing. Increased reliance on cognitive measures is related to a changed concept of the nursing profession.
- The criterion used in most studies is the GPA at the end of the first year. This criterion measures performance only in the basic sciences and/or in theoretical courses. Hence, selection is judged to be successful if students perform satisfactorily in theoretical/scientific courses.
- The best single predictor of first-year GPA in all professional programs is entry GPA, based on preprofessional grades.
- A variety of standardized achievement and scholastic aptitude tests, such as the SAT, SCAT, and ACT have been replaced by custom-made professional batteries, to improve prediction:
  1. The AHPAT was developed for allied health colleges, but its predictive value needs further studies. The AHPAT and the ACT seem to predict academic achievement equally well for mixed samples of allied health students in collegiate programs.
  2. The PCAT is used in pharmacy schools and, in general, the Reading subtest is the best predictor of first-year GPA. In some schools, the Chemistry or the Biology or the Quantitative Ability subtests improve prediction.
  3. The DAT has been used in dental schools for many years. The academic scores from the DAT have proved to predict grades in theory courses, but most researchers claim that the DAT predicts less well than entry GPA. For best results, both should be used. The Perceptual Motor Ability subtest score is a good predictor of grades in technique courses.
  4. The MCAT for medical school has been recently revised. The new MCAT's predictive value has been studied only in relation to first-year grades. Only two subtests contribute to prediction: the Science Problems and the Science Knowledge subtests. Scores from these subtests are substantially related to basic science grades.
- Clinical performance is much less predictable by currently available methods than academic performance. Standard academic predictors used to select students fail to predict clinical performance in all professions studied.
- Criterion measures of clinical performance include clinical ratings and clinical grades. The validity and reliability of these measures have been questioned by researchers, as well as faculty. Lack of predictability of clinical performance may be caused in part by inadequate criterion measures.
- Prediction of clinical performance has been studied most extensively in medicine. The ingredients of clinical performance have been defined as application of knowledge and interpersonal effectiveness with patients. Personality, value, and attitude measures show the most promise for predicting clinical performance.
- Although selection interviews do not predict achievement, they are likely to

continue to be used because admission committees have faith in them. They might be more useful if they were focused on assessing the applicant's knowledge about a career and a program, rather than his or her personality.

- Among the professions studied, attrition has been a serious problem only in nursing. About one-third of all entrants fail to graduate. Only 40 percent of the dropouts leave for academic reasons; 60 percent withdraw for a variety of personal reasons, mainly because they lose interest in nursing.
- No relationship has been shown in medicine and nursing between grades obtained in professional school and the quality of on-the-job performance. This finding suggests that the wisdom of relying exclusively on grades to validate selection is questionable.
- Personality and attitude measures are related to career choice, income, and attitudes toward medical practice twenty years after graduation. Academic achievement is not related to those outcomes.

### Implications and Recommendations

*Defining Minimal Cognitive Requirements.* Research on student selection for admission to a health profession program has been characterized mainly by refinements of cognitive measures during the past twenty years. Furthermore, these measures were validated in the majority of studies against grade point averages based on preclinical courses. Significant correlations between cognitive tests and first-year GPAs were used to justify selecting the students scoring highest on cognitive tests. This practice rests on a serious fallacy—students with the highest scores on cognitive tests and the highest GPA from college may not become superior health professionals. Other things being equal, a student with a GPA of 3.75 is not necessarily a better candidate than one with a GPA of 3.35. Similarly, a student with a score of 90 on a cognitive test may or may not perform better than a student with a score of 85 on the same test. Hence, with regard to cognitive tests, instead of selecting the highest scoring students, minimal entrance test scores should be defined by each school to satisfy academic requirements. Other qualities could then be taken into consideration to select the most suitable candidates from a larger pool of applicants.

*Developing Clinical Criterion Measures.* It has been taken for granted that the preclinical GPA is a valid criterion measure for performance in the health professions. However, it has been demonstrated in many studies that preclinical grades are unrelated to clinical grades or to professional performance. To validate selection procedures by using a criterion that reflects only superior classroom performance, as measured by written examinations, excludes from consideration student behaviors related to patient care. One reason why clinical performance has not been used more often as a criterion in research studies is the lack of adequate measures. One of the most important tasks of future research efforts is to develop multiple criterion measures, ranging from clinical application of knowledge to specific clinical skills. For example, measures of technical skills could be developed in dentistry, nursing, medical laboratory science, and physical therapy. Measures of interpersonal skills could be developed within the framework of patient interviews in nutrition, occupational therapy, and medicine. Without the development of sound clinical criterion measures, selecting students for clinical roles will remain largely speculative.

*Assessment of Nonacademic Characteristics.* Many research studies support the view that nonacademic qualities are better predictors of clinical performance than cognitive variables. Nevertheless, much less time, money, and effort have been exerted in their assessment than in the measurement of cognitive indicators. There are several possible reasons for this neglect. One may be the illusive and overwhelming nature of the task. Another may be that selection committees feel better prepared and more comfortable with data pertaining to abilities and achievements than with values and attitudes. However, there are at least two important issues to be dealt with in regard to nonacademic qualities: The first is the determination of those qualities that are likely to matter most in the clinical performance of health professionals; the second is the identification and/or development of methods for the valid assessment of selected qualities.

Regarding the first issue, numerous qualities have been suggested by different selection committees as important and/or desirable in a given profession. Some lists are so long that they discourage action. Some lists include both essential and marginally important qualities without prioritization. Most lists reflect the value judgments of selection committee members, mainly faculty and administration. It would be desirable to conduct critical incident studies to identify those nonacademic qualities that are seen by practitioners and consumers to contribute to satisfactory and unsatisfactory clinical performance. Such studies were recently conducted in nursing (Jacobs and others, 1978) and child psychiatry (McDermott, McGuire, and Berner, 1976) to define critical cognitive and skill requirements to be measured in board certifying examinations. The same technique could be used to define those nonacademic qualities that contribute to the affective aspects of clinical performance. If lack of time and money interfere with critical incident surveys, both practitioners and consumers could be asked to contribute to the selection of relevant nonacademic characteristics. These criteria should be specifically defined with relevance to the unique demand of the different professions. While many consumers cannot differentiate a more competent from a less competent dentist or nurse, they are well able to articulate qualities that impress them as being helpful or offensive.

Once the critical qualities have been determined, either by empirical means or by judgment, suitable methods of assessment need to be developed. Scores from standardized personality, value, and interest tests have shown significant correlations with clinical evaluations, but these correlations need to be improved if such tests are to be used. One strategy would be to use several formerly validated tests, hoping that multiple measures may increase correlations with multiple clinical criteria. Although interviews and letters of recommendation have been found wanting in the assessment of personal qualities, interviews could serve two important functions. First, they could be used to determine and clarify the extent and nature of applicants' nonacademic achievements, since interests and values, as manifested in both work and leisure activities, have been shown to play a major role in motivation. Second, they could be used to provide applicants with accurate information about the health professions, since misconceptions about a profession prior to entrance often result in loss of interest and subsequent failure or attrition.

*Manpower Projections.* In addition to their relevance for predicting clinical performance, it is important to pay attention to nonacademic qualities in selection in order to make better manpower projections. Questions relating to choice of specialty and practice location have not been significantly explained by variations in cognitive characteristics. At the same time, several studies suggest that work conditions, manpower factors, and, to a lesser extent, personal qualities are more predictive of career choices than differences in intellect or achievement in medical school (Hutt, 1976). Both general and family practitioners gravitate into locations where a physician shortage exists. "Person-oriented" specialties are more often chosen by students with personality needs that differ from those students who choose science or technique-oriented specialties. Although 50 to 70 percent of the students change their career goal between the freshman and senior year, "person-oriented" freshmen tend to shift from one social-centered to another social-centered goal (for example, from pediatrics to internal medicine). During the last decade, a commitment to primary care has been emerging, not only in underdeveloped countries but also in the United States. The willingness to provide primary care depends on personality, disposition, motivation, and interest rather than knowledge. Such motivation may be inferred from personality and interest tests, as well as work and leisure activities. The candidate's sex is also related to career choice. In medical school, for example, significantly more women than men express interest in pediatrics. Though some of them may shift their goals, women are more likely to select "person-oriented" specialties.

Regarding manpower distribution, there are two underserved areas in the United States: rural sections and inner-city areas in large metropolitan centers. Ex post facto studies of physicians practicing in rural areas suggest that they have grown up in rural environments and that their spouses prefer to live in small towns. Other factors that influence choice of practice sites are desire for social and cultural activities, the availability of clinical and institutional facilities, climate, and economic considerations. Both rural background and interest in family or general practice support choice of a rural practice; however, selecting students from rural areas will not guarantee their returning to small town practice, since large medical centers foster a shift in career choice toward secondary and tertiary specialties, and repeated longitudinal studies have shown that choice of location is significantly linked with specialty choice.

The need to provide more health personnel for the inner city, together with changes in prescribed social policy, has fostered the recruitment of minority students. Minority students have been encouraged to apply, entrance requirements have been made more flexible, and academic support services have been provided to remedy deficiencies. These policies should be continued and should be supplemented by additional efforts to increase retention. Merely admitting more minority students without bolstering retention is not likely to achieve either the goals of social policy or the production of manpower for the inner city.

*Self-Selection.* Even though applicants are technically selected by admissions committees, self-selection plays a major role. Although attrition for nonacademic reasons is a serious problem only in nursing, it is clear that many students who apply do not complete their professional training. In a profession where the shortage has been acute and is increasing, this is a serious problem.

Research has shown that in nursing, nonacademic withdrawal is caused mainly by loss of interest in the profession. Lacking more specific data regarding the reasons for that loss of interest, we can only speculate about the possible causes. Nursing faculty greatly modify the image of the professional nurse and place heavy emphasis on problem solving, leadership, and broader preparation in the sciences. At the same time, many students who enter nursing are motivated mainly by the desire to help and to have patient contact—"the Florence Nightingale image." Upon realizing that the requirements do not fit their expectations, these students lose interest. In two-year programs, where students are taught to perform concrete tasks in a service-oriented atmosphere, the dropout rate for nonacademic reasons is lower.

The above example from nursing was cited to underline the need students have for access to up-to-date health profession profiles, particularly when the profession is changing profoundly. Self-selection is also aided by knowledge of one's capabilities and limitations, as well as by knowledge of the program one wishes to enter. Occupational pamphlets give valuable but only limited factual information. Information about the emotional climate and environmental pressures inherent in a program is also essential to enable applicants to contemplate their ability and willingness to fit in with the climate and to cope with the pressures.

*Research Directions.* The findings summarized in this chapter point to the following directions for future research:

- Cognitive tests and grades determine admission to all health professions. It is assumed that the brightest student will perform best, but this assumption needs to be examined. What happens to students admitted with mediocre or lower intellectual qualifications? Do they graduate? Do they remain in the profession? More follow-up studies are needed to evaluate the legitimacy of present admissions requirements. *Minimal* cognitive requirements for entrance into different health professions should be identified. Lowering these requirements is likely to attract into some professions many students who bring other kinds of qualifications, perhaps as important as brain power or more so.
- The help of practitioners and consumers to identify essential noncognitive qualities for different health professionals should be enlisted. Involving practitioners and consumers is likely to reduce the discontinuity between education and practice.
- Major efforts should be directed toward the refinement and development of assessment methods designed to measure noncognitive characteristics and clinical performance. The latter needs to be developed to validate the contribution of noncognitive characteristics to clinical practice.
- Do selection procedures advance or frustrate selection policies? The relationship between stated selection policies and selection procedures should be studied.
- Do admissions practices contribute to manpower shortages? Do admissions practices encourage retraining and reward experience? The relationship between manpower projections and admissions practices should be explored.
- Do selection procedures lead to graduating health professionals who are satisfied and willing to work in patient-care settings where new graduates are needed? Are the graduates acceptable to the patients they are to serve? Studies of both provider and consumer satisfactions are needed.

When we know the answers to these questions, we will be in a better position to admit those candidates who not only can, but should, become health professionals.

## References

American Dental Association. *Dental Aptitude Test.* Chicago: American Dental Association, 1950.

American Dental Association. *Correlation Study: DAT and GPA vs. Sophomore Grades.* Dental Admission Testing Program Report no. 4, 1977/78. Chicago: American Dental Association, 1978.

American Dental Association. *Dental Student Attrition.* Supplement 5. Annual Report, 1978/1979. Chicago: American Dental Association, 1979.

Anderson, H. E., Jr., and Jantzen, A. C. "A Prediction of Clinical Performance." *American Journal of Occupational Therapy,* 1965, *19,* 76–78.

Association of American Medical Colleges. *New Medical College Admissions Test.* Washington, D.C.: Association of American Medical Colleges, 1977.

Association of American Medical Colleges. *AAMC Longitudinal Study of Medical School Graduates of 1960.* Publication no. (PHS) 79-3235. Washington, D.C.: U.S. Department of Health, Education, and Welfare, 1979.

Backman, M. E., and Steindler, F. M. "Let's Examine: Prediction of Achievement in a Collegiate Nursing Program and Performance on State Board Examinations." *Nursing Outlook,* 1971, *19,* 487.

Bailey, J. P., Jr., Jantzen, A. C., and Dunteman, G. H. "Relative Effectiveness of Personality Achievement and Interest Measures in the Prediction of Performance Criterion." *American Journal of Occupational Therapy,* 1969, *23,* 27–29.

Baker, E. J. "Associate Degree Nursing Students: Nonintellective Differences Between Dropouts and Graduates." *Nursing Research,* 1975, *24,* 42–44.

Baldwin, J. P., Mowbray, J. K., and Taylor, R. G., Jr. "Factors Influencing Performance on State Board Test Pool Examinations." *Nursing Research,* 1968, *17,* 170–172.

Barratt, E. S., and White, R. "Impulsiveness and Anxiety Related to Medical Students' Performance and Attitudes." *Journal of Medical Education,* 1969, *44,* 604–607.

Bartlett, J. W. "Medical School and Career Performances of Medical Students with Low Medical College Admissions Test Scores." *Journal of Medical Education,* 1967, *42,* 231–237.

Bell, J. A., and Martindill, C. F. "A Cross-Validation Study of Predictors of Scores on State Board Examinations." *Nursing Research,* 1976, *25* (1), 54–57.

Blaisdell, E. A., Jr., and Gordon, D. "Selection of Occupational Therapy Students." *American Journal of Occupational Therapy,* 1979, *33* (4), 223–229.

Bohan, K. M. *Performance Relationship: Nursing Student to Professional Nurse.* Washington, D.C.: Catholic University of America, 1966.

Boyd, M. A., Teteruck, W. R., and Thompson, G. W. "Interpretation and Use of the Dental Admissions and Aptitude Tests." *Journal of Dental Education,* 1980, *44* (5), 275–278.

Brandt, E. M., Hastie, B., and Schumann, D. "Predicting Success on State Board

Examinations: Relationships Between Course Grades, Selected Test Scores, and State Board Examination Results." *Nursing Research,* 1966, *15,* 62–69.

Brandt, E. M., and Metheny, B. H. "Relationship Between Measures of Students and Graduate Performance." *Nursing Research,* 1968, *17,* 242–246.

Chen, M. K., and Podshadley, D. W. "A Factorial Study of Some Psychological, Vocational Interest, and Mental Ability Variables as Predictors of Success in Dental School." *Journal of Applied Psychology,* 1967, *51,* 236–241.

Chissom, B. S., and Lanier, D. "Prediction of First-Quarter Freshman GPA Using SAT Scores and High School Grades." *Education and Psychological Measurement,* 1975, *35,* 461–463.

Clute, K. F. *The General Practitioner: A Study of Medical Education and Practice in Ontario and Nova Scotia.* Toronto: University of Toronto Press, 1963.

Cullen, T. J., and others. "Predicting First-Quarter Test Scores from the New Medical College Admissions Test." *Journal of Medical Education,* 1980, 55 (5), 393–398.

D'Costa, A., and Schafer, A. *Results of a Survey of Noncognitive Tests Used in Medical Schools.* Washington, D.C.: American Association of Medical Colleges, 1972.

Deardorff, M., Denner, P., and Miller, C. "Selected National League for Nursing Achievement Test Scores as Predictors of State Board Examination Scores." *Nursing Research,* 1976, *25* (1), 35–38.

Dubs, R. "Comparison of Student Achievement with Performance Ratings of Graduates and State Board Examination Scores." *Nursing Research,* 1975, *24* (1), 59–62.

Edwards, C. N. "Faculty Assessment of Medical School Criteria." In *Proceedings of Research in Medical Education Conference,* New Orleans, 1978. Washington, D.C.: Association of American Medical Colleges, 1978.

Elstein, A. S., and Teitelbaum, H. S. "A Systematic Evaluation of an Admission Process." In *Proceedings of the Thirteenth Annual Conference on Research in Medical Education,* Chicago, 1974. Washington, D.C.: Association of American Medical Colleges, 1974.

Erdmann, J. B. "Validating the MCAT." *Journal of Medical Education,* 1980, 55 (5), 463–464.

Erdmann, J. B., and others. "The Medical College Admissions Test: Past, Present, Future." *Journal of Medical Education,* 1971, *46,* 937–946.

Friedman, C. P. "A Nonlinear, Discriminant, Analytic Approach to Predicting Medical Student Performance." In *Proceedings of Research in Medical Education Conference.* Washington, D.C.: Association of American Medical Colleges, 1979.

Friedman, C. P., and Bakewell, W. E., Jr. "Incremental Validity of the New MCAT." *Journal of Medical Education,* 1980, 55 (5), 399–408.

Funkenstein, D. H. "Testing the Scientific Achievement and Ability of Applicants to Medical School: The Problem and a Proposal." *Journal of Medical Education,* 1966, *41,* 120–134.

Funkenstein, D. H. "Current Medical School Admissions: The Problems and a Proposal." *Journal of Medical Education,* 1970, *45,* 497–508.

Gellhorn, A., and Scheuer, R. "The Experiment in Medical Education at the City College of New York." *Journal of Medical Education,* 1978, *53* (7), 574–582.

Gordon, M. J., and Lincoln, J. A. "Family Practice Resident Selection: Value of the Interview." *Journal of Family Practice*, 1976, *3* (2), 175–177.

Gordon, T. L. "Study of U.S. Medical School Applicants, 1977–1978." *Journal of Medical Education*, 1979, *54*, 677–702.

Gough, H. G., and Hall, W. B. "Prediction of Performance in Medical School from the California Psychological Inventory." *Journal of Applied Psychology*, 1964, *48*, 218–226.

Gough, H. G., Hall, W. B., and Harris, R. E. "Admissions Procedures as Forecasters of Performance in Medical Training." *Journal of Medical Education*, 1963, *38*, 983–998.

Gough, H. G., Hall, W. B., and Harris, R. E. "Evaluation of Performance in Medical Training." *Journal of Medical Education*, 1964, *39*, 679–692.

Gough, H. G., and Kirk, B. A. "Achievement in Dental Schools as Related to Personality and Aptitude Variables." *Measurement and Evaluation in Guidance*, 1970, *2*, 226–233.

Hagarty, C. E. "Prediction of Nursing Competencies of Senior Baccalaureate Nursing Students." *Dissertation Abstracts International*, 1976, *37*, 1623B–1624B.

Hamberg, R., Swanson, A., and Dohner, C. "Perceptions and Usage of Predictive Data for Medical School Admissions." *Journal of Medical Education*, 1971, *46*, 959–963.

Holstrom, E. I. "Changing Characteristics of Students in Health Fields." *Journal of Allied Health*, 1975, *4*, 9–20.

Hood, A. B. "Predicting Achievement in Dental School." *Journal of Dental Education*, 1963, *27*, 148–155.

Hutcheson, J. D., Garland, L. M., and Lowe, L. S. "Antecedents of Nursing School Attrition: Attitudinal Dimensions." *Nursing Research*, 1979, *28* (1), 57–62.

Hutcheson, J. D., Garland, L. M., and Prather, J. E. "Toward Reducing Attrition in Baccalaureate Degree Nursing Programs: An Exploratory Study." *Nursing Research*, 1973, *22*, 530–533.

Hutchins, E. B. "Nonintellectual Factors in Selection." In M. A. Fruen and J. W. Steinen (Eds.), *Proceedings of the Fourth Panamerican Conference on Medical Education*, Toronto, Canada, 1972.

Hutt, R. "Doctor's Career Choice: Previous Research and Its Relevance for Policy Making." *Medical Education*, 1976, *10*, 463–473.

Ingersoll, R. W., and Graves, G. O. "Predictability of Success in the First Year of Medical School." *Journal of Medical Education*, 1965, *40*, 351–363.

Jacobs, A. M., and others. *Critical Requirements for Safe/Effective Nursing Practice*. Kansas City, Mo.: American Nurses' Association, 1978.

Jacoby, K. E., and others. "The Use of Demographic and Background Variables as Predictors of Success in Pharmacy Schools." *American Journal of Pharmaceutical Education*, 1978, *42*, 4–6.

Jiske, R. E., Ort, R. S., and Ford, A. B. "Clinical Performance and Related Traits of Medical Students and Faculty Physicians." *Journal of Medical Education*, 1964, *39*, 69–80.

Johnson, R. W., Arbes, B. G., and Thompson, C. G. "Selection of Occupational Therapy Students." *American Journal of Occupational Therapy*, 1974, *28*, 597–601.

Johnson, D. G., and Hutchins, E. B. "Doctor or Dropout? A Study of Medical Student Attrition." *Journal of Medical Education,* 1966, *41,* 1099-1274.

Johnson, R. W., and Leonard, L. C. "Psychological Test Characteristics and Performance of Nursing Students." *Nursing Research,* 1970, *19,* 147-150.

Jones, C. W. "Why Associate Degree Nursing Students Persist." *Nursing Research,* 1975, *24* (1), 57-59.

Katzell, M. E. "The Allied Health Professions Admissions Test." *Journal of Allied Health,* 1977, *6,* 14-20.

Keck, J. W., and others. "Efficacy of Cognitive/Noncognitive Measures in Predicting Resident-Physician Performance." *Journal of Medical Education,* 1979, *54,* 759-765.

Kegel-Flom, P. "Predicting Supervisor, Peer, and Self-Ratings of Intern Performance." *Journal of Medical Education,* 1975, *50* (8), 812-815.

Kelly, W. L. "Psychological Prediction of Leadership in Nursing." *Nursing Research,* 1974, *23,* 38-42.

Klahn, J. E. "Self-Concept and Change-Seeking Need of First-Year Student Nurses." *Journal of Nursing Education,* 1969, *8,* 11-16.

Knopf, L. *From Student to R.N.: A Report of the Nurse Career Pattern Study.* Publication no. (NIH) 72-130. Washington, D.C.: U.S. Department of Health, Education, and Welfare, 1972.

Knopke, H. J. "Predicting Student Attrition in a Baccalaureate Curriculum." *Nursing Research,* 1979, *28* (4), 224-227.

Korman, M., Stubblefield, R. L., and Martin, L. W. "Research in Medical Education: Patterns of Success in Medical School and Their Correlates." *Journal of Medical Education,* 1968, *43,* 405-411.

Kreit, L. H., and McDonald, R. E. "Preprofessional Grades and the DAT as Predictors of Student Performance in Dental School." *Journal of Dental Education,* 1968, *32,* 452-457.

Ledbetter, P. J. "An Analysis of the Performance of a Selected Baccalaureate Program in Nursing with Regard to Selected Standard Examinations." *Dissertation Abstracts International,* 1968, *29,* 3381A.

Leiken, A. M., and Cunningham, B. M. "The Predictive Ability of the Allied Health Professions Admissions Test." *Journal of Allied Health,* 1980, *9* (2), 132-138.

Levitt, E. E., Lubin, B., and DeWitt, K. N. "Attempt to Develop an Objective Test Battery for the Selection of Nursing Students." *Nursing Research,* 1971, *20,* 255-258.

Lewis, J., and Welch, M. "Predicting Achievement in an Upper-Division Bachelor's Degree Nursing Major." *Education and Psychological Measurement,* 1975, *35,* 467-469.

Liao, W. C., and Adams, J. P. "Methodology for the Prediction of Pharmacy Student Academic Success: I. Preliminary Aspects." *Journal of Pharmaceutical Education,* 1977, *41,* 124-127.

Litton-Hawes, E., MacLean, I. C., and Hines, M. H. "An Analysis of the Communication Process in the Medical Admissions Interview." *Journal of Medical Education,* 1976, *51* (4), 332-334.

Lowenthal, W., Wersin, J., and Smith, H. L. "Predictors of Success in Pharmacy School: PCAT vs. Other Admission Criteria." *American Journal of Pharmaceutical Education,* 1977, *41,* 267-269.

McCaulley, M. H. *Application of the Myers-Briggs Type Indicator to Medicine and Other Health Professions.* Center for Applications of Psychological Type, Monograph I. Gainesville: University of Florida, 1978.

McDermott, J. F., McGuire, C., and Berner, E. S. *Roles and Functions of Child Psychiatrists.* Evanston, Ill.: American Board of Psychiatry and Neurology, 1976.

McGuire, F. L. "The New MCAT and Medical Student Performance." *Journal of Medical Education,* 1980, *55,* 405–408.

Mann, W. C. "Interviewer Scoring Differences in Student Selection Interviews." *American Journal of Occupational Therapy,* 1979, *33,* 235–239.

Michael, W. B., Haney, R., and Jones, R. A. "The Predictive Validities of Selected Aptitude and Achievement Measures and of Three Personality Inventories in Relation to Nursing Training Criteria." *Education and Psychological Measurement,* 1966, *26,* 1035–1040.

Michael, W. B., and others. "The Criterion-Related Validities of Cognitive and Noncognitive Predictors for Nursing Candidates." *Education and Psychological Measurement,* 1971, *31,* 983–987.

Miller, M. H. "A Follow-Up of First-Year Nursing Student Dropouts." *Nursing Forum,* 1974, *13,* 32–47.

Molidor, J. B., and Elstein, A. S. "A Factor Analytic Study of the Old and New MCAT Examinations." In *Proceedings of the Eighteenth AAMC Conference on Research in Medical Education.* Washington, D.C.: Association of American Medical Colleges, 1979.

Morse, P. K. "The Interview as a Means of Assessing Personality Characteristics." In H. B. Haley, A. G. D'Costa, and A. M. Schafer (Eds.), *Personality Measurement in Medical Education.* Washington, D.C.: Association of American Medical Colleges, 1971.

Muhlenkamp, A. F. "Prediction of State Board Scores in a Baccalaureate Program." *Nursing Outlook,* 1971, *19,* 57.

Munro, B. H. "Dropouts from Nursing Education: Path Analysis of a National Sample." *Nursing Research,* 1980, *29,* 371–377.

Munson, J. W., and Bourne, D. W. "Pharmacy College Admissions Test (PCAT) as a Predictor of Academic Success." *American Journal of Pharmaceutical Education,* 1976, *40,* 237–239.

Murden, R., and others. "Academic and Personal Predictors of Clinical Success in Medical School." *Journal of Medical Education,* 1978, *53,* 711–719.

Nash, P. M. *Student Selection and Retention in Nursing Schools.* Publication no. (HRA) 78-5. Washington, D.C.: U.S. Department of Health, Education, and Welfare, 1977.

Nassif, J. Z. *Handbook of Health Careers.* New York: Human Sciences Press, 1980.

National League for Nursing. "NLN Survey." *Nursing Outlook,* 1981, *29,* 274.

Peterson, O. L., and others. "An Analytical Study of North Carolina General Practice." *Journal of Medical Education,* 1956, *31* (2), Part 2, 1–165.

Price, P. B., and others. "Measurement of Physician Performance." *Journal of Medical Education,* 1964, *39,* 203–211.

Psychological Corporation, Professional Examinations Division. *Handbook for the Pharmacy College Admissions Test.* New York: Psychological Corporation, 1975.

Raderman, R., and Allen, D. V. "Registered Nurse Students in a Baccalaureate Program: Factors Associated with Completion." *Nursing Research*, 1974, *23*, 71–73.

Rasmussen, R. H., and Boozer, C. H. "A Comparison of the Predictive Validity of Variables Used in the Selection of Students for Dental Schools, 1968–1976." *Journal of Dental Education*, 1978, *42*, 38.

Reeves, P. E. "The Selection Interview in the Assessment of Suitability for Nurse Training." *Journal of Advanced Nursing*, 1978, *3*, 167–179.

Rezler, A. G., and Buckley, J. M. "A Comparison of Personality Types Among Female Student Health Professionals." *Journal of Medical Education*, 1977, *52* (6), 475–477.

Rezler, A. G., and French, R. M. "Personality Types and Learning Preferences of Students in Six Allied Health Professions." *Journal of Allied Health*, 1975, *4*, 20–26.

Rezler, A. G., Manasse, H. R., and Buckley, J. M. "A Comparative Study of the Personality Types Attracted to Pharmacy and Medical School." *American Journal of Pharmaceutical Education*, 1977, *41*, 7–10.

Rezler, A. G., and Moore, J. "Correlates of Success in the Baccalaureate Education of Registered Nurses." *Research in Nursing and Health*, 1978, *1*, 159–164.

Rezler, A. G., Mrtek, R. G., and Manasse, H. R. "Linking Choice to Personality Types: A Preliminary Analysis of Pharmacy Students." *American Journal of Pharmaceutical Education*, 1976, *40*, 121–125.

Rezler, A. G., and Sinacore, J. Unpublished study, Center for Educational Development, Health Sciences Center, University of Illinois at Chicago, 1980.

Rhoads, J. M., and others. "Motivation, Medical School Admissions, and Student Performance." *Journal of Medical Education*, 1974, *49*, 1119–1127.

Roessler, R., and others. "Cognitive and Noncognitive Variables in the Prediction of Preclinical Performance." *Journal of Medical Education*, 1978, *53* (8), 678–680.

Ross, N. M. "Dental Aptitude Test Results and College Grades as Predictors of Success in a School of Dentistry." *Journal of Dental Education*, 1967, *31*, 84–88.

Rotenberg, A. "Attitudes and Beliefs Versus Study Results: Exemplified by Attrition in a School of Nursing in Israel During 1968–1974." *Journal of Advanced Nursing*, 1978, *3*, 427–432.

Rothman, A. I. "A Comparison of Persistent High and Low Achievers Through Four Years of Undergraduate Medical Training." *Journal of Medical Education*, 1973, *48*, 180–182.

Saffer, J. B., and Saffer, L. D. "Academic Record as a Predictor of Future Job Performance of Nurses." *Nursing Research*, 1972, *21*, 457–462.

Sanazaro, P. J., and Hutchins, E. B. "The Origin and Rationale of the Medical College Admissions Test." *Journal of Medical Education*, 1963, *38*, 1044–1050.

Schimpfhauser, F. T., and Broski, D. C. "Predicting Academic Success in Allied Health Curricula." *Journal of Allied Health*, 1976, *5*, 35–46.

Schofield, W. *Research Studies of Medical Students and Physicians Utilizing Standard Personality Instruments: An Annotated Bibliography.* Washington, D.C.: Association of American Medical Colleges, 1972.

Schwirian, P. M. *Prediction of Successful Nursing Performance.* Publication no.

(HRA) 77-27. Washington, D.C.: U.S. Department of Health, Education, and Welfare, 1976.

Schwirian, P. M., and Gortner, S. R. "How Nursing Schools Predict Their Successful Graduates." *Nursing Outlook*, 1979, *27* (5), 352-358.

Seither, F. F. "Prediction of Achievement in Baccalaureate Nursing Education." *Journal of Nursing Education*, 1980, *19* (3), 28-36.

Sherman, S. "Trends in Admissions Policies and Practices." In *Trends, Issues, and Implications in Student Selection*. Publication no. 23-1704. New York: National League for Nursing, 1978.

Smith, G. M. "The Role of Personality in Nursing Education: A Comparison of Successful and Unsuccessful Nursing Students." *Nursing Research*, 1965, *14*, 54-58.

Stefanu, C., and Farmer, T. A., Jr. "The Differential Predictive Validity of Science MCAT in the Admissions Process." *Journal of Medical Education*, 1971, *46*, 461-463.

Thurston, J. R., Brunclik, H. L., and Feldhusen, J. F. "The Relationship of Personality to Achievement in Nursing Education." Phase I. *Nursing Research*, 1965, *14*, 203-209.

Thurston, J. R., Brunclik, H. L., and Feldhusen, J. F. "The Relationship of Personality to Achievement in Nursing Education." Phase II. *Nursing Research*, 1968, *17*, 265-268.

Tidd, G. S., and Conine, T. A. "Do Better Students Perform Better in the Clinic?" *Physical Therapist*, 1974, *54*, 500-505.

Torosian, G., and others. "The Analysis of Admissions Criteria." *American Journal of Pharmaceutical Education*, 1978, *42*, 7-10.

U.S. Department of Health, Education, and Welfare, Bureau of Health Manpower. *Minorities and Women in the Health Fields*. Washington, D.C.: U.S. Department of Health, Education, and Welfare, 1978.

Waldman, A. M., and Leavitt, D. E. "Predicting an Applicant's Success in a Three-Year Professional Pharmacy Program." *American Journal of Pharmaceutical Education*, 1974, *38*, 23-27.

Warnecke, R. B. "Nonintellectual Factors Related to Attrition from a Collegiate Nursing Program." *Journal of Health and Social Behavior*, 1973, *14*, 153-167.

Weinstein, E. L., Brown, L., and Wahlstrom, M. W. "Selection Procedures and Attrition." *Journal of Nursing Education*, 1979, *18* (4), 34-86.

Weinstein, E. L., Brown, L., and Wahlstrom, M. W. "Characteristics of the Successful Nursing Student." *Journal of Nursing Education*, 1980, *19* (3), 53-59.

Williams, J. H., and others. "A Computer-Assisted Admissions Process." *Journal of Medical Education*, 1977, *52* (5), 384-389.

Wingard, J. R., and Williamson, J. W. "Grades as Predictors of Physicians' Career Performance: An Evaluative Literature Review." *Journal of Medical Education*, 1973, *48*, 311-322.

Wittmeyer, A., Camiscioni, J. S., and Purdy, P. A. "A Longitudinal Study of Attrition and Academic Performance in a Collegiate Nursing Program." *Nursing Research*, 1971, *20*, 339-347.

Wolfle, L. M., and Bryant, L. W. "A Causal Model of Nursing Education and State Board Examination Scores." *Nursing Research*, 1978, *27*, 311-315.

Wright, O. R., Jr. "Summary of Research on the Selection Interview Since 1964." *Personnel Psychology,* 1969, *22,* 391–413.

Yess, J. P. "Predictors of Success in Community College Nursing Education." *Journal of Nursing Education,* 1980. *19,* 19-24.

# 11

*Richard P. Foley*

# Instructional Media
# and Methods

One word—innovation—best characterizes the most popular topic of the research and writing on instruction in the health professions during the past two decades. Innovative techniques were developed in response to technological advances, the proliferation of knowledge, students' increasing dissatisfaction with their education, and a general questioning of the adequacy of the health care delivery system. During these years, computer-assisted instruction, simulation of portions of the body through electrical devices, and televised patient education programs were introduced. Meanwhile, we observed conventional instructional methods being challenged by self-instructional formats, standard curricula being rivaled by self-directed and problem-based learning programs, and nontraditional teachers, including housewives and actors, teaching basic skills to health professions students. Commenting on this flurry of activity, Trent and Cohen (1973) observed that: "Because of the almost relentless demand for educational innovations during the 1960's, however, the common tendency was to equate innovation with improvement without vigorously evaluating the effectiveness of each new program or instructional procedure" (p. 1024). This statement characterizing the research conducted in higher education is equally applicable to the work done in health professions education.

The bulk of the research on instruction in health professions education can be classified into two categories: research on instructional technology and research on instructional methods. These divisions are somewhat arbitrary, however, since many studies mixed both methods and media. This chapter begins by discussing studies in these areas, with a sharp look at the adequacy of the methodologies that were employed. Then it concentrates on some relatively new and promising work that involves the assessment of student learning preferences and styles, a neglected factor in the work on instructional methods and media. The chapter concludes with an analysis of current research in these areas and recommendations for new research directions.

## Instructional Technology

The 1960s began with the hope that technology would revolutionize education. Television, teaching machines, and multimedia programs were seen as ways of providing more efficient instruction, thereby freeing professors to spend more time with students in creative endeavors. As a result, the greatest portion of the research on media dealt with assessing whether one form was more effective or efficient than another. Some studies were of value, but others reported conclusions such as this: "The only significant finding regarding attitudes toward the three strategies was a preference for and greater interest in color videotapes than for black and white televised materials" (Moser and Kondracki, 1977, p. 26). Because of their special significance in the health professions, this discussion is limited to research carried out on three types of media: simulation, television, and self-instructional programs.

*Simulation.* Within the last ten years, the use of simulation in health professions education has increased as has its sophistication. A variety of simulation techniques has been developed, including paper-and-pencil constructions, usually dealing with patient management problems (McGuire, Solomon, and Bashook, 1976); actors who pose as patients (Barrows, 1971); computer-aided simulations (Harless and others, 1971); and three-dimensional models (Penta and Kofman, 1973). The merits of simulations are that they allow students to practice in a manner that does not affect actual patient care, provide them with immediate feedback concerning their performance, and generally permit individuals to proceed at their own rates. Since the most intriguing simulations are, perhaps, those replicating parts of the body upon which students can practice a variety of skills, several studies concerning this type are reviewed here.

Salvendy and others (1973) used electromechanical simulators to teach dental students the psychomotor skills required for cavity preparation. An experimental group of students using the simulator was compared with students learning with the conventional plaster model. The former group acquired the skills in half the time required by the other, and its work was of slightly better quality. Having made some changes that increased the efficiency of the devices, Salvendy and others (1975) repeated their study. While on this occasion no differences were noted in the quality of the work, the time spent learning the skills by the experimental group was one-third that of the control group. The magnitude of the time reduction was partially explained as resulting from the simulator's capacity to provide progressive part-training with instantaneous feedback. A related benefit was that the devices freed instructors for other teaching activities.

One of the earliest simulators in medicine was a manikin nicknamed Sim One. Lifelike in appearance and replicating indicators of such bodily functions as breath, heartbeat, pulse, and blood pressure, it allowed certain skills to be performed as they are in the operating room. Abrahamson, Denson, and Wolf (1969) gauged the effectiveness of Sim One in teaching residents endotracheal intubation. The experimental group that had access to the simulator was compared with the group that did not. Students in the experimental section achieved operating room proficiency levels in a smaller number of elapsed days and with fewer trials, thereby saving training personnel time and posing less threat to patient safety. Since the cost of constructing Sim One was approximately $100,000, Hoffman and Abrahamson (1975) analyzed its cost-effectiveness. On the basis of findings from fifteen studies conducted with a wide variety of health professionals over a two-year period, they concluded that decreased consumption of faculty and student time, gains in student performance, and the large number of personnel requiring training justified the expense within a short period of time. The development of Sim Two has subsequently been described by Abrahamson and Wallace (1980).

Simulators have also been reported to be effective in teaching physical diagnosis skills to medical students (Penta and Kofman, 1973) and in helping nursing students learn clinical observation skills (Jeffers and Christensen, 1979). In addition, teaching heart sounds by means of simulators has been successful (Aberg, Johansson, and Michaelsson, 1974; Sajid, Magero, and Feinzimer, 1977). The most recent, expensive, and, perhaps, impressive device is the Cardiology Patient Simulator (CPS), another manikin nicknamed Harvey, capable of duplicating most bedside findings of a wide variety of cardiovascular conditions. Gordon and others (1980) demonstrated that medical students in a CPS elective achieved significantly higher scores on written, CPS practical, and patient practical examinations than did a student group that experienced a conventional cardiology elective.

The research on the various mechanical simulation devices is especially encouraging in regard to student time savings and the apparent transfer of learning from the simulators to patients. Unfortunately, most studies merely related that those who used the simulators did better than those who did not. While the experimental and control groups usually received identical training, the former also had practice opportunities with the simulators that in some cases was an alternative to patient contact and in others an "add on." A much stronger case could have been made for simulations had students taught by conventional instruction also engaged in alternative activities designed to teach the particular skills under investigation. Furthermore, studies contrasting student performance and learning efficiency with different types of simulators could provide insight into certain nagging concerns, such as how sophisticated a device must be and what level of fidelity it must have. Is an extremely expensive heart sound simulator dramatically more effective than an audiotape and accompanying booklet that would also permit students to practice identifying auscultatory events? Since certain simulations now cost well over six figures, it is remiss not to investigate such issues.

*Television.* With the advent of videocassettes, closed-circuit television systems, cable television, and Telstar, television holds tremendous promise as an alternative medium for educating students, patients, and professionals. Within medicine, it was reported to be as effective as a lecture-demonstration and preferred by students for learning clinical signs in neurology (Cantrell and Craven, 1969). Continuing education telelectures were described to be as useful as workshops in meeting the professional needs of dietitians in remote locations (Spears, Moore, and Tuthill, 1973), and a slow-scan video system has been used in Canada on a regular basis for continuing medical education, graduate medical education, in-service education, and patient education programs (Dunn and others, 1980).

While much has been written about the merits of television, little has been done to assess its effects systematically. Marshall and Alexander (1976), in their review of studies on continuing medical education (CME) projects that utilized television, shed some light on the condition of this research. They concluded that the studies were so poorly executed that we learned little about the optimal uses of television or, in fact, whether it should be used at all. Ironically, they comment that "on the other hand, the success of traditional CME in altering physician behavior is so limited that it is perhaps inappropriate to expect more from television. In the absence of a standard of success, it is difficult to estimate the degree of television's failure" (p. 945). In the studies they reviewed, only one attempted an objective measurement of the impact of television on physician behavior, and this study failed because of unavailable or poorly maintained records. These authors believe that television is currently best utilized to motivate physicians to seek additional medical information through other formats, such as attending CME programs that follow television broadcasts, and that it should not be regarded as an educational end unto itself. They do suggest, however, a few promising areas for research. Using split cable, randomly assigned continuing education (CE) enrollees could receive different programs to determine physician receptivity and response to various presentations and formats. Careful studies comparing television-supplemented CE with other instructional formats could define the effectiveness of CE programs with and without television. Finally, research that is conducted should be assessed in terms of practitioner performance rather than by test scores or preferences.

*Self-Instructional Programs.* Self-instructional (S-I) programs have received by far the greatest attention among studies investigating the merits of instructional media. They encompass slide-tapes, computer-assisted instruction, programmed materials, audiotapes, videotapes, workbooks, and any combination of these, which are called multimedia. Regardless of the format, self-instruction generally allows students to proceed at individual paces, provides immediate performance feedback, and facilitates the learning of material that has been carefully organized and usually arranged in a logical sequence of steps. A good program includes a list of carefully defined behavioral learning objectives and pre- and posttests to measure mastery of the material. Typically, investigations have contrasted S-I programs with conventional modes of instruction and have examined one or more of these variables: knowledge acquisition, knowledge retention, the performance of various ability groups, student preferences for particular methods, student time spent studying, and the expenditure of faculty time.

In a comprehensive analysis of self-instructional programs reported in the dental literature between 1970 and 1979, Williams (1981) reviewed twenty-two articles. Of seventeen studies comparing S-I formats with conventional methods, thirteen reported that students acquired significantly more knowledge using the S-I format, while four reported no differences. One study not reported in Williams' review (Koch, Koch, and Tynelius, 1970) found the lecture to be superior to a slide-tape program for knowledge acquisition.

To determine whether Williams' findings were consistent with comparable studies in other health disciplines, I conducted a literature search for the same time period that produced twenty-five studies comparing S-I programs with conventional teaching in the fields of allied health, nursing, and medicine. This search revealed ten studies that described results indicating that self-instruction was significantly better than traditional instruction for knowledge acquisition by low-ability groups or on certain portions of achievement tests (Bogner, Sajid, and Ford, 1975; Davies, Gale, and Clarke, 1977; Huckabay and others, 1979; McCarthy, 1971; Myers and Greenwood, 1978; Munsick, 1975; Randels and others, 1976; Shafer, Weed, and Johnson, 1973; Stritter and others, 1973; White, Smith, and Sulya, 1973). Fifteen studies reported no differences in achievement (Arnold, 1978; Asklund, Brown, and Fiterman, 1976; Bickley, McDougall, and Pepe, 1973; deCarvalho and others, 1977; Kahn, Conklin, and Glover, 1973; Kao, Beeler, and Strong, 1978; Meyer and Beaton, 1974; Pensivy, 1977; Portnoy and Glasser, 1974; Roach and Wakefield, 1974; Rutan, 1973; Shafer, Johnson, and Weed, 1972; Stanley and Reich, 1974; Suess, 1973; Thompson, 1972). None of the studies analyzed reported a traditional teaching method to be superior to self-instructional programs.

These data suggest that S-I formats are equal or superior to conventional ones for teaching students cognitive information and, in some instances, even skills and attitudes. Yet, with our awareness of the forgetting curve, the ultimate test of the superiority of a particular method should rest with knowledge retention. Of the twenty-two studies in Williams' review, only two measured this factor, and no differences in retention were found. Among the articles I examined, only three (Asklund, Brown, and Fiterman, 1976; Meyer and Beaton, 1974; Thompson, 1972) investigated retention, and similarly no differences were reported. It is particularly interesting that four of the five retention studies compared an S-I format with the lecture. The tremendous knowledge loss six to eight weeks following a lecture is well-documented. Therefore, one would have expected students who learned material through S-I formats, which incorporated behavioral objectives, systematic feedback, and self-pacing, to have retained more information than those taught by lectures. Such was not the case, and as a result, we must be cautious of the unbridled enthusiasm for the teaching capabilities of this format.

Williams found eight studies that examined student performance in light of their GPA and/or dental admissions tests. Not unexpectedly, students in the high-ability groups in six studies performed significantly better than did students in the middle or low groups, irrespective of the instructional method. This finding was supported by two studies from other disciplines (Meyer and Beaton, 1974; Portnoy and Glasser, 1974). Bogner, Sajid, and Ford (1975), however, found that audio-based instruction was superior to the lecture only for the bottom quarter of medical students tested. It appears, then, that bright students will perform well no matter what the mode of instruction, whereas less able students may perform better with S-I formats.

Williams found ten studies that reported student preferences for the instructional modes employed, and S-I was highly favored. Students also tended to prefer self-instruction in the studies reviewed for this chapter. Unfortunately, however, in the studies reviewed students' opinions were often obtained by using dubious methods. Some investigators talked to students and summarized their impressions; in other instances, only S-I students were questioned. Only a small number employed course evaluations or attitudinal questionnaires, and these findings varied. Suess (1973) found that students favored conventional instruction over self-instruction, Roach and Wakefield (1974) found the opposite, and four other studies found no significant preferences (Asklund, Brown, and Fiterman, 1976; Huckabay and others, 1979; Rutan, 1973; Thompson, 1972). None of the studies controlled for ability level or prior experience. Consequently, the glowing reports of the strong student preference for self-instruction must be dimmed.

Of fifteen studies reviewed by Williams (1981), eleven indicated that students in S-I programs spent on the average one-third less time learning as much or more material than did the other students. Although less positive, the studies from the other health disciplines generally support this finding. This seems reasonable, since most S-I programs eliminate extraneous information and incorporate pre- and posttests that enable students to determine when they have mastered the required content, characteristics not usually associated with traditional instruction.

Too many studies on self-instruction referred to the investment of faculty time only as being substantial but worthwhile. Others implied that developmental costs would be offset by faculty time saved in contact with students. Shafer, Johnson, and Weed (1972) examined the faculty time expended in using a self-instruction program on which approximately 1,000 hours had been spent in its development. Instruction time spent per student with this program was thirty-six minutes, while faculty spent an average of fifty-five minutes per student teaching the same content through lectures and laboratories. On the surface, this appears to be a substantial savings, but these findings need further clarification. Not raised in the study was the fact that while nineteen minutes of faculty time per student were saved, 3,158 students would have to use the program to recoup the initial 1,000 hours spent producing the materials. If this many students use the materials at this institution, then the original investment will pay off. If not, the materials should probably be commercially distributed, if their cost is to be justified. The expense of producing such programs, faculty costs in developing and implementing them, projected student usage, and the feasibility of their being utilized in other settings must be weighed against student and faculty time savings in order to determine their cost-effectiveness.

Perhaps the most well-planned and widely disseminated project to introduce self-instructional materials into a curriculum is Project ACORDE (A Consortium of Restorative Dentistry Education), which developed twenty-six teaching modules comprised of a student syllabus, an instructor's manual, films, models, and methods and criteria for evaluating student performance. In order to evaluate the project, a national survey using questionnaires and site visits was conducted by Kress, Silversin, and Colenback (1979). Most dental educators queried were familiar with the materials, and approximately 36 percent of the dental students, 20 percent of dental hygiene students, and 6.5 percent of the accredited dental assistant students had been exposed to some part of the program. Of those surveyed, however, few nonusers planned to implement the program. The major reservations cited were uncertainties concerning the effectiveness of the materials, faculty reluctance to adopt standardized procedures, and faculty wariness of the concept of packaged instruction. These utilization figures are higher than those found in comparable surveys. In a survey of dental schools in the United States and Canada, Dowson and Engle (1973) found little use being made of S-I materials developed to teach endodontics, and similar findings were reported in a national survey examining the use of programmed instruction in the teaching of peridontics (Sturwold, 1973). A report from the Steering Committee for Cooperative Teaching of the Association of Professors of Gynecology and Obstetrics (1973) dealt with the impact of a teaching aids package sent to faculty at 116 medical colleges in North America. With a 75 percent return, respondents indicated that the materials were useful and more should be developed, but only 25 percent required students to use the packages.

In conclusion, on the basis of this review of S-I programs, it seems that in terms of student learning and satisfaction, this mode of instruction is an effective alternative to traditional methods, such as the lecture, the laboratory, and group discussion. Furthermore, it appears to be more efficient in terms of student time expended and may be particularly helpful to less able students. On the other hand, given the inordinate amount of research devoted to studying this medium, it is regrettable that we can say little more about it that is definitive.

## Instructional Methods

As with media, the research on instructional methods during the past twenty years has been primarily focused on comparing the effectiveness of one mode with that of another. The lecture method, always under attack as an inefficient way of presenting content, was the most popular foe in these comparative studies and is reviewed first. While teacher-centered instructional approaches were under fire, there were strong trends, particularly in the mid-sixties, to move toward introducing more student-centered modes of learning. These approaches ranged from students teaching each other in a course to curricula in which an individual's entire professional training was largely self-directed. Several of these methods and programs are also examined.

*Lecture.* " 'The lecture is the most inefficient method of diffusing culture. It became obsolete with the invention of printing. It survives only in our universities and their lay imitators, and a few other backward institutions.' Ever since B. F. Skinner made this statement, through his fictional character Frazier, the lecture has been under attack as the primary mode of presenting educational content'' (Fiel, 1976).

One way of testing this assumption has been to compare the lecture with other instructional formats. One study in nursing randomly divided staff nurses into groups taught by lecture, lecture and discussion, film, and film and discussion (Huckabay, Cooper, and Neal, 1977). The effects of these techniques were measured by an assessment of the nurses' cognitive learning, transfer of learning to new situations, and affective behavior. While no differences in cognitive learning or affective behavior were found, the film group was significantly more able to transfer learning than was the lecture group. Within medicine, Williamson and McGuire (1968) compared a series of consecutive case conferences with lectures to determine the effectiveness of each in improving physicians' clinical decisions. As measured by simulated patient management problems, neither the lectures nor the case conferences produced a significant change in clinical judgment.

In dentistry, two studies surprisingly reported the lecture to be superior to other formats. Gershen (1978) compared the effectiveness of minilectures to role play in a dental psychology course, and the lecture proved to be better in effecting student mastery of factual information. Taylor (1975) randomly assigned dental hygiene students who were learning how to scale teeth into groups taught by discovery, guided discovery, and rule-example (lecture and demonstration) and concluded that when initial learning is the criterion, the rule-example method of instruction is superior.

These studies all suffer from the same problem. Research has demonstrated again and again that certain methods are more effective than others in promoting particular learning outcomes. For example, Ellis (1965) demonstrated that films are better than lectures in aiding the transfer of learning when important aspects of learning are labeled and identified, and stimuli are made redundant by focusing and magnifying important features. Such was the case in the film used by Huckabay and her colleagues, and it is, therefore, no surprise that the film group was more able to transfer learning than their counterparts who learned through lecture. Likewise, Williamson and McGuire (1968) should not have expected the lecture to increase physicians' clinical judgment, since this ability involves problem solving, and the lecture is undoubtedly the worst method for promoting this aspect of cognition (Foley and Smilansky, 1980). That the lecture fared better than role play in Gershen's study (1978) is also predictable, since the goal was the mastery of factual information, that aspect of cognition the lecture best promotes. Finally, the students in Taylor's study (1975) had not previously been exposed to scaling procedures or the instruments involved, so it seems rather obvious that explicit teaching would be more helpful than guided discovery and, as was also found, that guided discovery would facilitate learning more than self-discovery without feedback. When comparing the effectiveness of instructional methods, the failure to match specific instructional techniques with their known learning outcomes is unfortunate and may account, in part, for the unsurprising findings in many of these studies. Would one expect a group of beginners to learn swimming better through a lecture or a series of supervised lessons with an instructor in the water?

## Instructional Approaches

Instructional approaches can be classified as teacher versus student-centered. As student activism grew in the 1960s and as educators were savoring *Freedom to Learn* by Carl Rogers, various self-directed and independent learning programs were established at all educational levels throughout the world. Within health professions education, this was epitomized by the McMaster philosophy (Neufeld and Barrows, 1974), a new problem-based approach to educating medical students. Since then several studies have compared student-centered teaching approaches with those that are teacher-centered.

*Students Teaching Each Other.* A few studies compared instruction delivered by students to instruction presented by faculty. Coppola and Gonnella (1968) reported that peer teaching was an effective alternative to lectures delivered by faculty in a third-year surgery clerkship. The bases for their conclusions, however, were highly subjective, and Flax and Garrard (1974) decided to test some of their hypotheses. In the latter study, five second-year medical students planned and facilitated a pilot course on patient interviewing and taking a medical history; a representative sample of first-year students took the pilot course, while the remaining freshmen took the standard course. The results indicated that students preferred the pilot course, completed more interviews with patients, and wrote up more histories than did those in the comparison group. No data were presented, however, as to how much these students learned in comparison to those in the teacher-led groups.

In a carefully planned study by Harvey, Chappell, and Ferguson (1970), dental students in a laboratory experience were divided into two groups, one taught by faculty and the other by students. In the latter format, a student was randomly chosen to function as teacher, which meant answering student questions and bringing unanswered ones to the faculty. After attaining high interrater reliability, faculty determined achievement by grading student laboratory projects according to well-defined criteria. Scores for both groups were comparable, but those in the student-run groups held their experiences in higher favor than did the others. VanDenBerg (1976) compared nursing students who studied patient care planning through the multiple assignment approach (peer teaching)—in which students collectively planned for the care of one patient—with students taught by the traditional assignment method—in which each planned for the care of at least one patient under an instructor's supervision. Results indicated that nursing students who learned from their peers were superior to the others in overall performance on tests of nursing knowledge, concept usage, and self-esteem.

In all these studies, it appears that students prefer their peers as instructors and learn as much or more from them as they do from faculty. Apart from the novelty of students' teaching each other and the possible accompanying halo effect, other questions remain. Are health professions students so bright that neither the instructional techniques used nor the presence of faculty is relevant, or are the instructors such mediocre teachers that they barely influence student learning? Furthermore, students are always teaching each other as they form study groups, prepare and sell well-deciphered lecture notes, and engage each other in games such as "name that disease." Perhaps, when permitted to teach each other in formal settings, students are merely being given the limelight for a role they already play.

*Independent Study Programs (ISP).* Independent study, another student-centered instructional approach, can be utilized in conjunction with other methods as part of a course or can form the basis of a student's entire curriculum. Most research has focused on independent study in this latter form. Geertsma and others (1977) studied ISP medical students and non–ISP students matched on the basis of certain admissions criteria, such as the Medical College Admissions Test. Comparison of mean scores on Part I of the National Board Examinations revealed no significant differences between ISP and non–ISP students, a finding also borne out at another institution (Korst, 1977). In Geertsma's work, non–ISP students did differ on certain personality measures. They showed greater timidity toward superiors, a willingness to accept blame and feel guilt, and also exhibited such traits as vying for the attention of others, eruditeness, and being especially personable in order to please. Conversely, ISP applicants expressed characteristics such as wanting to do new and different things, enjoying a wide range of experiences, and valuing esthetic experiences. In an analysis of the cost-effectiveness of this program, it proved slightly more expensive only in terms of study materials and laboratory supplies (that is, nonfaculty costs) and appeared to be a viable alternative to the traditional curriculum.

The long-range effects of the ISP format upon students are not yet known. One encouraging follow-up study of ninety-nine ISP graduates (Blumberg, Sharf, and Sinacore, 1982) compared them with their classmates and with national statistics on other physicians. They found ISP graduates selecting medical subspecialties at a much higher rate and engaging in more research, administration, and teaching than the comparison groups. More research of this nature would aid in assessing the overall value of independent study programs.

*Problem-Based Learning (PBL).* Problem-based learning, like independent study, can be used as an instructional technique or can provide the basis of an entire curriculum. Essentially, PBL encourages students to work with problems related to a patient or a clinical situation. Problems can be predetermined for students (Ways, Loftus, and Jones, 1973) or identified by the learner (Neufeld and Barrows, 1974) and are usually investigated in conjunction with small group tutorials. In 1969, McMaster University became the first health professions institution to establish problem-based learning as the primary approach for educating medical students. This curriculum represented a radical shift from other medical curricula and seems to have emerged as a result of dissatisfaction with the lack of responsiveness of the health care delivery system to societal needs. The shortage and maldistribution of health manpower, public discontent with the availability and quality of health care, and the lack of comprehensive care have also been cited as contributory factors.

As a curricular model, PBL draws upon the philosophy of John Dewey, the logic of the scientific method, and current knowledge of principles of adult learning; as an educational approach, it seems to make sense. Regrettably, little research documenting its efficacy, not even sound program evaluation, has been reported. The preliminary results of one study of McMaster graduates' clinical performance in postgraduate training showed them to be equal or superior to their counterparts elsewhere (Joorabchi, 1977). Another follow-up study of PBL graduates indicated that they were generally similar to graduates of the traditional curriculum and to graduates of other medical schools on conventional criteria (Richards and others, 1980). Students in this problem-based program, however, were noted for their openness regarding personal strengths and weaknesses, willingness to help each other improve, and greater sensitivity to the interpersonal needs and feelings of patients. Evaluating problem-based learning using simulated patients in a small group tutorial, Barrows and Tamblyn (1976) found that students taught in this way demonstrated greater skill in problem formulation than did those in a control group. Other more subjective evaluations of PBL include Ways, Loftus, and Jones (1973), who reported that the lack of teacher training might jeopardize the integrity of the small group tutorials, and Joorabchi (1979), who found that both faculty and students question the validity of tutors' evaluations of students' learning due to the potential biases that can develop while working so closely with student groups.

Since a tremendous amount has been written describing problem-based learning and because it is increasingly being incorporated into or replacing established health professions curricula throughout the world, further testing of its effectiveness is essential. Studies addressing major concerns, such as its cost or impact on patient care outcomes, have not as yet been reported.

*Summary Comments.* Regrettably, the investigations on methods in the health professions education literature have been misdirected. Most of the work continues to focus on trivial questions about the same tired issue of whether one method is superior to another; as was shown in the review of the lecture mode, it has not drawn upon findings from studies in general education. Conversely, little work has been conducted on such exciting concepts as problem-based learning and independent study programs that could, in fact, have a major impact upon the education of all health professionals.

On the other hand, credit must be given to those individuals who have conducted the research discussed in this chapter. Practically all the articles published on instruction are merely descriptive and, without adequate documentation, conclude that a new technique, course, or program was effective. An analysis of the literature on undergraduate clinical teaching in medicine brings this point home. Barzansky and Foley (1979) reviewed all articles published in the *Journal of Medical Education* from 1969 to 1978, and those on the clinical teaching of undergraduate medical students were identified. Of the 1,459 articles published during this period, 286 (19.6 percent) related to undergraduate clinical teaching; of these, only 10 percent included any program evaluation data beyond reports of student satisfaction. Sanson-Fisher, Fairbairn, and Maguire (1981) conducted a superb review of the methodologies used in studies designed to teach communication skills to medical students. Of the 46 reviewed between 1970 and 1979, 61 percent were descriptive and only 18 were experimentally oriented.

Unless effectiveness is demonstrated, the benefits of a new instructional medium or program are likely to fall the way of last year's fun fashions: popular at the time, probably expensive, and likely to be discarded since they were, after all, somewhat faddish to start with.

### Student Learning Styles and Preferences

Despite the lip service given to recognizing individual differences among students, little has been done to study the issue. In the numerous studies reviewed earlier in this chapter, a few looked at subgroups of learners with reference to aptitude, but none explored how learning styles might influence student achievement with, or preference for, a particular instructional technique. As Rosenshine and Furst (1973) point out, "Almost all the experimental and correlational studies have focused upon the relationship of teacher behavior to the class mean. Few investigators have focused on the personality or learning styles of subgroups of learners or have stratified classes according to the initial knowledge or aptitude of the student" (p. 173).

Within the last decade, efforts have been devoted to measuring student likes and dislikes regarding the learning process, primarily through the development of self-report instruments that assess learner tastes. Dubin and Taveggia (1968) defined learning style as an attribute of the individual that interacts with instructional circumstances in such a way as to produce differential learning achievement. Rezler and Rezmovic (1981) make a distinction between learning preference and *learning style*, the latter being the manner in which an individual perceives and processes information in learning situations. For example, Kolb's Learning Style Inventory (1976) purports to measure whether a learner perceives and processes information in an abstract, concrete, reflective, or experimental manner. Rezler and Rezmovic define *learning preference* as the choice of one learning situation over another. For example, two dimensions of the Learning Preference Inventory (Rezler and French, 1975) are Interpersonal and Independent. An individual who expresses a preference for interpersonal learning is likely to prefer a learning environment in which there are opportunities to work in groups or conduct projects with others. As more instruments measuring learning styles and preferences emerge, such definitions are essential.

In a concise comparison of the work of various learning style researchers, Dunn and others (1981) describe six self-report instruments. This thorough review does not include three other known self-report inventories (Friedman and Stritter, 1977; Rezler and French, 1975; Riechman and Grasha, 1974), and additional instruments may currently exist or be in developmental stages.

Three of the inventories reported have been used with health professionals. Using Kolb's instrument, Plovnick (1975) reported a relationship between medical students' learning styles and their specialty choice. This study was replicated with medical students and practicing physicians by Wunderlich and Gjerde (1978), and their findings revealed no relationship between specialty choice and learning style. Indeed, a factor analysis of the items comprising the inventory did not support Kolb's dimensions. Whitney and Caplan (1978) used the same instrument and found that family practice physicians preferred instructional formats for CME programs that correlated with their particular learning style. This study also lent weight to the work of Wunderlich and Gjerde, since no predominant learning style was found among the physicians sampled, suggesting again that learning styles, as measured by Kolb's questionnaire, are not associated with career choice. Furthermore, this instrument was used as a variable in assessing the characteristics of nursing students learning from a computer-assisted instructional program (Kirchhoff and Holzemer, 1979). Learning styles were not related to student achievement.

The Canfield-Lafferty Inventory was used at a national level to identify the learning preferences of almost half the students enrolled in the first year of the basic professional programs in physical therapy (Payton, Hueter, and McDonald, 1979). It was found that the typical student strongly preferred logical, clearly organized course work in which assignments and requirements were explicitly detailed. This typical student was not inclined to act independently, work alone, or compete with others but instead preferred to work with people. Generally, the individual preferred to learn by listening and through direct experience, having little interest in numbers, words, or reading.

The Learning Preference Inventory (LPI) has been used primarily with allied health and pharmacy students (Rezler and French, 1975; Rezler and Rezmovic, 1981) and yields six scores that indicate preferences for the following learning conditions or situations: Abstract, Concrete, Individual, Interpersonal, Student-Structured, and Teacher-Structured. Rezler found that the majority of allied health and pharmacy students tested preferred teacher-structured and concrete learning tasks and situations. In examining her sample of physical therapy students, for instance, the scales receiving the highest mean scores were Concrete,

Teacher-Structured, and Interpersonal, respectively. While a different instrument and sample were used, Rezler's findings with physical therapy students seemed to be affirmed by the previously discussed study by Payton, Hueter, and McDonald (1979), who found that physical therapy students preferred course work that is logically and clearly organized (that is, Teacher-Structured), learned it best through direct experience (that is, Concrete), and preferred working with people rather than alone (that is, Interpersonal).

As a whole, these data provide a generally precise profile of the learning preferences of physical therapy students. Further work to determine the preferences of other health professions students should be done. When it is, will we find that the majority of dental, nursing, and medical students also prefer a concrete and teacher-structured environment, or will other learning preferences emerge?

The learning preferences of health professions practitioners are virtually unknown. Studies in this area might identify the types of instructional formats that they would prefer in continuing education activities, and longitudinal studies could address whether professional practice influences learning preferences. Although her study was not longitudinal, Horton (1978) administered the LPI to 236 medical record practitioners whose experience ranged from less than one year to more than twenty-one. Mean scores were strikingly similar to those of beginning medical record students in Rezler and French's study (1975); again, the most preferred dimensions were Concrete and Teacher-Structured. Horton was not surprised by these results, since she sees this field as a concrete discipline dealing with technical processes from which other health professionals and civil and legal authorities demand precise information. She suggests, in fact, that learning preferences may have influenced these individuals' career choices. Studies comparing the preferences of students and practitioners in other professions might help us to determine whether specific disciplines attract students with particular learning preferences.

Dubin and Taveggia's (1968) definition of learning styles implies a relationship between a learner's reported preferences and differential achievement. While such relationships have been reported with airmen (James, 1962) and with community college students (Hunter, 1978), no published studies in the health professions education literature, save Kirchhoff and Holzemer (1979), have related learning preferences to academic achievement. Research regarding the predictive value of learning preferences scores is sorely needed. Studies examining the relationship among learning preferences, the relative effectiveness of different instructional methods, and learning satisfaction and achievement would add immeasurably to our understanding of the influence of learning preferences on the teaching-learning process.

Information with respect to the utility of learning preference scores in assisting student selection of programs, courses, and, possibly, teachers would also be useful. Rezler pointed out that while the majority of students she sampled preferred an environment in which the teacher was in control, many differed from this pattern. This was borne out in her study of the learning preferences of freshman pharmacy students (Rezler and Rezmovic, 1981). Those who elected to participate in an independent, self-study program preferred student-structured learning conditions more than those enrolled in the traditional lecture-laboratory curriculum. It would be of interest to see if this were also true of students who select independent study programs in other professional schools. Equally interesting would be studies that investigated the influences of a curriculum upon learning preferences. For example, would students who prefer teacher-structure at the time of enrollment in a problem-based curriculum prefer student-structure upon graduation?

Longitudinal studies such as those suggested here could help clarify whether learning preferences are relatively fixed dimensions of an individual's personality or whether they can be changed by educational or professional experiences. If they prove to be relatively fixed, matching students with teachers and learning environments that are compatible with their tastes could be justified. If learning preferences can be altered, however, educational interventions that facilitate individuals becoming more comfortable with varying learning conditions should be designed. If these and other issues are not explored, learning preference instruments may well fall the way of other descriptive profiles that are fun to take and worth little more.

## Recommendations for New Research Directions

Overall, the research that has examined various modes of instructional methods or media shows no, or at most only slight, differences among the formats investigated. When differences were found, they usually favored whatever had been labeled the experimental method. Insufficient information regarding the characteristics of the methods or media involved has been one acutely limiting factor in these studies, with the work comparing self-instructional formats to other modes of instruction being a case in point. In these studies, it was generally difficult to decipher the type of self-instructional program being tested and even more difficult to understand how the conventional instruction was carried out. It was not unusual, for instance, to find studies reporting only that the control group received a series of lectures. Therefore, identifying those discrete aspects of a method that made it superior or inferior to another was impossible, as would be replicating most of the studies.

Even if the investigators had been more careful in describing the variables involved, another flaw marred these studies since, in essence, it is not only the medium of instruction that is being tested. As Wallen and Travers (1963) caution, "All too often the unreasonable assumption is that because a teaching method has been described, corresponding patterns of behavior can be, or are, manifested by teachers" (p. 467). In some studies, the same instructor gave the lecture, ran the group discussion, and was the tutor for students working on a self-instructional program. To assume that this individual is equally qualified for all three endeavors is presumptuous. Teachers may favor or even value one method over another and cannot be expected to engage in all methods with equal effectiveness. Other studies used different individuals employing different methods to teach varying groups of students, thus confounding the issue even more. When reading the ensuing results, it is not as if we are dealing with actual teachers who approximate a particular method but rather with imaginary teachers who are a composite of a number of superb educators, each precisely implementing an instructional mode. It would have been refreshing to have found a study comparing self-instruction to the lecture in which the best lecturers, by whatever criteria employed, were used to teach the control group. Suppose also that the instructors had carefully constructed their speeches to incorporate the same objectives and materials covered by the other format and then had developed comparable pre- and posttests. The lectures would then have been rehearsed to ensure that the material was comprehensible, well-paced, and judiciously repetitious. In short, the study would guarantee that the lectures included all the components contained in a well-constructed self-instructional program. Ironically, researchers often bend backwards to be sure that they have carefully matched student groups, yet totally disregard assessment of the teachers who deliver the instruction.

Faculty preferences for certain teaching modes are also ignored in most of the research on instruction. Faculty often are expected to lecture, manage laboratories, run seminars, and hold tutorials, usually with little formal or informal background in education (Page, Foley, and Pochyly, 1975). Even if these skills were taught, a given teacher might detest lecturing and feel comfortable leading a seminar. Such preferences certainly influence how material is delivered and, probably, how well some students learn. Yet faculty preferences are not regularly considered in the research on teaching. In fact, in a national survey of undergraduate teaching in obstetrics and gynecology (Stenchever, Irby, and O'Toole, 1979), it was found that small group discussions, lectures, and professional patients were the preferred teaching modalities of faculty. The least preferred option was computer-assisted instruction, followed closely by programmed workbooks and other teaching aids. Data such as these might, in part, account for the figures noted earlier regarding the low utilization of self-instructional materials. Until faculty tastes are considered, we may continue to refine and research instructional strategies that faculty may rarely use.

Apart from the few studies that examined student aptitude in relation to achievement, most dealt with students as if they were carbon copies of each other and learned in exactly the same ways. Scant consideration has been given to student personality characteristics and how they might influence preference for, or performance with, a given method of instruction. This is equally true for student learning preferences. Would an enrollee in a self-instructional course who preferred to learn independently acquire more information intially, retain it longer, expend less time, and prefer self-instruction if compared with extroverted students who flourished in group learning situations? Less washout might result in studies that compare the effectiveness of various instructional techniques if such characteristics were taken into account.

Another concern about the existing research on instructional methods and materials is how program effectiveness is measured. Again, the work on self-instructional programs is illustrative. Regarding these programs, Williams (1981) notes, "We may appreciate the fact that the authors have developed a program that appears effective, but have they discovered any principles that might enable them (or us) to develop even better programs? Incidentally, how do we measure program effectiveness, by knowledge acquisition (short-term gain) or knowledge retention (how much, and after what length of time)? Once a promising program appears in the literature, it is seldom heard of again. Was it optimal the first time? What changes made it better? Why? These data must be examined if significant advances are to be made" (p. 297). True, the majority of studies have focused on cognitive achievement, and most of this work has looked at the simple recall of information. But Williams raises only a few of the issues. Granted, we have practically ignored knowledge retention, but we have paid even less attention to how a particular instructional format affects a student's ability to transfer the information learned to new situations. Studies exploring the relationship between an instructional intervention and higher-level thinking or affective and psycho-motor learning are rare. Equally rare are studies that examine the relationship between an instructional technique and its cost. While ward rounds are continuously criticized in the literature, as yet no studies have explored this experience in terms of student learning and its cost. Regrettably, research on the relationship of an instructional strategy to health care outcomes is also practically nonexistent. This may not be surprising, since the issue is even more complex than the measurement of knowledge retention that, to date, has been largely unproductive. Nonetheless, we have beaten to death the question of how a particular instructional technique affects short-term knowledge gains. It is time to change goals.

Furthermore, the era of comparing one instructional method or medium with another should be ended. Different teaching methods emphasize certain principles and do not address others. When the overall effects of teaching are appraised, it is unlikely that one method is superior to another; we can only expect, at best, that a particular technique may be most effective within very narrow aspects of the learning process. Rather than continue to belabor the merits of one method over another, it makes much more sense to examine larger sequences of instruction in light of principles of learning. For example, Hinkelman and Long (1976) designed a course in clinical operative dentistry, taking into account such principles of learning as prompting and feedback, principles that are relevant to learning an intricate psychomotor skill. Student learning in this course was then compared to that of a group who took the course as it is usually taught. The experimental group reached proficiency more quickly and retained their skills longer than did the other students. Similarly, Abou-Rass (1974) found that particular sequences of learning significantly influenced student performance in preclinical endodontics with respect to the length of time spent learning, the probability of error, and the transfer of learning.

It is time to explore which *mix* of techniques is the most efficacious in helping students learn the knowledge, skills, and attitudes that affect health care delivery. Courses or units of instruction should be studied in which the learning outcomes expected of students are identified and the corresponding criteria necessary for achieving them are clearly delineated. These outcomes should be more broadly formulated than behavioral objectives and should encompass the cognitive, affective, and psychomotor learning that students need to achieve them. If various alternative instructional sequences formulated upon sound principles of learning were then compared, data would be available concerning which sequence promoted the greatest amount of learning and satisfaction in the shortest time and at the least expense. Various sequences could be designed to explore specific effects, such as which ones resulted in preparing individuals who could conduct the most effective patient inteviews in twenty minutes or which sequences resulted in students ordering fewer unnecessary laboratory tests. If faculty preferences for certain teaching formats and student learning preferences were studied in conjunction with these sequences, we should have fascinating data that could substantially influence our present approaches to educating health professionals.

## References

Aberg, H., Johansson, R., and Michaelsson, M. "Phonocardiosimulator as an Aid in Teaching Auscultation of the Heart." *British Journal of Medical Education,* 1974, *8,* 262–266.

Abou-Rass, M. "Effects of Varying Sequence and Amount of Training on Learning and Performance in Preclinical Endodontics." *Journal of Dental Education,* 1974, *38* (5), 273–277.

Abrahamson, S., Denson, J. S., and Wolf, R. M. "Effectiveness of a Simulator in Training Anesthesiology Residents." *Journal of Medical Education,* 1969, *44,* 515–519.

Abrahamson, S., and Wallace, P. "Using Computer-Controlled Interactive Manikins in Medical Education." *Medical Teacher,* 1980, *2* (1), 25–31.

Arnold, J. A. "Let's Discuss Teaching Strategies." *Journal of Nursing Education,* 1978, *17* (1), 15–20.

Asklund, S., Brown, S., and Fiterman, C. "Slide-Tape Versus Lecture Demonstration Presentation of Thermal Agents in a Physical Therapist Assistant Program." *Physical Therapy,* 1976, *56* (12), 1361–1364.

Association of Professors of Gynecology and Obstetrics, Steering Committee for Cooperative Teaching. "Faculty Reactions to an Instructional Media Network in North America." *Journal of Medical Education,* 1973, *48,* 430–435.

Barrows, H. S. *Simulated Patients (Programmed Patients).* Springfield, Ill.: Thomas, 1971.

Barrows, H. S., and Tamblyn, R. M. "An Evaluation of Problem-Based Learning in Small Groups Utilizing a Simulated Patient." *Journal of Medical Education,* 1976, *51,* 52–54.

Barzansky, B., and Foley, R. P. "Clinical Teaching: A Content Analysis of the Literature." Unpublished paper, Center for Educational Development, Health Sciences Center, University of Illinois at Chicago, 1979.

Bickley, H. C., McDougall, M. S., and Pepe, S. H. "A Comparison of Programmed Learning and Conventional Lectures in the Teaching of General Pathology to Physical Therapy Students." *Physical Therapy,* 1973, *53* (7), 769–773.

Blumberg, P., Sharf, B. F., and Sinacore, J. M. "Impact of an Independent Study Programmed upon Professional Careers." *Medical Education,* 1982, *16,* 156–160.

Bogner, P., Sajid, A. W., and Ford, D. L. "Effectiveness of Audio-Based Instruction in Medical Pharmacology." *Journal of Medical Education,* 1975, *50,* 677–682.

Cantrell, E. G., and Craven, J. L. "A Trial of Television in Teaching Clinical Medicine." *British Journal of Medical Education,* 1969, *3,* 110–114.

Coppola, E. D., and Gonnella, J. S. "A Nondirective Approach to Clinical Instruction in Medical Schools." *Journal of the American Medical Association,* 1968, *205* (7), 487–491.

Davies, M. A., Gale, J., and Clarke, W. D. "Audiotape and Booklet Self-Instructional Materials in Physiology: An Evaluation of Their Effectiveness and Acceptability in the Preclinical Curriculum." *Medical Education*, 1977, *11*, 370–373.

deCarvalho, C. A. F., and others. "Comparative Analysis Between Guided Self-Instruction and Conventional Lectures in Neuroanatomy." *Journal of Medical Education*, 1977, *52*, 212–213.

Dowson, J., and Engle, D. "Survey of Instructional Materials Used in Teaching Endodontics." *Journal of Dental Education*, 1973, *37*, 47–48.

Dubin, R., and Taveggia, T. C. *The Teaching-Learning Paradox: A Comparative Analysis of College Teaching Methods.* Eugene: Center for the Advanced Study of Educational Administration, University of Oregon, 1968.

Dunn, E. V., and others. "The Use of Slow Scan–Video for CME in a Remote Area." *Journal of Medical Education*, 1980, *55* (6), 493–495.

Dunn, R., and others. "Learning Style Researchers Define Differences Differently." *Educational Leadership*, 1981, *38*, 372–375.

Ellis, H. C. *Transfer of Learning.* New York: Macmillan, 1965.

Fiel, N. J. "The Lecture: Increasing Student Learning." *Journal of Medical Education*, 1976, *51*, 496–499.

Flax, J., and Garrard, J. "Students Teaching Students: A Model for Medical Education." *Journal of Medical Education*, 1974, *49*, 380–383.

Foley, R. P., and Smilansky, J. *Teaching Techniques: A Handbook for Health Professionals.* New York: McGraw-Hill, 1980.

Friedman, C., and Stritter, F. "An Empirical Inventory Comparing Instructional Preferences of Medical and Other Professional Students." In *Proceedings of the Annual Conference on Research in Medical Education.* Washington, D.C.: American Association of Medical Colleges, 1977.

Geertsma, R. H., and others. "An Independent Study Program Within a Medical Curriculum." *Journal of Medical Education*, 1977, *52*, 123–132.

Gershen, J. A. "Comparing the Effectiveness of the Minilecture Technique to Role Playing in a Dental Psychology Course." *Journal of Dental Education*, 1978, *42* (8), 470–475.

Gordon, M. S., and others. "A Multi-Institutional Research Study on the Use of Simulation for Teaching and Evaluating Patient Examination Skills." Symposium presented at the 19th Annual Conference on Research in Medical Education, American Association of Medical Colleges, Washington, D.C., 1980.

Harless, W., and others. "CASE: A Computer-Aided Simulation of the Clinical Encounter." *Journal of Medical Education*, 1971, *46*, 443–448.

Harvey, W. L., Chappell, R. F., and Ferguson, D. J. "Teacher-Instruction and Student-Instruction Compared." *Journal of Dental Education*, 1970, *34*, 327–332.

Hinkelman, K. W., and Long, N. K. "Utilizing Learning Theory to Promote Effectiveness of Instruction in Preclinical Operative Dentistry." *Journal of Dental Education*, 1976, *40* (3), 154–157.

Hoffman, K. I., and Abrahamson, S. "The 'Cost-Effectiveness' of Sim One." *Journal of Medical Education*, 1975, *50*, 1127–1128.

Horton, E. "Learning and Teaching Preferences Among Medical Record Practitioners." Thesis, Center for Educational Development, Health Sciences Center, University of Illinois at Chicago, 1978.

Huckabay, L. M. D., Cooper, P. G., and Neal, M. C. "Effect of Specific Teaching

Techniques on Cognitive Learning Transfer of Learning, and Affective Behavior of Nurses in an In-Service Education Setting." *Nursing Research*, 1977, *26* (5), 380–385.

Huckabay, L. M. D., and others. "Cognitive, Affective, and Transfer of Learning Consequences of Computer-Assisted Instruction." *Nursing Research*, 1979, *28* (4), 228–233.

Hunter, W. E. "Noncognitive Factors and Student Success in College." *Community College Frontiers*, 1978, *u* (2), 44.

James, N. E. "Personal Preferences for Method as a Factor in Learning." *Journal of Educational Psychology*, 1962, *53*, 43–47.

Jeffers, J. M., and Christensen, M. G. "Using Simulation to Facilitate the Acquisition of Clinical Observational Skills." *Journal of Nursing Education*, 1979, *18* (6), 29–32.

Joorabchi, B. "The Maastricht Experiment." *Learner*, 1977, *4*, 4–9.

Joorabchi, B. "The Beginning Doctor: A Problem-Based Course for First-Year Medical and Dental Students." *Medical Education*, 1979, *73*, 10–13.

Kahn, R. H., Conklin, J. L., and Glover, R. A. "A Self-Instructional Program in Microscopic Anatomy." *Journal of Medical Education*, 1973, *48*, 859–863.

Kao, Y. S., Beeler, M. F., and Strong, J. P. "Comparison of the Conventional Lecture Method and the Self-Instruction Method for Teaching Clinical Pathology." *American Journal of Clinical Pathology*, 1978, *70* (6), 847–850.

Kirchhoff, K. T., and Holzemer, W. L. "Student Learning and a Computer-Assisted Instructional Program." *Journal of Nursing Education*, 1979, *18* (3), 22–30.

Koch, D. M., Koch, G. M., and Tynelius, G. M. "Comparison of Three Methods of Teaching Oral Hygiene to School Children." *Journal of Dental Education*, 1970, *34*, 98–104.

Kolb, D. *Learning Style Inventory: Technical Manual.* Boston: McBer, 1976.

Korst, D. R. "The Independent Study Program at the University of Wisconsin Medical School." *Journal of Medical Education*, 1977, *52*, 404–412.

Kress, G. C., and Jacobs, S. S. "Effects of Practice-Sequence Strategy on Cavity Preparation Skills." *Journal of Dental Education*, 1973, *37*, 20–31.

Kress, G. C., Silversin, J. B., and Colenback, P. R. "A Study of the Impact of Project ACORDE on Dental Education in the United States." *Journal of Dental Education*, 1979, *43* (4), 204–209.

McCarthy, W. H. "Improving Classroom Instruction: A Programmed Teaching Method." *Journal of Medical Education*, 1971, *46*, 605–609.

McGuire, C. H., Solomon, L. M., and Bashook, P. G. *Construction and Use of Written Simulations.* New York: Psychological Corporation, 1976.

Marshall, C. L., and Alexander, R. "Improving the Use of Television in Continuing Education." *Journal of Medical Education*, 1976, *51*, 945–946.

Meyer, J. A. H., and Beaton, G. R. "An Evaluation of Computer-Assisted Teaching in Physiology." *Journal of Medical Education*, 1974, *49*, 295–297.

Moser, D. H., and Kondracki, M. R. "Comparison of Attitudes and Cognitive Achievement of Nursing Students in Three Instructional Strategies." *Journal of Nursing Education*, 1977, *16* (1), 14–28.

Munsick, R. A. "Educational Methodology in an Obstetric and Gynecologic Medical School Curriculum: A Comparison of Self-Instructional with Traditional Methods." *American Journal of Obstetrics and Gynecology*, 1975, 900–906.

Myers, L. B., and Greenwood, S. E. "Use of Traditional and Autotutorial Instruction in Fundamentals of Nursing Courses." *Journal of Nursing Education,* 1978, *17* (3), 7-13.

Neufeld, V. R., and Barrows, H. S. "The McMaster Philosophy: An Approach to Medical Education." *Journal of Medical Education,* 1974, *49,* 1040-1050.

Page, G., Foley, R. P., and Pochyly, D. F. "A Survey of Interests in Teacher Training of Health Science Faculty." *British Journal of Medical Education,* 1975, *3,* 182-187.

Payton, O. D., Hueter, A. E., and McDonald, B. S. "Learning Style Preferences." *Physical Therapy,* 1979, *59* (2), 147-152.

Pensivy, B. A. "Traditional Versus Individualized Nursing Instruction." *Journal of Nursing Education,* 1977, *16* (2), 14-18.

Penta, F. B., and Kofman, S. "The Effectiveness of Simulation Devices in Teaching Selected Skills of Physical Diagnosis." *Journal of Medical Education,* 1973, *48,* 442-445.

Plovnick, M. S. "Primary Care Career Choices in Medical Student Learning Styles." *Journal of Medical Education,* 1975, *50,* 849-855.

Portnoy, A. L., and Glasser, M. "A Four-Year Experience with a Programmed Text in Clinical Pathology." *Journal of Medical Education,* 1974, *49,* 457-459.

Randels, P. M., and others. "Comparison of the Psychiatry Learning System and Traditional Teaching of Psychiatry." *Journal of Medical Education,* 1976, *52,* 751-757.

Rezler, A. G., and French, R. M. "Personality Types of Learning Preferences of Students in Six Allied Health Professions." *Journal of Allied Health,* 1975, *4,* 20-26.

Rezler, A. G., and Rezmovic, V. "The Learning Preference Inventory." *Journal of Allied Health,* 1981, *11,* 28-34.

Richards, R. W., and others. "The Upper Peninsula Medical Education Program: Educating Primary Care Physicians for Rural Areas." In Andrew D. Hunt (Ed.), *Medical Education Since 1960—Marching to a Different Drummer.* East Lansing: Michigan State University, 1980.

Riechman, S., and Grasha, A. "A Rational Approach to Developing and Assessing the Construct Validity of a Student Learning Style Scales Instrument." *Journal of Psychology,* 1974, *87,* 213-223.

Roach, F. R., and Wakefield, L. "Evaluating a Self-Instructional Module in Quantity Food Purchasing." *Journal of the American Dietetic Association,* 1974, *65,* 166-169.

Rogers, C. *Freedom to Learn.* Columbus, Ohio: Merrill, 1969.

Rosenshine, B., and Furst, W. "The Use of Direct Observation to Study Teaching." In R. M. W. Travers (Ed.), *Second Handbook of Research on Teaching.* Chicago: Rand McNally, 1973.

Rutan, F. M. "Comparison of Self-Instruction and Lecture-Demonstration in Learning a Physical Therapy Skill." *Physical Therapy,* 1973, *53* (5), 521-526.

Sajid, A., Magero, J., and Feinzimer, M. "Learning Effectiveness of the Heart Sound Simulator." *Medical Education,* 1977, *11,* 1-3.

Salvendy, G., and others. "Electromechanical Simulator for Acquisition of Psychomotor Skills in Cavity Preparation." *Journal of Dental Education,* 1973, *37,* 32-40.

Salvendy, G., and others. "A Second-Generation Training Simulator for Acquisition of Psychomotor Skills in Cavity Preparation." *Journal of Dental Education*, 1975, *79* (7), 466–471.

Sanson-Fisher, R., Fairbairn, S., and Maguire, P. "Teaching Skills in Communication to Medical Students: A Critical Review of the Methodology." *Medical Education*, 1981, *15*, 33–37.

Shafer, J. A., Johnson, W., and Weed, R. I. "Learning and Teaching RBC Morphology: Self-Instruction Versus Conventional Instruction." *American Journal of Medical Technology*, 1972, *38* (10), 394–400.

Shafer, J. A., Weed, R. I., and Johnson, W. "Evaluation of a Self-Instructional Program in Red Cell Morphology." *Journal of Medical Education*, 1973, *48*, 1133–1139.

Spears, M. C., Moore, A. W., and Tuthill, B. H. "Telelectures Versus Workshops in Continuing Professional Education." *Journal of the American Dietetic Association*, 1973, *63*, 239–247.

Stanley, J., and Reich, P. "Teaching Blood Morphology: Audiovisual Method Compared to Microscope Slides with Written Text and Instructor." *Blood*, 1974, *44* (3), 445–448.

Stenchever, M. A., Irby, D., and O'Toole, B. O. "A National Survey of Undergraduate Teaching in Obstetrics and Gynecology." *Journal of Medical Education*, 1979, *54* (6), 467–470.

Stritter, F. T., and others. "Documentation of the Effectiveness of Self-Instructional Materials." *Journal of Medical Education*, 1973, *48*, 1129–1132.

Sturwold, V. G. "Use of Audiovisual Materials in Teaching of Periodontics." *Journal of Dental Education*, 1973, *37*, 33–38.

Suess, J. F. "Teaching Psychodiagnosis and Observation by Self-Instructional Programmed Videotapes." *Journal of Medical Education*, 1973, *48*, 676–683.

Taylor, M. "A Comparison of Three Methods of Initial Presentation of Instrument Adaptation." *Journal of Dental Education*, 1975, *39* (3), 163–168.

Thompson, M. "Learning: A Comparison of Traditional and Autotutorial Methods." *Nursing Research*, 1972, *21* (5), 453–457.

Trent, J. W., and Cohen, A. M. "Research on Teaching in Higher Education." In R. M. W. Travers (Ed.), *Second Handbook of Research on Teaching*. Chicago: Rand McNally, 1973.

VanDenBerg, E. L. "The Multiple Assignment: An Effective Alternative for Laboratory Experiences." *Journal of Nursing Education*, 1976, *15* (3), 3–12.

Wallen, W. E., and Travers, R. M. W. "Analysis and Investigation of Teaching Methods." In N. L. Gage (Ed.), *Handbook of Research on Teaching*. Chicago: Rand McNally, 1963.

Ways, P. O., Loftus, G., and Jones, J. M. "Focal Problem Teaching in Medical Education." *Journal of Medical Education*, 1973, *48*, 565–571.

White, H. B., Smith, T. M., and Sulya, L. L. "Self-Instructional and Audiovisual Methods of Teaching Biochemistry Laboratory." *Journal of Medical Education*, 1973, *48*, 939–944.

Whitney, M. A., and Caplan, R. M. "Learning Styles and Instructional Preference of Family Practice Physicians." *Journal of Medical Education*, 1978, *53*, 684–686.

Williams, R. E. "Self-Instruction in Dental Education: 1960–1980." *Journal of Dental Education*, 1981, *45* (5), 290–299.

Williamson, J. W., and McGuire, C. "Consecutive Case Conference: An Educational Evaluation." *Journal of Medical Education,* 1968, *43,* 1068–1074.

Wunderlich, R., and Gjerde, C. L. "Another Look at Learning Style Inventory and Medical Career Choice." *Journal of Medical Education,* 1978, *53,* 45–54.

# Evaluation of Student and Practitioner Competence

Efforts to protect the public from incompetent health practitioners have a long and, for the most part, honorable history. Since ancient times, official permission to engage in the healing arts has been made contingent on an individual's ability to demonstrate completion of approved training and/or acquisition of requisite skills. Where practice of the profession was the monopoly of a priestly class, as in dynastic Egypt, the public could be assured that every healer had successfully concluded proper training and endured the rituals prescribed for graduation. The earliest known recorded specification that an entry-level health professional also demonstrate skills is to be found in the sacred books of the Parsis (the Avesta), which contained the interesting requirement that a worshiper of Mazda, aspiring to practice his healing art, first prove himself by "cutting with the knife" three worshipers of Daêvas. If all lived, the applicant had the right to apply his arts to worshipers of Mazda for all time; if none lived, he was forever prohibited from treating true believers, and the penalties for ignoring that prohibition were severe (Sigerist, 1935). Medical licensure as an institution became general in the West only during the Middle Ages.

The history of the evolution of that institution in Europe and America is a fascinating one. First, and most readily accommodated, was the control of surgeons who fitted neatly into the guild structure that dictated and supervised the conditions of their training and regulated the practice of their craft. But physicians, as members of a liberal profession, followed a different route; very early they began to organize themselves into faculties that ultimately became the grantors of

*Note:* Grateful acknowledgment is made for the able assistance in bibliographical research and literature review of Jo Ann Hartline, research associate in the Department of Medical Social Work, University of Illinois at Chicago.

licenses and the arbiters of standards of professional practice. The first European faculty to license physicians was the famous school at Salerno. The first European "medical practice act" was embodied in the complex codes of the Hohenstaufen emperor, Frederick II—the Constitutiones Imperiales—developed between 1231 and 1240. "The law required examinations under a regular teacher of medicine at Salerno and set forth educational standards in the form of three full years devoted to logic. In addition, the statute required that, 'after having spent five years in study, he (the physician) shall not practice medicine until he has during a full year devoted himself to medical practice under the direction of an experienced physician.' The Code also provided for severe punishment for violations and regulated ethical conduct by setting fees and requiring free care for the poor. Thus, the Code of Frederick II contained all the elements of the modern laws—educational standards, postgraduate education, evaluation by examination, and the requirement that the applicant be of good moral character" (Derbyshire, 1979, p. 263).

Some would argue that in the succeeding eight centuries, there has been little, if any, improvement either in the nature of the evaluation of professional competence or in its implementation, at least in this country (Sigerist, 1935). It was not until the late 1890s that most states had established medical boards for licensure to control discrepancies in performance of graduates from different schools (Samph and Templeton, 1979). Subsequent efforts to assure that physicians and, more recently, newer health care providers are qualified to render effective care have embraced two general types of regulation: (1) institutional accreditation guaranteeing that each health care provider receives approved training, and (2) individual certification testifying that each individual has reached an adequate level of proficiency. It is with this latter approach to quality assurance that we are primarily concerned in this chapter—specifically, with research on the purpose, nature, instrumentation, and interpretation of evaluations of professional competence in the health professions.

## Status in the 1960s

While most health professions invoke some kind of final certifying examination process for entry into the profession, in most instances testing at that point is only the last of many hurdles the aspiring professional must leap. For example, even after repeated examination by a medical faculty and one to three examinations by the National Board of Medical Examiners (NBME) and/or the Federation of State Medical Boards, most physicians are further subject to examination by specialty societies or specialty boards before they can expect to establish a genuinely independent practice and to obtain appointment to a hospital staff (Samph and Templeton, 1979). Nor does that end the process—for some, periodic recertification and/or relicensure by examination is required; for many, their work will be monitored by various hospital committees; and, for most, some form of ongoing peer review, such as the Professional Standards Review Organizations (PSROs), has been mandated by the federal government. Dentists, nurses, pharmacists, and allied health personnel undergo comparable assessment procedures at the undergraduate and licensure or certification points in their careers, though once licensed or certified they are less likely to face further mandatory personal evaluation. In short, until relatively recently, most professional schools have used examinations primarily for the purpose of ranking students and granting degrees. Most other examining bodies have used them exclusively for the purpose of granting licenses or specialty certificates, and most health care delivery or reimbursement agencies have used them for granting special privileges.

Individual assessment for these purposes has most often been based on a combination of written and oral or practical examinations, though the latter have gradually been abandoned for both technical and feasibility reasons. In the case of students, these methods have often been supplemented by instructors' evaluations of attitudes and day-to-day performance in the clinic. However, all these methods, as conventionally employed, measure primarily individuals' ability to recall fragments of information rapidly and under stress and their conformity to faculty/ examiner values (McGuire, 1968b). Scoring and grading have been essentially normative, with the passing level determined on the basis of an individual's performance relative to that of peers. The system differs only in detail among the several health professions.

Concern about deficiencies in this process of evaluating the professional competence of both students and practitioners led in the late sixties and early seventies to numerous innovations affecting almost all the individual elements of the system: the purpose for which evaluation was used, the techniques of defining the essential components of competence, the range of competencies actually assessed, the methods of evaluation employed, the approaches to scoring and reporting performance, and the criteria used in setting standards.

## Purpose of Evaluation

### Summative Evaluation

As we have seen, evaluation of professionals has in the past been undertaken primarily as an exercise in summative evaluation—that is, to certify that an individual has satisfactorily completed a certain stage in his or her training, ranks at a certain level among peers, or is eligible to be accepted as a member of the relevant community of professionals. No one questions that summative evaluation of competence at a state or national level is essential. The differential failure rates among graduates of different U.S. institutions and the significantly higher failure rates among foreign trained professionals, consistently revealed by twenty years of research on existing licensure and certification examinations, have merely reinforced the view that adequate methods must be found that will yield valid and reliable measures of professional competence for purposes of summative evaluation at all levels of professional training and practice.

More recently, two additional purposes of summative evaluation have surfaced in the health professions: Some of the allied health professions have argued for the use of a national equivalency or proficiency examination in order to open up training opportunities, even at advanced levels, to persons of unusual education and experience (Pennell, 1972). More common has been the pressure on all health professions to develop a sound means of assuring continued competence. But both of these developments represent merely extensions to preentry and posttraining of the traditional notion of individual evaluation for purposes of certification of competence.

## Formative Evaluation

In addition, a radically new set of purposes has emerged as increasingly important over the past twenty years. These new purposes can be broadly grouped under the term *formative evaluation*. As currently employed, the concept of formative evaluation embraces *diagnostic testing* (to diagnose an individual's strengths and weaknesses as a basis for recommending educational therapy), *needs assessment* (to determine educational priorities for individuals or groups), *student progress monitoring* (to assure that the student is progressing at a reasonable rate toward the institution's objectives), and *self-assessment* (to provide immediate feedback to individuals and to assist them in developing important self-critical skills). All types of formative evaluation—diagnostic testing, needs assessment, and student progress examinations—may be employed for purposes either of program development or of individual assessment; our concern here is with research on the latter—formative evaluation for purposes of assessing the individual.

At the undergraduate level, self-assessment is used primarily to allay anxiety, to assist the student in preparing for summative evaluations, and, most importantly, to develop the habits and skills necessary for continued, independent learning. Numerous studies of self-assessment at the undergraduate and first postgraduate year of training are consistent in finding that self-ratings and ratings by peers of specific competencies correlate highly with faculty or supervisor ratings, tending to be at least as rigorous, and often harsher than the former (Brehm, 1972; Kegel-Flom, 1975; Cochran and Spears, 1980; Barrows and Tamblyn, 1976; Linn, Arostegni, and Zeppa, 1975; Morton and Macbeth, 1977); the agreement between self-assessments and assessments by others tends to increase with experience (Cochran and Spears, 1980). Interestingly, Linn, Arostegni, and Zeppa (1975) also found that while self-ratings and ratings by peers have high reliability over time, factor analysis of the ratings of presumably independent characteristics yielded only two factors that they labeled interpersonal relationship and self-knowledge, both of which were significantly correlated with final grades.

In addition, self-assessment has been employed to enable students to monitor their own progress toward specified objectives. For example, Gurley and Blair (1975) devised an instrument that students were required to use monthly to assess their own progress on objectives related both to performance and to personal characteristics; in dentistry, Abrams and Kelley (1974) developed a similar device that students were instructed to use in evaluating their cavity preparations until each met the criteria, at which time the work was to be brought to the instructor for final grading.

Most recently, professional associations, particularly medical specialty societies, have increasingly made self-assessment exercises available to graduate trainees and to practitioners. Though at least one study by the American Board of Internal Medicine shows "that performance can be evaluated by having peers audit office records" (Rosenow, 1979, p. 216), this has not been the mechanism typically employed. For the most part, these self-assessment programs for advance trainees and practitioners have taken the form of lengthy multiple-choice examinations, in some instances supplemented with written simulations of clinical problems, as discussed later in this chapter, often with special emphasis on new knowledge. Feedback to participants may include not only an individual profile of test scores but also a syllabus with detailed discussion of each question and an annotated bibliography or other self-instructional materials (Rosenow, 1979).

## Conclusions

Many investigators report positive results from the increased emphasis on formative, in contrast to summative, evaluation; most report beneficial effects of stressing regular self-assessment activities; and virtually all report significant agreement between self-ratings and supervisor ratings and adequate rigor in the former, when *self-assessment is employed as one component in a program of formative evaluation.* While there is agreement that the habit of self-assessment should be encouraged, no one advocates it as a complete substitute for more formal assessment or for evaluation by others. Indeed, aside from the experience reported at McMaster University (discussed later in this chapter), no studies were found of the reliability and validity of self-assessments when these are incorporated as a part of the certifying process. While this might be an interesting area to explore, results from general studies of self-reports strongly suggest that their validity diminishes as their impact on career opportunities increases.

### Determining the Components of Professional Competence

In continuing efforts to develop more valid definitions of the essential components of professional competence, more systematic methods have been developed for the collection of expert opinion that itself has been increasingly supplemented by formal analysis of empirical data. (For an excellent compilation of approaches now employed by medical specialty boards, see American Board of Medical Specialties, 1979.)

### Methods Relying on Expert Opinion

In an attempt to rank order the variables that are "most meaningful in evaluating the performance of a first-year house officer on a clinical service," Wigton (1980, p. 207) employed a modified Delphi technique to obtain a consensus among full-time faculty, volunteer faculty, and residents. However, he found important differences among the three groups, as did Sweeney and Resan (1982) in an analogous attempt to have educators, employees, and new graduates define the essential skills for baccalaureate nurses.

On the assumption that "professional performance is socially determined by the situation in which it occurs," LaDuca, Engel, and Risley (1978, p. 150) developed a new model—the Professional Performance Situation Model (PPSM)—for utilizing expert judgment in defining requisite skills and knowledge. They found that for the three professions to which they applied the model, the total universe of professional situations could be defined in terms of three dimensions: setting, client, and problem. This universe could then be systematically and comprehensively sampled by developing a limited number of scenarios (15 to 25), from each of which an expert group could derive a detailed set of requisite knowledge and skill statements. Employing appropriate analytic techniques, statements in this set (which might number 2,000 to 3,000) could be aggregated and reduced to a manageable number (40 to 50) to define the components of competence within the field. The model was found to be appropriate both to patient-oriented professions, such as occupational therapy (LaDuca and others, 1980) or medical dietetics (Engel and others, 1980), and to laboratory-oriented professions, such as medical technology (Risley and others, 1980). The authors argue that the model is applicable to the health professions generally.

## Empirical Methods

Among the many possible empirical approaches to defining components of competence, the critical incident technique (Flanagan, 1954) has been most widely utilized in large nationwide studies. The technique requires the collection of detailed descriptions of specific, actual incidents in which a professional has behaved in an especially effective or especially ineffective manner. Categories of competence are empirically derived by classifying the incidents according to the essential element of competence demonstrated in each. In the medical (American Institutes for Research, 1960; Miller, McGuire, and Larson, 1965) and nursing (Fivars and Gosnell, 1966) specialties in which the technique has been applied, it has been found to yield unique definitions of the data-gathering, data-interpretation, data-synthesis, management, technical, and interpersonal skills required for the effective practice of the specialty.

Traditional task and activity analysis has not been extensively employed in the health professions as a basis for competency definition, though activity questionnaires and log-diary studies have been used to some extent. In one of the most comprehensive of the latter, Mendenhall, Girard, and Abrahamson (1978) developed a highly structured log-diary form to gather data on the activities and practice characteristics of generalists and specialists of different types; responses were analyzed to yield a unique practice profile in twenty-four specialties and subspecialties. Under the sponsorship of the Bureau of Health Manpower, the allied health professions have also made extensive use of activity questionnaires to obtain data from various level practitioners regarding the activities they *actually* perform and those they think they *ought* to perform. Results of such questionnaires are then combined in various ways with observations and expert judgment to yield a definition of the roles and functions of professionals at various levels. At the undergraduate level, responses to similar questionnaires from practitioners, educators, employees, and professional associations have been utilized to arrive at statements of behaviors thought to be related to performance as a professional (Lynch, 1977) or at a definition of core competencies essential for progression to entry level (Johnson and Hurley, 1976).

In an interesting combination of these various empirical methods, the Committee on Child Psychiatry of the American Board of Psychiatry and Neurology analyzed critical incidents obtained both from professionals in the field and from those who use their services (for example, juvenile court judges and teachers). This analysis was then combined with the results of an activity analysis based on questionnaire responses from practitioners and with expert opinion to yield a three-dimensional table of specifications of the roles and functions of child psychiatrists. The specifications include a definition (by examples) of effective and ineffective behavior in each skill domain, the "indicators of competence" in each, and the knowledge base essential to effective performance in each; it concludes with suggested methods of evaluating each domain (McDermott, McGuire, and Berner, 1976).

### Conclusions

Until the early 1960s, techniques of assessing professional competence were commonly based on the intuitive, and usually implicit, judgments of senior teachers, supervisors, and leaders about what was important in their respective fields. Clearly, such judgments varied widely among experts and were necessarily biased by the often narrowly focused interests and experience of each. Despite its advantages, each of the various remedial approaches subsequently taken has unique shortcomings. The critical incident technique does not supply information about the importance of a behavior in terms of the frequency with which it will be required. On the other hand, log-diary studies and task or activity analyses inform us only about what is, not about what ought to be; nor do they tell us which of existing activities really make a difference in health outcomes. The PPSM model, as it has been applied, relies only on the judgment of academicians and fails to incorporate more empirical data from practitioners. Finally, the costs of any technique, in terms of both time and money, need to be given serious consideration in choosing among available methods. Though we have not yet developed an adequate theory of the structure of professional competence nor a totally satisfactory method of defining its constituents, the increasing systematization of the process for utilizing expert judgment and for incorporating relevant empirical sources in defining its dimensions, which has occurred over the past twenty years, constitutes one of the most important developments leading to its more valid assessment.

### Research on Evaluation Instruments

Attempts to summarize and generalize findings from studies of various evaluation instruments in this field are particularly difficult, not only because of the breadth and diversity of sources and interests represented but also because much literature describes either purely developmental activity or, at best, applied research *with* tests designed to solve urgent practical problems rather than basic research *on* tests. Furthermore, the literature on tests is often limited to descriptive reports either of an instrument or, at most, of the results of its incorporation in individual school testing programs, from which it is especially hazardous to generalize. The problem is further compounded by the great variety of evaluation instruments now embraced by the health professions. For purposes of discussion, these diverse instruments are classified into the following categories: traditional tests—multiple-choice, essay, oral, and practical examinations; simulation exercises—written, computer, oral (role-playing), and multimedia formats; special techniques for assessing clinical performance, attitudes, and patient care (audits). (For comprehensive surveys of testing and evaluation instruments now used in medicine generally, see Barro (1973); for those used by medical specialty boards, see Lloyd (1981).)

## Research on Traditional Tests

Much of the research on tests and testing techniques conducted in the late fifties and early sixties simply confirmed in the health professions what had previously been well-documented in other educational settings: specifically, that conventional multiple-choice (MCQ) examinations were at best highly reliable but typically lacking in validity; that practical examinations tended to have the opposite characteristics—high face validity but low reliability; and that traditional essay and oral examinations were usually lacking in both reliability and validity (Cowles and Hubbard, 1952; Abrahamson, 1964; McGuire, 1966; Foster and others, 1969; Hubbard, 1971; American Board of Medical Specialties, 1975).

Studies designed to investigate the relationship between performances on purportedly comparable tests presented in different formats have tended to confirm the theory of most evaluators that it is not the *form* of a test but rather the *nature of the tasks* it sets that determines what a test measures. In applying this theory, however, one note of caution is necessary. Scores on free-response formats tend to be generally lower than scores on objective formats, and this difference seems to be most marked for less able students (Forsdyke, 1978; Newble, Baxter, and Elmslie, 1979).

Review of all types of examinations widely utilized in the health professions has led me, as well as many other evaluators, to conclude that, in addition to their technical deficiencies, these instruments focus primarily on assessment of general knowledge (McGuire, 1968b) and that they often fail to sample some of the most important behaviors relevant to the purported goals of professional education. Much research on traditional test formats has therefore been related to studies of modifications that would improve their technical quality and increase the range of competencies to which they are addressed.

*Free-Response Examinations.* Perhaps the most significant innovation has been the introduction of the Modified Essay Question (MEQ) and the Sequential Management Problem (SMP) formats. Tests in these formats are designed to assess clinical problem-solving skills by means of sequential presentation of a sometimes extensive data base about a particular case, accompanied at each stage by a very specific question (Feletti, 1980; Berner, Hamilton, and Best, 1974). Though provision of model answers and/or training of examiners to score papers consistently will always enhance interrater reliability, carefully constructed questions in these formats have been shown to produce high interrater agreement even in the absence of such safeguards (Wakeford and Roberts, 1979).

*Multiple-Choice Tests.* Here, the most important innovation has been the increasingly widely accepted practice of designing items to a table of test specifications that includes, preferably, both cognitive skill and content domains. Multiple-choice tests designed in this manner are regularly shown to assess a broader and more relevant range of competencies (Levine, McGuire, and Nattress, 1970; Chambers and Hubbard, 1978) and to distinguish in the expected direction among examinees at different levels of training and/or experience (Grosse, Croft, and Blaisdell, 1980; Lloyd, 1981; Maatsch, Munger, and Podgormy, 1983).

*Oral Examinations.* Aside from the increasing recognition of the importance of systematic examiner training in the administration and scoring of oral examinations, the single most important factor contributing to improvement has been the increased use of a structured oral examination in which examiners are provided with standardized case materials, detailed instructions for their use, and detailed checklists for rating examinee performance. The American Board of Orthopedic Surgery, which pioneered in introducing structured orals to test problem-solving, interpretive, and interpersonal skills, demonstrated convincingly that the new orals were more reliable and more valid for assessing a broader and more relevant range of competencies than were the conventional orals, in which each examiner quizzes a candidate within a general topical area (Levine and McGuire, 1970b; McGuire, 1975a).

*Practical Examinations.* While laboratory practicals have traditionally involved reasonably well-standardized problems and clear outcome criteria for scoring, such has not typically been the case of practical examinations involving a patient; the latter have consequently suffered from unreliability arising from both patient and examiner variability. The recently developed Objective Structured Clinical Examination (OSCE) represents an important new technique for retaining the face validity of the practical examination, while eliminating its major sources of unreliability. It accomplishes this feat by defining the components of the complex skill to be tested and testing one component only at each of a series of "stations" where examiners merely observe some clearly specified aspect of the examinee's interaction with the patient and/or confirm the accuracy of the findings he or she reports (Harden and Gleeson, 1979; Frejlach and Corcoran, 1971). Thus, not only are the main sources of unreliability due to lack of standardization eliminated, but the sampling reliability is also considerably elevated, since in a relatively short time each examinee can interact with not one or two but up to twenty or thirty patients.

*Summary.* Important steps have been taken to enhance the technical adequacy of conventional testing instruments and to extend the range of competencies that, by careful structuring, each can be made to assess. At best, however, they are still of limited usefulness as reliable measures of high-level problem solving, more complex technical skills, and subtle habits and attitudes; new approaches are required to meet these needs.

## Simulation Exercises

In this author's opinion the single most important development in the evaluation of professional competence in the health professions over the past two decades has been the application of simulation and gaming theory in the creation of a vast array of innovative types of test exercises, produced in oral, written, practical, and computerized examination formats.* Today, some form of simulation is being used either for formative or summative evaluation and/or for research purposes in the educational programs of medicine,** dentistry, nursing, pharmacy, and allied health. It is represented throughout the educational continuum—from undergraduate, through graduate, to in-service and continuing

---

*For a comprehensive description of the various forms of simulation exercises, see McGuire, 1977.

**For an excellent annotated bibliography of reports on the development and use of simulation for both instruction and assessment in medical education, see Maatsch and others, 1976.

education—and is employed for all purposes, from self-assessment to licensure and certification.

### Written Simulations—The PMP*

Patient Management Problems (PMP)—as written simulations are known—were introduced more or less simultaneously in the early sixties by the National Board of Medical Examiners and the University of Illinois College of Medicine (McGuire and Babbott, 1967; Hubbard, 1964). These PMPs and the various adaptations of them that followed have certain unique features, the most important of which is that through application of latent image printing technology, examinees are provided immediate feedback about each option they select. The feedback is presented either in the form of the data requested (for example, a laboratory report in response to an order for a diagnostic test) or in the form of the patient's response to an intervention (for example, the patient's vital signs in response to an order to administer adrenalin). Thus, a uniquely appropriate set of data obtained in response to earlier choices is available to each individual as a basis for further decisions about data gathering and/or intervention as the problem evolves. This technique almost immediately captured the imagination of examinees and examiners alike, but it also raised many new psychometric issues that have been the subject of intensive investigation.

*Validity Issues.* Of primary and continuing interest is the question of *validity*, defined in this context to refer to the congruence between decisions on written simulations and decisions in real life or in other simulated situations in which individuals must generate their own inquiries and interventions, rather than select them from a list, and record the results in the patient's records. Three approaches have been used to investigate this issue: (1) comparison of observed behaviors in a spontaneous situation with decisions made on corresponding PMPs (McCarthy, 1966; Page and Fielding, 1980), (2) comparison of findings and orders documented in patient records with inquiries and interventions selected on analogous PMPs (Williamson, 1965; Goran, Williamson, and Gonella, 1973), and (3) investigation of the extent to which performance on one or more PMPs distinguishes among different individuals or groups in the hypothesized direction (McGuire, 1968a; McIntyre and others, 1972; Palva and Korhonen, 1976; McLaughlin, 1978; Holzemer and others, 1981; Marshall and others, 1982; Maatsch, Munger, and Podgormy, 1983).

While there is some evidence of small positive correlation between PMP scores and some other criterion measures (Raffman, Tobias, and Speedie, 1980; Fielding and Page, 1978; Dincher and Stidger, 1976; Sherman and others, 1979), findings from detailed comparisons of decisions on PMPs and observed or recorded behavior on strictly comparable realistic situations reveal many discrepancies between the two, especially in data gathering. For example, virtually all researchers report that in the diagnostic workup of patients, more data are collected (particularly about historical and physical findings) in the written simula-

---

*For detailed instructions about the construction and use of various types of written simulations, see McGuire, Solomon, and Bashook, 1976; for examples of various types of patient simulations, see McGuire, Solomon, and Forman, 1977.

tion than are elicited in oral simulations or documented in the comparable real patients' records. Some investigators attribute this phenomenon, in part, to the cuing effects of providing long lists of inquiries in the PMP, from which the examinee can merely choose (McCarthy, 1966; Page and Fielding, 1980); if so, it appears most serious in the data-gathering sections and almost inoperative in the laboratory and management sections of branching PMPs (Martin, 1975). Other investigators attribute this particular discrepancy in PMP and observed behavior, in part, to structural deficiencies in the particular exercises studied and to systematic deficiencies in recording behavior (McGuire, 1968a; Williamson, 1965). Finally, some investigators (Williamson, 1976a; Templeton and others, 1977; Page and Fielding, 1980) have found that the situational constraints that exist in real life may cause performance on otherwise "identical problems" to vary with time and place to such an extent that multiple samples of real-life behavior are required in order to obtain a generalizable index of performance. If so, discrepancies between responses to written simulations and observed behavior or patient records may be in large measure a function of the inadequate sample of either or both.

Studies to determine the extent to which scores on PMPs distinguish between groups in the expected direction have been characterized by more variable findings and equally disparate interpretation. For example, some authors (Maatsch, Munger, and Podgormy, 1983, p. 203) report that "(medical) students perform about as well as board-eligible (emergency) physicians" on data acquisition sections of linear PMPs and that, overall, "PMPs were less sensitive to ability group differences than were . . . multiple-choice items." Other investigators have found meaningful differences in PMP scores that are positively associated with level of training (McGuire, 1968a; Palva and Korhonen, 1976) and/or amount of experience (McGuire, 1968a; McLaughlin, 1978; Holzemer and others, 1981). Interestingly, in studies of both physicians (McGuire, 1968a; Meskauskas and Webster, 1975) and nurses (Holzemer and others, 1981), performance appears to be associated with age, to peak with five to ten years' experience, and to fall off rapidly with less than two or more than fifteen years' experience.

Though significant differences in PMP total scores have been reported for groups at different levels of training and experience, in the limited studies currently available such differences have not usually been found between groups with different kinds of relevant training—for example, between baccalaureate and associate degree nurses of comparable experience (Goder, 1972) or between nurses and nurse practitioners (Holzemer and others, 1981) or between nurse practitioners and physicians (McLaughlin, 1978). However, meaningful differences of the expected type have been reported in the patterns of responses of such groups. For example, McLaughlin (1978) reports that in the assessment and management of a case of chronic obstructive pulmonary disease, physicians selected more pathophysiological items and interpreted them more accurately than did nurse practitioners, while the latter group selected more psychosocial items. In analogous studies of the relation between patterns of performance and levels of training and/or experience, most investigators concur in the finding that experienced groups extract less information than inexperienced groups (Marshall, 1977). In several studies of a number of different populations, McGuire (1968a) found repeatedly that in the diagnostic workup of simulated patients, the amount of data collected diminished with increased training, increased years of experience, and increased psychological distance from academic health care settings. At the same time, she found that scores on the laboratory workup and management sections of PMPs were closely and positively associated with amount of training, number of years of experience (up to ten to fifteen years postresidency), and closeness to an academic-type practice. This association was strongest on emergency problems and on problems requiring radical, definitive action, such as amputation.

In summary, it should be stressed that it is possible to assess the validity only of particular interpretations of specific tests; it is not possible to determine the validity of a generalized test format. The findings cited in this chapter are based on studies of many specific exercises that differ in type (for example, linear versus branched), quality (for example, length, complexity, and sophistication), and content (for example, nursing versus pharmacy, hypertension versus trauma, and the like). Thus, it is not surprising that results and their interpretation differ among investigators. Nonetheless, the findings do suggest some appropriate ways of utilizing this innovative approach when exercises are constructed so as to exploit fully its potential advantages and minimize its potential limitations.

*Reliability Issues.* A second major area of concern has focused on the *reliability* of written simulations, defined in this context to refer to the reproducibility of the scores that they yield. In studies of this issue three questions have been of particular concern to investigators: (1) To what extent do expert judges agree in categorizing the listed inquiries and interventions as lifesaving, important, nonessential, harmful, and life-threatening? (2) To what extent do variations in weights assigned each of these categories or the methods of combining them modify the rank order of respondents? (3) To what extent can performance on one or a few PMPs be generalized to a universe labeled problem-solving skills?

Investigations of these issues with many groups responding to quite varied PMPs in many fields have yielded remarkably similar findings. Much to the surprise of all the Cassandras who solemnly predicted that it would be impossible to get agreement among professionals on the approach to the workup and management of patients, researchers almost uniformly report close agreement (correlations or percent agreement ranging into the high nineties) among experts asked to classify the quality of a particular inquiry or intervention at a specified point in the workup and management of a clearly described patient (Lewy and McGuire, 1966; McLaughlin, Carr, and Delucchi, 1980; Fielding and Page, 1978). Similarly, within very broad limits, assignments of different sets of weights to the various categories of inquiries or interventions (for example, −1 to +1 versus −4 to +4, or −16 to +16) apparently does not alter the rank order of examinees significantly (Lewy and McGuire, 1966); however, altering the relative contribution of data gathering versus management decisions in the overall score does appear to do so (Marshall, 1977; Maatsch, Munger, and Podgorny, 1983).

Of much greater interest has been the almost universal finding that despite high test–retest reliability (McLaughlin, 1978), individual performance varies very significantly from problem to problem. Is this finding an artifact of the test format? A consequence of disease-oriented instruction rather than problem-based learning in professional schools? Or a fact of life? The first explanation can, for all practical purposes, be ruled out since the same phenomenon is reported on all types of simulation and even on audits of real patient care (discussed later in this chapter). The effects of different instructional methodologies on the generalizability of performance have not been thoroughly studied, but there are a few reports that suggest that students in problem-based curricula do not differ in this respect from students in more traditional programs. If we are forced eventually to conclude that "problem solving" or "clinical judgment," which written simulations are designed to measure, is merely a convenient but misleading construct, the implications are clear and of overriding importance for both instruction and evaluation—namely, both learners and examinees must be exposed to much larger numbers of much more systematically selected problems than we have heretofore thought necessary.

*Relation to Other Measures of Competence.* Finally, written simulations have also been studied to determine their *relationship to other measures of competence.* While the numerous studies of the relation between performance on PMPs and performance on MCQs are in general agreement in reporting, as would be expected, low positive correlations between the two (McGuire, 1968a; Templeton, 1979), more convincing evidence of the divergent and convergent validity of PMPs and of their cost-effectiveness compared to simpler techniques is to be found in the more sophisticated factor analytic and multitrait, multimethod studies conducted by a very few investigators. For example, Maatsch, Munger, and Podgormy (1983) found that conventional MCQs, MCQs with a visual stimulus, and linear PMPs all loaded on one factor that they labeled clinical knowledge and, as previously noted, that the PMPs were less able than the MCQs to distinguish among groups at different levels of education and/or training. Holzemer and others (1981) concluded that their multitrait, multimethod study (involving chart audits, self-evaluations, and peer evaluations, an MCQ and a PMP exam, and a demographic questionnaire of nurses and nurse practitioners) "provided minimal evidence to support the claim that the PMP simulation is a valid measure of the construct of clinical problem-solving" (p. ii). Three earlier studies came to almost exactly opposite conclusions: In a study of the relation between clinical ratings and written examination of physician assistants, Dowaliby and Andrew (1976) found that performance on each of three factors—data gathering and recording, interpersonal skills, and clinical judgment—on a carefully designed rating scale generally correlated with the appropriate examination score or subscore (that is, PMP scores correlating with clinical judgment). In a study of performance on three multiple-choice examinations (constructed by two different agencies—NBME and University of Illinois) and three PMP exams (one linear, constructed by NBME, and two branching, constructed by the University of Illinois) administered to each of three student populations over a three-year period, Nerenberg and others (1978) found that total scores on all MCQ examinations and on the linear PMP examination loaded on one factor (clinical knowledge), while the total score on the branching PMP examinations loaded on another (clinical judgment); further, subscores on the branching PMPs defined two general factors in the latter: "data gathering and management," which were stable over groups and over time (Juul, Noe, and Nerenberg, 1979).

How does one interpret these seemingly conflicting findings? One possibility is that "latent image doth not a problem make." There is growing evidence that at least some linear PMPs may simply be exotic-appearing forms of MCQs and that assessment of the rich complexity of problem-solving skills requires a format that permits examinees to demonstrate flexible, alternative strategies as well as tactics. Does the branching PMP format have that potential? The evidence supports a cautious yes. Is the evidence sufficient to justify the additional time and costs involved in utilizing a sophisticated PMP format to assess clinical problem solving rather than relying on the more economical but equally objective MCQ? Given the other beneficial side effects of the PMP—perceived relevance, enhanced learning, obvious focus on important objectives—it merits wider use.

*Computer Simulations.* It was inevitable that with the evolving capabilities of computers and the burgeoning interest in simulation, the two would come together in new forms of assessment exercises that attempted to exploit fully the exciting potentials of each. The disadvantages of cuing inherent in the written simulation are eliminated in the Computer *A*ssisted Simulated clinical *E*ncounter (CASE) that allows the examinee to address the computer in unconstrained natural language and to elicit realistic data about the patient (Harless and others, 1971). However, that form of simulation is essentially a diagnostic problem that does not make provision for the problem to evolve and for the patient's condition to change over time or in response to alternative interventions. These dynamic qualities of real life are more fully captured in the program for simulating the Patient-Physician Encounter (PPE), which includes built-in time and cost dimensions, both of which are used as criteria in evaluating the examinee's performance (Friedman, 1973).

The relative merits and feasibility of CASE, PPE, and other formats designed to minimize problems that older professionals have in interfacing with the computer have been studied in a long-term, large-scale project (the Computer-Based Examinations [CBX] Project) supported by the National Board of Medical Examiners and the American Board of Internal Medicine. The investigators conclude that while it is technically feasible to administer computer-based examinations on a national scale, the number of cases necessary to employ (reliability) and the relation between computer and real-life decisions (validity) still remain to be determined (Friedman, 1977). The feasibility of using computerized examinations for certification has been further documented in a limited Canadian trial (Taylor and others, 1976) and for recertification in an extensive study by the American Board of Internal Medicine (Webster and others, 1979). However, as of this date, computerized simulations are still being employed primarily for student self-assessment, not for certification, and there are relatively little data about their psychometric properties.

It is surprising that this should be so: The computer is a natural tool for creating an unlimited library of dynamic, technically sound, automatically debugged cases, thus virtually eliminating the burdensome and costly process of individual case-by-case authorship and the associated hazards of technical flaws inherent in that process. Its capacity for graphics means that it can more and more closely approximate reality. It can tirelessly examine and reexamine thousands of candidates on completely standardized, parallel exercises until each reaches the prescribed standard, and it can do so simultaneously in thousands of different sites or at one place on thousands of different occasions. It is the perfect slave for scoring, reporting, and providing instantaneous feedback and analysis to examinee and examiner alike. It is no longer an unfamiliar stranger that creates unnecessary apprehension in those of us who are required to approach it. Why have these overwhelming assets not been fully exploited in the assessment of professional competence? Is it that we lack the pathophysiological knowledge to create and program the basic models of human functioning and response to stress? Is it that we lack the imagination to apply what we know or to organize the required varieties of expertise into working teams? Whatever the cause, this is one area that merits major research and development support.

*Oral Simulations—Role Playing and Programmed Patients.* Limitations on the availability of real patients and variation in those available stimulated Barrows, a neurologist, and Abrahamson, an educator, to collaborate in their pioneer research on "the programmed patient." They concluded that simulated patients can overcome difficulties inherent in traditional oral and observational techniques in evaluating clinical competence (Barrows and Abrahamson, 1964).

While the technique is still not widely used for evaluating skills of physical examination, it has gained broad acceptance as a method of assessing interviewing and related interpersonal skills. Investigators routinely report high interrater agreement among examiners (for example, Levine and McGuire, 1970a; Hutter and others, 1977) and relatively high sampling reliability—that is, consistency of performance across simulated cases (for example, Levine and McGuire, 1970a; Sanson-Fisher and Poole, 1980). However, it is important to note that this consistency across cases is characteristic of simulated encounters that focus on the assessment of interpersonal skills; it has not been found true of those designed to assess broad skills of data acquisition, problem solving, and patient management (Levine and McGuire, 1970b; Maatsch, Munger, and Podgormy, 1983). In the latter type of simulated clinical encounter, performance appears to be problem specific, as has been repeatedly found in the use of written simulations.

Evidence of the concurrent validity of the technique is suggested in a small, well-controlled study in psychiatry designed to assess empathy of psychiatric clerks, in which no significant differences were found in the assessment of the students' performances with genuine and with simulated patients (Sanson-Fisher and Poole, 1980). Indirect evidence of the construct validity of the technique is suggested in a small, well-designed pediatric study using simulated mothers, in which it was found that an experimental group being taught interviewing skills showed significant gains on the fifteen-month evaluation and scored significantly higher than the control group on both process and content (Hutter and others, 1977).

Finally, despite interest (at least at the undergraduate level) in using simulated patients and the sensitivity of the health professions to the precautions necessary when conducting experiments involving human subjects, it is strange that no one has undertaken a comprehensive investigation of the effects on the *simulator* (that is, the actor-patient) of participating in such activities. In an admittedly small-scale and uncontrolled study, Naftulin and Andrew (1975) could detect no adverse consequences, but urge careful screening of potential subjects.

In summary, the use of role playing in the assessment of professional competence, although pioneered in the mid-sixties by the American Board of Orthopedic Surgery (ABOS), is still rare in licensure and certification examinations. While its introduction by the ABOS was based on a sound and continuing research effort, that body soon abandoned it and very few other licensing or certifying bodies have adopted it. Virtually all such groups have also eliminated the practical examination and all other opportunities to observe and assess clinician-patient interaction. Yet today there is both mounting evidence of the importance of these interactions for patient outcome and expressions of rising concern about them by professionals and public alike. Perhaps some form of role playing or other simulated clinical encounter could be used to resolve the dilemma. Surely it merits further research.

*Multimedia and Three-Dimensional Simulators.* There is now general recognition of the contribution that motion pictures and other visual or auditory stimuli can make in the assessment of skills involved in the application of knowledge and the interpretation of data (Felkner, 1973; Pearson, 1978; McGuire, 1977, 1980a). Where cost does not preclude it, this recognition has been implemented at all levels, in all professions, and for all purposes for which assessment of individual professionals is carried out. Beginning in the early sixties, developments of increasing numbers of three-dimensional manikins into which different pathologies could be inserted, for both instructional and assessment purposes, were at first greeted with enthusiasm. However, despite their high promise and the obvious benefits to be derived from the standardization of problems these manikins permit, they have proved to be of limited value in the assessment of skills of eliciting and interpreting physical findings, except at introductory educational levels. Perhaps this is because of the fact that, with the exception of the simulation device for ophthalmoscopy (Colenbrander, 1972), the crudity and relatively low fidelity of such simulators seem to restrict their usefulness with advanced students and practitioners.

Ultimately, of much greater potential value (but also incomparably higher costs) are the fully automated manikins capable of displaying a wide array of physical findings (Gordon, 1974) and of responding appropriately to various interventions (Abrahamson, Denson, and Wolf, 1969). The development of a whole family of high-fidelity, fully computerized manikins capable of displaying physical findings in several body systems simultaneously and of changing in response to various stimuli is, in principle, theoretically possible. However, whether such simulators could ever become cost-effective instruments for assessment is far less certain.

## Techniques for Assessing Clinical Performance

Though the Objective-Structured Clinical Examination and the various forms of simulation described in this chapter appear to constitute reasonable approaches to the assessment of certain aspects of clinical competence, evaluators continue to search for satisfactory methods of assaying that more general and somewhat more elusive characteristic (trait? achievement?) often referred to as clinical performance. As the term is used, it seems to combine elements of both cognitive and noncognitive skills and attitudes; it refers both to overall clinical competence and to competence in performing certain complex tasks—for example, interviewing or physical examination. (For detailed descriptions and illustrative models of a variety of instruments recommended for use in the health professions generally, see Katz and Snow (1980); Morgan and Irby (1978); for nursing, see Rezler and Stevens (1978); and for allied health, see LaDuca and others (1980); Engel and others (1980); Risley and others (1980).)

*Overall Competence.* Attempts to evaluate *overall clinical competence* are illustrated by the procedures instituted by training directors in response to the requirement of the American Board of Internal Medicine that they must evaluate and certify the overall clinical competence of trainees (including their relations to patients, as well as their history-taking, physical examination, record-keeping, and patient-management skills) as a condition for the latter's admission to the board examination. In an early survey of a 33 percent sample of approved programs Futcher, Sanderson, and Tusler (1977) found that 73 percent of the programs reported that they used a clinical exercise for this purpose. However, these investigators found that, in fact, rounds were used as the principal source of data in 85 percent of the reporting programs. Regrettably, no data about the validity and reliability of the resulting ratings are available from the large-scale survey. In the absence of such data, one must suspect a high level of observer error in global ratings based on these sources. Observer error on such relatively straightforward matters as interpretation of x-rays, electrocardiograms (ECGs), Pap smears, and serum drug assays has been found to range between 13 percent disagreement with oneself on some items to 50 percent disagreement between two experts on other items (Williamson, 1976a). Why should we expect any more accuracy on global ratings of complex human performance?

In an interesting departure from the usual reliance on audit and/or training directors' and supervisors' observations as a major source of data about overall competence or practitioner-patient interaction, Coarse and Kubica (1979) hypothesized that if pharmacists had done their job properly, their patients would be able to answer correctly a series of questions about their medications. To test this hypothesis, they designed an instrument to be administered to patients as a test of the practitioner's competence. Again, regrettably, no data from its administration are reported.

In the two situations just described, we see exemplified the two major approaches to assessing overall competence: *observation* of the candidate in many settings and *assessment of the outcomes* of his or her actions through patient interview or audit of some aspects of patient care. To date, we lack convincing evidence of the relative merits of these approaches, when each is used in a manner to exploit its maximum potential. Perhaps this is because we also lack a satisfactory construct of overall competence as discussed later in this chapter.

*Individual Task Performance.* Until we develop an adequate theory of clinical competence, we shall probably need to continue to employ various techniques to assess *individual task performance.* The individual tasks most often evaluated in the context of clinical performance include interviewing, physical examination, and complex technical procedures (for example, surgery, in the evaluation of physicians, or prosthesis construction, in the evaluation of dentists). Three accoutrements are now widely regarded as almost indispensable adjuncts of this process: detailed checklists, videotape, and descriptive rating scales.

Checklists have, of course, been around for a long time and, as is the case with other techniques, can be judged only on the basis of concrete manifestations whose psychometric characteristics will vary enormously depending on the skill and care with which they have been constructed and used. That the technique, when optimally managed, has high potential is convincingly documented in a well-designed study by Andrew (1977b) of the use of a checklist to assess the physical examination skills of physician assistants. She reports impressive inter-rater reliability ($r$ = .82 to .94), almost perfect internal consistency ($r$ = .95 using split-half technique), and promising indications of validity in distinguishing formally trained groups from those with exclusively on-the-job training and in assessing aspects of competence apparently not sampled on either MCQ or PMP examinations.

Not surprisingly, however, there is some evidence to suggest that performance on different tasks is not highly correlated (Dunn, 1970), that complete and correct procedure in performing a task (for example, a cardiovascular examination) is not necessarily correlated with accuracy of results (for example, elicitation, interpretation, or recording of auscultatory findings) (Aloia and Jonas, 1976), and that both process and outcome may be case-specific (Stillman and others, 1980). Until we know more about the cause of discrepancies, performance checklists should include both process and outcome criteria and, as long as either is case-specific, the number and variety of required observations must be given careful consideration.

Most investigators also report exceedingly high interrater reliability (in some cases exceeding .90) when trained examiners use detailed checklists to evaluate videotaped performance with real or simulated patients (Barnes and others, 1978). Assessments using these techniques are probably more rigorous (that is, scores are less inflated) and are certainly more objective and accurate than conventional overall ratings of clinical performance or grades in clinical courses (Richards and others, 1981).

Videotaped interviews conducted by a real or simulated provider of health care have been used by some investigators as a basis for multiple-choice or other objective-type questions, responses to which are interpreted as an indirect index of ability to perform certain tasks. Typically, the tape is divided into segments, each of which is followed by one or more sets of questions about the appropriateness of the provider's technique, its consequences, the findings that have been elicited, and/or the examinee's recommendation regarding next steps (Grayson, Nugent, and Oken, 1977; Stillman and others, 1977; Hyde, 1979; Andrew, 1977a). Investigators have been optimistic about this approach because they have generally found that, in addition to its obvious potential for yielding reliable (that is, internally consistent and reproducible) scores, it has also demonstrated high construct validity in that scores on such instruments differentiate groups at different levels of training in the expected direction (Stillman and others, 1977) and have only low correlations with scores on strictly cognitive examinations (Hyde, 1979).

Rating scales for evaluation of task, as well as overall, performance are also familiar. They have evolved in recent years from unidimensional, global scales with undefined points to, in some cases, very elaborate multidimensional scales, points along each dimension of which are defined and/or illustrated in detail. Though there is much support for the conventional wisdom that the latter type of scale yields more reliable evaluations (Gaines, Bruggers, and Rasmussen, 1974; Tower and Vosburgh, 1976; Dhuru, Rypel, and Johnston, 1978; Goepferd and Kerber, 1980), there are some discordant notes that suggest that scale elaboration beyond a certain point may be counterproductive. For example, O'Connor and Lorey (1978) found that using photographic slides of adequate preparations as a standard did not improve interjudge reliability in rating dental preparations;

Davidge, Davis, and Hull (1980) found that an elaborate fifteen-item scale for evaluating medical students actually reduced to two factors—problem-solving and interpersonal skills; Mayo (1973) found such high interscale correlations (.56 to .95, all significant at .01 level) in the rating of physical therapy students that she concluded that an eleven-dimension set of scales could readily be reduced to no more than four without losing any important information.

Similarly, expert opinion holds that training of examiners will enhance the accuracy and reliability of ratings, even to the point where paraprofessionals can be trained to rate at least some types of performance (Stillman and Sabers, 1978). Certainly, there is much support in the literature for the importance of rater training. But again there are a few discordant notes: Newble, Hoare, and Sheldrake (1980) found that training of experienced physician-examiners did not improve the reliability of their ratings (when using a precisely defined checklist) and concluded that some raters were inherently consistent, others inherently inconsistent, and training did not change the latter group. Fuller (1972) asserted that while there is no evidence of agreement between raters using traditional methods, there is no evidence that training or other aids improve interrater reliability in judging amalgams and fillings prepared by students. Houpt and Kress (1973) went even further in concluding not only that training of dental faculty was ineffective but also that evaluations of total performance on cavity preparations, for example, were more reliable than ratings on individual criteria.

Interestingly, most of these discordant notes come from studies of dental faculty ratings of student products. In most other professions, the evidence is overwhelming that, as compared with global ratings by untrained experts, rater training and the use of multidimensional scales or other aids increase the reliability of ratings of task performance. Why these differences between professions should exist is not clear, unless it is that in judging a physical product, the whole is more than the sum of its parts, and making a judgment on the basis of specific characteristics of the latter somehow distorts the process.

## Techniques for Assessing Attitudes

Clearly, an individual's attitudes influence his or her moral, ethical, and even legal behaviors. Nor does anyone any longer seriously doubt that professionals' attitudes toward themselves and their own professional development, toward their patients, toward each other, and toward their work and their field are strong determinants of the health of those they serve and, by extension, of the population at large. Nor is the influence of professional attitudes limited to their effects on patient outcomes; attitudes and the work styles associated with them exert subtle but nonetheless powerful control over the nature and organization of health services and the costs of providing them. For these reasons, educators and public alike have been concerned about the assessment and prediction of attitudes in the recruitment, selection, training, and licensure of health professionals.

The first obstacle researchers have encountered in trying to respond to these concerns has been their difficulty in identifying specific behaviors that reflect attitudes that "make a difference" and in distinguishing these from generalized traits that characterize "good guys and gals." The most promising methods for overcoming this barrier are the critical incident and related observational techniques that lead to concrete, precise statements that describe professional behavior (for example, "does not order costly, unnecessary tests" or "informs patients of, and makes arrangements for, alternative professional assistance during personal absences"). True, such specific behaviors are associated not only with what may be called professional values but also with such broader personality traits as rigidity, authoritarianism, social conformity, introversion, extroversion, aggression, self-confidence, cynicism, and self-esteem. However, for many reasons including their obvious lack of specific relevance and the legal pitfalls in basing decisions on them, measurements of such general traits have not been perceived as appropriate in selection and certification of professionals. Instead, most research and developmental activities have focused on techniques ranging from direct self-report on questionnaires, attitude scales, and the like, through indirect self-report forms based on responses about concrete situations, to long-term observation and analysis of clinical performance records. Rezler concludes that these methods are useful primarily for career guidance and formative evaluation; with minor exceptions, the state-of-the-art is not as yet sufficiently advanced for their inclusion in summative evaluation (Rezler and Stevens, 1978).

The minor exceptions include some data about attitudes toward patient risk and toward cost containment that can be derived from review of patient records and from analyses of responses to simulated clinical problems *when cost and risk factors have been built into the problem* (as discussed earlier in this chapter). Exceptions may also include data about attitudes toward patients derivable from observation of patient interviews and of role-playing simulations of clinical encounters *when the cognitive problem does not overwhelm the encounter.* However, data from both these sources are highly suspect in many quarters. The suspicion of observation in both real-life and simulated settings derives primarily from the artificiality of both and the fear that individuals will behave "as they think they should, not as they ordinarily do." Justification for this suspicion is to be found in the report from the Center for Disease Control that on a set of split specimens sent to laboratories for analysis, "a 4 percent deficiency rate occurred when the lab was aware it was being tested, whereas a 50 percent deficiency rate was found when the lab was not aware" (Williamson, 1976b, p. 26). To the extent that this is a general phenomenon, observation of "test" behavior in either real or simulated situations will not identify all those who regularly behave in an unacceptable manner. It will, however, identify at least those who don't know what the acceptable manner of behaving is (Levine and McGuire, 1970a); that, in itself, is no mean achievement.

Finally, in our increasingly litigious society, one of the most recalcitrant obstructions to wider use of attitudinal assessment has been the threat of legal action. Until such assessments can be made with a degree of accuracy "to stand up in court," it is not likely that they will be extensively used in summative evaluation.

## Assessing Habitual Performance

Educators and supervisors in all health professions have traditionally incorporated at least implicit evaluations of habitual performance in certification and promotion decisions about trainees and employees. What is becoming more common is their explicit inclusion in formative evaluation and systematic study of their reliability and validity in both modes (Levine and McGuire, 1971a). In general, however, progress in this area has been limited to the development of multidimensional rating scales that specify points on the scale in more descriptive terms and the use of chart audits to identify general behavior patterns.

## Chart Audits and Peer Assessment

Since the appearance of the problem-oriented medical record (POMR) and the advent of computerized medical records, chart audits have become ever more fashionable and increasingly mandated by third-party payers as part of their programs of quality assurance and cost containment. However, despite their promise as the ultimate tool for assessing professional competence, the results have been disappointing. Many methodological problems remain to be solved before audit can become a cost-effective technique for general use in the evaluation of individuals.

First, there is the problem of determining the *nature* of the standards to be used. For example, in an analysis of 296 records, Brooks and Appel (1973) found that only 1.4 percent met acceptable standards if process criteria were used, whereas 63.2 percent met such standards if outcome criteria were used. Similarly, Studnicki and Saywell (1978) found the correlations between a Physician Performance Index (proportion of recommended actions taken) and Flags (number of unjustified variations from accepted practice) to range from $r = -.88$ to a shocking $r = +.14$, depending on the diagnostic category being audited. Second, there is the question of the *criteria and level of standards* to be applied. In a review of 1,258 cases of obstetrical complications, Richardson (1972) found that in 33 percent of the cases, one of the three expert reviewers disagreed with the other two in categorizing care as satisfactory or unsatisfactory. Third, there is the question of the *number of records* that must be audited to get a reliable estimate of performance. In a very carefully designed study, Templeton and others (1977) concluded that it required ten records to get a relatively stable estimate of a given resident's performance in a particular setting (a single hospital service) with a given medical condition (diagnosis or syndrome). Knowing that performance on the same problem will vary even more in different settings (offices and hospitals and services) because of different situational constraints and that in the same setting it will vary from problem to problem, we simply have no idea what volume of records would be required to obtain a stable estimate of *overall competence*.

Even if some of these major methodological difficulties could be resolved, judgments based on audits will continue to require long-term observation of many patients (Samph and Templeton, 1979). Under these circumstances, it would seem that, promising as the technique of auditing real-life performance may appear, its use for the immediate future should probably be limited to the identification of that very small group of dangerous repeat offenders who exist in any profession and the discovery of specific breaches in quality that are fairly common to large groups of practitioners.

## Research on Scoring and Reporting Performance

Along with the study of new techniques of assessing professional competence, numerous efforts during the 1960s and 1970s were directed at modifying the scoring, grading, and reporting of performance and the setting of standards of adequacy. These efforts were stimulated both by the concern to increase the validity and utility of professional evaluation and by the desire to minimize its deleterious side effects. These concerns within the professions, together with the psychometric issues raised by newer assessment techniques, have led many institutions and certifying bodies to substitute a pass-fail system for the former system of ranking. While this reform may reduce the competitive atmosphere and allay some of the anxieties surrounding professional evaluation that entails ranking, it seriously limits the usefulness of the information derived from the whole evaluation process. To remedy this defect, there has been increasing pressure to introduce diagnostic, descriptive profile reporting to augment the single examination score characteristic of earlier periods or the simple pass-fail judgment typical of more recent times.

*Summarizing and Grading.* Despite mounting doubts about their validity, two methods of summarizing performance of both students and practitioners still predominate in health professions schools and in licensure and certification agencies. In one system, each test or performance measure is independently scored, and the weighted (or unweighted) scores on each are added together or are averaged to obtain a single "mark" for each individual. This mark is then compared with some set of standards to determine each individual's overall grade for a course or an examination. Despite both theoretical and practical problems, this system is still widely used in many educational institutions. Most licensure authorities and certifying bodies continue to employ a different but equally defective system in which each test or performance measure (that is, each written examination, each of the orals, and each practical examination) is treated as an independent measurement, and the candidate is required to obtain a passing score on every one in order to be admitted to the next level of the examination process and/or to be certified. In addition to their dubious validity, neither of these techniques of scoring and reporting performance supplies an operational definition of an individual's strengths and weaknesses in terms of the aspects of competence that are purportedly assayed by the set of instruments employed.

To minimize the inherent weaknesses in these prevailing systems, some authors recommend the use of a profile system in which no total score is obtained on any individual test or performance measure; rather, a set of *subscores*, representing the several aspects of competence sampled in each set of questions or exercises, is computed on each instrument; related subscores are then combined across tests and performance measures to yield an overall mark for each aspect of competence sampled in the entire test battery. When this system is employed, candidates are not required to meet a passing standard on the test battery as a whole, nor on any individual test in it; rather, they are required to perform satisfactorily with respect to each essential *component of competence* (Levine and McGuire, 1971b). Proponents of this method of summarizing performance argue that such a profile system (1) yields a more reliable estimate of achievement on each component of competence, since that estimate is derived from multiple measures; (2) results in a more valid judgment of readiness to practice, since an individual cannot compensate for real deficiencies in one area (for example, surgical skill) by outstanding performance in another (for example, cognitive knowledge); and (3) provides more informative feedback to candidates, examiners, and educators.

These advantages are based on certain assumptions about the interrelationships of skills and knowledge and will be realized only if those assumptions are met in a particular measurement situation. Specifically, it is assumed that a certain level of knowledge is a necessary but not a sufficient condition for adequate performance in a given situation and that the overall level of performance in a situation is determined by a combination of different and not necessarily highly correlated skills. Most researchers report that assessments directed at particular elements in complex situations do, indeed, meet the required assumptions. A possible exception is the recently reported finding by Maatsch, Munger, and Podgormy (1983) of one large general (competency) factor across a variety of test formats and content domains in emergency medicine. They also report that the descriptive profile is more consistent with concepts of mastery learning and is especially useful in diagnostic testing administered for purposes of self-assessment and of counseling students and/or practitioners. However, the issue cannot be fully resolved until we examine more carefully research on the structure of competence itself.

*Setting Standards.* Concomitant with the introduction of new techniques of assessing professional competence and new ways of scoring and reporting performance were varied attempts to introduce new methods of setting standards so as to reduce reliance on the performance of the particular group being evaluated. Such a movement represents a genuine revolution in the approach to standard setting since, until relatively recently, judgments about the adequacy of students' and practitioners' performance have been based almost exclusively on normative standards—that is, the individual's *rank* among peers. During the past twenty years, however, there has been increasing dissatisfaction with a system that inevitably results in the failure of approximately the same percentage of students or practitioners, irrespective of the quality of their performance. Further, over the past two decades it has become increasingly obvious that such a system necessarily encourages and rewards competitive isolation rather than cooperative learning.

For these two reasons, numerous attempts have been made to develop methods of setting performance standards that represent an independent judgment of mastery or adequacy, irrespective of the actual performance of any specific group. The main thrust, particularly in research, has been in the investigation of two major alternative approaches to setting standards on particular tests in advance of their administration: One utilizes empirical methods for deriving standards from the actual performance of some other well-defined population; the second is based on systematic application of expert judgment to define standards of mastery or of adequacy. In the former approach, tests are "normed" by prior administration to a criterion group previously judged to be adequate (Schoeff and Ciurczak, 1980) or are "validated" by prior administration to several groups representing different levels of education and experience. A standard is chosen that would result in the failure of most of those judged to have inadequate experience and the acceptance of most of those judged to be qualified (Maatsch, Munger, and Podgormy, 1983).

Several methodologies for utilizing expert judgment to establish standards have been investigated (Meskauskas, 1976). In the case of written tests, the two most widely studied methods of setting preestablished standards require expert judgments about each item comprising a test. In adaptations of the Nedelsky (1954) approach, each expert is asked to identify all those distractors in a multiple-choice question that the barely adequate student should be able to exclude. This procedure yields a minimum passing index (MPI) for each item, which represents the *probability* of a barely passing student's answering that item correctly; aggregation of these MPIs yields a minimum passing level (MPL) or acceptable level of performance (ALP) for the test as a whole (Center for Educational Development, 1967). Adaptations of the Ebel (1972) procedure require each judge to assign each item to a cell in a matrix, one axis of which represents various levels of relevance and the other various levels of difficulty, and then to judge the percentage of items in each cell that the minimally qualified examinee *should* be required to answer. Aggregation of these judgments yields a minimally acceptable passing score.

With few exceptions (Meskauskas and Webster, 1975), both the Nedelsky and the Ebel systems have been found to produce a high level of consensus among experts; however, judgments involving a probability estimate tend to produce lower standards than those involving a judgment of importance and difficulty (Andrew and Hecht, 1976). Studies of the use of standards based on the performance of a criterion group produce more diverse results, depending on the definition and selection of the group regarded as criterion, since this group might, for example, be selected samples of trainees, of practitioners, of examiners, or of super subspecialists.

*Conclusions.* Considerable progress has been made in sensitizing evaluators and those who use evaluation results to the most egregious errors frequently committed in connection with obtaining and massaging the numerical data that issue from their efforts. Nonetheless, research of the past twenty years has not succeeded in entirely eliminating the worst practices nor has it produced generally accepted alternatives that meet sound psychometric standards and that produce maximally useful information to decision makers—examiners, examinees, and educators. This is due, in part, to the fact that much of the research has limited generalizability because it has been done on highly variable instruments, administered on a one-time basis only to relatively small groups under unique circumstances for particular purposes. Perhaps what is now required is the codification of this research into some generally acceptable standards for achievement testing in the health professions.

## Research on the Structure of Professional Competence

A review of the studies of different instruments and of performance on them makes it at once apparent that researchers have often based their conclusions about the construct validity of individual instruments on certain assumptions about the structure of professional competence. Here, as a way of examining the validity of those underlying assumptions, we shall look at only a few studies that have involved multiple assessments of the same individuals, either at different points in time or by a variety of different methods at more or less the same time.

*Competence Over Time.* First, despite a few marginal successes, the evidence is overwhelming that there is little or no correlation between overall performance as it is conventionally measured during undergraduate training and performance in practice, whatever criteria are used to measure the latter (Price and others, 1971; Wingard and Williamson, 1973). Equally disturbing is the finding from studies of the relation between board certification and patient care that indicates that present procedures for certification cannot be validated against performance (Williamson, 1976b; Crocker, 1976) and that "there is less predictive validity in board certification than there is in having completed the training requirement for admission" (American Board of Medical Specialties, 1976, p. 5). Williamson (1976b) sums it up well when he says: "Certification results, whether based on professional performance, undergraduate grades, or medical specialty certification examinations, seem to have very little relationship to quality of subsequent professional performance" (p. 25).

Do individuals change so much over time that prediction of human behavior is subject to large error, or is this phenomenon an artifact of imperfect measurement? Certainly, individuals do change at different rates and in different directions, and this fact does place a limit on the accuracy of prediction. However, such change is not random: Evidence from the general study of human behavior makes it clear that the best predictor of performance in the future is current response to situations of the same type. This suggests that the lack of predictive validity of performance assessment is due not so much to the inherent nature of individual professional evolution as to the limited range of competencies sampled in most certification procedures. Some support for this view is suggested by the findings of Nerenberg and others (1978) that examinations using a varied or multicomponent format contribute more to the prediction of first-year postgraduate performance than do examinations with a more conventional or unidimensional format. Additional evidence is to be found in the study by Keck and others (1979) showing that a combination of cognitive and noncognitive predictor variables functions much better than any individual variable or any specific class of variables in predicting the clinical performance of residents, and the study by Dubs (1975) showing, not surprisingly, that cumulative grade point average and grades on theory courses were the best predictors of scores on state board examinations in nursing, whereas grades in nursing practice courses were the best predictors of supervisors' ratings of the R.N.s' subsequent performance on the ward. Whatever the explanation, it is clear that many of our summative evaluations lack predictive validity.

*Patterns of Competence.* Some evidence about patterns of competence is contained in the earlier discussion of the interrelations among assessment techniques. Here four comprehensive and well-designed investigations are cited as illustrative of the conflicting conclusions about patterns of competence to be derived from studies of multiple measures.

At the undergraduate level, O'Donohue and Wergin (1978) found, as expected, low correlations among three methods—written tests, oral examinations, and preceptor ratings of on-the-job performance. They had hypothesized that each of the three methods would provide independent data relating to overall performance, and so each was designed to address different aspects of competence. The results seemed to indicate that competence was composed of different elements and performance was format specific. In contrast, Maatsch, Munger, and Podgormy (1983) found very high intercorrelations between scores on MCQs, PMPs, and ratings of performance on simulated clinical encounters. The intercorrelations were so high that the investigators concluded that "the relationship between these formats can be represented by two underlying factors defined as clinical knowledge and clinical performance on simulated cases" (p. 216); however, "the correlations between the two factors ($r$ = an astonishing .92!) suggest a central underlying . . . *single general competence factor*" (pp. 217–218).

As noted earlier, still different results were obtained by Dowaliby and Andrew (1976) in their sophisticated analysis of the interrelations between ratings of clinical competence and performance on two written examinations, the MCQ and the PMP. In this study, the ratings were found to contain three factors—data gathering and recording, interpersonal skills, and clinical judgment; the MCQ examination contained four components—patient management, interpretation of physical findings, knowledge of clinical procedures, and interpersonal skills; and the linear PMP examination contained two components—data gathering and management. All intercorrelations between rating factors were less than .09, whereas generally significant correlations were found between each of the three rating factors and the appropriate written examination component, irrespective of format. What has happened to the format-specific effects found in the O'Donohue and Wergin (1978) study and to the general competence factor found in the Maatsch, Munger, and Podgormy (1983) study?

Finally, we shall examine the results of a large-scale multitrait, multi-method study (Webster and others, 1979) of the interrelationships among test formats (MCQs, multiple-true-false questions, written PMPs, and computer simulations) and of their respective correlations with, and contributions to, the variance on a criterion measure (a weighted checklist rating form completed by two colleagues and the chief of service for each practitioner-examinee). First, the investigators found that the individual traits rated on the checklist were so highly intercorrelated that it was possible to combine all scales and all judges into a single composite rating for each individual. However, performance on the tests was highly format-specific and even content- and skill-specific within formats. Very low correlations were found between scores on content-matched cases in written and computer format, between problems in the computer format, and between different components (data gathering, management, and so on) within a problem. Second, though correlations of the total score on each format with the criterion were positive and statistically significant (.28 to .30), altogether they accounted for only 14.2 percent of the variance in the criterion ratings. All this seems to suggest a general competence factor, or a halo effect, in at least some kinds of ratings, to which each examination format makes a tiny but not a unidimensional contribution.

What can be concluded from such disparate results? I feel that we can conclude very little about the "real" structure of competence and that, once again, we find we cannot infer what a test or a rating scale measures by looking at its format but only on the basis of a careful examination of the tasks it demands of the examinee. In short, unlike roses, a test is *not* a test is *not* a test; those that share the same formal structure may or may not belong to the same species and most certainly will not always function in the same way. Until we know more about both the structure of competence and the potential of different test techniques, we must, for purposes of triangulation, continue to use multiple methods implemented at the highest possible quality level to gather data that will assist us in making inescapable decisions about individual competence.

## Research on Innovation in the Overall System of Evaluation

The last two decades have seen a generally more systematic approach to the entire process of developing evaluation procedures for purposes of certification in all health professions—from more careful delineation of the competencies to be assessed, through the creation of a detailed "blueprint" that specifies the content and skill to be sampled in each instrument, to the ultimate summary and reporting of results. This process of systematization has certainly been facilitated by the establishment of sophisticated, computerized test item banks, capable of maintaining a large data base about the characteristics of each item and of responding to requests for items meeting specified criteria (Smith, 1977). In some instances, the reform has been part of, and supported by, a long-term research project, such as those following the Goals and Priorities (GAP) Report of the National Board of Medical Examiners and those conducted by the American Board of Orthopedic Surgery, the Committee on Child Psychiatry of the American Board of Psychiatry and Neurology, and, most recently, by the newly established Board of Emergency Medicine. The impact of the research conducted by these organizations has fortunately not been limited to them but has influenced general practice in the area of licensure and certification and has enhanced the potential for implementing more valid and reliable procedures throughout the field.

Sweeping changes in the evaluation system of individual training institutions are more rare, not only because so few can afford the costs of an expert support staff for evaluation research but also because of the entrenched interests and resistance to change in faculties whose primary expertise lies in other fields. However, two noteworthy revolutions in the entire system for student evaluation that are radically different from each other may be cited, not as representative but as examples of what a highly motivated faculty with a strong educational research unit can accomplish.

The first, initiated in the early sixties at the University of Illinois College of Medicine (McGuire, 1975b) came in response to the conviction shared by students and faculty alike that the then existing system of ranking and certifying students—on the basis of a combination of frequent quizzes, amateur examinations, and implicit, intuitive, individual faculty judgments—was a total disaster. It represented an abdication by the faculty of its corporate responsibility for setting standards and poisoned the learning environment by placing teachers in the unfortunate position of both mentor and judge. It forced students into a lockstep progression through the curriculum, distracted them from the main business of learning, caused them to focus on trivia, and exacerbated competition among them. Finally, it involved a great deal of time and effort without yielding useful information to either students or faculty.

The reform consisted of eliminating all summative evaluations by individual faculty or departments and establishing a representative faculty College Committee for Student Appraisal (CCSA), which was responsible for creating and administering two lengthy (twelve to fifteen hour) interdisciplinary, integrated, comprehensive examinations that yielded a detailed individual score profile for student guidance and counseling but required only an overall passing score for promotion and certification. At the same time, mountains of data about group strengths and weaknesses were made available to individual departments to assist them in instructional improvement. The CCSA was also made responsible for approving all skills examinations (also graded on a pass-fail basis) used in the certifying process, for creating a mechanism to collect valid data on professional habits and attitudes, and for forwarding to a Committee on Promotions information about each student's success in meeting preestablished (nonnormative) faculty standards in all three domains—cognitive, skill, and affective. The latter committee was given the ultimate responsibility for making the final judgment about the retention and promotion of each student. This certification procedure was to be accompanied by an expansion and upgrading of a system of formative evaluation to be administered by departments purely for purposes of student self-assessment. Though some details of the system were less effectively implemented than others and some changed over time, the main features remained in place for almost twenty years.

Did the institution of this system alleviate the "disaster" it was designed to correct? While no formal evaluation was ever prepared and disseminated, suffice it to note, first, that a considerable body of anecdotal information is available that strongly suggests that the feedback to students has helped them to clarify the important goals of the instructional program and that the character of the examinations has helped students to focus their attention on learning to apply the vast body of knowledge they are acquiring. In that sense, at least, perhaps it has been successful in developing a system of internal evaluation that corrects some of the limitations and deficiencies in the one that preceded it. Second, by relieving the instructor of an inherent conflict of interest and by creating a situation in which students' performance is compared not to that of their colleagues but to a preestablished standard that theoretically all can meet, the system has—in principle at least—removed some of the competitive pressures and some of the impediments to a mature and responsible relation among students and between students and their instructors. Third, the system has made it possible to collect exceedingly useful longitudinal and cross sectional data on the consequences of curricular change and to document improvement or its opposite, as these have occurred. Finally, without any sacrifice of quality control, the system has permitted increasing individualization of instruction for some students and greater curricular flexibility for all. Regrettably, however, no comparative data are available regarding the effects of the system on the pattern of professional competence of graduating students.

The second example is from McMaster University, whose faculty felt that the system of student evaluation typical of most medical schools was so totally incompatible with the basic tenets of their radically new curriculum—problem-based, small group learning, and self-assessment—as to jeopardize the entire system. In its purest form and as initially implemented, all formal, objective, summative evaluation of students by faculty was eliminated; in its place, small tutorial groups periodically devote a discussion session to sharing self-evaluations, as well as peer and tutor evaluations of each other, with special focus on each individual's group skills; summaries of the outcomes of these sessions are forwarded to the dean's office. This system too has evolved, and though there has been a gradual trend toward the incorporation of *some* formal evaluation exercises, the primary emphasis still remains on almost continuous, introspective self-evaluation and peer evaluation.

Has this system produced professionals who, when compared with the graduates of traditional programs, are better problem solvers, more skilled in and more disposed to self-criticism, and more likely to take personal responsibility for continued learning? Has it also avoided the danger of releasing on the public persons who, however qualified in their own and their peers' view, are on the basis of more objective evaluation not yet competent to practice their profession? Again, no definitive answers to these questions are forthcoming in the absence of further study. However, in a fascinating report on "The Hidden Curriculum of Professionalization in an Innovative Medical School Program," Haas and Shaffir (1982) sound certain cautions: First, they doubt the validity of self-evaluations and group evaluations because of an anticipated "gentlemen's agreement" and suggest that a subtle competitiveness develops based on interactional competencies to avoid being perceived as a threat by other students in the group. Further, they assert that the interactional evaluation combined with the absence of formal examinations and grades breeds uncertainty in which "rumor and gossip are common." Finally, they conclude that since the Canadian licensing examination is the exact opposite of the school's philosophy, "students' uncertainty about successfully meeting professionalizing expectations leads them to organize their behavior in accordance with the (licensure) mode of evaluation, even though they have adapted to a very different system during the past three years" (p. 148).

In short, we really know very little about the sequelae of system-wide changes.

### Directions for the Future

Throughout this chapter, specific recommendations for research and development have been offered. Here we shall focus on broad areas that require attention. First, despite the plethora of studies on individual issues and/or individual examinations, there is, as yet, far too little information available from the research of the past two decades about the consequences of system-wide modifications. For example, what has been the effect of reduced emphasis on examinations per se? What has been the result of introducing a pass-fail system as one means of reducing competition in the ranking of students? Has the shifting emphasis in the aspects of competence that are evaluated influenced the quality of health care actually delivered? If so, how and how much? These broad issues require serious study.

Second, while considerable progress was made during the sixties and seventies in introducing more reliable and more valid techniques of assessing professional competence, efforts to improve these must continue, and further developmental work, particularly in the area of audit and of computer-aided assessment, is critical if we are to meet the ethical and legal challenges to the evaluation of individuals for which reliable, valid, and relevant techniques are indispensable.

Third, after thirty years of research, we do not yet have a satisfactory methodology for evaluating professional habits and attitudes. Perhaps a radically new approach is required to achieve any progress in this arena.

Fourth, the problem of relating standards to realistic requirements derived from health care delivery settings is far from resolution. This issue requires considerably more investigation to assure that those who meet the standards are competent to practice.

Finally, work on the development of an acceptable theory or unifying conception of competence is urgent. Without this, neither instruction nor evaluation can proceed rationally.

## References

Abrahamson, S. "A Study of the Objectivity of the Essay Examination." *Journal of Medical Education,* 1964, *39,* 65–68.

Abrahamson, S., Denson, J. S., and Wolf, R. W. "The Effectiveness of a Simulator in Training Anesthesiology Residents." *Journal of Medical Education,* 1969, *44* (6), 515–519.

Abrams, R. G., and Kelley, M. L. "Student Self-Evaluation in a Pediatric-Operative Technique Course." *Journal of Dental Education,* 1974, *38* (7), 385–391.

Aloia, J. F., and Jonas, F. "Skills in History-Taking and Physical Examination." *Journal of Medical Education,* 1976, *51* (5), 410–415.

American Board of Medical Specialties. *Proceedings of a Conference on the Oral Examination.* Evanston, Ill.: American Board of Medical Specialties, 1975.

American Board of Medical Specialties. *Conference on Extending the Validity of Certification.* Evanston, Ill.: American Board of Medical Specialties, 1976.

American Board of Medical Specialties. *Definitions of Competence in the Specialties of Medicine.* Proceedings of conference, September 19, 1979. Evanston, Ill.: American Board of Medical Specialties, 1979.

American Institutes for Research. *The Definitions of Clinical Competence in Medicine: Performance Dimensions and Rationales for Clinical Skill Areas.* Palo Alto, Calif.: American Institutes for Research, 1960.

Andrew, B. J. "Objective Assessment of Interpersonal Skills." In J. P. Hubbard (Ed.), *An International View of Qualification for the Practice of Medicine.* 1976 annual conference of the National Board of Medical Examiners. Philadelphia: National Board of Medical Examiners, 1977a.

Andrew, B. J. "The Use of Behavioral Checklists to Assess Physical Examination Skills." *Journal of Medical Education,* 1977b, *52* (7), 589–591.

Andrew, B. J., and Hecht, J. T. "A Preliminary Investigation of Two Procedures for Setting Examination Standards." *Educational and Psychological Measurement,* 1976, *36,* 45–50.

Barnes, H., and others. "Senior Medical Students Teaching the Basic Skills of History and Physical Examination." *Journal of Medical Education,* 1978, *53* (5), 432–434.

Barro, A. R. "Survey and Evaluation of Approaches to Physician Performance Measurement." *Journal of Medical Education,* 1973, *48* (11), 1045–1093.

Barrows, H. S., and Abrahamson, S. "The Programmed Patient: A Technique for Appraising Student Performance in Clinical Neurology." *Journal of Medical Education,* 1964, *39* (8), 802–805.

Barrows, H. S., and Tamblyn, R. M. "Self-Assessment Units." *Journal of Medical Education*, 1976, *51* (4), 334–336.

Berner, E. S., Hamilton, L. A., Jr., and Best, W. R. "A New Approach.to Evaluating Problem Solving in Students." *Journal of Medical Education*, 1974, *49* (7), 666–672.

Brehm, T. W. "Peer Evaluation of Fixed Partial Dentures in a Preclinical Course." *Journal of Dental Education*, 1972, *36* (2), 54–55.

Brooks, R. H., and Appel, F. A. "Quality of Care Assessment: Choosing a Method for Peer Review." *New England Journal of Medicine*, 1973, *288* (25), 1323–1329.

Center for Educational Development, Evaluation Section. *Setting Standards of Competence—The Minimum Pass Level.* Chicago: Center for Educational Development, University of Illinois, 1967.

Chambers, M. J., and Hubbard, R. M. "Assessing Achievement for Minimum Academic Competency: I. Instrument Development; II. Validity and Reliability." *Journal of the American Dietetic Association*, 1978, *93* (1), 27–39.

Coarse, J. F., and Kubica, A. J. "Objective-Focused Approach for Appraising the Performance of Institutional Pharmacists." *American Journal of Hospital Pharmacy*, 1979, *36* (12), 1676–1682.

Cochran, S., and Spears, M. C. "Student Self-Assessment and Instructors' Ratings: A Comparison." *Journal of the American Dietetic Association*, 1980, *76* (3), 253–257.

Colenbrander, A. "Simulation Device for Ophthalmoscopy." *American Journal of Ophthalmology*, 1972, *74* (4), 738–740.

Cowles, J. T., and Hubbard, J. P. "A Comparative Study of Essay and Objective Examinations for Medical Students." *Journal of Medical Education*, 1952, *27*, 1–4.

Crocker, L. M. "Validity of Certification Measures for Occupational Therapists." *American Journal of Occupational Therapy*, 1976, *30* (4), 229–233.

Davidge, A. M., Davis, W. K., and Hull, A. L. "A System for the Evaluation of Medical Students' Clinical Competence." *Journal of Medical Education*, 1980, *55* (1), 65–67.

Derbyshire, R. C. "State and Local Agencies." In T. Samph and B. Templeton (Eds.), *Evaluation in Medical Education: Past, Present, and Future.* Cambridge, Mass.: Ballinger, 1979.

Dhuru, V. B., Rypel, T. S., and Johnston, W. M. "Criterion-Oriented Grading System for Preclinical Operative Dentistry Laboratory Course." *Journal of Dental Education*, 1978, *42* (9), 528–531.

Dincher, J. R., and Stidger, S. L. "Evaluation of a Written Simulation Format for Clinical Nursing Judgment: A Pilot Study." *Nursing Research*, 1976, *25* (4), 280–285.

Dowaliby, F. J., and Andrew, J. B. "Relationships Between Clinical Competence Ratings and Examination Performance." *Journal of Medical Education*, 1976, *51* (3), 181–188.

Dubs, R. "Comparison of Student Achievement with Performance Ratings of Graduates and State Board Examination Scores." *Nursing Research*, 1975, *24* (1), 59–64.

Dunn, M. S. "Development of an Instrument to Measure Nursing Performance." *Nursing Research*, 1970, *19* (6), 502–510.

Ebel, R. L. *Essentials of Educational Measurement.* Englewood Cliffs, N.J.: Prentice-Hall, 1972.

Engel, J. D., and others. *Competence in Clinical Dietetics.* Chicago: Center for Educational Development, University of Illinois, 1980.

Feletti, G. I. "Reliability and Validity Studies on Modified Essay Questions." *Journal of Medical Education,* 1980, *55* (11), 933-941.

Felkner, L. L. "Development and Evaluation of a Standardized Measure for Assessing Diagnostic Skills." *Journal of Dental Education,* 1973, *37* (3), 26-33.

Fielding, D. W., and Page, G. G. "Development and Validation of Written Simulation Problems for Pharmacy." *American Journal of Pharmaceutical Education,* 1978, *42,* 270-280.

Fivars, G., and Gosnell, D. *Nursing Evaluation: The Problems and the Process.* New York: Macmillan, 1966.

Flanagan, J. C. "The Critical Incident Technique." *Psychological Bulletin,* 1954, *51,* 327-358.

Forsdyke, D. R. "A Comparison of Short-Answer and Multiple-Choice Questions in the Evaluation of Students of Biochemistry." *Medical Education,* 1978, *12,* 351-356.

Foster, J. T., and others. "Analysis of an Oral Examination Used in Specialty Board Certification." *Journal of Medical Education,* 1969, *44,* 951-954.

Frejlach, G., and Corcoran, S. "Measuring Clinical Performance." *Nursing Outlook,* 1971, *19* (4), 270-271.

Friedman, R. B. "A Computer Program for Simulating the Patient-Physician Encounter." *Journal of Medical Education,* 1973, *48* (1), 92-97.

Friedman, R. B. "Computer-Based Examinations (CBX)." In J. P. Hubbard (Ed.), *An International View of Qualification for the Practice of Medicine.* 1976 annual conference of the National Board of Medical Examiners. Philadelphia: National Board of Medical Examiners, 1977.

Fuller, J. L. "The Effects of Training and Criterion Models on Interjudge Reliability." *Journal of Dental Education,* 1972, *36* (4), 19-22.

Futcher, P. H., Sanderson, E. V., and Tusler, P. A. "Evaluation of Clinical Skills for a Specialty Board During Residency Training." *Journal of Medical Education,* 1977, *52* (7), 567-577.

Gaines, W. G., Bruggers, H., and Rasmussen, R. H. "Reliability of Ratings in Preclinical Fixed Prosthodontics: Effect of Objective Scaling." *Journal of Dental Education,* 1974, *38* (12), 672-675.

Goder, V. "The NPSI: A Nursing Performance Simulation Instrument." In E. Jacobi and L. E. Natten (Eds.), *American Nurses' Association Eighth Nursing Research Conference.* Washington, D.C.: American Nurses' Association, 1972.

Goepferd, S. J., and Kerber, P. E. "A Comparison of Two Methods for Evaluating Primary Class II Cavity Preparations." *Journal of Dental Education,* 1980, *44* (9), 537-542.

Goran, M. J., Williamson, J. W., and Gonella, J. S. "The Validity of Patient Management Problems." *Journal of Medical Education,* 1973, *48,* 171-177.

Gordon, M. S. "Cardiology Patient Simulator." *American Journal of Cardiology,* 1974, *34,* 350-355.

Grayson, M., Nugent, C., and Oken, S. L. "A Systematic and Comprehensive Approach to Teaching and Evaluating Interpersonal Skills." *Journal of Medical Education,* 1977, *52* (11), 906-913.

Grosse, M. E., Croft, G. E., and Blaisdell, F. W. "The American Board of Surgery In-Training Examination." *Archives of Surgery*, 1980, *115* (5), 654–657.

Gurley, L. T., and Blair, T. E. "Criteria-Referenced Approach to Clinical Practicum." *Radiologic Technology*, 1975, *47* (2), 63–72.

Haas, J., and Shaffir, W. "Ritual Evaluation of Competence: The Hidden Curriculum of Professionalization in an Innovative Medical School Program." *Work and Occupations*, 1982, *9* (2), 131–153.

Harden, R. M., and Gleeson, F. A. "Assessment of Clinical Competence Using an Objective Structured Clinical Examination (OSCE)." *Medical Education*, 1979, *13*, 41–54.

Harless, W. G., and others. "CASE: A Computer-Aided Simulation of the Clinical Encounter." *Journal of Medical Education*, 1971, *46* (5), 443–448.

Holzemer, W. L., and others. *Patient Management Problems for Nurse Practitioners*. Washington, D.C.: Division of Nursing, Bureau of Health Manpower, U.S. Department of Health and Human Services, 1981.

Houpt, M. I., and Kress, G. "Accuracy of Measurement of Clinical Performance in Dentistry." *Journal of Dental Education*, 1973, *37* (7), 34–46.

Hubbard, J. P. "Programmed Testing." In *Examinations and Their Role in the Evaluation of Medical Education and Qualification for Practice*. Philadelphia: National Board of Medical Examiners, 1964.

Hubbard, J. P. *Measuring Medical Education*. Philadelphia: Lea and Febiger, 1971.

Hutter, M. J., and others. "Interviewing Skills: A Comprehensive Approach for Teaching and Evaluation." *Journal of Medical Education*, 1977, *52* (4), 328–333.

Hyde, C. E. "The Use of Television in the Assessment of Home and Foreign Postgraduate Groups During an Introductory Course in Psychiatry." *Medical Education*, 1979, *13*, 209–216.

Johnson, L. C. A., and Hurley, R. S. "Design and Use of an Instrument to Evaluate Students' Clinical Performance." *Journal of the American Dietetic Association*, 1976, *68* (5), 450–453.

Juul, D. H., Noe, M. J., and Nerenberg, R. L. "A Factor Analytic Study of Branching Patient Management Problems." *Medical Education*, 1979, *13*, 199–203.

Katz, F. M., and Snow, R. *Assessing Health Workers' Performance: A Manual for Training and Supervision*. Public Health Paper no. 72. Geneva, Switzerland: World Health Organization, 1980.

Keck, J. W., and others. "Efficacy of Cognitive/Noncognitive Measures in Predicting Resident-Physician Performance." *Journal of Medical Education*, 1979, *54* (10). 759–765.

Kegel-Flom, P. "Predicting Supervisor, Peer, and Self-Ratings of Intern Performance." *Journal of Medical Education*, 1975, *50* (8), 812–815.

LaDuca, A., Engel, J. D., and Risley, M. E. "Progress Toward Development of a General Model for Competence Definition in Health Professions." *Journal of Allied Health*, 1978, *7* (2), 149–156.

LaDuca, A., and others. *Competence in Occupational Therapy*. Chicago: Center for Educational Development, University of Illinois, 1980.

Levine, H. G., and McGuire, C. H. "The Use of Role Playing to Evaluate Affective Skills in Medicine." *Journal of Medical Education*, 1970a, *45* (9), 700–705.

Levine, H. G., and McGuire, C. H. "The Validity and Reliability of Oral Examinations in Assessing Cognitive Skills in Medicine." *Journal of Educational Measurement*, 1970b, 7 (2), 63–74.

Levine, H. G., and McGuire, C. H. "Rating Habitual Performance in Graduate Medical Education." *Journal of Medical Education*, 1971a, *46* (4), 306–311.

Levine, H. G., and McGuire, C. H. "Use of Profile System for Scoring and Reporting Certifying Examinations in Orthopedic Surgery." *Journal of Medical Education*, 1971b, *46* (1), 78–85.

Levine, H. G., McGuire, C. H., and Nattress, L. W. "The Validity of Multiple-Choice Achievement Tests as Measures of Competence in Medicine." *American Educational Research Journal*, 1970, 7 (1), 69–82.

Lewy, A., and McGuire, C. H. "A Study of Alternative Approaches in Estimating the Reliability of Unconventional Tests." Presented at the annual meeting of the American Educational Research Association, February 18, 1966, Chicago. Chicago: Center for Educational Development, University of Illinois, 1966. (Mimeographed.)

Linn, B. S., Arostegni, M., and Zeppa, R. "Performance Rating Scale for Peer and Self-Assessment." *British Journal of Medical Education*, 1975, *9* (2), 98–101.

Lloyd, J. S. "Survey of Member Board Evaluation Procedures: Review and Critique." In *Board Evaluation Procedures: Developing a Research Agenda*. Proceedings of conference, September 17, 1980. Evanston, Ill.: American Board of Medical Specialties, 1981.

Lynch, B. L. "A Behaviorally Anchored Rating Scale for the Evaluation of Student Performance." *American Journal of Medical Technology*, 1977, *43* (1), 54–63.

Maatsch, J. L., Munger, B. S., and Podgormy, G. "On the Reliability and Validity of the Board Examination in Emergency Medicine." *Emergency Medicine Annual*, 1983, *1*, 183–222.

Maatsch, J. L., and others. *A Study of Simulation Techniques in Medical Education*. Contract no. N01-LM-5-4752. Washington, D.C.: National Library of Medicine, 1976.

McCarthy, W. H. "An Assessment of the Influence of Cuing Items in Objective Examinations." *Journal of Medical Education*, 1966, *41* (3), 263–266.

McDermott, J. F., Jr., McGuire, C. H., and Berner, E. S. *Roles and Functions of Child Psychiatrists*. Evanston, Ill.: Committee on Certification in Child Psychiatry, American Board of Psychology and Neurology, 1976.

McGuire, C. H. "The Oral Examination as a Measure of Professional Competence." *Journal of Medical Education*, 1966, *41* (3), 267–274.

McGuire, C. H. *A Summary of the Evidence Regarding the Technical Characteristics of Patient Management Problems*. Chicago: Center for Educational Development, University of Illinois, 1968a. (Mimeographed.)

McGuire, C. H. "Testing in Professional Education." *Review of Educational Research*, 1968b, *38* (1), 49–60.

McGuire, C. H. "The Oral Examination Revisited." Paper presented at the Conference on Oral Examinations of the American Board of Medical Specialties, Chicago, March 19, 1975a.

McGuire, C. H. "The University of Illinois System of Internal Institutional Evaluation." Paper presented at the 1975 Annual Invitational Conference of the National Board of Medical Examiners, Philadelphia, March 13, 1975b.

McGuire, C. H. "Simulation as an Evaluation Technique." In J. P. Hubbard (Ed.), *An International View of Qualification for the Practice of Medicine*. 1976 annual conference of the National Board of Medical Examiners. Philadelphia: National Board of Medical Examiners, 1977.

McGuire, C. H. "Assessment of Problem-Solving Skills: Part 1." *Medical Teacher*, 1980a, *2* (2), 74–79.

McGuire, C. H. "Assessment of Problem-Solving Skills: Part 2." *Medical Teacher*, 1980b, *2* (3), 118–122.

McGuire, C. H., and Babbott, D. "Simulation Technique in the Measurement of Problem-Solving Skills." *Journal of Educational Measurement*, 1967, *4* (1), 1–10.

McGuire, C. H., Solomon, L. M., and Bashook, P. *Construction and Use of Written Simulations*. New York: Psychological Corporation, 1976.

McGuire, C. H., Solomon, L. M., and Forman, P. M. *Clinical Simulations: Selected Problems in Patient Management*. 2nd ed. New York: Appleton-Century-Crofts, 1977.

McIntyre, H. M., and others. "A Simulated Clinical Nursing Test." *Nursing Research*, 1972, *21*, 429–435.

McLaughlin, F. E. *Primary Care Judgments of Nurses and Physicians*. Division of Nursing, Bureau of Health Manpower, U.S. Department of Health, Education, and Welfare. San Francisco: Veterans' Administration Hospital, 1978.

McLaughlin, F. E., Carr, J. W., and Delucchi, K. L. "Selected Psychometric Properties of Two Clinical Simulation Tests." *Journal of Medical Education*, 1980, *55* (4), 375–376.

Marshall, J. "Assessment of Problem-Solving Ability." *Medical Education*, 1977, *11* (5), 329–334.

Marshall, J. R., and others. "Pilot Study on the Use of PMPs." *Medical Education*, 1982, *16*, 365–366.

Martin, I. "Empirical Examination of the Sequential Management Problem for Measuring Clinical Competence." *Proceedings of Fourteenth Annual Conference on Research in Medical Education*. Washington, D.C.: Association of American Medical Colleges, 1975.

Mayo, M. J. "Reliability of a Method of Evaluating the Clinical Performance of a Physical Therapy Student." *Physical Therapy*, 1973, *53* (12), 1298–1306.

Mendenhall, R. C., Girard, R. A., and Abrahamson, S. "A National Study of Medical and Surgical Specialties." *Journal of the American Medical Association*, 1978, *240*, 848–852, 1160–1168.

Meskauskas, J. A. "Evaluation Models for Criterion-Referenced Testing: Views Regarding Mastery and Standard Setting." *Review of Educational Research*, 1976, *46* (1), 133–158.

Meskauskas, M. S., and Webster, G. D. "The American Board of Internal Medicine Recertification Examination: Process and Results." *Annals of Internal Medicine*, 1975, *82* (4), 577–581.

Miller, G. E., McGuire, C. H., and Larson, C. B. "The Orthopedic Training Study—A Progress Report." *Bulletin of the American Academy of Orthopedic Surgery*, 1965, *13*, 8–11.

Morgan, M. K., and Irby, D. M. (Eds.). *Evaluating Clinical Competence in the Health Professions.* Saint Louis, Mo.: Mosby, 1978.

Morton, J. B., and Macbeth, W. A. A. G. "Correlations Between Staff, Peer, and Self-Assessments of Fourth-Year Students in Surgery." *Medical Education,* 1977, *11* (3), 167-170.

Naftulin, D. H., and Andrew, B. J. "The Effects of Patient Simulations on Actors." *Journal of Medical Education,* 1975, *50* (1), 87-89.

Nedelsky, L. "Absolute Grading Standards for Objective Tests." *Educational and Psychological Measurement,* 1954, *14*, 3-19.

Nerenberg, R. L., and others. "Prediction of Graduate Clinical Performance Ratings from Multicomponent Medical School Examinations." In *Seventeenth Annual Conference on Research in Medical Education.* Washington, D.C.: Association of American Medical Colleges, 1978.

Newble, D. I., Baxter, A., and Elmslie, R. G. "A Comparison of Multiple-Choice Tests and Free-Response Tests in Examinations of Clinical Competence." *Medical Education,* 1979, *13*, 263-268.

Newble, D. I., Hoare, J., and Sheldrake, P. F. "The Selection and Training of Examiners for Clinical Examinations." *Medical Education,* 1980, *14*, 345-349.

O'Connor, P., and Lorey, R. E. "Improving Interrater Agreement in Evaluation in Dentistry by the Use of Comparison Stimuli." *Journal of Dental Education,* 1978, *42* (4), 174-179.

O'Donohue, W. J., and Wergin, J. F. "Evaluation of Medical Students During a Clinical Clerkship in Internal Medicine." *Journal of Medical Education,* 1978, *53* (1), 55-58.

Page, G. G., and Fielding, D. W. "Performance on PMPs and Performance in Practice: Are They Related?" *Journal of Medical Education,* 1980, *55* (6), 529-537.

Palva, I. P., and Korhonen, V. "Validity and Use of Written Simulation Tests of Clinical Performance." *Journal of Medical Education,* 1976, *51* (8), 657-661.

Pearson, B. D. "Evaluation of the Nursing Processes Through Visual Motion Media." *International Nursing Review,* 1978, *25* (4), 119-120.

Pennell, M. Y. "Certification and Licensing in the Allied Health Professions." *Journal of Dental Education,* 1972, *36* (8), 10-16.

Price, P. B., and others. *Measurement and Prediction of Physician Performance: Two Decades of Intermittently Sustained Research.* Salt Lake City, Utah: Lynn Lloyd Reid Enterprises, 1971.

Raffman, D. S., Tobias, D. E., and Speedie, S. M. "Validation of Written Simulations as Measures of Problem Solving." *American Journal of Pharmaceutical Education,* 1980, *44* (1), 16-24.

Rezler, A. G., and Stevens, B. S. (Eds.). *The Nurse Evaluator in Education and Service.* New York: McGraw-Hill, 1978.

Richards, A., and others. "Videotape as an Evaluation Tool." *Nursing Outlook,* 1981, *29* (1), 35-38.

Richardson, F. M. "Peer Review of Medical Care." *Medical Care,* 1972, *10* (1), 29-39.

Risley, M. E., and others. *Competence in Medical Technology.* Chicago: Center for Educational Development, University of Illinois, 1980.

Rosenow, E. C., Jr. "Medical Specialty Societies." In T. Samph and B. Templeton

(Eds.), *Evaluation in Medical Education: Past, Present, and Future.* Cambridge, Mass.: Ballinger, 1979.

Samph, T., and Templeton, B. *Evaluation in Medical Education: Past, Present, and Future.* Cambridge, Mass.: Ballinger, 1979.

Sanson-Fisher, R. W., and Poole, A. D. "Simulated Patients and the Assessment of Medical Students' Interpersonal Skills." *Medical Education,* 1980, *14,* 249–253.

Schoeff, L., and Ciurczak, F. "Construction and Validation of an Equivalency Examination for an MLT/MT Career Mobility Curriculum." *American Journal of Medical Technology,* 1980, *46* (1), 51–57.

Sherman, J. E., Miller, A. G., Farrand, L. L. and Holzemer, W. L. "A Simulated Patient Encounter for the Family Nurse Practitioner." *Journal of Nursing Education,* 1979, *18* (5), 5–15.

Sigerist, H. E. "The History of Medical Licensure." *Journal of the American Medical Association,* 1935, *104,* 1057–1060.

Smith, D. E. "Computerized Test Item Library." In J. P. Hubbard (Ed.), *An International View of Qualification for the Practice of Medicine.* 1976 annual conference of the National Board of Medical Examiners. Philadelphia: National Board of Medical Examiners, 1977.

Stillman, P. L., and Sabers, D. L. "Using a Competency-Based Program to Assess Interviewing Skills of Pediatric House Staff." *Journal of Medical Education,* 1978, *53* (6), 493–496.

Stillman, P. L., Sabers, D. L., Redfield, D. L., and Stewart, D. "Testing Physical Diagnosis Skills with Videotape." *Journal of Medical Education,* 1977, *52* (11), 942–943.

Stillman, P. L., Ruggill, J. S., Rutala, P. J. and Sabers, D. L. "Patient Instructors as Teachers and Evaluators." *Journal of Medical Education,* 1980, *55* (3), 186–193.

Studnicki, J., and Saywell, R. O. "Comparing Medical Audits: Correlations, Scaling, and Sensitivity." *Journal of Medical Education,* 1978, *53* (6), 480–486.

Sweeney, M. A., and Resan, P. A. "Educators, Employees, and New Graduates Define Essential Skills for Baccalaureate Graduates." *Journal of Nursing Administration,* 1982, *12* (9), 36–42.

Taylor, W. C., and others. "The Use of Computerized Patient Management Problems in a Certifying Examination." *Medical Education,* 1976, *10,* 1–4.

Templeton, B. "The National Board of Medical Examiners and Independent Assessment Agencies." In T. Samph and B. Templeton (Eds.), *Evaluation in Medical Education: Past, Present, and Future.* Cambridge, Mass.: Ballinger, 1979.

Templeton, B., Erviti, V. F., Bunce, J. V., and Burg, F. D. *Medical Audit of Pediatric Resident Performance.* Final Report to Maternal and Child Health and Crippled Children's Services, Grant no. MC-R-420310. Washington, D.C.: U.S. Department of Health, Education, and Welfare, 1977.

Tower, J. B., and Vosburgh, P. M. "Development of a Rating Scale to Measure Learning in Clinical Dietetics. I. Theoretical Considerations and Method of Construction. II. Pilot Test." *Journal of the American Dietetic Association,* 1976, *68* (5), 440–449.

Wakeford, R. E., and Roberts, S. "A Pilot Experiment on the Interexaminer Reliability of Short Essay Questions." *Medical Education,* 1979, *13,* 342–344.

Webster, G. D., and others. "Symposium: Results of a National Study of a Computer Simulation and the American Board of Internal Medicine's Recertification Examination: The MERIT Project." In *Proceedings, 18th Annual Conference on Research in Medical Education.* Washington, D.C.: Association of American Medical Colleges, 1979.

Wigton, R. S. "Factors Important in the Evaluation of Clinical Performance of Internal Medicine Residents." *Journal of Medical Education,* 1980, *55* (3), 206–208.

Williamson, J. W. "Assessing Clinical Judgment." *Journal of Medical Education,* 1965, *40,* 180–187.

Williamson, J. W. "The Product of Our Medical Schools." In *Academic Decision Making, Issues, and Evidence,* proceedings of the Association of American Medical Colleges 1975 Council of Deans spring meeting. Washington, D.C.: Association of American Medical Colleges, 1976a.

Williamson, J. W. "Validation by Performance Measures." In *Conference on Extending the Validity of Certification,* March 24, 1976. Evanston, Ill.: American Board of Medical Specialties, 1976b.

Wingard, J. R., and Williamson, J. W. "Grades as Predictors of Physician's Career Performance: An Evaluative Literature Review." *Journal of Medical Education,* 1973, *48* (4), 311–322.

*Frank T. Stritter*

# 13

# Faculty Evaluation
# and Development

The definition of teacher suggested by McNeil and Popham (1973, p. 219) as "a person engaged in interactive behavior with one or more students for the purpose of effecting change in those students" serves as an appropriate point of departure for this chapter. Green's (1971) conceptualization adds to the definition by dividing that change into the "transmission of knowledge" and the "formation of behavior." One can infer from Rippey (1980) that faculty evaluation includes some type of judgment concerning a teacher's skill in effecting that change, with the eventual goal of improving the interaction between teacher and student. Faculty development is the process of assisting teachers to improve that skill. According to Bergquist and Phillips (1977) and Gaff (1975), that process includes consideration of the personal needs of the instructor, the instructor's professional responsibilities, and the organizational context in which that instructor functions. Any improvement in instruction might, therefore, involve personal, technical, and/or situational assistance.

As Miller (1980) has indicated, medical school teachers in particular and (by inference) instructors in the several health professions generally receive little or no preparation for the task they accept or are assigned. Yet teachers are regularly evaluated and often rewarded, based on someone's perception of their success in teaching.

## Faculty Evaluation and Faculty Development

Faculty evaluation and faculty development mean different things to different people. However, systematic faculty evaluation necessarily involves collecting and analyzing data concerning an individual's teaching, rendering a value judgment about that teaching, and suggesting ways of improving it. Systematic faculty development necessarily entails the design and implementation of a program intended to develop and/or improve the skills necessary for instructors to carry out their teaching responsibilities. The two processes should be inextricably intertwined and interdependent, but they seldom are. They should be complementary: Faculty evaluation should be employed to diagnose a teacher's problems and needs in teaching, in the same way that a physical examination is used to diagnose a patient's medical problems; faculty development should be designed to assist an instructor in improving instructional problems, in the same way that therapy or medication is prescribed as a remedy for a patient's medical problems. In actuality, however, this is seldom how the process works. Most often, the two functions are undertaken separately, each occurring in isolation from the other.

Teachers can improve their interactions with their students. They can modify their instructional practices so that students develop better attitudes toward instruction and learn more from that instruction. Levinson-Rose and Menges (1981) have documented three stimulants to such improvements: (1) feedback from students alone, (2) feedback from students coupled with professional interpretation of the data, and (3) feedback from students coupled with participation in some ongoing faculty development activity. They suggest that the probability that any improvement will occur and the amount of that improvement vary with the extent to which the instructor is personally involved in the evaluation and/or change process. It would, therefore, seem appropriate and worthwhile for an institution to organize both faculty evaluation and faculty development activities and to encourage its faculty members to participate. This would facilitate the establishment of a link between evaluation and development.

Centra (1976) has classified faculty development activities into four categories: (1) individual assistance, (2) group activities that entail high faculty involvement, (3) traditional faculty support practices, and (4) faculty assessment procedures. In the first category, a specialist in the teaching process or in educational technology works with individual faculty members to assist in diagnosing and remedying teaching problems. The second category embraces workshops, seminars, conferences, and other similar means by which colleagues learn from and with each other about instruction, evaluation, student advising, and students in their role of developing professionals. The third category refers to visiting scholar programs, sabbaticals, teaching awards, work load reductions, and travel funds for conferences. The last category includes all the activities in which instructors are evaluated or rated in some way, utilizing self, students, peers, or administrators as sources of information. The first two categories differ from the third in that they stress technical assistance or interaction with colleagues concerning information about teaching and/or learning, while the third provides time and money to obtain more information about the content of one's discipline or professional field. All three differ from the fourth, which is based on the collection and interpretation of information from a variety of sources about an individual's performance as an instructor. It does not necessarily include follow-up assistance to the instructors who need it or request it.

This chapter describes representative activities and approaches that have been employed in faculty development projects in the health professions. While the focus is on an analysis and synthesis of the literature from those professions, occasional reference is made to broader studies in the general field of education. However, it is noteworthy that few references could be located that met the following criteria for research on the effects of faculty development activities, as set forth by Levinson-Rose and Menges (1981):

- The independent and dependent variables of a study are statistically related
- The statistical relationship between an independent and dependent variable is a causal one
- The statistical and causal relationship is generalizable to more abstract concepts
- The construct relationship is generalizable to other persons, settings, and times
- The evidence of an intervention is its impact on students
- Randomized studies using two or more groups are preferable.

Table 1 summarizes the approaches to faculty development that have been employed in the health professions, under three broad categories adapted from Centra's (1976) classification scheme. The categories—technical assistance, high faculty involvement, and assessment—refer to teaching style and its components, that is, the art and science of teaching, not to an instructor's command of his or her discipline. These are the approaches usually employed in faculty development programs in the health professions. Each is discussed in detail and recommendations for its use are made. These three categories just named are the categories of faculty development for which a body of literature exists. The literature summarized in this chapter is largely from the health professions. However, reference is made to studies in the general field of education as relevant. A bibliography keyed to the categories used in Table 1 is also included at the end of this chapter.

## Technical Assistance

Technical assistance includes all those activities in which a specialist in the teaching process or in some phase of educational technology works with instructors in an individualized or small group setting. Usually this educational specialist joins with the subject matter instructor in developing a specific instructional project or in addressing a particular problem with that faculty member's teaching. Thus, technical assistance embraces both consultation with educators and collaborative educational research. Miller (1980) reports that as of 1977, seventy-two medical schools had established some type of identifiable unit that had the capacity of providing such educational expertise to faculty members. At other medical schools, individual departments often employed individuals to provide that type of resource, and at some schools it was furnished by individuals who were not members of identifiable units. Similarly, nearly all dental schools have at least one individual, if not a unit, who can work with dental faculty members in this manner. Comparable figures are not available for other types of health professions institutions; however, instructors in many schools of nursing and allied health have demonstrated interest in the educational process and have access to an educational resource of some type. Many instructors in these latter two types of institutions themselves possess advanced degrees in education and, therefore, provide perhaps an even more valid educational presence.

Table 1. Types of Faculty Development in the Health Professions.

| Approach to Faculty Development | Representative Description | Effect | Citation |
|---|---|---|---|
| **Technical Assistance** Consultation with Educators (Ia) | Faculty members meet with educational consultant individually or in small groups, for the purpose of resolving a perceived need, usually self-determined. | Increased use of objectives, improved testing procedures, more effective presentation techniques, and the like. | Carrier, 1980 Irby and others, 1976 Foley and others, 1976 |
| Collaborative Research (Ib) | A question concerning education is formulated by a health professional and an educational professional. A research project is then designed and conducted jointly to answer the question. | Raises health professionals' awareness of educational issues and concerns. Aids them in the development of research skills in the social science areas; most take on new projects. | Stritter, 1980 Connell, Alberti, and Piotrowski, 1975 |
| **High Faculty Involvement** Extended Programs (IIa) | Increased satisfaction with preparation to teach, increased number of trained instructional personnel, the development of trained educational leaders in the health professions. | Participants develop educational skills and presentation techniques. Participants often become models. Awareness is stimulated. professions. | Holcomb and others, 1980 McGaghie and others, 1981 |
| Short Programs (IIb) | A list of objectives is arrived at either by needs assessment or by consultation with professional educators. A series of sessions is then planned to address these objectives. Some form of post-course evaluation is undertaken to determine if objectives have been met. | Participants develop educational skills and presentation techniques. Participants often become models. Awareness is stimulated. | Bland, 1980 Stritter and Hain, 1977 Farr and Heider, 1974 |

**Table 1. Types of Faculty Development in the Health Professions, Cont'd.**

| Approach to Faculty Development | Description | Effect | Representative Citation |
|---|---|---|---|
| Structured Institutional Approaches (IIc) | A system is established for evaluating all faculty members within the institution. The evaluation is carried out by a team and shared with the faculty member. Some form of remediation is then agreed upon and steps are taken to improve the process. The evaluations are often shared with the tenure and promotions committee. | All participants in the system are involved, including a high level of involvement by administration. Faculty members become aware of the necessity for good teaching and of methods to improve their own skills. | Lindquist, 1978 Sibley, 1980 |
| Assessment Self-Evaluation (IIIa) | A system is developed to aid faculty members to evaluate their own teaching behaviors (questionnaires, checklists, observation charts, etc.) through self-report, videotapes. Faculty members then devise their own approaches to improve teaching. | Faculty members can self-evaluate in a nonthreatening environment and choose their own approaches to improvement. | Bronstein, 1978 Schaffer, 1980 |
| Peer Evaluation (IIIb) | A department sets standards that all faculty agree on. Faculty members are then evaluated by peers according to standards previously set. Videotape is often used to allow faculty members to rate themselves and determine if they agree with peer evaluation. Remedial activities are left to the individual faculty members. | Faculty are involved in the setting of standards and thus become more aware of the teaching process. Peer pressure is introduced into the instructional setting; peers often improve as well. | Sauter and Walker, 1976 Skeff, 1981 |

Table 1. Types of Faculty Development in the Health Professions, Cont'd.

| Approach to Faculty Development | Description | Effect | Representative Citation |
|---|---|---|---|
| Student Evaluation (IIIc) | A system is developed by which students evaluate instruction on prescribed variables. These evaluations are compiled and shared with the faculty members. They are also used by promotion and tenure committees in some systems. | Faculty are given the opportunity to check their perceptions about their instruction. Students are allowed input into the instructional system. | Sall and others, 1976 Rippey, 1975 |

*Consultation with Educators.* This type of institutional support is the major one available to health professions faculty; it usually takes the form of an individual or unit within the institution who provides assistance to instructors, individually or in small groups, to develop or improve some aspect of the teaching process. Such consultants generally work with instructors in diagnosing teaching needs, in designing new approaches to instruction, and in developing or improving a skill and in evaluating its effectiveness. They may also provide help in designing and validating measures of student performance and give advice on the selection and use of various instructional media. The instructors who take advantage of this opportunity generally volunteer to do so, their numbers are usually small, and the areas they can improve in this manner are usually limited to the instructional component of their professional responsibilities. In health professions institutions, little overt attention seems to have been devoted to personal needs and organizational components, as suggested by Bergquist and Phillips (1977).

Schein (1969) has described three different but related structures in which a consultant can function: the dyadic relationship, observation of the work situation, and a small group. Carrier (1980) describes the procedures in these three settings as follows: *Individual consultation* is a one-to-one dyadic relationship between a faculty member and an educational expert in which they function as equals, sharing expertise to resolve an instructional question. The consultant's task is to collect information about the problem before using that information to assist the instructor in its resolution. *Observation* of a teaching segment can be conducted by a consultant functioning as an expert, followed by feedback delivered to the instructor specifying salient behaviors and suggesting alternatives. A *seminar* is a small group that allows a consultant to model teaching behavior for instructors and facilitates their discussion of teaching and learning issues with one another.

In a University of Illinois program (Foley and others, 1976) designed to improve the lecturing skills of medical faculty, consultants observed videotapes of instructors' lectures and then met in small group sessions with each participating department to discuss the lectures that had been presented. Irby and others (1976) used a slightly different approach at the University of Washington. Individual faculty lectures were observed in person by consultants, who provided immediate verbal and written feedback to instructors. Subsequent follow-up observations were made; improvements were noted and comments furnished about them. Both these approaches resulted in demonstrated improvements. Kohler (1981) describes a complex program, entitled "Advanced Instruction in Medical Settings (AIMS)," developed at the University of Kentucky. Although AIMS is not limited to lectures, its steps are somewhat similar to the Washington program: (1) interview interested faculty members, (2) develop contracts with faculty members, (3) make preliminary observations of instructor performance, (4) review instructional materials used by the instructor, (5) conduct detailed assessment of teaching skills, (6) review results of assessment with instructor, (7) suggest alternative teaching approaches, and (8) interview instructor on results. While this type of consultation could take any of a number of directions, its essential characteristic is that it is individualized and targeted to a specific faculty member's self-identified teaching problem. From their experiential involvement with many instructors, Wergin, Mason, and Munson (1976) derived an excellent set of guidelines for use in the consulting process; they conclude that two distinct phases of a consulting relationship exist, in which the process moves from a professional-expert phase to a personal-collaborative phase.

Based on the conclusions of these reports, relevant discussions with colleagues, and personal experience as a consultant, the following suggestions are offered for maximizing the effectiveness of the consultation process. First, the consultant must be open, flexible, and adaptable to the needs of a particular client(s); a rigid, dogmatic approach is usually doomed to failure. Consultants learn as much as the instructor(s) with whom they work, and each must be prepared to modify emphases and interventions rapidly, based upon what he or she learns. Second, the consulting process must often be both long-term and intensive, the length and quality of the interaction being directly related to the quality of the instructional change that results. Consultants should not be satisfied with a speedy or one-time interaction. Third, the consulting process must be individualized, depending on the particular instructional situation encountered; no single approach is appropriate to all problems. Theories of teaching and learning should be adapted to a particular instructor or instructional problem in a way that represents a unique application in each situation. Fourth, action plans can profitably include a contract that specifies goals, tasks, responsibilities of participants, and target dates for completion of tasks. Leaving any of these to chance or to informal agreements will often result in their being ignored. Fifth, the consultant must consider the organizational context in which the instruction occurs, as well as the individual responsible for it. Unless the context, as well as the individual, is open to change and supports it, the individual instructor will usually be able to modify performance only slightly, if at all. Sixth, consultants should acquire personal skill in individual interaction, organizational analysis, and adaptation of innovations. One who endeavors to intercede with only technical expertise will often not be sufficiently sensitive to stimulate productive change. Finally, consultants must realize that a few instructors' practices can be improved through consultation, but the process is difficult and time-consuming. It can, however, be extremely rewarding.

*Collaborative Research.* Collaborative educational research can be defined as cooperation between an educational researcher and a health professions instructor in the conduct of an applied educational study. It is not addressed to the acquisition of particular skills or knowledge but rather to the discovery and articulation of dissatisfaction with a specific instructional problem. It necessarily entails study of some aspect of the problem.

The first indication of the use of this approach was the establishment of the Division of Research in Medical Education at Western Reserve University in 1958. The founder, T. H. Ham, based the development of that unit almost entirely on an experimental research model, in contrast with the action-oriented teaching and consulting units that were then developing at other medical schools (Miller, 1980). Ham's unit provided a place where faculty members could turn to reflect upon and study their educational problems (Ham, 1975). Palmer, O'Leary, and Sterling (1967) describe their discussion of a joint study by engineering and medical faculty at Tufts. In that project, the medical group defined problems while the engineering group suggested solutions, and both participated in joint discussions and work sessions to study and resolve the problems. Connell, Alberti, and Piotrowski (1975) refer to this idea as the "educational inquiry approach," in which participating faculty develop an experimental set regarding their educational responsibilities. That set includes: (1) analyzing one's personal teaching style to identify aspects likely to inhibit goal achievement, (2) developing alternative ways of working with students, (3) anticipating the consequences of each alternative, (4) choosing and testing the best alternative, and (5) studying the consequences of implementation. Connell's data indicate that faculty development programs that cultivate an inquiry set can be developed and that students taught by faculty using that set improve in their own abilities to engage in inquiry.

At the University of North Carolina, individual educational research faculty, based in the health professional educational research and development unit, work jointly with individual medical school faculty who have a significant question(s) about some aspect of their instructional responsibilities. Both agree to study the question systematically, basing their mutual work on the criteria of educational research and/or evaluation (Stritter, 1980). The two individuals participate on a collegial basis, the educational faculty member learning more about medicine and the medical faculty member learning more about education. The intended result is a jointly authored paper that can be presented at educational meetings by the educator and at medical conferences by the medical faculty member and/or that can be submitted for publication. Any particular project is considered additionally successful when the medical faculty member (1) communicates the results of the study to colleagues either locally or nationally, (2) feels comfortable in cooperating with and seeking additional help from educators, and (3) reflects the results in his own instruction or in that of his department. Of ten individual medical faculty collaborators studied at North Carolina, all reported significant outcomes of one type or another, while five were in the process of conducting additional studies with educational colleagues (Stritter, 1980).

Grimes and others (1975) report on a case study at North Carolina in which a medical resident, pursuing an academic career, and an educational researcher collaborated. The resident participated in a three-month elective in which he interacted extensively with the educational researcher. They studied an instructional problem that the resident had identified but that was also of interest to the educator. The resident undertook library research, conducted a major portion of the study, assisted in the data analysis, collaborated in writing the paper, and presented the results at selected meetings. The paper (Stritter, Hain, and Grimes, 1975) served in part to launch the resident on an academic career and as a basis for many other studies in the important area of clinical teaching.

The effects of collaborative educational research on faculty development are mixed. Such research is, unfortunately, not valued to the same extent by all academic departments; some include it in the criteria for faculty promotion while others do not. It is extremely time-consuming since, at any one time, only a few health professions faculty members can collaborate with a small educational research unit. Frequently, those who participate in one study return to initiate other studies, thus making it difficult to expand the pool of faculty members with whom the educational researcher can work effectively. Those instructors most in need of studying and improving their own teaching rarely participate; those who do and who are good collaborators are, most often, already good teachers. However, the impact on the health professions faculty members who do elect to participate can be staggering. They all demonstrate learning about selected instructional issues and become sensitive to the complexities of educational research. Many become concerned about broader instructional problems, and some even become educational leaders in their departments and schools. Collaborative educational research as an alternative to other forms of faculty development is well worth the investment of time and resources.

### High Faculty Involvement

This category is comprised of all those faculty development activities that take a concentrated period of faculty time and in which faculty colleagues explore instructional issues with one another's assistance. It includes three specific types of faculty development activities: (1) extended programs, such as degree programs and fellowships; (2) short programs, such as workshops, seminars, and short courses; and (3) structured institutional approaches. Such programs are usually highly structured, heavily dependent on discussion among the participants, and not necessarily developed to address the specific problems of the participants. They are generally under the leadership of an individual who has engaged in professional study of the educational process. Programs in this category have been sponsored by a variety of entities: occasionally by entire institutions, sometimes by specific academic departments, and most often by the type of educational development unit described by Miller (1980).

*Extended Approaches.* These programs normally take the form of a long-term (for example, one-year) fellowship or of formal study for a degree in education. Participants in the latter are usually either persons just beginning academic careers who have chosen not to pursue advanced degrees in their own fields (for example, nurses and allied health personnel) or those who find themselves assuming significant educational responsibilities in the middle of their academic careers. One of the best examples of the degree program is the project supported by the W. K. Kellogg Foundation for the educational preparation of academic personnel for allied health (W. K. Kellogg Foundation, 1977). In that project, the Kellogg Foundation provided funds, beginning in 1968 and ending in 1977, to eight university-based regional centers for the preparation of allied health instructors and educational program directors. Each of the centers (1) coordinated a regional faculty preparation program, (2) selected trainees, (3) counseled students, (4) developed curricula, (5) arranged learning experiences and practice teaching, (6) offered a general seminar for all trainees, (7) arranged career placement of graduates, and (8) provided continuing education for instructors already teaching in health-related programs. At the program's conclusion in 1977, the participating universities had graduated 541 individuals: 41 at the doctoral level, 279 at the master's, 101 at the baccalaureate, and 119 at the certificate. Holcomb and others (1980) surveyed the 94 graduates of the Texas center and found that they were (1) from a variety of allied health fields, (2) all in faculty or administrative positions in allied health, (3) from several minority groups, (4) living in the southwest region, and (5) largely satisfied with their preparation for the roles they had assumed.

Louisiana State University School of Dentistry and the University of New Orleans College of Education cooperated in a somewhat similar program for dental educators (Boozer and others, 1977). These institutions offered a master's degree in education with a strong educational research component. The program was designed to promote self-directed learning and improvement of dental education through systematic educational research and evaluation. One of the most widely known degree programs is that offered by the Center for Educational Development at the University of Illinois Health Sciences Center. Approximately twelve mid-career professionals are admitted each year to a program of study in administration, educational change, instructional methods, course planning, test construction, educational technology, and program evaluation. Since its inception in the late 1960s, that program has graduated approximately 150 health professionals. In addition to a large number of fellows sponsored by the World Health Organization (WHO), many of the early participants were American physicians funded by the federally supported Regional Medical Program; more recent participants have included allied health professionals, as well as physicians in academic medicine from foreign countries.

Other long-term fellowship programs have enrolled many different types of health professionals. In 1977, the W. K. Kellogg Foundation sponsored the establishment of the Kellogg Center for Advanced Studies in Primary Care at McGill University and the Montreal General Hospital. This center annually provides postresidency and/or advanced education for eleven to fifteen family physicians and ambulatory care nurses who have confirmed future faculty posts in university faculties of medicine or nursing. The participants are enrolled in a degree program that includes study of teaching methods, investigative principles, biomedical communications, and management of community health care facilities; they are expected to apply what they learn during periodic rotations to satellite community-based teaching practice units, in both urban and rural areas (Spitzer, 1978).

The federal government has also funded a number of faculty development efforts. One of the largest was the Regional Medical Program Fellowship program (RMP) of the National Institutes of Health. Between 1967 and 1972, it funded one-year fellowships for approximately one hundred health professionals and others pursuing careers in health education at the Universities of Illinois, Southern California, Washington, Michigan State, and Ohio State. The programs were designed to help participants integrate educational science in planning and conducting programs in continuing medical education (Miller, 1980). Beginning in 1978, the Bureau of Health Professions of the U.S. Department of Health and Human Services financed several university projects in their program of Faculty Development in Family Medicine. In one of these, the fellowship program at the University of North Carolina, young faculty members are enrolled in a year-long program in which they spend approximately 20 percent of their time in the program and the remaining 80 percent in their normal professional duties. The program goals relate to the full scope of their responsibilities, not only to the teaching and research components. Among the features of the program reported as most significant by the participants are the interdisciplinary team approach to teaching, the "learn and work" concept, and the applied nature of the material taught. One unanticipated outcome has been the establishment of an informal professional network among graduates. By interacting with each other, they have obtained reinforcement for their concerns and valuable feedback on the projects they undertake. This network, although difficult to evaluate, may be a much more valuable outcome than any individual skills participants may develop (McGaghie and others, 1981).

Although the overall results of extended programs are extremely difficult to document, participants regularly report that they have had significant personal impact. Unfortunately, however, only a relatively small number of individuals can devote the time necessary to complete such a program. On the negative side, there is also danger that the concepts dealt with in the courses are not relevant to the participants' specific job contexts; special efforts must be made to avoid this potential problem.

*Short Programs.* This approach is certainly the most common, appearing in the form of workshops, short courses, or seminars sponsored by professional associations, institutions, departments, or entrepreneurial individuals (Bergquist and Phillips, 1975). Such offerings are generally of four types: (1) longer residential programs of five days to two weeks in which objectives tend to be broad; (2) short-term residential programs of two to four days in which objectives tend to be highly specific; (3) extended on-site programs of three to twelve hours in which objectives tend to be specific and that enable participants to learn at home; (4) brief on-site programs of one to two hours focusing on a limited number of very narrow objectives.

Beginning in the mid-1950s, the Association of American Medical Colleges offered such programs to its members. Other associations such as the American Association of Dental Schools, the American Society of Clinical Pathologists, the Association of Schools of the Allied Health Professions, the Association of Hospital Directors of Medical Education, and the Society of Teachers of Family Medicine have sponsored workshops as part of their annual meetings or have offered short residential programs from time to time. Such programs have tended to be one-time efforts with little or no follow-up undertaken by the sponsors of the programs. In a comprehensive study of four workshops conducted by the Society of Teachers of Family Medicine (Bland and others, 1979), participants reported increased ability to perform faculty functions; both immediately after the workshops and nine months later, participants indicated that they were significantly more knowledgeable about the topics addressed in the workshops. This study led to the development of a comprehensive guide to planning and conducting workshops (Bland, 1980).

The literature includes many references that describe various short-term programs at specific institutions. Wergin, Mason, and Munson (1976) summarized the "do's and don't's" derived from offering several different types of workshops to a variety of health professions faculty members. Prentice and Metcalf (1974) report a twelve-week course for medical faculty and students that met for two and one-half hours twice per week. Littlefield (1979) describes another eight-unit course of a self-instructional nature designed for dental faculty. Meleca and Schimpfhauser (1976) report a somewhat similar self-paced course on instructional materials and microteaching, designed for medical residents. Stritter and Hain (1977) describe a one-day workshop on clinical teaching; the workshop employed discovery learning as a method and was adapted for several different health professions. Papers from nursing have described short courses on instructional topics for faculty, based on the premise that multiple, brief, activity-oriented sessions would be of the most benefit to the most people (Gerber, 1980; Leichsenring, 1972). Such descriptive references were informative but provided little documentation as to the effects of these efforts, other than an occasional mention of positive participant attitudes.

Though hardly classifiable as research, selected papers have included limited evidence about the specific outcomes of particular programs. For example, Donnelly and others (1972) found positive cognitive outcomes on an objective test and positive attitudinal outcomes on a questionnaire, following six weekend workshops. Koen (1976) reported gains in participants' self-perceptions following a twelve-week seminar series with preset goals. Farr and Heider (1974) found that five to fourteen weeks after a three-day workshop, 55 percent of the participants reported that they had changed in four of five areas of teaching behavior emphasized in the program. A majority of nursing educators who participated in a workshop on the Keller Plan conducted in England agreed to test the Keller Plan in their instruction (Sheahan, 1979). (The Keller Plan combines individualized instruction with the principles of operant learning.) In their follow-up of participants in a three-day session, Jedrychowski and Galligani (1978) found a significant retention and increase of knowledge about instruction but noted that changes in teaching behavior were insignificant, both six months and one year after the course.

Research on the effect of short programs as a faculty development strategy is sparse indeed. Based on personal experience and on impressions obtained from the reports that were available, it can be concluded that participants' knowledge about the topic(s) under discussion can be increased. However, changing behavior over a period of time is another matter; something in addition to the program is definitely needed to stimulate and reinforce a change. There are, however, some helpful guides to planning and conducting short programs that can be gleaned from the experiences and perceptions reported. First, consult with participants in planning the program so that specific needs relating to perceived problems are addressed. Second, focus on a limited number of goals that can realistically be accomplished during the program. Third, ensure that instruction in the program is based on practical examples and that participants can perceive an obvious positive return for their efforts. Fourth, build in active participation so that brief presentations, focused discussions, relevant practice of new skills, and focused feedback from both program leaders and peers are all systematically included. Finally, determine the effect of the program so that necessary revisions in strategy can be implemented prior to its next administration.

Structured Institutional Approaches. Many programmatic efforts to improve instruction, such as those previously described, fail, not because they are planned improperly or are ineffective but because the participants' institution does not really support instructional improvement. The organizational climate prevailing in the institution can provide subtle but significant indications that it opposes the expenditure of faculty time in this endeavor. Instructors are often rewarded more for success in other aspects of their faculty roles; instructional innovators may actually be penalized rather than encouraged. Time is not made available to develop new instructional ideas or improve old ones. Institutional leaders often feel that they have attended to instructional needs by sponsoring some type of instructional or faculty development unit, but they fail to provide a climate that encourages their faculty to use that unit as a resource.

This condition leads to a need for institutional or organizational development to create a climate favorable to instructional improvement. Applied behavorial science theories and procedures that underlie management consultation in business and industry can be used to improve organizational functioning in educational institutions in the health professions. Such approaches make it possible for individuals in an institution to work together in identifying and reducing obstacles to institutional support for improving instruction (French and Bell, 1973).

Although Bergquist and Phillips (1977) discuss the necessity for an institutional focus, there is little evidence regarding the application or the success of such programs. On two separate occasions in the past twenty-five years, the Association of American Medical Colleges (AAMC) has attempted formal programs of an institutional nature, but both efforts flourished for only a few years (Miller, 1980). The first was the teaching institute program that began in the mid-1950s and extended through the early 1960s. That program provided a series of opportunities for medical school faculty and administrators both to learn about and to discuss instructional issues. The second was the establishment of the Division of Faculty Development in 1974, which lasted only through 1978. That division had responsibility for identifying faculty instructional needs, implementing short-term workshops, creating long-term fellowships for selected participants, developing instructional packages, disseminating information, stimulating instructional activity, and providing consultation. Activities related to the first responsibility led to a major study (Jason, Slotnick, and Lefever, 1977) that, in addition to identifying specific faculty needs, provided some indication of a general improvement in the institutional climate in support of instructional development. Both efforts required medical schools to participate with the AAMC as institutions, but their failure to survive is one indicator of the difficulties in implementing such an approach. Unfortunately, no analysis of the life history or the outcomes of either program is available to aid future efforts.

Buckner (1974) describes how a faculty development program can be institutionalized in a nursing department and concludes that a faculty coordinator can work effectively with various individuals in meeting their goals. Schaffer (1980) proposes a model that entails individual "growth contracts" as an institutional approach for schools of allied health; however, it has yet to be tested in a health professions institution. Certainly the most significant effort representative of institutional approaches to date is located at McMaster University (Sibley, 1980). This approach is based in a matrix form of administration that has the following characteristics: (1) departments are faculty resource centers with department chairmen serving as career development officers and resource managers; (2) educational program chairmen (for example, undergraduate medicine) coordinate their assigned programs and report directly to the Associate Dean for Education; (3) the various program chairmen contract for teaching services of individual faculty members from specific departments and then evaluate those services, using both students and other faculty members as information sources; (4) both the Associate Dean for Education and the department chairmen receive the results of the evaluation, on the basis of which they may (a) strongly recommend any of several appropriate faculty development activities, and/or (b) communicate the results to the Faculty Promotion and Tenure Committee for use in promotional decisions. As a result of the institutional nature of the program, individual faculty members see how important good teaching is to the institution and how helpful faculty development can be in improving that teaching. Although no empirical evidence has been reported regarding the success of the McMaster system, the interest in and concern about teaching that characterize it are known throughout the world, and it has been an influential model in the development of new institutions in several countries. This is an intangible result that documents the success of an institutional thrust.

It is, indeed, unfortunate that more attention has not been paid to institutional approaches similar to McMaster's or to organizational development, in general. It is extremely unlikely that extensive and ongoing improvement in teaching will occur unless an institution supports it in ways that are very evident to its faculty. Though evidence of the impact of institutional approaches is limited to experiential reports, Lindquist (1978) and Bergquist and Phillips (1977) have eloquently advocated consideration of this issue in higher education generally. Both Lindquist (1978) and Sikes, Schlesinger, and Seashore (1974) provide valuable information about initiating institutional programs that support improved teaching.

## Assessment

This cluster of activities can be defined as including those in which the instructor is evaluated or rated in some way. Because evaluation of an individual's professional performance is often perceived as threatening, this series of approaches is probably less effective in accomplishing teaching improvement than those previously detailed. However, they can be helpful and should be considered as one viable strategy in any instructional improvement effort.

Assessment and/or evaluation necessarily involves the collection and sub-sequent interpretation of information about an individual's performance. Information about teaching performance can come from any of a variety of sources: the individual using a set of teaching criteria as a guide, students responding formally or informally to specific questions, and faculty peers and administrators responding to similar questions. Rippey (1980) has provided extremely comprehensive instructions for such evaluation efforts. While this chapter draws heavily upon that source, it takes a slightly different perspective, examining the various assessment techniques primarily from the point of view of their influence in improving teaching.

*Self-Assessment.* In the self-assessment model proposed by Schaffer (1980) for schools of allied health, the process begins by having a faculty member evaluate himself or herself against a consensually agreed-upon set of instructional standards in order to determine specific areas of strength and weakness. The individual then identifies areas in need of improvement, articulates the means for evaluation of any improvement that does occur, and develops a "growth contract" with a supervisor. The contract is then implemented and individual progress monitored. Although this proposal has theoretical support, it has not been tried in a health setting and no documentation of its effectiveness in improving instruction is, therefore, available.

In the early 1970s, the federal government, through the Bureau of Health Manpower, funded development of the Instrument for a Comprehensive and Relevant Education (ICARE) system and a corresponding set of workshops to teach its use (Bronstein, 1978). A variety of health professionals, mostly from nursing and allied health, learned how to use ICARE in evaluating and improving their own teaching. A self-reported follow-up survey indicated that most participants (1) used self-assessment to analyze their teaching; (2) used ICARE or some modification of it; and (3) improved their instruction by increasing their use of objectives and by implementing new student activities, different instructional methods, improved communication approaches, and improved student evaluation techniques.

Although self-ratings do not correlate with those completed by peers, administrators, and students (Clark and Blackburn, 1978), Centra (1972) reports that self-assessments used in conjunction with student evaluations increase the impact of the student evaluation in subsequently improving teaching. Irby's (1978) research also suggests that self-evaluation can be coordinated with that of educational consultants and/or students, and Adams and others (1974) describe a project in which self-assessment has been successfully combined with colleague discussions to improve teaching. In the latter project, several clinical instructors agreed, after completing an extensive self-assessment based on a common set of criteria, to meet weekly to discuss their teaching. The group sessions revealed the strength and impact of individually held ideas of good teaching, and the self-assessment facilitated the development of consistent and flexible teaching behaviors.

Rippey (1980) concludes that self-assessment, though fraught with methodological problems, can be useful in improving instruction. In the long run, it is probably the only really effective way for an individual to improve. One will not improve until he recognizes his own deficiencies and internalizes the necessary changes. In summary, self-assessment is recommended for any program designed to improve teaching, but it should be undertaken in conjunction with assessment from students, peers, administrators, and/or educational consultants. Further, the criteria for self-assessment should be specific, preset, and agreed to by the instructor doing the assessing.

*Peer Evaluation.* Peer evaluation of one type or another has occurred for years. Various analyses of its effectiveness, validity, and reliability did not, however, begin to appear in the literature until the 1970s and then mostly in non-health-related educational programs (for example, Clark and Blackburn, 1978). Most of the studies report that this process is characterized by weak validity and reliability; in general, they are descriptive in nature and provide no evidence regarding associated improvement in teaching.

Nonetheless, it seems clear that colleagues in the same department can help one another to improve, by observing each other's teaching and by reviewing each other's instructional materials (including course or program objectives, syllabi, manuals, reading lists, tests, and audiovisual aids). After the observation and/or review, some type of evaluative feedback can be provided to the instructor along with suggestions for alterations and improvement. Rippey (1980) indicates that both the instructor and the evaluator generally benefit from this type of process.

Miller (1980) describes one such program, developed at the University of Saskatchewan in 1958, in which an instructor was observed by both a faculty colleague and an educator, followed by a critique with all members of the department present. The discussion of teaching that ensued was evaluated positively by the participants; however, the effort ended when its originator left the institution. Lazerson (1972) reports a project in one department in which medical residents were assisted in developing teaching skills by having fellow residents and faculty members observe and comment upon their classroom teaching. Highly positive comments from all participants suggested that their teaching styles had improved and that even faculty had benefited from involvement by being stimulated to analyze their own teaching. Gorecki (1977) describes a process in which participant trust was first developed, criteria for review of teaching were agreed upon, and teaching reviews were conducted. The process began with a self-assessment, moved to a one-on-one evaluation by a peer, and concluded by sharing observations with the faculty of the entire department. Results were positive in that participants identified improvements they had made in their own teaching as a result of the program. Sauter and Walker (1976) propose a model for peer evaluation of instruction based on specific criteria embodied in an objective scale. They conclude that each faculty participant should be involved in developing the evaluational approach and the criteria, that the validity of the criteria should be continually investigated, and that the interpretation of the reviewer's results to each participant should be nonpejorative.

The most comprehensive and best-researched approach to peer review was undertaken by Skeff (1981). In that study, a member of a department of medicine reviewed videotapes of clinical teaching with each faculty participant in a nonthreatening manner and provided extensive individual feedback on the basis of preset criteria. The study was conducted in this manner because it had been assumed that participants would prefer to receive assistance in improving teaching from another member of the department, rather than from an outside expert in teaching. The effectiveness of the procedure was evidenced by the fact that participants viewed the intensive feedback as clearly beneficial, and participants' subsequent teaching, as measured by additional ratings of videotaped teaching segments, was significantly improved from the earlier tapes.

In summary, it appears that peer evaluation of teaching can be helpful in improving teaching. As Rippey (1980) emphasizes, however, its notorious unreliability limits its usefulness in *assessing* teaching performance. Certainly, it would seem logical to suppose that an individual could learn from evaluating someone else's teaching as well as his own and that both could gain from discussing conclusions with each other. Any approach of this type, therefore, requires participant agreement and mutual trust, a mutually approved set of criteria for effective teaching, and someone to facilitate the process.

*Student Evaluation.* The most typical approach to assessing an instructor's teaching performance is to request all or some portion of that instructor's students to complete a questionnaire at the conclusion of the instruction. That questionnaire can be constructed either intuitively or empirically, and the technical properties of the instrument may or may not be determined, depending on the instructor's preference. The process does not stop there, however. In my view, if improvement is to occur, it is essential that the instructor receive the results of the evaluation, accompanied by some interpretation; that is, feedback is regarded as a necessary impetus for changed teaching. This definition corresponds with the formative evaluation concept advanced by Scriven (1967), which requires that an evaluation be conducted while the course/program is in progress so that necessary modifications can be made prior to its conclusion. This assumes that instructors can improve their teaching when confronted with evaluations. It also assumes, at least in the case of student evaluation, that teachers can improve on the basis of the feedback they receive from a systematic survey of their students. This view has received some support (Centra, 1973), but only in those cases where the initial student ratings are lower than the instructor's self-rating.

Research on student ratings shows that they can be reliable, valid, and useful but that they have limited generalizability (Costin, Greenough, and Menges, 1971; Rippey, 1975; Rippey, 1980). Instruments on which to obtain those ratings can be developed empirically for specific faculty groups employing relevant criterion variables and appropriate statistical methods (Purohit and Magoon, 1977; Kotzan and Entrekin, 1978), or they can be developed using a more generalizable format. Illustrative of the latter is the Purdue University "cafeteria" system that permits individual instructors to select those criteria on which they are to be rated (Derry and others, 1974). Student ratings employing such instruments are used extensively in medical schools (Lancaster, Mendelson, and Ross, 1979) and in dental schools (Chambers, 1977). In nearly all the medical schools responding to the Lancaster survey, student ratings were used to provide feedback to faculty; 86 percent of the schools used them in curriculum development, 51 percent in designing faculty development activities, and only 43 percent in promotional decisions.

It is not clear whether student assessment alone can lead to improved teaching; the evidence is conflicting. It can be argued that, as the ultimate consumers, health professions students are in an advantageous position to judge whether a particular instructor's efforts are effective. It can also be argued that written assessments can provide feedback that students might be unwilling to furnish in a face-to-face confrontation. However, Rotem and Glasman (1979) concluded from an extensive literature review that student feedback at the university level generated minimal effect in improving teaching. This conflicts with the results reported by Rous and others (1972) in a study of sixteen medical faculty who demonstrated significant improvement on reevaluation following student evaluation. Skeff (1981) also observed a greater change in an experimental group of attending physicians receiving feedback from trainee evaluations than in a control group receiving no feedback. He concluded that, although all the members of his study group did not find the evaluative feedback beneficial in making improvements, enough did to justify its use.

When students' evaluations are followed by some type of systematic technical assistance in interpreting the results and in suggesting areas for improvement, instructors do seem to modify their teaching, as measured by subsequent evaluations (Jacoby, 1977; Erickson and Erickson, 1979). A faculty committee can also occasionally facilitate marked improvement by consulting with colleagues (Sall and others, 1976). In facilitating changes in teaching, personal, verbal feedback from consultants that can be mutually discussed seems better than printed feedback alone (McKeachie and Lin, 1980).

In summary, student evaluations alone, however obtained, are generally not sufficient to facilitate teaching improvement by the instructors who solicit or otherwise receive them. This may occur because some instructors feel that the ratings generated by students have questionable validity and are, therefore, not meaningful. Some variation of the comment "How do learners really know what they need?" has often been heard in the halls of medical centers and other health institutions. Conversely, health professions students are generally adult learners who must find their teaching meaningful and relevant to their current and perceived future needs in order to learn, retain, and use what is being taught. In addition, they are the only ones who know whether the instruction that they are experiencing is actually helping them to learn. It would, therefore, seem to follow that evaluations by students do have a function in the instructional improvement process. However, the effectiveness of that function is enhanced when student evaluations are coordinated with a faculty or instructional development activity in which instructors have consultative assistance, either from their colleagues or from educational specialists. Such assistance can aid them in progressing from the assessment to the design of a remedial program and, ultimately, to improved practice.

### Conclusions and Recommendations

This chapter was undertaken to determine implications for policy with respect to instructional development and evaluation of health professions faculty. It was somewhat surprising to find that while much has been written descriptively about the topic, there are few quality studies to document the effectiveness of the various approaches discussed. It obviously follows that more and better research must be conducted in the health professions environment, to guide those devoting their professional careers to improved instruction in that arena. The few empirical reports that are available do, however, support my personal bias that individual instructors can improve their teaching. The improvement that does occur aids both teachers and learners—by helping the former to derive greater pleasure from their instructional responsibilities and the latter to attain more positive attitudes and higher achievement.

As we have seen, faculty development and faculty evaluation activities utilized in recent years can be grouped into three categories. First is *technical assistance*, in which a specialist in educational process, technology, or research works with an individual instructor in either a consultative or a collegial manner to study or improve some aspect of instruction. Second is *high faculty involvement*, in which faculty colleagues learn with and from each other about such topics as teaching methods, learning, evaluation, and advising. This approach includes short courses and seminars, workshops, or extended programs, such as degree programs or fellowships. Third is *assessment*, in which an instructor's teaching performance is evaluated using himself, his students, and/or his colleagues as sources of information to provide feedback with a view to improving performance.

The findings of studies of these approaches can be summarized as follows:

- *Consultation* has extremely individualistic outcomes, based on the nature, needs, and characteristics of both parties. To have maximum results, it should be flexible, long-term, individualized, based on a contract, and take the organizational context into consideration.
- *Collaborative educational research*, in which the instructor and the educator interact as colleagues studying an educational problem, can change the behavior of the instructor significantly but is time-consuming for all.
- The results of *extended approaches* are difficult to document, but they may have the greatest impact of any of the types reviewed. Such approaches as fellowships and degree programs can facilitate professional development, but only a small number can devote the time necessary to participate.
- *Short programs*, the most common type, can increase knowledge, motivate interest in change, and raise levels of awareness. Lasting change is not likely to result, however, unless some type of skill practice sessions, accompanied by specific feedback, continue after the program's conclusion.
- *Structured institutional approaches* indicate in very evident ways to the faculty that the institution supports good teaching. It is difficult for an individual to work in such an environment without being, or working on becoming, a good teacher.
- To be most effective, *self-assessment* must be based on specific criteria (as opposed to general) and used in concert with assessment from some other source, such as educational specialists, peers, and/or administrators. Some type of self-assessment must occur, however, if an individual is to recognize his or her own deficiencies and work toward realistic improvements.
- *Peer assessment* can be helpful in improving teaching if participants evaluate each other and then discuss conclusions with one another. However, it must be nonthreatening and it should be based on agreed-upon specific evaluative criteria, characterized by understanding and trust between the participants, and facilitated by a leader.
- Feedback based on *student assessment* alone is generally not sufficient to facilitate improvement on the part of the instructors who receive it. Coordinated with a faculty or instructional development activity in which personal consultative assistance is provided, it can help to improve instruction.

In addition to these conclusions, my personal experience leads to several related recommendations.

- Faculty members should understand why participation in any program is advantageous—that is, an acceptable rationale should be developed for them.
- Both responsibility and authority for planning an activity must be assigned to an individual or group who has the time and resources for the task.
- Faculty members who are potential participants in the activity must be actively involved in the planning.
- As no one approach will fit the needs of every constituent, flexible alternatives should be provided.
- Participation must be voluntary. Development efforts are most effective when professionals who participate do so because they feel a personal need to learn what the program has to offer, not because someone tells them they should.
- There must be adequate administrative support, such as audiovisual, typing, and other services available to those participating in the program.
- Those who participate or otherwise undertake projects should be rewarded in some way. The nature of the rewards should be negotiated with participants prior to the program so that degree of success, criteria, and other conditions will be understandable to all.
- Adequate publicity should inform all faculty about the program, its content, methods, and potential results.
- The results of any program should be evaluated so that future offerings can be improved. Wergin (1977) provides an excellent model for evaluation of a program, although he does not document the effectiveness of his proposals. Nevertheless, common sense dictates that such a plan be undertaken.

### Future Research

These conclusions and recommendations cannot be offered, however, without indicating the need for more study of the entire process. Although more research is obviously necessary, it is equally clear that the analytical methods currently available are not adequate for the task. Most studies are forced into an experimental or comparative design that simply cannot address all the important questions. Conclusions are based on what can be measured objectively, quantified, and analyzed statistically. This orientation leads to an oversimplification of a very complex process, with many important issues being sidestepped or overlooked because they do not lend themselves to analysis by quantitative methods. The advice of Shulman (1981) should be heeded, and alternative approaches to examining the phenomena in question should be developed. Levinson-Rose and Menges (1981) suggest as qualitative approaches that might satisfy this concern, ethnographic methods, disciplined class studies, and structured clinical interviews. Weinholtz's (1981) doctoral dissertation is an excellent example of an ethnographic study. He examined teaching rounds in a university hospital, a process that was time-consuming for the researcher but much more illuminating for the questions it addressed than a quantitative approach would have been. It is not that quantitative, comparative approaches are unsatisfactory for studying instructional problems; rather, they can and should be complemented with qualitative approaches. The question for the researcher then is: What new approaches can be developed and adapted for use in studying the entire arena of instruction in health professions education, in general, and approaches to instructional improvement, in particular?

A related issue is that there does not seem to be one overall faculty development and/or evaluation strategy that is effective in all cases or even in a majority of cases. Certain personal characteristics make some instructors more promising candidates for instructional improvement than others. This observation may also apply to groups of instructors or even to departments as a whole. Is there some way that this susceptibility might be identified, so that the effectiveness of faculty development efforts can be maximized? The average faculty or instructional developer can work with only a small number of instructors at any one time, and it would seem prudent to use that time as productively as possible. The question for the researcher then is: What characteristics of individuals and departments correlate most significantly with desire and capability to improve, and which types of approaches work best with each?

A final concern pertains to the inadequacy of criteria to determine the effect of any intervention. For the most part, criteria used in health professions educational research are instructor knowledge—as assessed by short posttests—and instructor attitude toward a variety of topics—as assessed by self-reports. Improved or modified instructional behavior and sensitivity are critical goals of most faculty development activities and, therefore, should be addressed in both objective and subjective ways. The final question for the researcher then is: What additional approaches and/or criteria can be developed to measure instructional behaviors and thus document the effect of various faculty development efforts? It appears that the efforts of faculty evaluation and development are worthwhile, but that conclusion is, as yet, somewhat difficult to document.

## References*

Adams, W. R., and others. "Research in Self-Evaluation for Clinical Teachers." *Journal of Medical Education*, 1974, *49*, 1166–1174. (IIIa)

Bazuin, C. H., and Yonke, A. M. "Improvement of Teaching Skills in a Clinical Setting." *Journal of Medical Education*, 1978, *53*, 377–382. (Ia)

Bergquist, W. H., and Phillips, S. R. *A Handbook for Faculty Development*. Vol. 1. Washington, D.C.: Council for the Advancement of Small Colleges, 1975. (IIb)

Bergquist, W. H., and Phillips, S. R. *A Handbook for Faculty Development*. Vol. 2. Washington, D.C.: Council for the Advancement of Small Colleges, 1977. (Ia, IIc)

Bland, C. J. *Faculty Development Through Workshops*. Springfield, Ill.: Thomas, 1980. (IIb)

Bland, C. J., and others. "Effectiveness of Faculty Development Workshops and Family Medicine." *Journal of Family Practice*, 1979, *9*, 453–458. (IIb)

Boozer, C. H., and others. "Formal Training in Education for Dental Educators: A Pilot Program." *Journal of Dental Education*, 1977, *41*, 248–252. (IIa)

*Numbers and letters in parentheses at ends of bibliographical entries refer to categories in Table 1.

Bronstein, R. A. *Teacher Evaluation in Health Professions Education: A Study of the Impact of ICARE.* Denver, Colo.: Association for Continuing Medical Laboratory Education, 1978. (ED 190 586) (IIIa)

Buckner, K. E. "Continuing Education for Nurse Faculty Members." *Nursing Forum*, 1974, *13*, 393–401. (IIc)

Carrier, C. A. *Consulting with University Faculty: A Model for Teaching Improvement.* Unpublished manuscript, University of Minnesota Instructional Systems, 1980. (Ia)

Centra, J. "Two Studies on the Utility of Student Ratings for Improved Teaching." In *SIR Report No. 2.* Princeton, N.J.: Educational Testing Service, 1972. (IIIa, IIc)

Centra, J. "Effectiveness of Student Feedback in Modifying College Instruction." *Journal of Educational Psychology*, 1973, *65*, 395–401. (IIIc)

Centra, J. *Faculty Development Practices in U.S. Colleges and Universities.* Princeton, N.J.: Educational Testing Service, 1976.

Chambers, D. "Faculty Evaluation: Review of the Literature Most Pertinent to Dental Education." *Journal of Dental Education*, 1977, *55*, 290–300. (IIIc)

Clark, M., and Blackburn, R. *Assessing Faculty Performance: A Testing Method.* Presentation to the American Educational Research Association annual meeting, Toronto, Canada, March 31, 1978. (IIIa, IIIb)

Connell, K. J., Alberti, J. M., and Piotrowski, Z. H. "What Does It Take for Faculty Development to Make a Difference?" *Educational Horizons*, 1975, *5*, 108–115. (Ib)

Cosbergue, J. "Role of Faculty Development in Clinical Education." In M. K. Morgan and D. M. Irby (Eds.), *Evaluating Clinical Competence in the Health Professions.* St. Louis, Mo.: Mosby, 1978. (IIc)

Costin, F., Greenough, W. T., and Menges, R. J. "Student Ratings of College Teaching: Reliability, Validity and Usefulness." *Review of Educational Research*, 1971, *41*, 511–535. (IIIc)

Derry, J. O., and others. *The Cafeteria System: A New Approach to Course and Instructor Evaluation.* West Lafayette, Ind.: Purdue University, 1974. (IIIc)

Donnelly, F. A., and others. "Evaluation of Weekend Seminars for Physicians." *Journal of Medical Education*, 1972, *47*, 184–187. (IIb)

Erickson, G. R., and Erickson, B. L. "Improving College Teaching Evaluation of a Teaching Consultation Procedure." *Journal of Higher Education*, 1979, *50*, 670–683. (IIIc)

Farr, W. C., and Heider, M. "Medical Education Workshops: A Case Study of Their Influence on the Teaching Behaviors of Medical College Faculty." *Ohio State Medical Journal*, 1974, *70*, 102–105. (IIb)

Foley, R., and others. "A Departmental Approach for Appraising Lecturing Skills of Medical Teachers." *Medical Education*, 1976, *10*, 369–373. (Ia)

French, W., and Bell, C. H., Jr. *Organizational Development.* Englewood Cliffs, N.J.: Prentice-Hall, 1973. (IIc)

Gaff, J. G. *Toward Faculty Renewal: Advances in Faculty, Instructional, and Organizational Development.* San Francisco: Jossey-Bass, 1975.

Gerber, R. M. "The Mini Workshop." *Nursing Outlook*, 1980, *28*, 126–127. (IIb)

Gorecki, Y. "Faculty Peer Review." *Nursing Outlook*, 1977, *25*, 439–442. (IIIb)

Green, T. *The Activities of Teaching.* New York: McGraw-Hill, 1971.

Grimes, D. A., and others. "A Residency Elective in Medical Education." *Journal of Medical Education*, 1975, *50*, 365–370. (Ib)

Ham, T. H. *The Student as Colleague*. Ann Arbor, Mich.: University Microfilms, 1975. (Ib)

Holcomb, J. D., and others. "Preparing Faculty for the Allied Health Professions: A Follow-Up Study of a Program's Graduates." *Journal of Allied Health*, 1980, *9*, 41–49. (IIa)

Irby, D. "Clinical Faculty Development." In C. E. Ford (Ed.), *Clinical Education for the Allied Health Professions*. St. Louis, Mo.: Mosby, 1978. (Ia, IIIa)

Irby, D., and others. "A Model for the Improvement of Medical Faculty Lecturing." *Journal of Medical Education*, 1976, *51*, 403–409. (Ia)

Jacoby, K. E. "Behavioral Prescriptions for Faculty Based on Student Evaluation of Teaching." *American Journal of Pharmaceutical Education*, 1977, *41*, 8–13. (IIIc)

Jason, H., Slotnick, H. G., and Lefever, R. D. *Faculty Development Survey: Final Report*. Washington D.C. Association of American Medical Colleges, 1977. (IIc)

Jedrychowski, J. R., and Galligani, D. J. "Longitudinal Evaluation of a Teacher Education Course Presented by Dental Faculty." *Journal of Dental Education*, 1978, *42*, 579–583. (IIb)

Kellogg Foundation, W. K. *Action Programs for Developing Allied Health Educators*. Battle Creek, Mich.: W. K. Kellogg Foundation, 1977. (IIa)

Koen, F. M. "A Faculty Education Development Program and an Evaluation of Its Evaluation." *Journal of Medical Education*, 1976, *51*, 854–855. (IIb)

Koffman, M., and Theall, M. *Instructional Development Activities in a Faculty Development Program*. Presentation at American Educational Research Association annual meeting, Boston, April 10, 1980. (ED 185 937) (IIc)

Kohler, C. L. *Advanced Instruction in Medical Settings*. Unpublished manuscript, College of Medicine, University of Kentucky, 1981. (Ia)

Kotzan, J. A., and Entrekin, D. N. "Development and Implementation of a Factor-Analyzed Faculty Evaluation Instrument for Undergraduate Pharmacy Instruction." *American Journal of Pharmaceutical Education*, 1978, *42*, 114–118. (IIIc)

Lancaster, G. J., Mendelson, M. A., and Ross, G. R. "The Utilization of Student Instructional Ratings in Medical Colleges." *Journal of Medical Education*, 1979, *54*, 657–659. (IIIc)

Lazerson, A. J. "Training for Teaching: Psychiatry Residents as Teachers in an Evening College." *Journal of Medical Education*, 1972, *47*, 576–578. (IIIb)

Leichsenring, M. "Teaching Seminars for New Faculty." *Nursing Outlook*, 1972, *20*, 528–531. (IIb)

Levinson-Rose, J., and Menges, R. J. "Improving College Teaching: A Critical Review of Research." *Review of Educational Research*, 1981, *51*, 403–434.

Lindquist, J. (Ed.). *Designing Teaching Improvement Programs*. Berkeley, Calif.: Pacific Soundings Press, 1978. (IIc)

Littlefield, J. *University of Texas Health Science Center at San Antonio Faculty Development Teaching Skills Program*. Paper presented at the American Educational Research Association, San Francisco, April 8, 1979. (IIb)

McGaghie, W. C., and others. "A Multicomponent Program to Increase Family Physicians' Faculty Skills." *Journal of Medical Education*, 1981, *56*, 803–811. (IIa)

McKeachie, W. J., and Lin, Y. G. "Using Student Ratings and Consultation to Improve Teaching." *British Journal of Educational Psychology*, 1980, *50*, 168–174. (IIIc)

McNeil, J., and Popham, W. "The Assessment of Teacher Competence." In R. Travers (Ed.), *Second Handbook of Research in Teaching*, Chicago: Rand McNally, 1973.

Meleca, C. B., and Schimpfhauser, F. *A House Staff Training Program to Improve the Clinical Instructor.* Paper presented to Conference on Research in Medical Education, Washington, D.C., Nov. 13, 1976. (IIb)

Miller, G. E. *Educating Medical Teachers.* Cambridge, Mass.: Harvard University Press, 1980. (I, Ib, II, IIa, IIb, IIc, IIIb)

Palmer, J. D. K., O'Leary, J. P., and Sterling, H. M. "Interfaculty Research-Training Crossover: An Experiment in Medical Education." *Journal of Medical Education*, 1967, *42*, 1096–1100. (Ib)

Patridge, M., Harris, T., and Petzel, R. "Implementation and Evaluation of a Faculty Development Program to Improve Clinical Teaching." *Journal of Medical Education*, 1980, *55*, 711. (Ia)

Prentice, E. D., and Metcalf, W. K. "A Teaching Workshop for Medical Educators." *Journal of Medical Education*, 1974, *49*, 1031–1034. (IIb)

Purohit, A. A., and Magoon, A. J. "Critical Issues in Teaching and Student Evaluations." *American Journal of Pharmaceutical Education*, 1977, *41*, 317–325. (IIIc)

Rippey, R. M. "Student Evaluations of Professors: Are They of Value?" *Journal of Medical Education*, 1975, *50*, 951–958. (IIIc)

Rippey, R. M. *The Evaluation of Teaching in Medical Schools.* New York: Springer, 1980. (III, IIIa, IIIb, IIIc)

Rotem, A., and Glasman, N. S. "On the Effectiveness of Student Evaluative Feedback to University Instructors." *Review of Educational Research*, 1979, *49*, 497–511. (IIIc)

Rous, S. N., and others. "The Improvement of Faculty Teaching Through Evaluation: A Follow-Up Report." *Journal of Surgical Research*, 1972, *13*, 262–266. (IIIc)

Sall, S., and others. "Improvement of Faculty Teaching Performance in a Department of Obstetrics and Gynecology by Student Evaluation." *American Journal of Obstetrics and Gynecology*, 1976, *124*, 217–221. (IIIc)

Sauter, R. C., and Walker, J. K. "A Theoretical Model for Faculty Peer Evaluations." *American Journal of Pharmaceutical Education*, 1976, *40*, 165–166. (IIIb)

Schaffer, D. R. "A Faculty Growth Contracting Model for Allied Health Schools." *Journal of Allied Health*, 1980, *9*, 233–241. (IIc, IIIa)

Schein, E. J. *Process Consultation: Its Role in Organizational Development.* Reading, Mass.: Addison-Wesley, 1969. (Ia)

Scriven, M. *The Methodology of Evaluation.* AERA Monograph Series on Curriculum Evaluation, No. 1. Chicago: Rand McNally, 1967, 39–83. (IIIc)

Sheahan, J. "An Evaluation of a Workshop for Teachers of Nursing on an Individualized Teaching and Learning Strategy." *Journal of Advanced Nursing*, 1979, *4*, 647–659. (IIb)

Shulman, L. "Disciplines of Inquiry in Education: An Overview." *Educational Researcher*, 1981, *10*, 5–12.

Sibley, J. C. "Faculty Development: The Interface Between Assessment, Improvement, and Promotion of Teaching Excellence." A special session at the Association of American Medical Colleges annual meeting, Washington, D.C., Oct. 27, 1980. (IIc)

Sikes, W., Schlesinger, L. E., and Seashore, C. N. *Renewing Higher Education from Within: A Guide for Campus Change Teams*. San Francisco: Jossey-Bass, 1974. (IIc)

Skeff, K. M. *Evaluation of a Method for Improving the Teaching Skills of the Attending Physician*. Unpublished doctoral dissertation, Stanford University, 1981. (IIIb, IIIc)

Spitzer, W. O. "A New Advanced Studies Program for Faculty Development in Primary Care." *Journal of Family Practice*, 1978, *6*, 1053–1057. (IIa)

Stritter, F. T. "Collaborative Research as Faculty Development." A special session at the Association of American Medical Colleges annual meeting, Washington, D.C., Oct. 27, 1980. (Ib)

Stritter, F. T., and Hain, J. D. "A Workshop in Clinical Teaching." *Journal of Medical Education*, 1977, *52*, 155–157. (IIb)

Stritter, F. T., Hain, J. D., and Grimes, D. A. "Clinical Teaching Reexamined." *Journal of Medical Education*, 1975, *50*, 876–882. (Ib)

Weinholtz, D. *A Study of Instructional Leadership During Medical Attending Rounds*. Unpublished doctoral dissertation, University of North Carolina at Chapel Hill, 1981.

Wergin, J. F. "Evaluating Faculty Development Programs." In J. A. Centra (Ed.), *Renewing and Evaluating Teaching: New Directions for Higher Education*. Vol. 17. San Francisco: Jossey-Bass, 1977.

Wergin, J. F., Mason, E. J., and Munson, P. J. "The Practice of Faculty Development: An Experience-Derived Model." *Journal of Higher Education*, 1976, *47*, 289–308.

Westberg, J., and Jason, H. "The Enhancement of Teaching Skills in U.S. Medical Schools: An Overview and Some Recommendations." *Medical Teacher*, 1981, *3*, 100–104. (IIIa, IIIb, IIIc)

*Richard M. Caplan*

# 14

# Continuing Education and Professional Accountability

Many of the large issues that cluster around continuing education relate to general philosophical, social, and economic changes—changes that impinge not only on physicians but on those in all health disciplines and, for that matter, on essentially all professional and quasi-professional groups in modern American society. These issues include the knowledge explosion, the knowledge delivery explosion, public clamor for assurance of competence and high-quality performance, increasing regulation and monitoring by various levels of government, improvements in educational methods, questions of professional image and turf, evaluation of effectiveness, and many others. In my view, the similarities of the issues among the health-related professions are far greater than the differences. The majority of the research in continuing *health* education, however, has been done in the "laboratory" of continuing *medical* education.

George Miller's article "Continuing Education for What?" (1967) proved to be not just a milestone to mark distance but a signpost that pointed a new direction. Its major emphasis on competence and performance, not just acquisition of knowledge, and on continuing learning, not just continuing instruction, have guided the thinking and direction of the continuing health education (CHE) movement ever since. That frequently cited article proclaimed that "we have been educating for the wrong thing" (p. 326) and must turn to a *process* model rather than a *content* model of education. Also in that article, Miller cited the comic strip character, Pogo, whose line "We have met the enemy and they are us" has continued to echo loudly through the literature of CHE. George Miller was a crucial figure in the kind of development that the historian of science, Thomas Kuhn (1970), has termed "a scientific revolution." Miller persuaded others to look at health education in a different way. By asking a new set of questions, he sensed puzzles and contradictions that needed solutions. That caused educators to adopt new basic assumptions and turn in a different direction. He urged the use of the scientific method to study the totality of medical education, and he developed the necessary climate and training base to prepare large numbers of enthusiastic disciples in a new paradigm. In his latest book (Miller, 1980), however, he begins to caution against the narrowness of the experimental science paradigm (see discussion of *paradigm* in "Summary and Recommendations" section of this chapter).

Houle (1980, p. 3) states that "every profession now has members who vigorously oppose what they regard as the excessive promotion of continuing education." If continuing medical education (CME) is defined as Hubbard (1978, p. 190) did—"keeping up with advancing knowledge and the ability to apply advancing knowledge through improved skills and techniques"—and if our society considers education in general to be good rather than bad, then how can we account for those to whom Houle refers? This chapter will attempt to answer that question as it explores and comments upon the assessment of health care practices in relation to the rise of continuing education (CE) over the past twenty years.

An alternative definition of CME is the one adopted in July 1979 by the American Medical Association's House of Delegates: "Continuing medical education is composed of any education or training which serves to maintain, develop, or increase the knowledge, interpretive and reasoning proficiencies, applicable technical skills, professional performance standards, or ability for interpersonal relationships that a physician uses to provide the service needed by patients or the public" (Council on Medical Education, 1979, pp. 140-141). This definition is important because it establishes what sorts of activities may be counted as CME when a physician applies for the Physician's Recognition Award of the American Medical Association. That, in turn, has large practical consequences, because the award has utility in meeting many CME requirements now faced by a great many American physicians.

It is historically inaccurate to call the concept of "life long learning" a *new* replacement for the notion that education is the preparation for a lifetime of doing. Socrates and Plato, for example, recognized that education is a lifelong process and clearly favored it. Osler was a modern eloquent proponent of this view. Many developments within Western civilization since the Renaissance have led to an accelerating desire to maximize the growth and development of individual talents. The economic and social shock waves that accompanied the Industrial Revolution have provided greater leisure and affluence in developed nations to allow the luxury to promote such individual fruition. Any idea that the information and skills obtained during one's formal education would suffice throughout a career has surely evaporated in the years since World War II. Few practitioners remain active today who have a static conception of the corpus of knowledge they would need. The growth of specialism since World War II also fostered the changing attitude.

A development of monumental importance in the CE world, parallel to the growing acceptance of the concept of lifelong learning, is the fecund notion that the learning of adults is qualitatively different from the learning of children. Credit for that development goes especially to Houle and to Knowles. Knowles' (1970) conceptual framework of androgogy (the teaching of adults) in contrast to pedagogy (the teaching of children) has many vital implications: the independent maturity of adults, their focus on realistic problem solving for practical and immediate ends, their base in their own rich life experiences, their ability to learn from each other, and their tendency to learn once their needs become clear to them through opportunities for self-assessment and other feedback. This androgogic perspective has painted an exciting vista of the future, as well as stirred deep discontent with the conceptions, methods, and results of millennia-old approaches to instruction.

In biomedical science and health care, the cliché "knowledge explosion" is part of the basis for the immense growth of the "CE industry." Ruhe (1980) has described the continuing evolution of all three levels of medical education (undergraduate, graduate, and continuing) but observes that "the rate of change is much faster in CME because it is the newest and least well-defined area." He also adds, "It is common to speak of the chaotic condition of continuing medical education. Those who view this with alarm and would attempt to set things in order immediately should understand that a certain amount of time is required for maturation and definition of a new component of the total lifetime learning of the physician. . . . Quick resolution of all of the problems and standardization of all of the activity is not only impossible but also undesirable at this stage in the evolution of the field" (p. 95).

Only an awakening Rip Van Winkle who had not yet visited a health science library could think to deny the present prodigious annual increase of new biomedical information—much of it even new knowledge, some of it probably even truth. For example, a recent ten-year review of the medical literature on the single subject of hepatitis yielded over 16,000 citations. Such impressive development has led to an often-heard cliché that the half-life of such information is five years—or some other small whole integer—as if such a numerical statement were a measured truth rather than simply an attractive metaphor. Whether metaphor or not, the concepts of the "knowledge explosion" and the "half-life of knowledge" have proved yeasty, and the subsequent ferment has contributed to the growth of the CHE industry. Even George Miller (1967) himself may have fanned this fire of "galloping obsolescence": "there is little dissent from the view that the world of medicine is changing so rapidly as a result of contemporary research that what is current today will be dated in a few months and obsolete in a few years" (p. 320).

### Growth of the CE Industry

Felch (1981b) submits the splendid notion "that CME is a mindset more than an activity. Doctors with a real bent for learning approach each patient as an intellectual challenge, so that anything out of the ordinary will trigger off the reflex to look it up, ask a colleague, seek a consultation. It's the attitude, we believe, that makes for useful learning, not the scheduling of episodic educational activities. Physicians having the right mindset—the unremitting attitude of intellectual curiosity—practice medical education that is truly continuing" (p. 3). Nevertheless, CE has become at the same time an industry, a word laden with the evil connotations of ugliness, commercialism, pollution, and exploitation, mixed inextricably with the virtuous intimations of progress, advance, improvement, well-being, and utopia. The very growth in numbers of CE offerings and enrollments, if it did not suggest the growth curve of a flourishing industry, might suggest at best a rapidly developing infant, or at worst a malignancy. Whether one counts the formal courses, or any of the local or regional options, or home study activities, or new-technology apparatus as a conduit to receive information, the growth of CE has been stunning. In addition, one may think of growth as implied in the term *knowledge explosion*, in the emphasis on lifelong learning, in the clarification of adult learning principles, and in the concepts involved in diffusion of knowledge. And, of course, one may consider and be awed by growth in terms of its economic consequences. (For an extensive presentation of the historical development of contemporary continuing medical education, the reader should consult the excellent monograph by Richards [1978a].)

L. A. Miller (1979) attempted to translate all this activity into a dollar value. His earlier estimate of 2 billion dollars annually for CME has been widely quoted, and in 1979 he published an updated figure of 3.6 billion dollars, including income lost when physicians are away from practice for educational reasons. Richards (1981) has argued, however, that CME is integral to the practice of medicine and no more warrants being considered as time "lost" from practice than the time one spends in examining a patient or performing a procedure. Furthermore, Miller's computation related principally to formal course enrollments, that is, to that portion of the activity sometimes called the tip of the CE iceberg. This iceberg metaphor envisions a far greater amount of below-the-surface individualized activity taking place in community hospitals and local organizations and then still greater learning from trial-and-error, peer conversations, and, of course, reading. Among the many formats of CME proposed in many surveys made over the past twenty years, reading the medical literature wins regularly in expressions of interest, value, and frequency (Caplan and Yarcheski, 1974; Stinson and Mueller, 1980).

**Personal Motivation**

Growth of the continuing education industry has naturally focused some scholarly inquiry on the motivation of practitioners to engage in any of these activities. A factor-analysis performed by Burgess (1971) on responses from 1,046 persons identified seven factors that described respondents' motivations for participating in group educational activities. More recently, two studies have reported similar analyses. Cervero (1981) reported on a factor-analytic study of responses from 211 practicing physicians who completed a thirty-four-item Participation Reasons Scale. He found four major categories of reasons for participating in CME: (1) to maintain and improve professional competence and service to patients; (2) to understand oneself as a professional; (3) to interact with colleagues; and (4) to enhance personal and professional position. He properly observes that "to evaluate the total impact of CME, unanticipated outcomes as well as stated program goals should be assessed" (p. 34). Those who think evaluation can be performed *only* in terms of stated objectives will clearly miss important arenas of evaluation and outcome. Richards and Cohen (1981), in reviewing the motivation literature, classified physicians' motivations for CME attendance into five categories: (1) as an integral part of professionalism; (2) as a result of interest in topical subjects; (3) as a means of validating or modifying prior learning and behavior; (4) as a means of obtaining an identified learning or behavioral objective; and (5) as a change of pace from practice routine and an opportunity for social contact with other physicians. These two lists reveal motivations that should be considered appropriate and necessary for both personal and patient care reasons, even though a strict behavioralist interpretation would not grant value to some of these motivations on the technical grounds that, by definition, they produce no observable change in the learners. Rubenstein (1973, p. 911) enunciated an important justification for continuing education in somewhat different language in his Back-to-Medical-School Program: "The goals of this project are the improvement of health care *and the invigoration of the intellectual pursuits of practitioners*" (emphasis added). The vigor of intellectual pursuits may be a soft concept for measurement, but to deny its importance is folly. Perhaps it can be considered a component of what Cervero (1981) describes as "understanding oneself as a professional" and what Richards and Cohen (1981) call "an integral part of professionalism."

## The Demand for Accountability

Houle (1980) provides an introduction to the demand for accountability—a general social phenomenon that has mushroomed in the past twenty years and obtains nurturance from such related developments as consumerism, back to basics, behavioralism, management by objectives, and widespread disaffection with, or even distrust of, all professionals and elites. We can wonder with him whether our society has oversold the value of education or the educational process: "As the amount of educational services has increased, following the general principle that 'more is better,' so has the skepticism of at least some highly qualified observers. . . . In profession after profession . . . efforts at teaching and learning seem to have had too little effect upon practice. A sense of despondency is sometimes expressed even by those who have devoted much of their careers to the process of lifelong learning" (p. 4).

The concepts of Brown and Uhl (1970) and their "bi-cycle approach"—an attempt to relate carefully planned educational effort to detailed study of patient care—have been powerfully influential and fruitful. The growing cadre of CME professionals has been weaned on the logic of those ideas and guided by the related urging that measurable change in process and outcome of health care is the only issue that matters in CME. It is further implied that CME providers who cannot demonstrate objective evidence of such change in behavior or health outcome should feel themselves to be at least inept and perhaps useless. However, many studies (as well as common sense) force our admission that a "physician's knowledge is not necessarily related to his actual performance" (Sanazaro, 1976, p. 247). Sanazaro also observes that "some physicians look upon (traditional) CME as an educational exercise somehow divorced from their actions in treating patients" (p. 247). Nonetheless, it seems unreasonable to protest against the desire to relate CME to actual patient care and to use it directly in the process of care and in the effort to improve health outcomes. George Miller, Sanazaro, Brown, and others have been valuable prods, and they have been effective, even if results have been less rapid and pervasive than they might wish.

The public clamor for the accountability of physicians has been a component of the similar clamor for accountability of every member of our society unto every other member. In America, litigation constitutes a major form of accountability. American law now requires that physicians be current in their knowledge and practices (Corbett, 1979). Hospitals, other health workers, counselors, even clergymen and attorneys are at risk. The huge increase in malpractice actions in the 1970s has added greatly to the sense of apprehension about competent practice. The pressure for accountability has been felt not only in the increasing instances of litigation and the various responses made to it but through multiple avenues of regulation. Physicians encounter societal controls through the states' authority over licensure and relicensure. The federal government exercises controls on physicians' behavior through its handling of payment mechanisms, through the activities of health planning agencies, and through the Professional Standards Review Organization (PSRO) mechanism. The Joint Commission on the Accreditation of Hospitals (JCAH) imposes many rules on applicant hospitals, which in turn exert pressure to influence physicians who hold staff privileges. Such pressure molds what shall be done as an institutional effort in CE and how the quality of care is to be monitored and modified. Some hospitals have seen fit to impose on their medical staffs their own CME requirements for continuing staff privileges. State medical societies—some fifteen of them in January 1981—require CME as a condition of continued membership. Some specialty societies as well, starting in 1947 with the American Academy of General (now Family) Practice, require CME as a condition of continuing membership; still others offer voluntary "certificate-of-accomplishment" programs modeled after the American Medical Association's Physician Recognition Award. Many medical specialty boards now have mandatory or voluntary processes of recertification.

Among the most powerful and worrisome of the pressures related to accountability has been the mandating of CE requirements by state governments as a condition of annual relicensure. Once again, Richards (1978a and 1978b) has chronicled well the history of this development in medicine. The debate about mandatory CE has continued for over a decade—ranging from persuasive anti-mandatory arguments, such as those of Brown and Uhl (1970), to positive arguments, such as those of Derbyshire (1979). For example, Derbyshire reported with satisfaction that New Mexico's experience led to the discontinuation of 256 medical licenses, 73 held by practitioners in New Mexico. About half the states had accepted the arguments favoring mandatory CME when the "bandwagon" wave of legislation ceased in 1979. A factor fostering the legislative inclination toward mandatory CME for relicensure was its support by groups of physicians and organized medicine, partially out of conviction that the practice would be meritorious. Partially, however, that support was conceived as a defense against potential legislative intrusion into the actual arena of patient care, with its prospect of legislative inspectors checking patient interview videotapes, reading patient records, requiring practicing physicians to pass pencil-and-paper examinations, and so on. The fear of the state's intervention (a la George Orwell's *1984*) seemed sufficiently great to make some leaders recommend mandatory CME as a pacifier or gesture of appeasement.

### Confusion of Education with Quality Assurance

Much of the argument about mandatory CE centers on the question of how effective CE can be in keeping good things good while purging the system of its weaknesses or evils. It seems easier now than a decade ago to recognize not just the similarity and overlap of education with quality assurance practices but the distinctions that should be made between them. As Thompson (1981) puts it: "Quality assurance is an aid to continuing education. It is a way to identify teaching topics and to make them relevant. It can also be an effective way to assess the impact of continuing education sessions. But not all continuing education has to relate to quality assurance activities. Likewise, not all quality assurance activities are educational" (p. 5).

But this distinction has not always been clearly made. A large educational effort is needed to clarify what is knowledge, what is competence, and what is high-quality performance. I believe, however, that more educators—as well as physicians, licensure boards, legislatures, and the public—may be starting to perceive this more clearly. Several recent examples from the literature may be helping to reinforce what one might have thought was obvious enough. Essentially confirming the classic Rockford study of Williamson, Alexander, and Miller (1967), Wigton and others (1981) employed reminders about anemia in patients' charts when the patient's hemoglobin level fell more than 1 gm below the hospital's "normal" limits. Even with the reminders, 16 percent were missed or ignored by both "control" and "educated" groups. The authors refer to the "regular and reproducible phenomenon of overlooked abnormal laboratory results." Once again, it was demonstrated that educational effort does not assure quality performance. Wilbur (1978) asserts that "although one cannot practice competently without knowledge, one certainly can practice incompetently with knowledge. . . . Accumulating evidence that what the physician learned improved his knowledge, competence, and performance and benefited his patients will be enormously costly. Moreover, the evidence will, at best, be difficult to evaluate scientifically." Mazmanian and others (1979, p. 379) put it: "CME can contribute to the improvement of patient care, but CME alone cannot guarantee it. Nor can the public, educators, or physicians act alone in transforming the delivery of health care through continuing education." Gonnella and Storey (1981, p. 14) have been forceful and helpful in striving to "point the direction out of the present chaos, and to restate reasonable boundaries for 'continuing' medical education." They lash out at "the tendency . . . to confuse intermediate educational objectives with long-term patient care objectives" and issue a clear call for requiring physicians to "provide proof that they continue to upgrade their knowledge and skills, and maintain the proper attitudes which will result in good patient care. . . . To reassure the public by using CME credits as an indication of competence is misleading" (p. 14).

A study by Weinberg and others (1977) asked physicians to estimate the scores they would likely attain on tests of knowledge and skill during an advanced course on cardiac life support. Their subjects were relatively successful at predicting correctly their own knowledge level but tended to overestimate their skills considerably. Their postcourse predictions were more accurate than precourse estimates of both knowledge and skills, and both showed improvement. This study showed that discrepancies may exist between knowledge and competence (ability to perform). But then, who really doubted that it could or would be so? Almost all the research designed to demonstrate the existence of such an incongruity has been successful. Furthermore, Weinberg's study did not measure long-range retention, but studies that attempt it show a decline in retention unless some sort of reinforcing experience intervenes. But again, who would not predict that? Is it necessary to continue to *prove* that Ebbinghaus's classical curve of forgetting can be believed?

A recent article by Farrington, Felch, and Hare (1980) compares and contrasts three widely used methods of assessing physician competence: CME participation, board reexamination, and performance monitoring. Their description emphasizes again the distinctions among knowledge, competence, and performance and how they might be assessed. These authors are optimistic that performance monitoring—via inpatient audit at the hospital and outpatient audit at the office—will yet prove feasible. They refer to "the medical profession, apparently obsessed with the need to prove itself" and consider that obsession as part of the response to the public and professional clamor for accountability.

Many vocal CHE professionals seem to be perfectionists, zealots with a great sense of mission. They argue that if the major goal of CHE is to improve patient care, then any apparent failure to demonstrate improved patient care is properly interpreted as a failure of the educational effort. Greenburg, Bruegel, and Peskin (1977) ask "how does one go about defining an effective (educational) experience in methodology to assure (that) the primary objective, improved patient care, is attained?" (p. 708). This question and others of its type seem to place on the educator the burden of *delivering education that assures improved patient care*. The time has come, I believe, to assert that *such an assurance is not the proper charge to educators or to education alone*. It is proper for educators to work toward practical and patient-oriented goals, but they should no longer docilely accept blame and develop feelings of guilt when their educational labors cannot be shown in every instance to have produced the desired perfection in the process or outcome of care. To try to use the educational effort as a springboard to better care and outcome is noble; but when inadequacies of measurement, multilevel politics, shortages of funds, and society's habits and inertia all impede the outcome, educational effort should not be made the whipping boy for the resulting frustration.

### Assessment of Care Practices

Reasonable it is, and consonant with principles of adult learning, that identification of a "need to know" or a "need to be able to do" would be a proper first step in developing a rational and effective CE effort. The renaissance of the medical audit during the past fifteen years has been viewed as a method par excellence to determine what needs to be learned. The "bi-cycle" concepts of Brown and Uhl (1970) describe a system for deriving educational needs from the study of patient care data. A great deal of enthusiasm greeted these ideas in some quarters, and in the past decade the compelling logic of the "bi-cycle" formulation seems to have become well-known and well-accepted. The JCAH and PSRO requirements that hospitals perform medical care evaluation studies arose in the context of "bi-cycle" interest. The *potential* impact on quality of care seemed great. But panaceas are hard to come by. Although the basic logic of the "bi-cycle" system seems impeccable, time has led to a decreased enthusiasm and a more temperate expectation about what peer review and medical audit can contribute to needs assessment. Nelson (1976) expressed frustration at all the data accumulated in the audit process, so little of which seemed able to work its way back into the educational loop of the "bi-cycle" process. With huge numbers of such audits being performed during the past decade, immense labor and expense have indeed produced immense amounts of data, but few workers have reported any impressive success in translating the findings of deficiency into CE programmatic effort. Perhaps many small successes occur in community hospitals, as they should, without making their way into the scientific literature. Part of that paucity of reported success may be explained by the findings of Ashbaugh and McKean (1976), who performed fifty-five audits on thirty-seven topics involving 5,499 patient records. Of the deficiencies disclosed, only 6 percent were thought to be due to lack of knowledge or to be the sort of problem amenable to an educational remedy. The other 94 percent of deficiencies were performance deficits, and their correction had to depend upon administrative maneuvers and attempts to motivate individuals to behave in ways they already knew how to behave. However, their study did provide two examples of effectiveness of CME efforts addressed to the 6 percent educational gap: a decreased incidence of removal of normal appendices during primary appendectomy and a desirably increased use of packed blood cells rather than whole blood for transfusion.

Why are so many audits less fruitful than their logic and proponents seem to promise? These may be some of the reasons:

- Too few persons involved really understand the language and logic of the audit process; therefore, the data they generate and the interpretations they make may well be inaccurate or inadequate.
- Audits often attempt to be too comprehensive, causing the amount of labor and data to become staggering. This problem is aggravated in multihospital or regional audits.
- The "wrong" topics are audited—for example, uncommon diseases, routine problems in which little goes awry, extremely difficult problems where medical knowledge and methods of treatment are insufficient.
- We may audit the wrong steps; that is, we too often study process activities that are not significantly related to the more important aspects of care or outcome.
- The word *audit* is still surrounded by negative connotations and arouses negative attitudes (perhaps through association with procedures of the Internal Revenue Service) and what Thompson (1981) calls: "a narrow negative definition. The emphasis was on meeting requirements, rather than on a wide range of substantive and productive activities. When we began to conduct patient care evaluation studies, we followed the didactic, absolute approach. We did 'audits' to find 'deficiencies' and to take 'corrective action' against 'deviant' people. . . . It has been difficult to integrate quality assurance findings with continuing education programs for a fundamental reason: continuing education traditionally has focused on health care professionals' knowledge and technical skills, while quality assurance activities have discovered the need for improvement in attitudes, clinical judgment, and communication skills" (p. 4).

Experience teaches that medical care evaluation studies identify real educational needs only if very competently performed and only for very limited purposes. Among other things, this suggests that shared medical care evaluation studies, as may be done throughout an entire PSRO, will not likely yield much substantive information that can lead either to useful education or to targeted remediation. That is because the large number of persons and institutions involved, with their highly variable approaches to the audit process, yields a large amount of noncomparable data. Drawing composite conclusions and attempting to prescribe effective remedies for such a diverse universe fall short of the necessary precision and individuality. Occasional studies look directly at individual physician performance. Two recent examples illustrate the use of performance data to tell us something clearly valuable. Manning and others (1980) developed a system for reviewing duplicates of prescriptions written by cooperating physicians. By studying the prescriptions, an "expert panel" was able to discern seven types of problems. The authors observed such a wide variety of prescribing practices that they concluded "that typical continuing medical education courses based on group trends in drug therapy may be an inadequate method for meeting the individual needs of practicing physicians" (p. 1114). Instead, the investigators designed individual learning packages that were returned to the participating practitioners. This was clearly an imaginative attempt to link CME to actual behavior in clinical practice. Unfortunately, no follow-up study has been reported, so we do not as yet know whether the effort produced a change in behavior of the target learners. In a second example, Linn (1980) used algorithms and treatment outcomes to judge quality of care for burn patients treated in hospital emergency rooms. He showed that mortality, morbidity, compliance with treatment regimens, and satisfaction with care were all significantly correlated with the process of care and were improved by their educational approach.

The National Board of Medical Examiners has expended much effort in recent years attempting to develop satisfactory measures of competence. Whether using pencil-and-paper format, latent image methods, or computer technology, patient management problems seem to have much promise, but the developmental work is slow, difficult, and expensive. Simulated patients, either live, filmed, or computerized, and monitored directly or via computer, also seem to offer long-range potential (Barrows, 1981). Until such methods provide us a more reliable, valid, and inexpensive way to monitor clinical performance, we will probably continue to be saddled with litigation, occasional peer intervention, and complaints made to boards of licensure, as our principal techniques for coping with seriously unsatisfactory performance. Some might not view such an arrangement as unreasonable, arguing that education—even preventive education or computer-diagnosed and administered education—ought not to be considered the proper avenue for dealing with lapses that arise largely from such "noneducational" events as physician debility (alcohol, drugs, age, illness), cupidity, or maladroitness in human relations.

The American Board of Family Practice has pioneered the use of office-record audits as a component of their mandatory recertification process. The American Society of Internal Medicine is also breaking ground with regard to office-audit techniques for monitoring care practices and identifying educational deficiencies or other kinds of lapses. And one must give credit to the visionary work of Weed (1969) in developing the problem-oriented medical record and integrating it with a computerized system of "self-correcting" and "self-educating" medical practice. One would have to be remarkably inattentive or reactionary to doubt that these applications of computers and other information technology will enter increasingly into the monitoring and guidance of the future practice of health care professionals.

Licensure by specialty is another administrative mechanism that some believe might help assure competence and excellent performance. The idea has had its proponents for decades; so far, our society has not deemed it wise. Until human beings and their manifold problems and illnesses can be categorized into mutually exclusive compartments, licensing by specialty would create an unenforceable and ineffectual fiasco. Likewise, highly controversial is the suggestion that a professional license should be granted from a national rather than a state agency. Such an approach rests on the hope that a national system of setting standards, monitoring practice, and judging individual practitioners would better achieve a perfection we now lack. The prospect for national licensure relates closely to the development of national health insurance. As the federal government pays more of health care costs, there develops a correspondingly greater pressure for control of all other aspects of the system. Richards (1978a) cites a prediction, made in 1938 by an influential senator during a speech given to the American Medical Association, that every doctor in America would soon need to pass a federal examination because of the inexorable movement of the federal government into so many other aspects of health. I think that predicted requirement less likely now than in 1938, but should that lawmaker ultimately prove prescient, I would predict more undesirable than desirable outcomes.

### Growth of CE in Community Hospitals

As formally identified CE became more abundant in the late 1960s and then became obligatory for many professionals during the 1970s, it was felt to be increasingly necessary to provide CE that was close to home and thereby less expensive, less time-consuming, and quickly available in response to a need to solve actual patient care problems. In retrospect, at least, it seems easy to see that CE at local hospitals would be likely to grow, and indeed it has. For example, each year since 1969 the annual course listings in the *Journal of the American Medical Association* show more and more CME programs being sponsored by local hospitals. Correspondingly, the proportion provided by medical schools has decreased, even though the actual numbers have increased. Many medical schools have spent great energy and much federal, state, and private money to promulgate such local activity. Overall, those stimulatory efforts are successful. In addition, over the past twenty years the occupational category "Director of Medical Education" has been instituted in many teaching hospitals, and those officers are often charged with trying to stimulate local efforts in CME. Another inducement came as medical malpractice decisions began to hold hospitals, as corporate entities, legally responsible for some aspects of care rendered in them. And still another prod in this same direction came when the JCAH established CE requirements for hospitals that desired its accreditation.

Greater ease of travel and the use of technical aids (telephone and radio conferences, videotape, telecommunication satellites, and so on) have made possible the "bringing" of experts into every community hospital. To the extent that

CE involves dissemination of information and interaction with experts, much progress has occurred in bringing biomedical advances quickly to the health professional, sometimes even before proper validation of the advances. Recognizing the importance of these activities and acknowledging the growth of assessment of care practices, quality assurance, and CE efforts in hospitals, Williamson (1977) published a prodigious effort of bibliographic scholarship to facilitate access to the relevant literature. But even with the aid of computers, the process of publication was slow. The reviewed articles in that impressive tome date only through 1972.

Pohlmann (1980), writing from the perspective of the community hospital, identifies four levels of educational need that those responsible for local educational planning can use to develop structured programs that are uniquely appropriate to the local situation:

- "automatic deficits" that arise because of advances in biomedical knowledge
- collective problems in diagnosis or treatment discovered through audits or record reviews (the "bi-cycle" model functions here)
- observed individual deficiencies that may be suspected to be index cases of a general lack of knowledge or skill
- problems that surface during periodic review of local clinical experience, such as complications, deaths, tumor boards, and so on

For example, in an illuminating study of hospital activity and the relationships between peers and authority, Munster (1978) constructed a set of "correct" answers prepared by an "expert committee" (not a peer group) regarding fourteen surgical procedures and the use of prophylactic antibiotics. He then gathered data from the chief of surgery at 133 of a possible 135 Veterans' Administration hospitals and reported that the overall "correct test score" averaged only 62 percent. Furthermore, he found that the chiefs of service were not monitoring staff performance to assure implementation of their own philosophies of care, nor did they generally even know what their individual staff members thought or did in this regard. Laissez-faire autonomy, not just the prerogative of private practice, was thus shown to be present in a large, bureaucratic medical system.

Neither professional schools, national and state or regional specialty societies, nor private entrepreneurs have ready access to patient care data at local hospitals. Clearly then, hospitals are playing and will continue to play a vital role in any CE of the future that relates closely to inpatient care. Not only that, but the hospital is the major locus for peer interaction, where clinically oriented conversation and the example of "educational influentials" (Hiss, MacDonald, and Davis, 1978) will continue to take place. Group practice settings increasingly help provide more such opportunity to physicians, but CME in the office, though rich in potential, remains largely unexplored and undeveloped.

### Criticism of CHE and Critique of the Criticism*

The present world of CHE certainly merits the wonderful descriptive phrase of William James: "a buzzing, booming confusion." Watts (1981) has well

*This section might perhaps be dubbed—with proper thanks and apology to Immanuel Kant—"A CRITIQUE OF (IM)PURE REASON(ING)," for it seems that much of what is unwarranted in the criticism stems from failure of precise thinking. The errors of reasoning are relatively simple ones, of the kind described in most introductory texts of logic.

described the complexities of the entire system. As one reads the literature, attends meetings, and listens to formal and informal speakers talk of CHE, one hears much critical comment and relatively little praise for the total entreprise. Comments like these are rampant:

- "There is little evidence that continuing education [courses] changes the behavior of doctors" (Stead, 1981, p. 2).
- "There has been a growing concern about the efficacy of many continuing medical education programs of conventional design" (Erviti and others, 1977, p. 85).

Such comments and others like them tend to convey the impression that "nobody ever got anything worthwhile from CHE." Such sweeping generalities are especially surprising when they come from individuals trained in the methods of logical scientific thinking and careful statement. An example of overgeneralizing and imprecise meaning can be found simply by asking, "What is *traditional* CHE?" I believe it cannot now be clearly defined—not regarding format, mode of transmission, site, or characteristics of teacher or learner. Perhaps at some earlier time, such as 1950, it was capable of crisp definition. But now the many kinds of instruction, their juxtaposition, and quality are so variegated that we do not communicate meaningfully when we use the phrase "traditional CHE." We would benefit by speaking more specifically about the kind of CHE we are discussing.

Recognizing how painfully seldom schemes of classification appeal to anyone but the originator, I have nonetheless grouped the criticisms of CHE into seven categories, about which I offer comments in an effort to help identify some lines of thought and research that are worth abandoning and others that are worth pursuing. The seven types of criticism I will address are these:

- CHE needs assessment is inadequate.
- CHE puts too much effort into attempts to transmit information and not enough into solving real problems.
- CHE is too didactic, that is, lecture-bound.
- There is no proof—no solid research to show—that CHE makes any difference.
- CHE fails to assure competence and proper performance.
- CHE is too expensive.
- Even if CHE has value, it doesn't do enough good.

**Adequacy of Needs Assessment**

Much of the criticism of CHE's needs assessment is justified if we are speaking of small groups of homogeneous learners, and especially if our $N = 1$. To the extent that CHE issues are chosen for an $N > 1$, then—practically by definition—content will be presented that will to some degree be inappropriate. If the group of learners is large, then surveys, grouped data, audits of practice, and analysis of health and illness trends will all yield wide variations of either felt or demonstrated needs. If the number of intended learners is large, then a committee representative of the intended learners, or even a committee of experts, will probably estimate the needs about as accurately as would more formal and "objective" means; this is because many planners and representatives are in tune with their constituencies.

When the group of learners is large and diverse, any method of choosing issues for the curriculum will necessarily fail to "hit the mark squarely" for a substantial number. To insist on any particular technique of needs assessment, especially the surveying of a large group, borders on fetishism. An enlightened and well-motivated teacher/planner may often do as well or better, if he or she is willing to validate the ideas with a small group of reactors from the potential learning audience. That planner must ultimately exercise substantial creativity, for no amount of needs-assessment data can in itself produce an educational effort of merit. The empathic and imaginative program planner can do wonders without the necessity of much *formal* inquiry into needs as long as there is effective communication with content specialists.

**Transmitting Information Versus Solving Problems**

Good health care practice requires large amounts of information that is constantly being modified, substantiated, or replaced. In any case, information is necessary and means are needed to convey it. Lectures, audiovisual packages, colleagues, and computers can all perform this function. What is essential is assurance that the methods for transmitting the information are *good.* A colleague assisting on an individual patient's problem may teach, or at least model, clinical problem solving; but that effort may help with only one problem. Efforts to obtain data about a physician's behavior over time—such as those entailed in a practice audit, in the analysis of duplicate prescriptions (Manning and others, 1980), or in the creation of a personal practice profile (Sivertson and others, 1973)—are laudable, but are currently very expensive and not totally reliable. Gradual improvement in technology, coupled with gradually expanding willingness to employ it, will increasingly permit the immediate application of pertinent information to the solution of problems.

**Overdependence on Lectures**

While some lectures and lecturers may deserve the criticism frequently leveled at them, lecturing can be a marvelously effective and inexpensive way not only to transmit information but also to demonstrate organization and selection, clarify confusing concepts and emphasize the more important ones, and provide orientation, motivation, enthusiasm, even inspiration. Miller (1980), himself an excellent lecturer, has tried to clarify his own criticism of lectures so that it pertains not to lecturing as a method or to any individual who employs it but to a *system of education that depends too heavily on lectures.*

**Proof of Impact**

The charge that there is no evidence that CHE makes any difference is a very serious and frequently heard accusation—one that I believe to be thoroughly false. The time has come to muster a rebuttal so that CHE can desist from its guilt inducing and wasteful quest for the "Holy Grail of Proof" that its efforts produce effects. There are several lines of argument.

*Observation and Common Sense.* Most physicians not fresh from medical school are practicing medicine in ways that differ significantly from what they learned in their undergraduate or graduate training. For example, older surgeons are replacing hip joints, inserting vascular grafts, and replacing opaque vitreous humor; new drugs are prescribed by essentially all practitioners; old procedures for laboratory and x-ray examinations are regularly replaced by superior methods; and doctors participate in many relatively new practices, such as peer review, medical audits, and patient education. All this change and the fact that so many doctors are doing things they did not learn in the years of formal training are evidence that they have obviously learned—and the total *system* must be given the credit.

*The Summit of the S-Shaped Curve.* As Miller (1967) observed about CME, we do our striving near the top of an s-shaped curve in a system with a great amount of excellence. Huge educational effort can therefore produce only small amounts of further improvement, in contrast to that which could be obtained in the steeper part of the curve (Figure 1). This contributes to the difficulty of demonstrating change.

*What the Literature Now Contains.* It is simply no longer true that the scientific literature contains no evidence that CHE efforts have been useful. Investigations by Talley (1978), Hein, Christopher, and Ferguson (1975), Mahan, Phillips, and Costanzi (1978), Klein, Charache, and Johannes (1981), Paino, Cline, and Demarest (1979), Wirtschafter and others (1979), Christiansen and Weinberg (1977), Pinkerton and others (1980), Linn (1980), and the eight studies summarized by Stein (1981) are all examples that provide such evidence. True, the effects reported in these studies were not always as great as the authors hoped, and there are many other studies whose authors report no effect of a particular CHE effort. However, to generalize about so multifactorial a world as CHE from particular failures is dangerous, especially when one considers how situation-specific educational interventions are, and how near to impossible is our ability to control so many of the variables, especially when we are concerned with long-range effects.

A major logical difficulty arises when we try to prove in the usual scientific way that any *one limited effort* makes a big difference, or even a statistically significant difference. The difficulty is illustrated by Goldfinger (1982), who, in responding to the study by Sibley and others (1982), makes an excellent case for "contamination" in his description of the necessarily multiple ways in which physicians learn. Further, just as we do not see an electron but can know its presence by its tracks in a bubble chamber, so we may not see the outcome of any single CHE activity, but its effect may appear in a different way, place, or time, and the connection to the original may be lost. Much mischief results from people's failure to understand or remember that something may be significant, that is, important or valuable, without being *statistically* significant. Another point frequently overlooked is that in *almost all instances* the measuring instruments available to CHE research are unquestionably inadequate to the task. No measurement can be better than the yardstick used to make it; yet we attempt, with grievously defective tools, to measure groups that are diverse in age, experience, and practice setting and location, and we further attempt global, statistical descriptions of that extremely heterogeneous population. The inevitably contaminated laboratory, the permanently uncontrollable variables, and the nongeneralizability of results

**Figure 1. Relationship of Effort to Benefit in Continuing Health Education.**

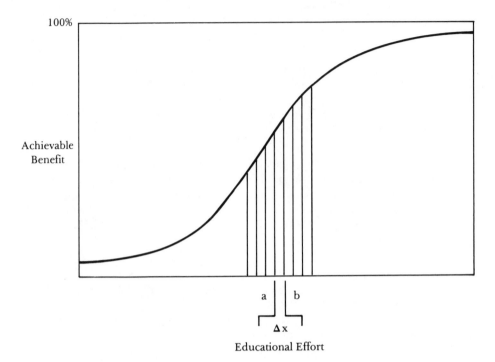

Educational Effort

will continue to characterize most CHE research. We must be more willing to trust our students and distrust our measuring instruments and experimental designs.

Much criticism has been aimed at CHE for years as a result of studies like that of Lewis and Hassanein (1970) that failed to show, for example, short-term improvement in the infant mortality rate in Kansas even though 7 percent of Kansas practitioners attended obstetrical and pediatric short courses at the University of Kansas. It should be obvious that infant mortality, if not irrelevant, is certainly a grossly insensitive measure of the many bits of pediatric and obstetrical learning acquired by the small proportion of Kansas physicians who attended those courses. Yet this study and others with similar large methodological flaws have been cited repeatedly to buttress the assertion that traditional CHE accomplishes nothing. When the research looks for specific and limited results of instruction that was tailored to a clear purpose, as in the many studies cited earlier, favorable results have been shown.

*The Test of Statistical Significance.* Investigators have naturally tried to use the mensurational tools of science, including statistical techniques, to judge whether control and experimental *populations* differ from each other. Such tests of significance deal with numerical values treated collectively. The meaning in human terms of each number in the data is of no consequence whatever to the mathematical computations, but it may matter immensely to an individual. Consider a clinical example: If in one hundred cases of anemia (8 gm of hemoglobin/100 ml of blood), ninety-nine of the patients have an iron deficiency and one has pernicious anemia, and if all are treated with nothing but therapeutic injections of vitamin $B_{12}$, then only the one patient with pernicious anemia will respond favorably and show a normal posttreatment hemoglobin. When ninety-nine patients with hemoglobin of 8 gm/100 ml and one with hemoglobin of 14 gm/100 ml are then compared to the initial population, there will be *no statistically significant difference* in the two *populations.* Yet consider the significance, the *clinical meaning,* of the difference to that one patient who was helped.

Now look at an educational example: Consider a population of nineteen individuals measured on some usual scale, for example, test scores, lives saved, or patients diagnosed or treated properly. The results of the measurement are depicted as outline symbols in Figure 2. Then consider an educational intervention and a subsequent remeasurement of those same individuals, with the postintervention results depicted by the dark symbols in Figure 2. Assume that due to the educational effort, the two lowest scorers on the initial measurement made a sizable true gain. Assume that as measured by a reliable and valid instrument their scores moved from 3 to 12 while those of everyone else remained the same. Though these two individuals showed marked, demonstrable improvement, indicating that they learned a substantial amount, the two populations are not significantly different (t-test at the 5 percent level of probability). Compare the foregoing with the situation illustrated in Figure 3, in which the three initially lowest scorers improve to score 12 on the second measurement. Now the two populations have become significantly different. Consider a similar array of data, as shown in Figure 4. This time, the five at the top of the initial distribution improve their score to 12 while all other scores remain the same; the statistician must once again report no statistical difference. However, if six of the original high scorers show

**Figure 2. Results of Hypothetical Experiment I.**

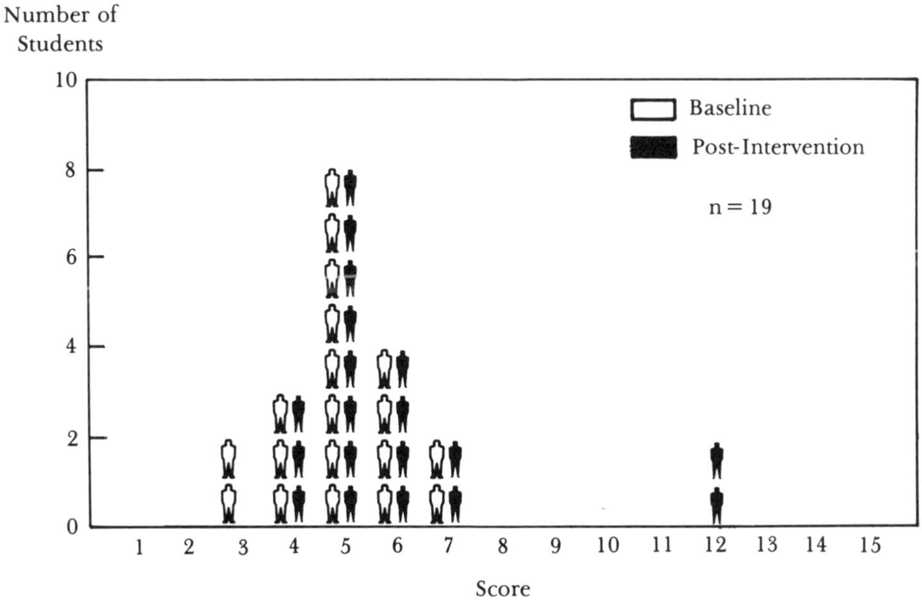

**Figure 3. Data from Hypothetical Experiment II.**

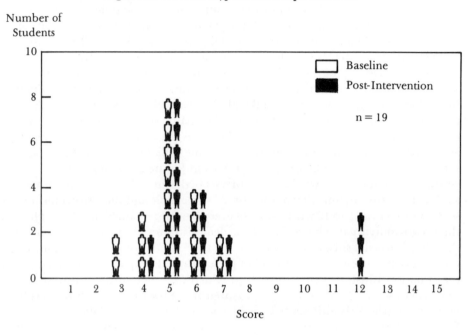

**Figure 4. Data from Hypothetical Experiment III.**

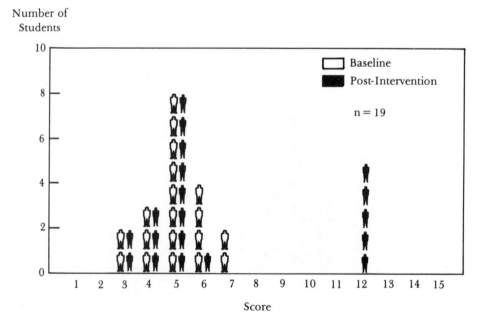

**Figure 5. Data from Hypothetical Experiment IV.**

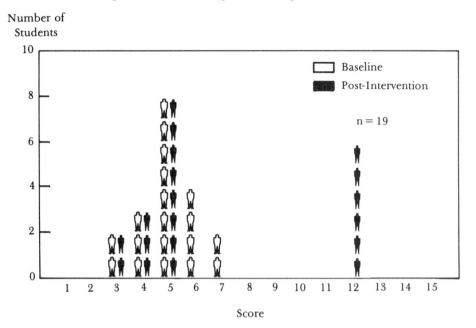

improvement to a score of 12 (Figure 5), now at last the statistician can report a significant difference in the two populations.*

Educators should acknowledge at least some measure of success upon help-ing even one person to achieve learning. To argue that the effort has not produced a statistically significant change in the data array for an entire population is to overlook individuals and to forget human meaning while searching for statistical significance. Just as we must remember that statistically significant changes may have no clinical importance whatever, we must likewise remember that impor-tant, valuable differences may be concealed by statistical nonsignificance.

We must learn how to value the individual, the anecdote, the $N$ of 1. There can be no sure way to foretell when and under what circumstances knowledge will prove useful. Reports from practitioners about how a particular bit of learning or insight obtained during CHE proved useful to a patient months or years later are legion. We must understand that these practitioners are telling us something crucial about the value of the CHE enterprise, even if we do not know how to give proper weight to the anecdote in postconference scores, structured audits, or other means yet to be devised. The learning and progress of one individual must be prized, even if it cannot generate a reliability coefficient. If we indeed value the individual human personality and personal experience—as our credo as adult educators requires—then what happens to one learner or one patient matters, whether or not it can be summed with other persons or anecdotes to be useful in a research project. The CHE investigator who says, in effect, "I'd give up my rever-

*Statistical assistance was kindly provided by Mark Albanese, Ph.D.

ence for individual accomplishment in order to justify my efforts by scientific proof" is like the person who says, "I'd give my left arm to be ambidextrous."

*Value of Small Victories.* I argue here that small victories are worthwhile. They may be almost the only real victories we do attain in CHE. Our efforts may be considered inefficient or expensive, but that is true for all education. Small victories that may seem individually unimportant can be summed to impressive totals. Another mathematical illustration may help. Consider the problem of measuring the area under a curve—for example, the area from $a$ to $b$ in Figure 1. Using integral calculus, we can discover the area by adding together the areas represented by "rectangles" of tiny width $\Delta x$, each so narrow, in fact, that it seems ultimately to have no width—that is, the width approaches zero. The area of an individual rectangle of near zero width cannot be distinguished from zero; yet if we sum an infinite number of such rectangular areas, we discover that there is indeed an area. Furthermore, it may be impressively large, even though its individual components were so small that they seemed to be zero when we tried to measure them individually.

*Evaluation Fetish.* "Nothing is good unless some formal evaluation study is undertaken." Those who make this mistake in reasoning fail to distinguish between the outcome in a learner and an assessment of that outcome. As a teacher, I may do things daily that affect students, for good or ill, but whether I or anybody else succeeds in measuring, or even *attempts* to measure, that effect does not change the reality: I produced an effect. The practical result of this error appears as an almost compulsive need to evaluate (Greenburg, Bruegel, and Peskin, 1977; Lloyd and Abrahamson, 1979; Bertram and Brooks-Bertram, 1977), ignoring at times how much effort and cost can be expended to indulge the fetish of evaluation. Often the data or conclusions serve only as proof of our compulsiveness or our enslavement to the Janus-god of "accountability" and "significance." A related error is to confuse *evaluation research*—that is, the testing of hypotheses in search of new knowledge—with *program evaluation*—that is, the gathering of data to guide practical judgments about planning and implementing future learning activities.

*Evaluation Without Objectives.* "No evaluation is possible unless specific and measurable objectives are declared in advance." I make no objection to stating objectives or trying to state them, *when feasible.* There are, however, many instances in which we do not or cannot state them. To argue that no evaluation is possible or meaningful in their absence misunderstands the word *evaluate*, which means "to place a value upon, or to judge the worth of." One of the oldest, most profound instances in our civilization of an evaluation with no predetermined objectives may be read in Chapter 1 of the Book of Genesis, where the Lord created the earth "and He saw that it was good." We find no indication of the goal, purpose, or objective, and certainly no specification of behavioral, measurable outcomes. Still other examples come to mind, whose many ultimate outcomes could not have been specified: the Lewis and Clark expedition, the discovery of x-rays, and many others. Evaluation of a fait accompli is possible and useful; we should stop telling ourselves it isn't.

*Hazard of Scientific Narrowness.* "Nothing is good unless it can be proven with the statistical tools of experimental science." Questions of goodness or value are ultimately and always subjective. If we think not—because we try to quantify the judgment with numerical data or say an effort was valuable if it met the predetermined objective—we delude ourselves, for the choice of either the numbers on our measurement scale or the predetermined objective was itself a subjective decision. *The methods of science do not answer value questions.* Stoeckle (1979, p. 270) states: "(medical) education is falsely rationalized as scientific when it is only technological." He goes on to warn against the "narrowness of spirit that characterizes those out to 'scientize' all of medicine by rejecting any knowledge or skill unless it has scientific provability." George Miller (1980) recommends the acceptance of systematic studies of rigor that are descriptive or analytical, and he eschews the demand for the experimental model in all instances. In other words, the model of pure experimental science is often inappropriate to CHE research; to attempt it may be like trying to divide an equation by zero—it may *seem* like a reasonable thing to do, but it can produce bizarre conclusions.

    *Proof-of-Failure Fallacy.* "Failure to prove is not proof of failure." Evidence of ignoring this truth appears often in the literature. As mentioned earlier, inadequacy of technique, insensitive or inappropriate measuring instruments, the contaminated laboratory, the fallacies involved with the notion of statistical significance, and many other limitations may account for the failure to prove that something valuable has happened.

## Competence Assurance

    The statement that CHE fails to assure competence and proper performance is correct. Unfortunately, however, many commentators seem to find in it the implication that CHE *should* assure competent performance. Pochyly (1978) has stated the expectation thus: "Because of the nature of societal forces, it is likely that CME planners will experience increased pressure to document that their educational programs are an effective means of maintaining physician competence" (p. 44).

    Yet even in 1967, George Miller urged the distinction between assuring continuing competence and participating in traditional CHE. Clearly, knowledge is a necessary precursor of competence and performance but never can be, and should not be, considered congruent with them. Fully competent practitioners make independent decisions about their behavior, decisions governed by a multitude of personal and environmental circumstances that do not now and never will lie within the control of the educators or the educational process. Such circumstances include, for example, the pressure of patient volume and the gravity of illness, the availability of certain equipment, the presence and strength of diverse distractions, the quality of helping personnel, the professional's personal health or fatigue, the nature of the reward system, and many others. Since such powerful determinants of behavior never will be under the direct control of the educators, we must avoid unwarranted expectations of what CHE can reasonably do and not use it as a scapegoat when the inappropriate expectations remain unfulfilled. Suter and others (1981) offer a useful conceptual model of CME and a comprehensive list of elements of quality that seek to reduce the gap between CME and effective health care.

If we subscribe to the principles of adult education, we must grant that our learners are mature, responsible, and professional, meaning that they must therefore accept fully their own responsibility for competent performance. For continuing educators to think themselves (or be thought) responsible for the ultimate behavior of the learners is to trample this most hallowed principle of adult education. We cannot have it both ways—either practitioners are responsible professionals accountable for their own performance, or else CHE behaves in loco parentis and can therefore be held accountable for inadequate performance of practitioners who participate in CHE. The latter view is not logical, feasible, or acceptable without rejecting the bedrock principle of adult education or the spirit of freedom that otherwise governs American society.

Perhaps we should consider the application of principles of adult learning as a goal and try to work toward it rather than decree that such principles are now operative and suffer the resultant frustration. Jean Piaget, the seminal educational psychologist and philosopher, implies in his developmental theory (as described in Bringuier, 1980) that the status of an adult learner may be attained but that possibly not everyone can or will reach that level. We must understand that many of our learners are not yet adults in this sense; therefore, we must be willing to accept and employ some of the methods of pedagogy, at least until the learners clearly demonstrate themselves to have moved beyond adolescence to the developmental level of true adult learners.

## Cost of CHE

Even if we could agree on what CHE really costs and whether we should or shouldn't include "opportunity costs" in the computation, the question remains a value issue about which there will inevitably be different opinions. Since assigning the dollar value of well-being, comfort, freedom from illness and worry, or of life itself by any ratiocinative process will be forever beyond our grasp, we remain at the mercy of the political process for such a determination. The argument about expense seems to suggest that we ought to be able to make some modest investment in CHE that should suffice to produce much permanent change. Such a simplistic idea violates the spirit of the laws of thermodynamics, which describe the inevitable "running down" of any system unless new energy is added to it, and the psychological counterpart, Ebbinghaus's law of forgetting. Finally, reflect on the wisdom of the saying, "If you think education is expensive, try ignorance."

## Value of CHE

It is often argued that even if CHE has value, it doesn't do enough good. However, the question of "How much is enough?" is another fruitless issue to debate. Health professionals should not carry the blame for the ill effects due to patients' harmful life-style choices. Those inside and outside CHE must accept that the world is imperfect and should desist from the constant flagellation of the CHE enterprise because of those imperfections. Why should we expect one or two days or weeks of lectures, workshops, reading, home study courses, or any other learning activity to bring about full understanding, permanent retention, and ever-competent performance? Our collective expectations of the overall CHE system have been excessive. Continuing education must be *continuing* and *repetitive* and, therefore, intrinsically "inefficient."

## Summary and Recommendations

The young world of CHE is attaining maturity but not by crossing some clearly identifiable boundary. Rather, we have come to an inflection point—a new paradigm is appearing. The term *paradigm* is used here in the sense described by Kuhn (1970) in his important book, *The Structure of Scientific Revolutions.* Kuhn describes the progress of any scientific discipline as dependent upon a growing dissatisfaction with the state of knowledge and its basic assumptions. In his perception, the accumulation of anomalies and contradictions leads to a radically different conception of the discipline. A questioning and ultimate rejection of one or more basic premises leads to a new fundamental proposition that motivates much new work, which he calls "normal science," "mopping up," or "filling in the details." Copernicus, in reasserting the heliocentric nature of our solar system and providing persuasive evidence, did away with all manner of cycles and epicycles that had to be invented by earlier astronomers to explain observed phenomena.

In attempting to draw an analogy between the growth of CHE research and Kuhn's conception of the growth of science, I do not suggest a single, fundamental premise or notion that will demolish many old beliefs and serve as *the* base for all new fruitful effort. I do believe, however, that we can now reject many widely held notions. Not all of them can be proved incorrect (as the nonexistence of phlogiston remains unproven), but they can still be rejected because they hold little further promise or lead only to confusion. I will therefore enumerate beliefs and types of research that I think are no longer worth pursuing. Then I will describe types of research or development that I feel offer promise of a productive new direction for CHE.

### Beliefs and Types of Research That Deserve Abandonment

"CHE has merit only if we can prove its usefulness." Felch (1981a, p. 2) has said: "Why not just accept the a priori belief, based on empirical evidence of doctors using CME, that CME does have intrinsic worth? We don't need double-blind studies to prove penicillin works, so why should we need control groups to establish the merit of CME? . . . As long as there are still significant numbers of people who have lingering doubts about the usefulness of CME, we conclude—somewhat reluctantly—that there is need to prove it once and for all." Richards (1978a, p. 87) states: "Methods . . . must also be developed and large-scale studies conducted if we are to reach any definite conclusion about the efficacy of CME." I believe the combination of common sense and experience is sufficient, now that they are backed by numerous studies that have shown beneficial effect, when the issues were limited and sharply enough drawn to be examined meaningfully by our impoverished techniques. More effort to prove globally and once and for all to everyone's satisfaction that CHE makes a difference would be as unfulfilling and unnecessary as an all-out attempt to demonstrate the characteristics of phlogiston.

"Further demonstration is needed to prove that knowledge is not synonymous with competence, and competence does not assure high-quality performance." Both common sense and adequate research are persuasive; further such studies are unnecessary and would only deplete available time and money. Correspondingly, I think no further studies are needed to help "prove" that mandatory CHE does not guarantee high-quality medical practice. Studies like those of Williamson, Alexander, and Miller (1967), Pinkerton and others (1980), and Wigton and others (1981), for example, demonstrate this point very well indeed.

"Lectures are bad and should not be used." Only bad lectures and lectures inappropriately chosen for a particular task are bad. Lectures have been shown to be as effective as, and less expensive than, computer-assisted instruction or small group discussions (Plotz and others, 1978; Thies and others, 1969; Gauvain and Walford, 1965). Research on lectures must be done with particular lectures, and little transfer can properly be made to lectures in general. Further research to generalize along these lines is fruitless.

"Traditional CHE is a meaningful term." I argue that it is vague and its use leads to mischief. It should be used in the future only if sharply defined.

"CHE efforts (as on any one day, for example) should be expected to produce measurable impacts on all the intended learners and on the operation and outcomes of the health system." For reasons given earlier, we may not be able to make those measurements. Further expensive labor to provide post hoc justification for small CHE activities will continue to be largely wasteful. As Richards (1978a, p. 183) puts it, "CME is an educational support system, not a determinant of practice."

"An anecdote (because the N is only 1) tells us nothing that matters or can be believed." As I have argued, we simple need a methodology for dealing with unique but important events.

"There is a best way to provide CHE." For example, Senior (1978, p. 14) laments that "We do not yet know the best way that continuing education programs can be used to disseminate new information and help practitioners use it best." Until humans become totally standardized, diverse approaches will be needed. Such pluralism should not be struggled against—it is the glory of the human condition.

"Technology will permit us to do away with personal interactions and expert teachers." Fear not. If for absolutely nothing else, experts will always be needed to write computer programs.

"Needs assessment surveys among my clientele will be useful to others." The more widespread the effort and study population and the more conglomerate the data (Brandt, 1975; Tye, Hartford, and Wallace, 1978), the further removed will be the results from the needs of individual learners, and, therefore, the less will be the utility to them of efforts derived from such data. Surveys done on more limited populations, although perhaps useful in guiding program development for that group and assisting the purveyor's marketing needs, likewise have little generalizability to other groups. In my opinion, editors would do well to reject further manuscripts of this type.

"CHE, in contrast to all other educational efforts the world has ever known, should be inherently inexpensive and produce prompt, large benefits that last indefinitely." Research or evaluation based on such patently false premises cannot yield useful results.

"Independent learning means solitary learning; people gathered in groups, especially in a pleasant place, will not learn actively or out of individual initiative." Those who repeat this curiosity of logic may be prompted less by good sense or educational research than by punitive puritanism.

"That 'continuing education must be accountable' (Houle) means that rigorous and extensive evaluation efforts must be applied to each and every instructional effort." I submit that Houle's comment refers not to each effort but to the total enterprise of continuing education. In the case of CHE, the evidence of change and benefit lies all about us.

"All CHE learners are adult learners and should be dealt with according to the principles of adult learning." Not all have reached "adulthood" yet. Efforts to force on them the implications of that generalization will sometimes go awry. Conversely, many "adult educators," no matter what their academic background or professional identification, do not always behave in a truly adult relationship with their learners. Instead, they behave parentally and try to decree what is best for that individual adult. "I am here only to facilitate your learning" becomes too easily transformed into directives and stern judgments. A clear parental example occurs when adult educators try to assume unto themselves far more responsibility for the outcome of their efforts than they would ever be entitled to on the basis of adult learning theory.

"CHE can be truly effective only to the extent that it arises from the professional's actual problems and contemporaneous responsibilities, for no learning can occur except in response to a question." Acceptance of this view would mean that no CHE would be meritorious unless it would relate to, and perhaps monitor, the day-to-day activities of the professional in office or hospital. Learning "by accident" would be defined, bizarrely, as impossible. It would also follow that the more distant purveyors, such as professional schools and specialty societies, could have little meaningful role to play. To the contrary, pluralism of methods, sites, issues, and purveyors is to be desired, not eschewed.

"The health care audit will be a panacea for identifying educational needs and correcting the ills of the health care system." Its effectiveness is proving about the same as all other low-grade panaceas. But this is not to deny its usefulness when done well by willing participants in an adequately limited setting.

"Mandatory CHE is a good (or bad) thing." It indeed offers no assurance of quality performance. On the other hand, it seems to be doing little clear harm, at least in the very small quantities now mandated. Perhaps it even does some good occasionally. The popularity of this debate will wither, but probably not because proponents will be dissuaded from their subjective attitudes on the subject. Those formerly outraged at the philosophical denial of freedom of action and by the imposition of a record-keeping nuisance seem less outraged now.

"There is no evidence that CHE is beneficial." On the contrary, this analysis and the many other reviews of the literature demonstrate otherwise.

### Beliefs and Types of Research That Merit Further Effort

The following issues cannot be claimed to be new, but they seem to be directions that merit further investigation, where research and development would probably justify the investment:

*Using the "Educational Influential."* Hiss, MacDonald, and Davis (1978) and Stross and Bole (1980) describe a number of developments growing out of work on the diffusion of innovation (Gordon and Fisher, 1975). These efforts make use of the "educational influential" by targeting instruction on community role models, gaining their commitment, and using their talent as teachers and disseminators. The approach has not only face validity and research evidence but also centuries of practical politics and salesmanship to support it. It is worth pursuing.

*Maximizing Individualization.* Genuine individualization requires multiple types of learning experiences. Both teachers individually and "the system" collectively will need to provide such multiple modalities. Individual learners who behave as truly adult learners must be allowed maximum choice, not only choice of modality of instruction but also great freedom in the choice of content. For example, a urologist attempting to learn about the immunologic factors affecting graft rejection—whether via a lecture given by an internist or a self-study module prepared by a microbiologist—should be allowed to exercise personal, independent judgment as to whether it is worth "credit" for him or her. For others to make the determination that it is an appropriate subject for that person to study would violate individual freedom, the spirit of professionalism, and the principles of adult learning. If you are working with true adult learners, don't get in their way!

*Matching Educational Needs to Patient Care Needs.* The ultimate in matching the individual professional's educational needs with patient care needs will come via the instant algorithms and monitoring that computer technology, as pioneered by Weed (1969), can bring to us. Further development of this important aid merits serious efforts.

*Improving Competency Measures.* Patient management problems (paper/pencil or computer interaction) or simulated patients (Barrows, 1981) appear to show great potential. However, the complexities of the methods, the uniqueness and unpredictability of the clinical interchange and therefore the limitations on the reliability of the measuring instruments, and the costs of their development are impediments to their becoming as widely employed as some of the enthusiasts would wish. Nonetheless, developmental work on modifications, abbreviations, and mass production appears to be worthwhile.

*Helping Learners to Become More Sophisticated.* Participants in CHE require assistance in enhancing their understanding of needs assessment, in becoming acquainted with new learning aids (for example, new video formats, computer-assisted methods, literature searches), and in gaining confidence and greater self-determination in their learning activities. Rather than attempting to use the CHE system to increase regulation and supervision of health care practice, enlightened educators of the future will work to heighten motivation and modify in a positive direction such factors as work load, availability of support personnel and facilities, mental and emotional health, and information management—all of which play so vital a role in influencing clinical judgment.

*Employing "Inquiry" Methods.* CHE should experiment with greater use of the "inquiry" mode of learning. Stimulating a sense of the "need-to-know" will serve the educational enterprise best. Persistent behavioral change can be accomplished by group methods or by one-on-one educational work (preceptorpreceptee or mentor-student relationship of mutual respect). Change can also result from modifying the administrative or physical circumstances so as to shape the desired behavior. All reasonable avenues toward developing a spirit of inquiry in practitioners should be pursued.

*Utilizing Multiple Motivations.* It is time that we acknowledge that participation in CHE is motivated by the expectation of benefits other than its direct contribution to improved care. Continued study in the intellectually based professions should not be reduced only to its mechanistic core of problem solving, important though that is. CHE must also serve many intellectual and psychosocial needs of the learner, not just the immediately goal-oriented ones related to patient care (Richards ãnd Cohen, 1981; Cervero, 1981).

*Understanding Creativity.* It is important that we investigate the determinants of curiosity, flexibility, and creativity in both the adult teacher/facilitator and the adult learner. This effort could play a major role and may even alter drastically our methods of student selection, instructional implementation, and evaluation of learners and programs.

*Characterizing the Effective Participant.* We need a better understanding of the characteristics of the effective CHE learner and teacher. We need to find ways to identify and nurture those characteristics.

*Developing Computer Literacy.** Acquaintance and facility with new methods of information processing are essential. Success in this area of effort will greatly benefit our learners and those they serve.

## Coda

The educational process, like clinical practice, is yet more art than science. Whoever attempts to understand education solely as science will not only fail to be an effective teacher but will sully the good repute of education. Practitioners of CHE should be moderate in their tendency to indulge compulsively in rigid approaches to needs assessment, behavioral objectives, and evaluation busywork. We need to remain humble as well, and forgo the arrogance often adopted as a defense against ignorance. The sculptor Rodin said, "In art, to admit only what one understands leads to impotence." I think it is true for education and science, too.

Ellis (1978, p. 513) cited Sir George Pickering who believes that "loss of scholarly habits is the central tragedy of contemporary medical education. Such habits have made medicine into a highly respected learned profession and only the possession of such habits will keep it so." Ellis adds that while Sir George "despairs of teachers, he does not despair for the future. As he says, 'while there is death, there is hope': while today's teachers may be immutable, they are not immortal."

Most of us who follow the George Miller model take ourselves and our work very seriously. We strive compulsively at it and are unforgiving of ourselves when our grasp does not equal our reach. The time is at hand to winnow out some unproductive and self-flagellating aspects of our own behavior. Let us work dili-

*For an extended discussion of this topic see Chapter 21.

gently, spend less time cursing the darkness, and accede to the wisdom expressed by Will Durant (1961, p. xv): "We are all imperfect teachers, but we may be forgiven if we have advanced the matter a little, and have done our best. We announce the prologue, and retire; after us better players will come."

## References

Ashbaugh, D., and McKean, R. "Continuing Medical Education: The Philosophy and Use of Audit." *Journal of the American Medical Association,* 1976, *236,* 1485-1488.

Barrows, H. S. *American Medical Association Continuing Medical Education Newsletter,* 1981, *10,* 5-7.

Bertram, D., and Brooks-Bertram, P. "The Evaluation of Continuing Medical Education: A Literature Review." *Health Education Monographs,* 1977, *5,* 330-348.

Brandt, E. N., Jr. "Preferences of Family Physicians for Subject Matter in Continuing Medical Education." *Journal of Medical Education,* 1975, *50,* 395-398.

Bringuier, J. C. *Conversations with Jean Piaget.* Chicago: University of Chicago Press, 1980.

Brown, C., Jr., and Uhl, H. "Mandatory Continuing Education: Sense or Nonsense?" *Journal of the American Medical Association,* 1970, *213,* 1660-1668.

Burgess, P. "Reasons for Adult Participation in Group Educational Activities." *Adult Education,* 1971, *22,* 3-29.

Caplan, R. M., and Yarcheski, T. "Survey of Continuing Medical Education in Iowa." *Journal of the Iowa Medical Society,* 1974, *64,* 159-166.

Cervero, R. M. "A Factor Analytic Study of Physicians' Reasons for Participating in Continuing Education." *Journal of Medical Education,* 1981, *56,* 29-34.

Christiansen, C. H., and Weinberg, A. D. "The Effects of a Geographic Continuing Education Program on Physician Behavior: An Unobtrusive Study." In *Proceedings of the 16th Annual Conference on Research in Medical Education.* Washington, D.C.: Association of American Medical Colleges, 1977.

Corbett, T. "The Impact of Continuing Medical Education on Quality of Care: Implications of the Continuing Medical Evaluation Literature." In P. LeBreton and others (Eds.), *The Evaluation of Continuing Medical Education for Professionals: A Systematic View.* Seattle: University of Washington, 1979.

Council on Medical Education. *Proceedings, House of Delegates, 128th Annual Convention of the Council on Medical Education,* July 22-26, 1979, Chicago, Council on Medical Education, Report C, pp. 140-141.

Derbyshire, R. C. "Let's Be Fair." *West Virginia Medical Journal,* 1979, *75,* 215-216.

Durant, W. *The Story of Philosophy.* 2nd ed. New York: Washington Square Press, 1961.

Ellis, J. R. "The Pickering Survey." *Lancet,* Sept. 2, 1978, pp. 512-513.

Erviti, V., and others. "Development of a Medical Record Audit for Continuing Medical Education." In *Proceedings of the 16th Annual Conference on*

*Research in Medical Education.* Washington, D.C.: Association of American Medical Colleges, 1977.

Farrington, J. F., Felch, W. C., and Hare, R. L. "Quality Assessment and Quality Assurance: The Performance-Review Alternative." *New England Journal of Medicine,* 1980, *303* (3), 154–156.

Felch, W. C. "CME and Research: Some Reflections." *Alliance for Continuing Medical Education Almanac,* 1981a, *3* (7), 2–3.

Felch, W. C. "CME or EME?" *Alliance for Continuing Medical Education Almanac,* 1981b, *3* (4), 3.

Gauvain, S., and Walford, J. "An Experiment in Postgraduate Education to Evaluate Teaching and Examination Techniques." *Journal of Medical Education,* 1965, *40,* 516–523.

Goldfinger, S. "Continuing Medical Education: The Case for Contamination." *New England Journal of Medicine,* 1982, *306,* 540–541.

Gonnella, J. S., and Storey, P. B. "Continuing Medical Education and Clinical Competence: A Matrix Approach to a Complex Problem." *American Medical Association Continuing Medical Education Newsletter,* 1981, *10,* 3–15.

Gordon, G., and Fisher, G. L. *The Diffusion of Medical Technology: Policy and Research Planning Perspectives.* Cambridge, Mass.: Ballinger, 1975.

Greenburg, A. G., Bruegel, R. B., and Peskin, G. W. "Surgical Continuing Medical Education: Format and Impact." *Surgery,* 1977, *81,* 708–715.

Hein, H. A., Christopher, M. C., and Ferguson, N. N. "Rural Perinatology." *Pediatrics,* 1975, *55,* 769–773.

Hiss, R. G., MacDonald, R., and Davis, W. L. "Identification of Physician Educational Influentials in Small Community Hospitals." In *Proceedings of the 17th Annual Conference on Research in Medical Education.* Washington, D.C.: Association of American Medical Colleges, 1978.

Houle, C. O. *Continuing Learning in the Professions.* San Francisco: Jossey-Bass, 1980.

Hubbard, J. P. "Profiled Continuing Education." *Transactions and Studies of the College of Physicians of Philadelphia,* 1978, *45,* 190–196.

Klein, L. E., Charache, P., and Johannes, R. S. "Effect of Physician Tutorials on Prescribing Patterns of Graduate Physicians." *Journal of Medical Education,* 1981, *56,* 504–511.

Knowles, M. S. *The Modern Practice of Adult Education.* New York: Association Press, 1970.

Kuhn, T. S. *The Structure of Scientific Revolutions.* 2nd ed. Chicago: University of Chicago Press, 1970.

Lewis, C., and Hassanein, R. "Continuing Medical Education: An Epidemiologic Evaluation." *New England Journal of Medicine,* 1970, *282,* 254–259.

Linn, B. S. "Continuing Medical Education: Impact on Emergency Room Burn Care." *Journal of the American Medical Association,* 1980, *244,* 565–570.

Lloyd, J. S., and Abrahamson, S. "Effectiveness of Continuing Medical Education: A Review of the Evidence." *Evaluation and the Health Professions,* 1979, *2,* 251–280.

Mahan, J. M., Phillips, B. U., and Costanzi, J. J. "Patient Referrals: A Behavioral

Outcome of Continuing Medical Education." *Journal of Medical Education,* 1978, *53,* 210–211.

Manning, P. R., and others. "Determining Educational Needs in the Physician's Office." *Journal of the American Medical Association,* 1980, *244,* 1112–1115.

Mazmanian, P. E., and others. "Perspectives on Mandatory Continuing Medical Education." *Southern Medical Journal,* 1979, *72,* 378–380.

Miller, G. E. "Continuing Education for What?" *Journal of Medical Education,* 1967, *42,* 320–326.

Miller, G. E. *Educating Medical Teachers.* Cambridge, Mass.: Harvard University Press, 1980.

Miller, L. A. "$3.6 Billion a Year for CME—Is It a Good Investment?" *Alliance for Continuing Medical Education Almanac,* 1979, *1,* 22.

Munster, A. M. "Teaching Surgeons the Correct Use of Prophylactic Antibiotics." *Helvetica Chirurgica Acta,* 1978, *45,* 471–473.

Nelson, A. R. "Orphan Data and the Unclosed Loop: A Dilemma in PSRO and Medical Audit." *New England Journal of Medicine,* 1976, *295,* 617–619.

Paino, S. E., Cline, D. W., and Demarest, L. "Using Audit as a Needs Assessment and Evaluation for a Continuing Education Program." In *Proceedings of the 18th Annual Conference on Research in Medical Education.* Washington, D.C.: Association of American Medical Colleges, 1979.

Pinkerton, R. E., and others. "Resident Physician Performance in a Continuing Education Format: Does Newly Acquired Knowledge Improve Patient Care?" *Journal of the American Medical Association,* 1980, *244,* 2183–2185.

Plotz, C. M., and others. "Clinical Learning in Respiratory Disease: A Comparison of Computer-Assisted Instruction and Lecture Method." In *Proceedings of the 17th Annual Conference on Research in Medical Education.* Washington, D.C.: Association of American Medical Colleges, 1978.

Pochyly, D. F. "Measuring the Effectiveness of Continuing Medical Education." *Proceedings of the Institute of Medicine of Chicago,* 1978, *32* (3), 43–44.

Pohlmann, G. P. "Continuing Medical Education in the Community Hospital." *Wisconsin Medical Journal,* 1980, *79,* 23–27.

Richards, R. K. *Continuing Medical Education: Perspectives, Problems, Prognosis.* New Haven, Conn.: Yale University Press, 1978a.

Richards, R. K. "Past History and Future Trends in CME." *Quality Review Bulletin,* 1978b, *4,* 8–11.

Richards, R. K. *American Medical Association CME Newsletter,* 1981, *10,* 10.

Richards, R. K., and Cohen, R. M. *The Value and Limitations of Physician Participation in Traditional Forms of Continuing Medical Education.* Kalamazoo, Mich.: Upjohn Co., 1981.

Rubenstein, E. "Continuing Medical Education at Stanford: The Back-to-Medical-School Program." *Journal of Medical Education,* 1973, *48,* 911–918.

Ruhe, C. H. W. "Seventy-Five Years of American Medical Education: Perceptions and Reflections." *Connecticut Medicine,* 1980, *44,* 95–99.

Sanazaro, P. M. "Medical Audit, Continuing Medical Education, and Quality Assurance." *Western Journal of Medicine,* 1976, *125,* 247–252.

Senior, J. R. "The Learning Point." *Quality Review Bulletin,* 1978, *4* (3), 14–15.

Sibley, J. C., and others. "A Randomized Trial of Continuing Medical Education." *New England Journal of Medicine,* 1982, *306,* 511–515.

Sivertson, S. E., and others. "Individual Physician Profile: Continuing Medical Education Related to Medical Practice." *Journal of Medical Education*, 1973, *48*, 1006-1012.

Stead, E. A. "The Patient as a Teacher for Continuing Medical Education." *American Medical Association Continuing Medical Education Newsletter*, 1981, *10*, 2-7.

Stein, L. S. "The Effectiveness of Continuing Medical Education: A Research Report." *Journal of Medical Education*, 1981, *56*, 103-110.

Stinson, E. R., and Mueller, D. A. "Survey of Health Professionals' Information Habits and Needs Conducted Through Personal Interviews." *Journal of the American Medical Association*, 1980, *243*, 140-143.

Stoeckle, J. D. "The Tasks of Care: Humanistic Dimensions of Medical Education." In W. R. Rogers and D. Barnard, *Nourishing the Humanistic in Medicine.* Pittsburgh, Pa.: University of Pittsburgh Press, 1979.

Stross, J. K., and Bole, G. G. "Evaluation of a Continuing Education Program in Rheumatoid Arthritis." *Arthritis and Rheumatism*, 1980, *23*, 846-849.

Suter, E., and others. "Continuing Education of Health Professionals: Proposal for a Definition of Quality." *Journal of Medical Education*, 1981, *56* (Supplement), 687-707.

Talley, R. C. "Effect of Continuing Medical Education on Practice Patterns." *Journal of Medical Education*, 1978, *53*, 602-603.

Thies, R., and others. "An Experiment Comparing Computer-Assisted Instruction with Lecture Presentation in Physiology." *Journal of Medical Education*, 1969, *44*, 1156-1160.

Thompson, R. E. "Relating Continuing Education and Quality Assurance Activities." *Quality Review Bulletin*, 1981, *7*, 3-6.

Tye, J. B., Hartford, C. E., and Wallace, R. B. "Survey of Continuing Education Needs for Nonemergency Physicians in Emergency Medicine." *Journal of the American College of Emergency Physicians*, 1978, *7*, 16-19.

Watts, M. S. M. "An Anatomy of Continuing Medical Education." *Möbius*, 1981, *1*, 5-15.

Weed, L. L. *Medical Records, Medical Education, and Patient Care.* Cleveland, Ohio: Case Western Reserve University Press, 1969.

Weinberg, A. D., and others. "Perceived Ability Versus Actual Ability: A Problem for Continuing Medical Education." In *Proceedings of the 16th Annual Conference on Research in Medical Education.* Washington, D.C.: Association of American Medical Colleges, 1977.

Wigton, R. S., and others. "Chart Reminders in the Diagnosis of Anemia." *Journal of the American Medical Association*, 1981, *245*, 1745-1747.

Wilbur, R. S. "Mandatory Continuing Education: A Liability." *Quality Review Bulletin*, 1978, *4*, 12-13.

Williamson, J. W. *Improving Medical Practice and Health Care: A Bibliographic Guide to Information Management in Quality Assurance and Continuing Education.* Cambridge, Mass.: Ballinger, 1977.

Williamson, J. W., Alexander, M., and Miller, G. E. "Continuing Education and Patient Care Research: Physician Response to Screening Test Results." *Journal of the American Medical Association*, 1967, *201*, 938-942.

Wirtschafter, D. D., and others. "Continuing Medical Education: An Assessment of Impact upon Neonatal Care in Community Hospitals." In *Proceedings of the 18th Annual Conference on Research in Medical Education.* Washington, D. C.: Association of American Medical Colleges, 1979.

# Part Three

Forces for Change
in Health Professions
Education

# Introduction:

# New Realities
# and Responsibilities

## Alan Gorr

In Part Three an interdisciplinary team of scholars reviews the impact of the current state of the world upon health care professionals. The areas of concern include environmental, economic, demographic, and technological perspectives. Because health care delivery is a societal response that is highly conditioned by ethics and politics and by health planning on an international level, chapters are devoted to these concerns as well. The scholars represented here are keenly aware of the great interplay among their disciplines and write with that in mind. They are noteworthy not only for their experience and expertise in the areas about which they write but also for their boldness in being willing to be juxtaposed to one another and to allow their observations to be validated by the flow of events.

The chapters in Part Three look to the future against the background of the last century. The last hundred or so years have seen several waves of scientific advancement in health care. Each of these waves has unlocked great professional, economic, and political energies so that society might maximally benefit from new developments. But every advance has its own limitations, and in recent years, we have become accustomed to the possibility that an advance in health care may have a considerable number of negative effects that accompany its therapeutic benefits.

It is not historically accurate to speak about discrete periods of scientific and technical advancement, as there are many overlapping and separable trends in both spheres. But it can be fairly said that in the advanced, industrialized countries of the world, both scientific advancement in health care and widespread economic commitment to the expansion of health care services have continued without respite since World War II. The post–World War II era in the United States, represented a time when an undefined, yet positive view that extension of the doctor-patient relationships, together with adequate and accessible hospital facilities, would enhance the health of the public. At the same time, the general standards of housing, nutrition, and sanitation were rising. Subsequently, the condition of health and longevity of the American population did, in fact, improve. But the question of which change or set of changes in medical care or in living standards caused the improvement in health is still not determined.

While the evidence is mounting that the period of unbridled expansion has ended, the widely heralded period of contraction has not yet taken place. Therefore, speculation concerning how society will set its priorities in a period of economic retrenchment is based upon projections of current realities that have not actually been fully experienced.

It is often recommended that we place greater reliance upon health and patient education as an alternative to some kinds of medical intervention. Yet even in an expanding market, health and patient educators have not been able to enlarge their share of the health care dollar substantially, and they are often first to go when economic belt tightening is required. Similarly, it seems to be an unquestioned truism that preventive medicine and occupational and environmental health should have a larger role, even in a period of reduced health care services. Yet, to date, each economic shudder that sweeps through the health care delivery system hits these very areas first and hardest.

Nonetheless, the system of health care delivery is faced with perplexities that do seem to make limitation of services inevitable. First, unlike other industries, medical services do not seem to benefit from economies of scale, at least in the care of the acutely ill. On the contrary, aggregations of the seriously sick in large hospitals make feasible the use of technologically advanced techniques, which while practicable only in large-scale usage may be marginal in the amount of relief they afford the patient, relative to the time and expense they entail. Second, "hands-on" health care, whether by physicians or other personnel, has become an ever more expensive part of the health care bill. The cost for direct services in the health care sector has risen much more steeply than that for the general economy. Thus while the outcome of impending cutbacks may be questioned, the possibility of such cutbacks cannot be seriously doubted.

While the authors come from widely differing orientations, all are acutely aware that we are moving into an era when success or failure will be judged as much by the making of wise choices as by the employment of scientific medicine. They are aware that the nature of health care delivery is a reflection of the values that a society sets for itself, as well as the technologies and the economic resources available to implement new approaches. All the authors realize that the burden of curative medicine could be substantially lessened by the improvement of environmental and workplace conditions. The health of individuals could be greatly enhanced by better habits of hygiene, nutrition, and physical conditioning. Were health care providers to attend to more preventive measures, substantial benefits would accrue to the entire population. Finally, health care in an era of constraints must reflect equity of access for the public it serves.

The interactive nature of the sectors involved in health and health care is a point that is understood well by each of the authors. Many of the elements that run through these chapters derive from this understanding, and the reader may partake of a lively debate on the following questions:

- *Rational process:* To what extent are the current dilemmas in health care the result of the failure to define terms, rationally analyze data, and seek solutions geared to the problems as they have been defined?
- *Curative medicine:* What are its limits, and what are the possibilities of preventive medicine?
- *Health needs:* How are these defined and by whom?
- *Political will:* How have changes in political consensus signaled changes in public policy? How does public policy in turn reflect the values of society?
- *Allocation of scarce resources:* On what basis can this be done? What are the ethical and economic considerations that govern this?
- *Cost effectiveness:* How would the picture of health care delivery differ if this were the prime concern?
- *Role of the academic health center:* What shall its posture be during the coming decades? To what extent should it be a leader or a follower of trends in the health care delivery system?

The chapters in Part Three are intended to provide a logical sequence of concerns without necessarily reflecting a unified point of view. They begin with a chapter by Edmund Pellegrino whose view of health care services derives from the understanding that our attitudes toward the sick are a reflection of our deepest values as a society. Thus, in trying to make health professions education and all of health care delivery responsive to societal values, we must come to common agreement on such key terms as *health* and *medicine* and then determine the extent to which our society will employ biomedical, social, or ethical models to develop services. In this context, will the role of the physician be narrowly or broadly defined? Will the physician be responsible solely for the treatment of disease and leave the questions of health to others? Or will the treatment of disease be but one aspect of the physician's duties? Pellegrino provides a method by which societal demands, needs, and expectations may be sorted out and acted upon.

The chapters by Herbert Klarman, Julius Richmond and Milton Kotelchuck, and Jack Hadley provide the reader with basic insight into the economic and political processes that give rise to health policy and to which the academic health centers must respond. Klarman's analysis to primarily economic and, based upon current trends, he is able to make projections and draw implications for health manpower needs. Richmond and Kotelchuck's approach is primarily a political and historical analysis of the development of health care policy in the United States. Using a model that accounts for public policy on the basis of a knowledge base, the political will, and a social strategy, they show how these elements may be brought to bear on the future of health care delivery. The chapter by Jack Hadley reveals the implications of current proposals for health care funding. He meticulously leads the reader through the implications of capped and

uncapped reimbursement approaches and analyzes their consequences for financing of academic health centers and thus for the education of health care professionals. The educational effects of these changes may lead, as Klarman speculates,
to a decline in minority enrollment or, as Hadley sees it, toward more community-
based clinical experiences. Richmond and Kotelchuck see the probability of prospective budgeting and prospective medicine as having a substantial impact on
the education of health care professionals.

The next three chapters deal with the demographic, environmental, and
technological developments that will alter the health care picture in the coming
decades. Chapter Nineteen by Warren Winklestein provides an illustration of how
systematic thinking might bring about a reordering of health care priorities and
how such a reordering might provide dramatically better health for one segment
of the population, the elderly. Using the methodology of the demographer and the
epidemiologist, he delineates fundamental gaps in health care that would be
immediately cost-effective to fill. This chapter is meant to be illustrative of how
such an approach could benefit all segments of society and, by implication, how
it should alter the training of health professionals.

The following chapter by Raymond Suskind considers the environment as
a large determinant of health. He sets forth the many dimensions of environment,
such as the land, air, and water, the community, the workplace, and the goods and
services we use. Each of these influences our health. Suskind discusses the educational policies that an environmental perspective suggests.

The chapter by Duncan Neuhauser takes a futuristic look at health care
delivery. Such an understanding truly extends beyond the boundaries of a single
chapter, so he concentrates on the computer revolution as it applies to health care.
This technology, as do other technologies, gives direction and form to health care
delivery. The data processing revolution, unlike earlier revolutions, will have an
impact on the most basic element of the health sciences, the professional mind. It
has the potential to so alter reasoning and memory that health professions education in the coming decades may scarcely resemble the now established programs.

The final chapter by Tamás Fülöp supplies the international context
within which our own national health policies must be planned. The policies
adopted in the United States and those of other nations profoundly affect each
other. It is crucial, therefore, that the goals of nations be simultaneously tailored
to their own needs, yet be part of a larger global strategy. Fülöp explicates the
World Health Organization's (WHO) goal of "health for all by the year 2000."
Within this context, the foregoing chapters may be seen as a specific national
example of a larger health care picture that recognizes that each country must
develop its own health care system based upon the resources and expectations of
its people and their government, but the effectiveness of the policies that are derived will depend on adherence to several principles. First, like Richmond and
Kotelchuck, Fülöp stresses the necessity of developing a political will to bring
about the needed changes and of expressing it through a rational, systematic, and
broad-based process. The health care policies that emanate from the government
should be intersectorial in nature and should aim at the basic health care needs of
the population. These needs should be addressed by primary health care delivery,
and the professionals who provide such care should be trained with these specific
functions in mind. Planning and targeted production of human and material

resources are the two focuses of this approach. For the training of health care professionals, Fülöp recommends that their future functions be determined in the broad-based planning effort he espouses and that educational programs be designed around these primary care functions that he foresees.

Fülöp's chapter points to the far-reaching social, scientific, economic, and political implications of WHO's goal. It specifies the roles of both the developed and developing countries in this scheme. For that reason, his chapter serves to integrate the various aspects of health care planning and the education of health professionals that are explored in the previous chapters in Part Three.

# 15

*Edmund D. Pellegrino*

# Social Values

## Articulating Public Need and Educational Policy

The human being is uniquely a valuing animal. We choose among alternatives those we think most worthwhile. In those choices we reveal ourselves by what we value—the things we will work and suffer for, the things we will pay for and even die for. Our values define what we think is good for the kind of society in which we want to live.

Nowhere is this truer than in a society's policies toward the sick and the needy, those whose only remaining claim on us is their humanity. Much is revealed about our society in the sharp shift in values now occurring in our national health policy. In just a few years, we have turned from a concern with equity, social need, and health care as a civic right to an intense preoccupation with cost, competition, and health care as a commodity. Critical reflection has focused more on political exigencies than on what kind of society is likely to emerge. How much of what is revealed by our policy shifts do we really want to accept?

Considering the extent of the value shifts, public debate has been scanty and sporadic, pointed more to political philosophies than to the values they presuppose. Notably absent are the voices of the academic health centers, the indispensable producers of future health professionals. The present shifts in public policy will in turn require equally fundamental shifts in educational policy. The number and kind of health professionals must, after all, have some congruence with public policy.

Should those who prepare future health professionals accept the ethos of competition as the determinant of educational policy? What should be the relationship between educational purpose and social and public policies? In the previous few decades, the academic centers largely accepted the need for closing perceived gaps in equity of distribution, access, availability, and quality of medical and health services. As a result, they initiated programs dedicated to primary care and family medicine, team care and physician extenders, and minority recruitment. The number of places in medical schools was virtually doubled. Now, with the exception of family medicine, most of these programs are being curtailed. The academic health sciences centers already seem to be accommodating all too readily to what may be very profound changes. Does this imply agreement with the value presuppositions on which these changes are founded? Do academic centers accept the implied transformations of the relationships between patient and health professionals and the nature of the professions themselves?

Academic health centers are indispensable to the achievement of whatever national goals we set for health and medical care. Health policies are part of the social fabric, and therefore social and educational policies must bear some close relationship with each other. How academic health centers respond to current realities, such as the physician surplus, a changed economic philosophy, or the ethos of competition, will determine in part what kind of society will emerge. Academic health centers have a responsibility, therefore, that goes beyond mere adaptation and compliance. They must examine the values that underlie policy decisions.

Theoretically, educational policy and societal need are closely related. In actuality, there is always a certain inherent tension between them. Most academics would agree that their efforts ultimately must be for society's benefit, but they also feel that society's best interests are served if the academic world sets its own policies and priorities. Policy makers, on the other hand, see educational institutions, particularly in the health field, as instrumentalities of social purpose. There is real danger to both society and educational institutions if this tension ends in capitulation in either direction. In a democratic society, the relationship must always be a dynamic one, the university protecting its role as social critic, society its role as determinant of public policy. In the recent past, society exerted its influence through governmental regulation and incentives. In the immediate future, we are tending to a free-market determination of goals and priorities. While this may afford greater freedom to educational institutions, that freedom will have to be modified by something more than market considerations. If the equilibrium between the number and kinds of health professionals academic centers produce gets too far out of balance with the needs of society for its utilization of health professionals, the temptation to enact another round of governmental regulation will be difficult to resist.

This tripartite equilibrium between production, need, and utilization must be balanced, whatever economic philosophy is dominant. That balance is always beset by serious incongruities that promise to multiply. For one thing, the terms in the equation—medicine, health, needs, and reasonable cost—remain unclear and hotly debated. For another, past efforts to plan "rationally" have not been notably successful. Moreover, the present trend toward deregulation is hostile to all planned approaches. Finally, there is no reliable way, as yet, to ascertain or quantitate what society wants, needs, expects, or values in its medical and health care system. We are forced to rely on surveys of dubious provenance or the pronouncements of politicians, economists, medical educators, polemicists, and consumers—each with a ready remedy for the dysphoria they consider the most urgent. Even our best projections are extrapolations of present-day usages. These will undoubtedly change unpredictably so that all our projections run the risk of perilous imprecision. The question of numbers of health professionals, their distribution across professions, and their professional functions will depend on the extent to which we can agree on what we mean by medicine and health, what we agree to label as needs, and what values we want to optimize. While we cannot hope for unanimity in these definitions, it is important to reflect on the implications for policy making that reside in our competing definitions.

## What Is Health? What Is Medicine For?

What we think medicine is shapes what we ask of it. After so many centuries, we are still unclear about what we mean by medicine and what the physician's responsibilities should be in society. There exists a wide range of definitions of medicine, health, disease, and illness (Caplan, Engelhardt, and McCartney, 1981). Each definition generates a different form of practice, ethics, and public policy. But don't all agree that medicine is what doctors do? However, doctors do all sorts of things that fit some, and not other, definitions. The question is whether society should support all of them. As a result, there is growing debate both within and outside medicine on just what the boundaries of medicine should be. How can we design the education of health professionals if we are not certain of the limits of medicine? How do we educate nurses, dentists, and other health professionals without knowing what segment of health needs they are to fill? What responsibility for health should be left to each individual?

Some hold that modern society is overmedicalized and that health should become increasingly the individual's responsibility. Others would have the physician be all things to all men, the guarantor of human happiness: physical, mental, emotional, and even spiritual. Still others would restrict medicine to applied biology, defining its boundaries as those illnesses susceptible to cure, prevention, or amelioration by scientific and technological means (Seldin, 1981; Engel, 1977; Allen, Bird, and Herrmann, 1980). Those with restrictive views would limit medical care, as well as the doctor's role, to those technical things medicine now does reasonably well. The expansionists emphasize that most morbidity, mortality, and disability result from deleterious habits, disorders of family life, or sociopathology that are not susceptible to technological solution.

Each philosophy of medicine defines health as its goal, but each defines health and illness differently. What is illness for some counts as disease for others, and for still others they are the same. We are as unclear about the meaning of health as we are about medicine. Yet it makes a very real difference what philosophy we espouse, for each translates into a different form of medical practice, a different set of ethical obligations, and a different range of services.

The impact on the education of health professionals is clear. If medicine is technologically conceived as applied biology, then it is logical to train specialists almost exclusively, to select students with strong scientific and technological interests and abilities, and to emphasize tertiary care, radical cure, and research. The residuum of ordinary ills—the 85 percent, more or less, of self-limited disorders that require reassurance and relief of anxiety—would be undertaken by less technically trained professionals. According to this formula, fewer physicians and a larger number of nurse clinicians, physician's assistants, pharmacists, or psychologists must be produced. Such a division of labor might be cost-effective and better fitted to the epidemiology of illness. It might also be more realistic than expecting the scientifically educated physician to embrace the lesser ills of mankind, either efficiently or enthusiastically.

In a strictly biomedical model of medicine primary care, prevention, and health education and promotion would be assigned to nurse practitioners and physician's assistants. Working under prescribed protocols, they could meet the demands for primary care on a twenty-four hour, seven-day-a-week basis. Through telecommunication linkages, they could have ready access to consultation with specialists at secondary and tertiary care centers, assuring the quality and safety of the care they provide. The proportion of physicians and their functional relationships to other health professionals would differ greatly from the present.

Yet a different pattern emerges if we accept the more comprehensive views of medicine that embrace not only the whole realm of human ills but also prevention, behavior modification, and patient education. The divergence between generalists and specialists would continue to be accentuated. There would be two kinds of physicians: physician-technicians, whose domain would be that of biological and specific cure, and physician-generalists, whose concern would be with all the broader psychosocial, educational, and counseling needs of individuals, families, and communities.

From the expansionist viewpoint, many more generalists would be needed; the number of nurse practitioners and physician's assistants would be reduced, and their "extension" into medical care limited proportionally. The tendency to medicalize every untoward event in daily life would accelerate. The number of physicians needed might absorb the surplus predicted by the Graduate Medical Education National Advisory Committee (GMENAC) report (1980).

But a shift in public policy to a really comprehensive, holistic view of medicine would call for a drastic increase not only in the numbers of physicians but also in the breadth of their training. No medical school today prepares students with the range of competence encompassed in the biopsychosocial or holistic models of patient care. Even if they did, physicians would find themselves impinging on the domains of clinical psychology, nursing, social work, and the ministry. Emphasis would have to shift from the biological to the social and behavioral sciences. A passing acquaintance with these fields superimposed on a primarily scientific education, as is now the case with the primary care specialties, would not suffice. Different types of students would have to be selected, and different curricula provided for the generalists and technical specialists. For the former, we would need to attract new types of students since even the more broadly trained of today's primary care physicians would resist the dilution of their technical and scientific orientation that the new model would require.

Neither the extreme restrictionist nor expansionist view of medicine is likely to gain unqualified public or professional acceptance. We seem to prefer oscillations between them, without optimizing any one model. Hovering over the debate is still the romanticized notion of the superphysician who is simultaneously a scientist, social scientist, and humanist—a genie educators still hope to coax into appearance by rubbing the magic lamp of curricular reform.

The difficulties do not absolve us from answering the central question: How do we articulate public, social, and educational policies? That question still underlies those other critical questions about cost-effectiveness, patient and professional satisfaction, and curricular design. Sooner or later, we must arrive at some operating definition of the boundaries of medicine and, with it, of the other health professions as well.

In that definition, we cannot avoid the further question of who decides— the public or the profession? Even the more liberal thinkers who invite patients and society to negotiate this issue place the ultimate definition of health, illness, and medicine in the hands of the physician (Siegler, 1981; Engel, 1980). Increasingly, those who are outside medicine would made the definition of health or illness a matter of social, personal, or ethnocultural determination (Whitbeck, 1981; Fabrega, 1972).

Even if some agreement were possible, we would still lack a formula for telling precisely what numbers would be needed. It is clear that within certain limits, there is no strict correlation between the number of health professionals and the health of a nation or the distribution of its health services. Short of some requirement of mandatory national service, the distribution of health professionals will be only loosely related to their supply. How we use them could, however, alter markedly the way they distribute themselves.

A few years ago, state legislators often argued that there should be a sufficient number of places available in medical schools to satisfy all who were qualified to study medicine. Many of the new state schools were established to meet this demand. Now, as the costs of operating these schools become painfully obvious, there is the real possibility of either reduction in the number of these schools or their amalgamation with larger schools of longer standing. Now that the number of entering places in medical schools has increased to the point that a surplus of physicians is threatened, the immediate temptation is to reduce class size. Before the next cycle is initiated, we might try to answer some of the questions we have been discussing here. Approximate answers are all that are likely to result, but they are preferable to the experience of the 1970s when we went from a presumed deficit of 50,000 physicians to a presumed surplus of like size predicted for the end of the 1980s. Educators, practitioners, and policy makers desperately need some mechanism through which to negotiate some agreement on where medicine begins and ends.

### Needs, Demands, and Expectations

No small part of the frustrations about the definition of medicine's boundaries and what we expect of it rests with differences in perception of need. The topography of needs is an intricate nexus of conjectures about individual and social good. Needs are defined in ways that overlap and interrelate in the most complex way. Are needs what professionals deem desirable? Is a need the same as a desire, or is it a perceived lack, insistent enough to become a demand? Is it a disparity between services available to one segment of society and not to another?

How do these several senses of need relate to what some would call *real need*—the requirement for some service or object, the absence of which materially damages or discomfits some individual or group? Are not the weaker senses of need just as real to those who perceive them as the strong sense of real need? I have paraphrased here, and later in this chapter, the simple but useful taxonomy of needs suggested by Jonathan Bradshaw (1972).

The taxonomy of health or medical needs of individuals and societies involves a complicated matrix of interacting forces—desires, perceptions of inequities, demands, real needs, and expectations ranged against services, numbers and kinds of personnel, costs, efficiency, and effectiveness. The difficulties of reaching some agreement in the face of such a multicelled matrix are formidable. Still, without some operating definition of categories of need, no priorities among competing demands and no equilibrium between social goals and educational policy can be established. Like the limits of medicine, needs must be operationally defined in some orderly and cooperative way involving educators, practitioners, policy makers, and the general public. It is in the definition of needs that the most difficult obstacles to agreement are encountered. What we consider needs are, in truth, expressions of what we value, what we consider worthwhile and in our best interest. The unfortunate fact is that the values of the major participants in decision making may differ very markedly. Patients, physicians, hospitals, governments, and academicians each hold to different value systems. Each seeks something different from the medicine and health care system. It is the confrontation of these expectations that we should examine next.

### Value Systems in Confrontation

First is the patient. The things sought from the medical and health care system vary with an individual's life situation. If poor, the patient concentrates on relief from the grosser discomforts and disabilities of physical disease—mostly emergencies, acute conditions, or debilitating chronic disorders that interfere with work or accustomed activity. If affluent, the patient's level of tolerance for discomfort is much lower. Medical treatment will be sought for minor and even trivial problems. The patient will demand relief from small discomfort or anxiety, personal contact with the physician, assistance in prevention, education about health, and luxury items such as elective cosmetic surgery.

Patients look upon physicians as public servants who should assure quality care, be accountable, charge reasonable fees, provide answers to questions about illness in the terms the patient can understand, and meet needs as the patient defines them. Patients expect the hospital to be available twenty-four hours a day, seven days a week. They want someone they can trust, whose competence is assured and whose personal interest in the patient's good is sincere.

Doctors' value systems are perhaps the most important of all by virtue of their control of medical resources. They expect patients to make medical care one of their prime values and to define health in medical terms. Physicians are available for emergencies, but their conception of an emergency is not necessarily the same as the patients'. Doctors measure quality by access to and availability of the best facilities, the latest instruments, and the most skilled laboratories and consultants. They prefer to work with interesting and challenging diseases, not high-volume demands for the care of minor disorders. Mortality and morbidity are their measures. They believe that their knowledge makes them the best judge of what the patient needs and, therefore, that they should control the delivery system.

Physicians also value freedom to make their own decisions and to earn what they consider a justifiable income on a fee-for-service basis. They expect freely to choose where, what, and how to practice. They want a stimulating environment and not too many patients; they expect patients to be cooperative; they want opportunities for continuing education and a position of influence on decision making in all health care institutions.

A third set of values is held by the hospitals and health care institutions, often in tension with values of both the patient and the doctor. Community and university hospitals ordinarily subscribe to different values. Today both are driven by economic and fiscal concerns. They skew their services to those who can pay their bills. Occupancy, bed utilization, efficiency in billing and collection, the demands of physicians, image in the community, and staying ahead of competitors are significant driving forces. In the competitive climate, economics, marketing, and profit will assume even more prominent places in the administrator's value system. Indeed, to an increasing extent, university and community hospitals will become competitors with each other, especially for the secondary and tertiary care patient.

University and teaching hospitals have traditionally pursued scientific and technological excellence, clinical research, teaching, and care of the poor and less affluent. Fiscal constraints, together with a decrease in support for education and research, will force them to adopt values not very different from the larger community hospitals. Clinical faculties must now support themselves through clinical practice. The care of those at the margins of society, the "losers" in the game of competition, is already being deemphasized. A service and education-oriented value system is being replaced by a practice and profit-oriented one. As more nonprofit hospitals become proprietary, these pressures on the teaching hospitals are sure to increase.

Until recently, government assumed responsibility for equilibrating supply and need for health professionals, equity of access, availability, and quality control. Now these responsiblities are being thrust on local governments unprepared to assume them. While the national goal is still, ostensibly, high quality care at a cost we can afford, it is now to be achieved by competition between providers and through the operation of the magic of the marketplace. The thesis of the proponents of competition is that government regulation and intervention have escalated costs and fostered overuse of medical services. However, there is no evidence, as yet, that competition will not produce other deleterious effects; what is certain is that with deregulation, profit will become a dominant value, with results yet to be evaluated.

In the coming era of competition, the values of the marketplace and its criteria of success—profits, efficiency, return on investment, market penetration, capitalization potential, productivity, managerial efficiency, and bond ratings—will dominate. No one can say what effects the conversion of medical care to a commodity transaction will have. Some sectors of the health care field have always looked at the world this way. Now this is to be the sanctioned, even the encouraged, value system. We simply do not know what its effects will be on the quality of care, the compassion with which it is dispensed, or the tranformations it may induce in the healing relationship. One salubrious result will be the necessity to face the value questions more directly than ever before. In a time of plenty, the commercial aspects of medical care could be submerged. But in an era of competition, Bernard Shaw's *Doctor's Dilemma* is no longer denied but exalted and heralded as the road to both cost containment and quality care. (Shaw's play, and especially his introductory essay, scathingly portray the professions as conspiracies against the public. The play shows how subtly, and not so subtly, the physician's financial self-interest may color his decisions. While the "dilemma" is never completely eradicable, it is sure to be enhanced by an ethos of competition. The only check is a continual reemphasis on the moral grounding of all medical actions.)

The values of academic medicine constitute an identifiable ethos quite at odds with some of the values of patients, practitioners, and community hospitals. This ethos has been expressed usually in the Flexnerian doxology: Medicine is essentially a scientific endeavor, best taught by full-time academic clinicians who are primarily scholars, specialists, and nonpractitioners. The place for medical teaching is the university-controlled tertiary care hospital. Scientific method and problem solving are best taught there. The dominant values are faith in the rational, objectivity, competence, and dedication to the community of science—a dedication transcending personal interest.

In this view, medicine has a prime responsibility to eradicate disease through an attack on its causes. Palliation and caring functions that do not demonstrably change the natural course of an illness are acknowledged, but since they are not yet susceptible to scientific resolution, they are not intrinsic to medicine. Social and community responsibilities likewise dilute the physician's proper concentration on cure of individual patients.

In the last few decades, community and patient needs of a broader kind have been advanced as a complementary ordering of principles for medical education. In this view, the majority of physicians should be trained specifically to meet a nation's needs, giving special attention to the demographic, socioeconomic, and cultural sources of ill health. Technological medicine is applicable only when it benefits wide segments of the community and not a select few. Primary care, prevention, and health promotion should take precedence as the prime mission for medical education. This latter view is usually promulgated by those who prescribe for the developing nations, though it is not necessarily shared by those who live in those countries. Even those who think scientific medicine is too narrow will rarely extrapolate their view to its logical conclusion.

Undoubtedly, the most drastic value shift of all may come from the ruling of the Federal Trade Commission (FTC) stating that medicine is a trade and that its ethical code is a self-serving device. The 1980 case of the *American Medical Association* v. *Federal Trade Commission* upheld the claim of the FTC for jurisdiction over the AMA, at least with regard to "advertising, solicitation, and contractual relationships" (United States Court of Appeals, Second Circuit, October 7, 1980). The Supreme Court affirmed the decision without opinion March 23, 1982. "Justice Blackmun took no part in the consideration or decision in this case." While the issue here has been the AMA's interdiction against advertising, the issues are much more profound, touching directly on the intent, validity, and probity of professional ethical codes (see FTC Order and Opinion 94 FTC Rep. 701). This recent four-four decision of the Supreme Court to uphold the FTC opinion does more than leave the question moot. The fact of a split vote on a question of such importance reflects a deep-seated change in society's view of medicine and, indeed, of the whole idea of a profession as a distinct social calling.

If medicine is indeed only a trade and a commercial transaction, its values and ethics become those of business and commerce. This view will firmly reinforce the procompetition thrust of public policy and the inclinations of those physicians who have always wanted medicine to be a business and nothing more. The supporters of the FTC ruling see it as a breakthrough against the privileges medicine has unfairly claimed; to others, it is a potential disaster. For a vigorous statement of the competition ethos in health care, see Stockman (1981) and Havighurst (1981). For a balanced analysis of the implications of competition and the applications of antitrust law to medical affairs, see Marmor, Boyer, and Greenberg (1981). For the moral and ethical implications, see Pellegrino (1981b and 1983).

We are in something close to a neurosis about our health care system. We have the capability for the first time in history to make a fuller measure of health available to all people. In developed countries, even in the present gloomy economic climate, we command the resources to make this possible. Yet despite expenditures of great magnitude, the goal seems to recede. We lack agreement on what is the common good and what priority we should place on things we value when they come into conflict with each other. As we make our policies, we must reflect more critically on the values they revere and the kind of society those values will shape. In that examination, the academic health centers have an obligation they seem not to be assuming at present.

## What Does the Future Portend?

This selective look at the taxonomy of competing values illustrates the difficulties of any attempt to articulate social need and educational policy in the production of future health professionals. Certainly, we can never expect to reach a final resolution that for all time will harmoniously link a national health policy with a national educational policy. But we can, however, hope for some better mechanisms for airing the debate, for involving more of the public, and for defining the value presuppositions that undergird policy formation. We can come closer than we have to deciding what we want from our health and medical care expenditures, what we expect physicians and health professionals to do for us, what we are willing to sacrifice, and what we must retain from our traditional medical practices. We cannot decide how much of that society we want to accept unless we are familiar with the values that will emerge.

Americans are practical people, problem solvers more than ideologues. If a crisis becomes acute enough, compromises are always possible. Admittedly, there is a greater polarization at present than we have experienced in recent years, largely because of the recent reversal of political and economic philosophies. Can these conflicting value systems be subjected to some fundamental ordering principle that will arrange them in a system of logical priority? I think they can. But I do not think it will come about until we have purged ourselves of the newest panacea—the competition ideology. Its proponents are vocal, assured, and a bit triumphant over the evident failures of the regulation ethos. Obviously, they offer a change and in this there is always hope. Without hoping for disaster, I believe competition will soon exhibit its own damaging effects. When they become apparent, there will be an outcry for a return to regulation, this time for much greater control than we have yet experienced. Since we have already been down the regulation pathway, I hope we will pause before plunging into it again.

Perhaps at that point we will step back and begin from ground zero, from the fundamental human needs that medicine and the whole health care apparatus are supposed to serve. Therein lies the only morally defensible ordering principle, since it is based on needs we all share as humans. The restoration of reason to our debates rests on a restoration of the moral credibility of medicine and the other health professions. If the FTC is right, then morality beyond the minimalist ethics of business has little place; if, as I believe, the FTC is wrong, then we must restore our moral standing. This we can do only by redeeming the service element of our health professions. The choice is ours and society's, but it ought not be made by default.

We must start again from the obvious—the fact that the health professions exist because humans fall ill and need to be cured, healed, and cared for. Health is indispensable for the good life, no matter what other values one may esteem. The health professions are ordained specifically to help society attain these ends. This is the only justification for any privileges they may hold and for the support they receive. To acknowledge these obligations is the first step in regaining moral credibility.

Schools for the health professions are society's only means of assuring a continuing supply of competent practitioners. Society grants these schools a monopoly because they are essential for the good of all. This is the source of their moral mandate. To recognize that mandate is the first step in resolving the dilemmas of values we have been discussing.

If the health professions accept the proposition that they are commercial enterprises, if their work does not transcend self-interest, and if profit is their motive, then the FTC is right. The health professions cannot then claim the privileges of discretionary space or self-determination. Medicine and all the professions are forced by the FTC decision to examine what makes them different from business and the trades.

That difference will be found only in the social/moral obligations incurred by a profession that offers to help as well as to act competently. Illness is a state of special vulnerability, and healing requires a relationship of trust. Trust by its very nature cannot be assured by contract. Indeed, contracts exist because the parties cannot trust each other.

All the helping professions—medicine, law, ministry, teaching—must work through a fiduciary relationship, because in each instance the person to be served is in a special state of need and vulnerability. That need arises out of the condition of being human; it is usually not elective, and a person is usually not free to ignore that need as one might ignore the "need" for beer, a new suit, or even a vacation. In the helping professions, there is an expectation of trust. It is this expectation that distinguishes them from business and the trades where the self-interest of the tradesman is expected to dominate his actions. The sick person is in pain, suffering, and facing disability and death. He trusts the healer to recognize his vulnerability and not take advantage of it. This is what separates medicine from a business transaction where both parties can be trusted only to act in their own self-interest. Vulnerability in business is an advantage to be exploited, not the restraint on the practitioner's self-interest that it must be in a helping profession.

The patient's need, arising out of the fact of illness, is the ordering principle required to sort out the various categories of need with which society is faced in allocating limited resources. For example, the first needs to be satisfied might be those that, if left unattended, would result in serious damage—what has been defined as "real" need. Included would be those specific cures and preventions that demonstrably alter the natural history of disease. Following this might be the needs of those with chronic or serious illnesses for which we have no cure but that can be contained or ameliorated. In the last category might be needs arising in disorders that are self-limited or minor in their discomfort, whose remedies are desirable but whose absence would produce little or no discernible damage. These might be "relative" needs. Another way to look at priorities from the point of view of those who are ill would be as follows: emergency medicine first, followed by elective treatment for curable disorders, then treatment for catastrophic illnesses, and finally treatment for the self-limited less serious illnesses that may produce discomfort but relatively little impairment of function.

I am not suggesting either of these schemes as guidelines for insurance coverage or for setting priorities in resource allocation. This is what must be debated publicly. I am merely illustrating a way we might approach the setting of priorities based on some categorization of common human needs that arise when any of us becomes ill.

The order of priorities that would emerge from such a categorization will differ from that which might result from treating medical care like any other commodity transaction where consumers and providers "freely" negotiate demands and supplies. How free, indeed, we are in our consumer transactions is a moot point. We need only look at our current marketplace with its deceptive advertising, shoddy products, illusory warranties, and promotional chicanery. Does a competitive market offer "free" choices of the kind we want to make? Without some moral imperative and some ordering principle that transcends profit, we are likely to experience the same moral depreciation in the medical and health market. When the principle of "caveat emptor" replaces that of "primum non nocere," then the person who is ill is without protection. Lawsuits are ex post facto remedies that cannot restore lost lives. My purpose here is not to castigate competition; it has not yet been tested as a dominant principle in health care. But its dangers are substantial without the restraints of a moral ordering principle to contain them.

What I am suggesting is that we approach the question of what we want from our health care system in a modular and stepwise fashion based on a priority ranking of categories of need: real needs first; normative needs next; then perceived, comparative, and expressed needs, in that order. How far down the list any nation goes would depend upon the percentage of its gross national product it wishes to put into medical and health care. That decision involves how we value health against other competing good things. Obviously, as new treatments become available, they would be assigned a position in this schema.

Another example of a very basic real need that all humans share is for access to primary care in some proximity to where they live, twenty-four hours a day, seven days a week. I refer here to the restricted sense of primary care, that is, a system of first contact service that enables the patient to receive prompt advice on what should be done for some new medical event. Under such circumstances, most humans need to transfer some of their anxiety, to find out if the event is serious and whether it needs referral to a more advanced facility or can be treated promptly in a primary care facility. Freedom from the anxiety of being able to find help in an emergency is so fundamental to a civilized society that it must qualify as an obligation of the promise such a society makes to its citizens to be a concerned society.

Beyond this category of real needs, there is a wider latitude of choices between comparative, perceived, and expressed needs. The order of needs we select will depend upon which conception of medicine we accept, how much of life we wish to medicalize, and how much we wish to allocate to medicine and health as opposed to other things good for society and individuals.

This approach assumes that medical care is a necessary condition for a free life, that it has an intrinsic value, that without it the other privileges of a free society cannot be fully enjoyed, and that we share a corporate responsibility as citizens to assure ourselves and our fellow citizens of some definable range of services. Health needs cannot be defined globally; no society can afford to meet all categories of need without seriously compromising other things valued as good. By assuring real needs first, at least the most disadvantaged members of any society can have access to relief of remediable conditions. Meeting these needs—however far into the list a society chooses to go or can afford to go—becomes the end for which health professionals are educated and by which their functions are defined.

No element in the balance between educational and social policy can be treated in isolation from the others or permitted to function totally independently. Self-regulation requires a degree of ethical sensitivity rare even in the most enlightened societies. Some regulation will always be necessary. Reality demands that some mechanisms specifically designed to effect a coordinated effort be established. The partitioning of functions and responsibilities between academic institutions, the government, providers, and consumers cannot be effected otherwise.

Resolution of the dilemma of conflicting interests requires at least the following mechanisms: First, it requires a mechanism for examining the focal questions in the realm of public policy. Those questions cannot be answered by regulatory agencies, professionals, or consumers acting alone. To be rational, response must be based on factually reliable input. However, the fact and value issues must be disentangled or the self-interests of one or another group of experts will dominate.

Thus the value we place on health, how much to spend on it, how much on other social needs, and what uses we wish to make of medicine and health professions are matters of public and not professional decision. If public choices are to be informed, they must be based upon technically reliable information about what medicine can and cannot do, which treatments are effective, what is required to train one kind of health worker versus another, and what resources are requisite. Academicians and practitioners have a special responsibility to answer such questions with honesty, accuracy, and reliability. They cannot, however, assume that technical expertise confers authority on the value issues. On that score, professionals do not differ from their fellow citizens. Though they may presume otherwise, they are not experts in values, only in facts. I have argued elsewhere for both value and fact panels to help policy makers examine those two realms of decision making more explicitly than is now the case (Pellegrino, 1981b).

If we can decide what we wish from the health care system, then we can determine how many and what kind of health professionals we need. These questions are of a technical nature, and they can be most effectively addressed by the health professions. No single health profession can act in isolation from the others or consider itself automatically in a more authoritative position. Specifically, this means that physicians should take their place in the discussion with all the other health professionals. By virtue of its long history and its broad knowledge, medicine has a major contribution to make to the dialogue, but it is not necessarily or always the most authoritative contributor.

The health professions acting together can recapture some of their moral credibility. To do so, they must submerge their territorial disputes and take some steps such as the following: For one thing, there needs to be some common agreement on what is known and not known about a specific issue, at least factually. Nothing creates more confusion for policy makers than conflicting and contradictory statements of fact by different "experts." Separating the certain from the uncertain, the partial from the whole truth, and opinion from fact is a responsiblity we could mutually share. The same cooperative effort is required in defining which profession is best qualified to carry out the many functions required in a health care system. One profession cannot decide by itself what functions it arrogates to itself and which it relegates to others. This is the common practice, and much of the din is about territorial imperatives rather than how genuinely to meet the needs of patients and society.

This effort would be greatly enhanced if the professional associations were guided by some prioritized list of needs developed in a public forum outside the professions, with their participation but not final determination. With the help of such a list, the associations might more profitably determine how to partition the functions among them to meet the prescribed needs. If this were done, it could obviate the need for the development of new categories of health manpower. A more careful redistribution of functions among existing health manpower would suffice in most instances to meet most of the unmet needs in society today. The question would be not who is doing this function now or who has done it traditionally, but who can do it with some change or extension of existing function?

Ultimately, such an effort would result in a coalescence and condensing of the kinds of health professionals and the eventual formation of perhaps two to three general category health professions. The health professions are now headed in precisely the opposite direction of fragmentation, divergence, and conflict. Nonetheless, by concentrating on the question of what patients need and what societies need, the divisive and divergent tendencies might possibly be reversed.

A major responsibility of the health sciences centers is to develop new models of providing health care. These models are the testing ground for the decisions that must ultimately be made as to role realignment and reassignment, for evaluations of the efficiency of team care, and for assessing both cost-effectiveness and patient satisfaction. The elaboration and testing of such models is greatly facilitated when education of the various health professions is conducted at a multidisciplinary, multischool academic health center.

Perhaps the most specific challenge for the academician is to reexamine the presuppositions upon which the current value system of medical education is based. What are the purposes of education in the health professions? What obligations does an educational institution incur by virtue of the expectations of it that it permits society to entertain? Why do certain functions have to be assigned to certain professions? How closely does the theoretical content of a profession correlate with its manipulative functions? These questions expose a host of academic assumptions that need careful inquiry. The academic setting is the place for such explorations, provided they are carried out critically and objectively. If not, we can expect public interest to intrude with necessarily increasing vigor, as the gap widens between the systems of education, utilization, and need for future health professionals.

The split decision of the Supreme Court means that the question of the propriety of FTC jurisdiction over the medical profession will be decided by Congress. That decision will occur just as we are moving into an era of competition in the health care field, an era in which the antitrust laws are being applied to the medical profession. It is an era in which the traditional concept of a profession is being seriously eroded. How responsibly the health professions conduct themselves in the next few years will determine whether or not society will give up the idea of professions entirely. Are there human activities that are distinguished by motives that transcend personal interests, or is there nothing beyond business and the trades in the world of human services?

The values that underlie our public decisions will reveal a great deal about the kind of society we have become or want to be. Before society gives up the idea of professions, it is imperative that all of us ponder the implications. In that pondering, the academic health centers have more than a role of acquiescence. They stand at the junction between society's needs and the provision of the personnel who can respond to those needs. They must be both critics and servants of the public good.

## References

Allen, D. S., Bird, L. P., and Herrmann, R. L. *Whole Person Medicine*. Downers Grove, Ill.: Intervarsity Press, 1980.

Bradshaw, J. "A Taxonomy of Social Needs." In G. McLachan (Ed.), *Problems and Progress in Medical Care: Essays in Current Research*. London: Oxford University Press, 1972.

Caplan, A. J., Engelhardt, H. J., and McCartney, J. J. *Concepts of Health and Disease*. Reading, Mass.: Addison-Wesley, 1981.

Engel, G. "The Need for a New Medical Model: A Challenge for Biomedicine." *Science*, 1977, *196*, 129–136.

Engel, G. "The Clinical Application of the Biopsychosocial Model." *American Journal of Psychiatry*, 1980, *137* (5), 535–544.

Fabrega, H. "Concepts of Disease: Logical Features and Social Implications Perspectives." *Biology and Medicine*, 1972, *1* (4), 538–617.

Graduate Medical Education National Advisory Committee. *Summary Report to the Secretary, Department of Health and Human Services.* Vol. 1. Washington, D.C.: U. S. Government Printing Office, 1980.

Havighurst, C. C. "Competition in the Health Services: Overview, Issues, and Answers." *Vanderbilt Law Review,* 1981, *34* (4), 1117–1158.

Marmor, T. R., Boyer, R., and Greenberg, J. "Medical Care and Pro-Competitive Reform." *Vanderbilt Law Review,* 1981, *34* (4), 1003–1028.

Pellegrino, E. D. "Competition and Commerce or Covenant and Care: The Ethical Fallout of Pro-Competitive Policies in Medical Care." 1981 Esselstyn Lecture, Yale University, New Haven, Conn., April 1981a.

Pellegrino, E. D. "Optimizing the Uses of Medical Knowledge." In *Proceedings of the Symposium on the Optimum Utilization of Knowledge,* Academy of Independent Scholars, University of Massachusetts in Amherst, November 1981b, in press.

Pellegrino, E. D. "Pro-Competition Legislation: The Moral Dilemmas of Untested Assumptions." *Journal of Family Practice,* 1983, *16* (1), 17–19.

Seldin, D. W. "The Boundaries of Medicine." *Transactions of the Association of American Physicians,* XCIV 1981, LXXV-LXXXVI.

Siegler, M. "The Doctor-Patient Encounter and Its Relationship to Health and Disease." In A. Caplan, H. Engelhardt, and J. McCartney, *Concepts of Health and Disease.* Reading, Mass.: Addison-Wesley, 1981.

Stockman, D. A. "Premises for the Medical Marketplace: A Neoconservative's Vision of How to Transform the Medical Marketplace." *Health Affairs,* 1981, *61,* 5–18.

Whitbeck, C. "A Theory of Health." In A. Caplan, H. Engelhardt, and J. McCartney, *Concepts of Health and Disease.* Reading, Mass.: Addison-Wesley, 1981.

*Herbert E. Klarman*  $16$

# Economic Trends

## Reassessing Health Care and Manpower Needs

To help guide the reader, the conclusions I draw from the evidence and opinions to be presented are shown at the outset, and expressed in the form of four propositions.

*Proposition One.* The concept of health care needs, though widely employed in the rhetoric of health care, poses difficulties on several grounds, including those of reliability, validity, and feasibility of implementation. Indeed, the concept of need is neither operational nor would it be useful for formulating health manpower policy if it were.

*Proposition Two.* To plan for health care services, it is pertinent to focus on a population's use of services (past and present), on gaps and duplication in existing services, and on the population's ability and willingness to pay for the services. For reasons to be enumerated, I have come to believe that past trends in health care spending are not likely to continue in the foreseeable future. Rather, future increases in the amount of health care spending will be smaller than formerly, because they will be restrained.

*Proposition Three.* How health care spending will be restrained is problematic. The contents of health care legislation still to be enacted—whether financial, regulatory, or procompetition—are unknown. Employing the annual congressional budget resolution as a vehicle for changing the formula for reimbursing hospitals under the Medicare program, as happened in 1981, adds an element of caprice. Even if the forms of market competition that will emerge were known, the forms that will prosper are not known. Moreover, how the various categories of health manpower will adapt to the new constraints adds another element of uncertainty, given the lack of prior, analogous experience.

*Proposition Four.* As for the implication of restraint on health care spending for the education of health professionals, the association between the two is not one-to-one. Nonfinancial returns to an occupation relative to its financial returns have different degrees of importance.

For example, it can be asserted with confidence that, for the foreseeable future, the demand for admission to medical schools will continue to exceed by far their stated capacities. Within a wide range, expected health care spending will have no relationship to the number of Americans who wish to become physicians. True, a marked rise in medical school tuition or a reduction in student aid is likely to cause some changes in the composition of the student body. However, the total number of physicians trained will remain at the level of total medical school capacity, as long as the latter falls short of the number of applicants.

In some health professions, in which nonfinancial rewards like prestige and autonomy are not important, a lower rate of increase in spending for the services of those occupations may lead to a drop in average earnings as the total numbers increase, and then to a decline in school enrollment. For a profession like registered nursing, it is difficult to foresee the outcome of interplay between changes in the financial and nonfinancial rewards of the occupation and in the forces impinging on this occupation that originate within the health care industry and the forces that originate in the economy and society at large. Accordingly, ranges in projections of registered nurse employment and school enrollment are wide. The uncertainty is heightened by continuing shifts in the site of nurse training and by well-founded speculation about the direction of the trend in the capacity of the nation's short-term hospital system.

In dentistry, two new forces are likely to compete for dominance. One, increasing the amount spent and raising the demand for services, is the emergence and growth of dental care insurance. The other, reducing the financial attractiveness of the occupation, is the increase in the cost of training to the student, as governmental subsidy declines.

As usual, let me declare that the preceding propositions, as well as the arguments to be adduced in their behalf, represent but one economist's viewpoint. Health economists are known to differ not only in how they explain past events but also in how they perceive them. Indeed, the same individual may hold different views of events, depending on his or her current responsibilities as academician and detached observer or as public official and advocate of specific policies.

## Conventional Formulation of Health Manpower Needs

It is helpful to begin with a conventional formulation of the supply and need for a particular health care occupation, as typically found in the health care literature. This establishes a point of departure for appraisal and criticism. In typical health care usage, the supply of an occupation is the number of persons actively working in it at a given time. It is not the economist's more conditional notion of a supply function, which relates the number offering their services to a price. Sometimes the term *requirements* is employed, as a somewhat neutral (or perhaps ambiguous) proxy for the term *need*.

Several sources of official figures are now available on projected health manpower availabilities (supply) and needs (or requirements), all of them incorporated in fairly sophisticated models. Some models aim directly at fashioning manpower policy, while other models employ manpower data and equations for the purpose of projecting health care expenditures. Projections from the Bureau of Health Manpower of the U.S. Department of Health and Human Services (1980), by Stambler (1979), and by the Graduate Medical Education National Advisory Committee (1980) exemplify the former; projections from the Health Care Financing Administration (Freeland and Schendler, 1981) exemplify the latter. The models that aim directly at manpower policy yield figures of surplus or shortage by simple subtraction of the projected numbers working from the projected numbers required. It has long been a constant source of wonder to me that the estimates of surplus or shortage invariably apply to one or more future years and never to the past or present. Indeed, when applied to the past, as by the Graduate Medical Education National Advisory Committee (1980), the figures are generated by an admittedly oversimple extrapolation backward of a future forecast.

It is but a simple step, one that does not call for a behavioral model, to translate figures on net manpower requirements (gross requirements less availabilities) into figures on educational capacity requirements. Involved here is an arithmetic identity, that is, an estimate of the annual requirement for replacements if the profession were in a steady state, plus or minus an allowance for the profession's projected expansion or contraction from its current baseline. The size of this allowance is judgmental, depending on how quickly the steady-state goal is to be reached.

The preceding discussion of arithmetic details presupposes that the projections of availabilities and requirements derive from the same source or at least that the assumptions underlying them are mutually consistent. Not all the figures have to be published, however, since professional standards of courtesy ensure the release of unpublished worksheets to other scholars. More and more, it is fair to say, the task facing the educational planner has become one of choosing among alternative models and their sets of projections rather than one of reconciling inconsistent assumptions or contradictory data. Without a doubt, our technical capability has improved over time. As assumptions have become specified and made explicit, the feasibility of replicating results has become virtually assured. All this notwithstanding, the usefulness of the output of formal models for policy formation has not improved to a corresponding degree, if at all. This I shall now try to demonstrate.

## Concept of Need

When the criterion of need is made operational, it usually lacks reliability in the statistical sense. That is, different sets of experts facing the same data on the occurrence of illness will arrive at different estimates of health manpower needs (Klarman, 1951, 1977). In addition to different ideas on the appropriate numbers of physician visits, different ideas on the proper length of the visit, on the length of the physician's workweek, and on the length of his vacation are conducive to divergent estimates.

It also happens that the same experts who espouse teamwork in staffing health care will, with no awareness of apparent inconsistency, estimate separately the need for each category of health manpower. The latter procedure implies, of course, that health manpower ratios are in constant and unalterable proportion to one another. Yet the concept of fixed staffing ratios is invalidated by the changes in staffing that have taken place over time and by the variations in staffing that prevail at a given time. My own review of the literature on ambulatory care indicates that the delegation of functions by physicians to auxiliary workers varies to a large extent with local market conditions (Klarman, 1970).

In dentistry, employment of auxiliary workers is widespread. Even so, I know dentists in New York City who work alone, without any assistants. In hospitals in New York City, the ratio of bedside registered nurses to practical nurses has varied inversely with their respective salary ratios, which vary in turn with hospital ownership (Klarman, 1963). Moreover, within the same institutions, the tasks permitted to a practical nurse seem to vary by time of day.

One can anticipate a reasonable rebuttal to the preceding line of argument. It is only to be expected that an economist would invoke market conditions and occupational earnings. However, this economist does so with full awareness of the traditional, widely held view in this country that health care should be available to all persons who need it, regardless of individual ability to pay for it (Klarman, 1951). Such a benevolent attitude toward the provision of health care commands support from a wide range of political sentiment, from right to left, and clearly antedates the 1960s claims to health care as a right. This special attitude toward health care helps explain why the provision of health care to the poor antedates cash benefits and why health care is often given free to the medically indigent.

The laymen—businessmen, lawyers, bankers, and politicians, as well as community activists—who serve on the boards of directors of voluntary, nonprofit hospitals and community service agencies with the aim to do good rely on health care experts to instruct them as to what to do. Lay board members expect the experts to know how to measure the need for health care, to measure it with precision, to infer findings on the extent of unmet need, and to prepare recommendations for filling it.

In the same spirit, commission reports, statutes, regulations, and health plans refer to need as if it were a self-evident, objective, and measurable standard of the amount and types of services that a community should have. When measured need is combined with an estimate of availabilities, the net balance is seen as providing simply and directly a basis for acting to overcome the impending shortage or surplus of health manpower.

This is not the place to review the evidence as to whether American society's performance measures up to its professed aspiration to provide health care to all persons who need it, regardless of individual ability to pay for it. By such a standard, virtually every society is bound to fall short. What is fair to note in the present context is that if the criterion of need is taken seriously and made operational, it accords to health care and to each of its components an absolute priority of claim on resources. If so, it follows that this standard affords no practical guidance in allocating resources to and among health care programs and, hence, to and among health care occupations. Under the criterion of need, as formulated in the classic study by Lee and Jones (1933), individuals are deemed to need care even when they do not know it, do not want care, or refuse to seek it at the designated site, so long as health care experts believe that such care is appropriate according to prevailing standards of good medical practice. One possible result of allocating resources on the basis of need is a waste of resources if patients fail to use them for any of the above reasons.

It is tempting to account for departures from the criterion of need by pointing to the professional prerogatives of physicians and to their financial self-interest. However, there is ample evidence that the use of health care, though heavily influenced by the presence of illness, is also influenced by other consumer characteristics, such as income, health insurance status, age, sex, marital status, travel distance from a provider, educational level, and personal health practices. Prices too influence use, and the price of health care may extend beyond the patient's out-of-pocket charges to include the value of travel time and waiting time (Newhouse, 1978).

The above observations raise questions about the very validity of the criterion of need, that is, whether it measures what we should like to measure. Indeed, is the criterion of need useful in forming health care policy, except for the extreme case of a medical emergency? Other approaches are necessary, and they are not simple (Klarman, 1974, 1979). Nor are they totally dependent on data, devoid of value judgments.

## Outlook for Health Care Spending

My most serious reservation about the usefulness of the criterion of need is that society is expected to implement it, regardless of the aggregate financial ability of its members to support the implied expenditures. This criticism of the criterion of need warrants elaboration, since in the foreseeable future the availability of requisite funding for health care, regardless of the amount, can no longer be taken for granted, if it ever could be.

Not so long ago, health care providers served also as philanthropists. Physicians scaled their fees in relation to patients' incomes, and voluntary nonprofit hospitals furnished free care to the poor and part-pay care to the working poor. These pricing practices have been undermined by the growth of voluntary health insurance and other sources of third-party payment. As the measure of an individual's ability to pay for health care shifted from income to health insurance status, the old method of distributing health care in a community—rationing by providers—became obsolete.

Moreover, following World War II, while the dollar amount of philanthropic contributions to health care increased, their proportion of total health care expenditures fell drastically (Klarman, 1981). Increasingly, philanthropic monies received by hospitals have been diverted from defraying the cost of free care to other, special purposes, such as providing seed money for research projects or for employing full-time clinicians. The charge structure adopted by Medicare has enabled physicians to charge more to all their patients, even as the program reduced the claim by the aged to free or part-free care. The result is that today the availability of health care to an individual depends much more than formerly on the presence of an identifiable source of funds to pay for it.

It is well-known that expenditures for health care have increased substantially in the past generation or two. A brief summary of trends in health care spending will suffice (Gibson and Waldo, 1981; Klarman, 1981). Between 1950 and 1980, health care expenditures in the United States rose twentyfold. Expressed in constant dollars, health care expenditures increased 5.5 times between 1950 and 1980. Expressed as a ratio of the gross national product (GNP) health care expenditures have more than doubled between 1950 and 1980, from 4.4 to 9.5 percent. According to Gibson (1982), the figure for 1981 was 9.8 percent.

In all these figures, the upward trend has accelerated since 1965, when the Medicare and Medicaid programs were enacted. In my judgment, these past increases in health care spending lie at the root of future restraint on such spending and are reinforced by our perceptions of the low value received for the money spent.

One reason for this judgment is that the current baseline ratio of health care expenditures is much higher than the 1950 ratio. I borrow from Fuchs (1982) this simple exercise in the arithmetic of compound interest. When the annual rate of increase in health care expenditures exceeds the annual rate of growth in GNP, a differential in these rates of two percentage points a year, when extended over ten years, raises the ratio of health care spending to GNP to 6.1 percent from an initial baseline of 5.0 percent but to 12.2 percent from a baseline of 10.0 percent.

A second reason for anticipating restraint on health care spending lies in the labor-intensive nature of the health care industry. In an expanding economy, such an industry lags in productivity gains behind the economy at large. At the same time, in a mobile economy the health care industry must match the average increase in real wages in the economy at large. In consequence, the unit cost of health care increases. Health care expenditures will increase disproportionately in an expanding economy, even if the total volume of health care services is constant, unless some countervailing action is taken.

Economic growth does enable some sectors to expand by absorbing increasing shares of the growth in GNP, without taking anything away from other sectors. Between 1950 and 1966, health care took 7 percent of the increment in GNP, and between 1966 and 1980, 11 percent. Between 1979 and 1981, the corresponding figure was 14 percent (Gibson, 1982).

Such an increase in the unit cost of health care can be avoided if there is no lag in productivity gains, but this is most likely to occur in a stagnant economy. To increase the volume of health care services, however, it becomes necessary to divert resources from other sectors of the economy. Similarly, to raise average wages in health care, it becomes necessary to lower them elsewhere. The result is conflict over who gets how much; that is a conflict among producers, which is usually contested much more vigorously than an assertion of consumers' interests.

A third source of probable constraint on spending for health care is the change in status of the social security fund. Voting for increases in social security cash benefits is no longer automatic, as it formerly was. Even funding for Medicare is at risk today.

A fourth possible source is legislation to limit the amount of the employer contribution to health insurance premiums excluded from taxation to the individual employee. Such a limit is expected to lead to restraint on the part of employees in purchasing comprehensive health insurance and uninsured health care. I believe that another effect, surely unintended, may be a decline in health insurance enrollment by low-earning employees.

Our perceptions, valid or not, of the value received for the money spent on health care represent a fifth source of future restraint on health care spending. For example, research findings on hospital use in prepaid group practice lay virtually unnoticed for twenty years, until they were unearthed to serve as the supporting data for the first procompetition intiative in health care, the Health Maintenance Organization. A seed was sown for the idea that more hospital use is not necessarily better. It reinforced another intellectual position, namely Roemer's, that asserts that under conditions of prepayment, a wide range of hospital bed to population ratios exists, while bed occupancy rates are uniform (Shain and Roemer, 1959; Roemer, 1961). In time, recognition has been given to the availability effect, which is a medical corollary of Roemer's law. Whether and how the availability effect operates is a matter of controversy among economists, just as Roemer's law is. My own view is that physicians can and do influence their patients' demand for procedures and visits, because they know so much more about diagnosis and treatment, while the range of appropriate care for the individual patient is wide.

Another example pertains to the perception that health care spending is futile. One argument is that halfway technology is expensive; it would be better to wait for more effective and less costly technology, as developed by research. Another argument is pervasive and more influential, since it is associated with such leading experts in health care as Cochrane (1972) and McKeown (1976) and White (1973) in the United States. The position of these researchers is that the vastly increased health care expenditures have yielded no significant improvement in health status. Owing to the ready availability of mortality statistics, changes in health status are typically measured by changes in death rates. Fuchs allowed for the possibility of a small contribution, since health care may have compensated for the deleterious changes in life-style that are often associated with a rise in income.

Today we know that mortality rates have fallen appreciably in the United States. In the decade of 1968 to 1978, the overall age-adjusted death rate from all causes declined 19 percent. For stroke, the reduction was double this figure—38 percent. It was also sizable for heart disease—23 percent (Kleinman, Fingerhut, and Feldman, 1981). The fact is that most of us do not examine raw data or read tables. Rather, we rely on articles, many of which continue to refer to the uselessness of health care spending, given the stable death rates that prevailed in the preceding generation. It is also true that the causes of the appreciable decline in death rates remain unknown. Amidst such uncertainty, virtually any explanation commands attention, and most explanations tend to reflect the predilections of their adherents.

Meanwhile, the caring function in health care tends to be neglected. The penultimate chapter in Cochrane's (1972) otherwise influential book has gone unheeded in this country, while the Medicaid program has quietly, almost surreptitiously, taken over responsibility for financing long-term nursing home care from the Medicare program, which moved early to limit extended care benefits to a short period of posthospital recovery. The need for health care by long-term patients is especially difficult to measure operationally, since a patient's condition can fluctuate even in a short interval; situations at patients' homes vary; and the range of professional opinion, which in this case crosses professional disciplines, is wide. Indeed, there is often a tendency to regard some types of care for long-term patients as essentially social services, thus putting them outside the bounds of health care concern, health care spending, and health care policy.

Another reason for lag in support for financing long-term care is lack of confidence that expansion of one service will necessarily lead to the contraction of another, presumably substitute, service. Even when one service, such as home care, is demonstrably more cost-effective (less costly) for a given population cohort than another service, such as institutional care, expansion of the former service may still lead to a rise in total spending if the pool of clients is enlarged. The latter may happen due to the sheer availability of the service or the removal of obstacles to receiving it.

True, a few sources of possible increase in the future health care spending do come to mind. One is the continuing diversity in the sources of financing health care in this country. Such diversity tends to hinder the adoption and pursuit of large-scale policies to restrain health care spending. Increases in expenditures are less visible than they would be under a single source of financing, and there is no focal point of responsibility. Moreover, it takes longer to agree on what is going awry and even longer on what to do about it. Concerted action is certainly delayed, if not blocked.

Another possible source of future increase in the ratio of health care spending to GNP is associated with a decline in the rate of inflation in the economy at large; for reasons that are not clear, a high rate of inflation is often associated with a lower ratio of health care expenditures to GNP (Klarman, 1975). As the rate of inflation declines, the higher ratio of health care spending to GNP may serve as a deterrent to increases in the amount of health care spending.

I conclude that in the foreseeable future, increases in health care spending are likely to be of smaller magnitude than indicated by extrapolation of past trends. This conclusion is independent of the particular mix of policies and practice on health care competition, regulation, planning, and financing that may emerge over the next decade or two. Although a breakthrough in the diagnosis and treatment of a particular disease may be expected to attract additional funding, the health care sector as a whole will, I submit, be subjected to spending restraint, somehow.

The key word is "somehow." The forms of restraint on health care spending that prove to be politically acceptable and will be adopted are by no means evident. To begin with, there is the tendency for any organization or agency to concentrate on its own budget, to the virtual disregard of professed principle. It is not astounding that leading figures in the promarket Reagan administration threaten to impose regulatory controls if the rate of increase in spending by federal health care programs does not decline.

Even if the measures to be adopted were evident, I should still be inclined to caution in predicting a particular outcome. Major changes in programs are likely to yield major effects, only some of which are expected (Klarman, 1974). Among the great changes that have occurred in health care in this country over the past generation or two, some were altogether unexpected. Examples would include:

the expansion in enrollment in voluntary health insurance plans, which was expected to reach a plateau at 40 percent of the population; the post–World War II increase in health care spending in most countries, despite the scholarly finding that the amount of health care spending is governed everywhere and at all times by a universal constant of 4 percent of the national income; the marked and continuing rise in the unit cost or price of health care in the United States after the enactment of Medicare and Medicaid in 1965; the large and consistently underestimated expansion of the number of physicians, in the face of the medical schools' assertion that their capacity was fixed; persistence to the present of a sense of shortage of registered nurses in hospitals, despite sizable increases in the number graduated from nursing schools; and the appreciable decline in death rates, discussed earlier in this chapter.

Despite our inability to predict, I do believe that we know some of the areas of health care spending that we may wish to contract. What is not so well-known is that certain areas of health care have already been shrunk, sometimes with a reduction in spending and sometimes without. For example, in the state of New York in the late 1970s, almost 10,000 beds in short-term community hospitals were eliminated (Klarman, 1979); this happened in the face of early studies that found regulatory action in this area to be ineffectual. I do not mean to suggest that the total reduction was accomplished according to plan, with forethought and deliberate implementation. I do, however, insist that a sizable reduction in bed capacity was possible, as evidenced by the achievement. Conversely, spending in the state's mental hospitals, which it owns and operates, continues at a high level, despite a drastic decline in patient census. It appears easier for the state of New York to exert decisive influence on other people's hospitals. Continuation of a high level of spending in the state's own hospitals has prevented a sizable increase in spending for community health programs, a policy for which widespread agreement exists. Increased funding is a necessary, if not sufficient, condition for expanding the latter services.

### Implications for Health Manpower

What are the implications for health manpower and for health manpower education of the preceding discussion of the probable path of health care spending, as well as the difficulties posed by the criterion of need?

*Dentistry.* I believe that the demand for dental care is likely to increase, because dental insurance has begun to grow rapidly. The future trend in the nation's per capita real income will be another important factor, since expenditures for dental care are sensitive to changes in income. However, the substantial rise in dental school tuition, now under way, may deter entry into dental school. Finncial returns are more important in recruiting college graduates to dentistry than to medicine, because the nonfinancial returns, such as prestige and high sense of healing mission, are smaller. Possibly the combination of higher demand for dental care and lower output of dentists will eventually lead to an increase in the employment of auxiliary dental personnel.

*Medicine.* It is reasonably certain that the number of physicians in this country will continue to increase at an appreciable rate (U.S. Department of Health and Human Services, Bureau of Health Manpower, 1980). Indeed, it would only repeat past experience if current projections fell short of the actual numbers. Despite recent restrictions on immigration, foreign physicians are likely to enter in appreciable numbers, for the United States remains an attractive haven to foreign physicians in search of training or careers. More important, the children of American middle-class families continue to press for admission to medical school in numbers that far exceed the stated capacity of the schools.

True, average physician earnings have declined slightly and may decline even more if total health care spending is restrained. If the short-term hospital system contracts, the amount of effort a physician must exert to earn a given amount of net income will increase disproportionately, since the dollar earned in inpatient care takes the least time and effort by the practicing physician and is least encumbered by his own expenses. Conversely, as a result of the significant increase in stipends for trainees, the period in which earnings are postponed after graduation from medical school is not nearly so long as it was but a generation ago.

If market forces prevail, they will induce not only a reduction in net earnings but also a wider geographic distribution of physicians (Schwartz and others, 1980; Fruen and Cantwell, 1982). Notwithstanding, it is well to recall that geographic mobility is not a recent development for physicians. Their practice locations ultimately reflect their responses to a bundle of financial and nonfinancial rewards, and some of the latter may be changing as well (Klarman, 1965).

Likely to offset somewhat the downside forces in total demand for physicians is the growth of several new medical specialties, such as sports medicine, emergency medicine, and geriatric medicine; persistence of high prestige for medicine as the key healing profession; and continued acceptance by the patient of the physician's role as his agent amidst uncertainty and dependence. I am suggesting that physicians will be able, with additional effort, to continue to influence the demand for their services (Klarman, 1969).

If the financial subsidy to medical education declines, the cost of such education falling on the student will increase. Assumption of heavy debt during training may produce undesirable social consequences, including a decline in minority enrollment, but the reserve of applicants to medical school who are turned away is large. A drop in enrollment can be ruled out, unless it is accomplished by federal fiat. The sizable number of American citizens who attend medical school abroad lends support to this belief.

In my opinion, this country will continue to find means to pay for the services of physicians at an ample level, if not at the level to which physicians have become accustomed in the Medicare era. Currently, physicians receive a little less than one-fifth of the health care dollar (Gibson and Waldo, 1981); the fact that they exert influence over other, much larger expenditures, including hospital care and drugs, is not relevant in the present context.

The educational structure in medicine may change, but I should be hard put to gauge the form or direction of change. Any attempt toward training of a more general character seems to be accompanied by an increase in its duration. In the past, a broad, general practice has also run counter to the physician's important role in the hospital that rewards specialization. Curtailing the hospital system in the future may weaken the influence of the latter factor, just as expanding prepaid group practice serves to enhance the importance of the primary care physician. Nevertheless, the nonfinancial rewards of medical specialization—in terms of superior prestige and status—combined with the felt difficulty of mastering the growing body of complex preclinical information, point to the persistence of medical specialization, offset somewhat by an increasing tendency for specialists to spend some of their time in primary care practice.

*Nursing.* Since World War II, we have witnessed several episodes of shortage of registered nurses in hospitals. During much of this period, students of the profession from the inside have tended to emphasize the increase in demand for care, while hospital administrators, who are the principal employers of registered nurses, have continually pressed for increased output by schools of nursing. By contrast, economists have emphasized and endeavored to explain the profession's low earnings (Yett, 1975). The fact is that today, after a period of total reconstruction of the educational system and a shorter period of catching up in salaries in the 1960s, the cries of dissatisfaction among registered nurses sound louder than ever. Despite the absence of systematic data, most close observers believe that the real earnings of registered nurses working in hospitals lagged in the 1970s (Aiken, Blendon, and Rogers, 1981; Sloan and Steinwald, 1980). Even so, the complaints voiced by nurses and the efforts of some to move out of clinical nursing seem to reflect intensified concerns over burnout and mandatory shift rotation. It is well to note that these complaints arise in a climate of enhanced opportunities for women to pursue various careers.

For many hospitals, the result is once again an appreciable shortage of registered nurses. Sizable boosts in salary may serve to mitigate the shortage here and there and may not be required in a recession, but in the long run and for the country as a whole, this profession's nonfinancial disadvantages loom so large that financial remedies are likely to afford insufficient relief. This is my reading of Aiken's presidential address to the American Academy of Nursing (Aiken, 1981).

In any event, it is doubtful that the manifold problems facing the nursing profession will be solved in the educational setting. As for the numbers of registered nurses to be trained, I take solace in the empirical observation that the capacity of schools is much more flexible than deans or faculty acknowledge. The recent contraction in enrollment is modest (Institute of Medicine, Committee for a Study of Nursing and Nursing Education, 1981).

### Epilogue

For conclusions, I refer the reader to the four propositions that opened this chapter. I concede that none has been established conclusively and certainly not to everyone's satisfaction; I believe, however, that each is a reasonable inference from the available evidence. Finally, it is evident that I eschew forecasts, many of which are bound to be mistaken. I prefer to rely on flexibility in the design and operation of programs acting on information gathered by close and continuing monitoring of such programs, as well as of health care problems, policies, and trends (Klarman, 1976).

### References

Aiken, L. H. "Nursing Priorities for the 1980s: Hospitals and Nursing Homes." *American Journal of Nursing*, 1981, *81* (2), 324–330.

Aiken, L. H., Blendon, R. J., and Rogers, D. E. "The Shortage of Hospital Nurses: A New Perspective." *Annals of Internal Medicine*, 1981, *95* (3), 365–372.

Cochrane, A. L. *Effectiveness and Efficiency.* London: Nuffield Provincial Hospitals Trust, 1972.

Freeland, M. S., and Schendler, C. E. "National Health Expenditures: Short-Term Outlook and Long-Term Projections." *Health Care Financing Review*, 1981, *2* (3), 97–138.

Fruen, M. A., and Cantwell, J. R. "Geographic Distribution of Physicians: Past Trends and Future Influences." *Inquiry*, 1982, *19* (1), 44–50.

Fuchs, V. R. *Who Shall Live?* New York: Basic Books, 1974.

Fuchs, V. R. "Comment on Health Care as a Public Service." In C. R. Rorem, *A Quest for Certainty.* Ann Arbor, Mich.: Health Administration Press, 1982.

Gibson, R. M. "National Health Expenditures, 1981." *Health Care Spending Bulletin.* Washington, D. C.: Health Care Financing Administration, U. S. Department of Health and Human Services, July 21, 1982.

Gibson, R. M., and Waldo, D. R. "National Health Expenditures, 1980." *Health Care Financing Review*, 1981, *3* (1), 1–54.

Graduate Medical Education National Advisory Committee. *Summary Report to the Secretary, Department of Health and Human Services.* Vol. 1. Washington, D. C.: U. S. Government Printing Office, 1980.

Institute of Medicine, Committee for a Study of Nursing and Nursing Education. *Six-Month Interim Report.* Washington, D.C.: National Academy Press, July 1981. (Mimeographed.)

Klarman, H. E. "Requirements for Physicians." *American Economic Review*, 1951, *41* (2), 633–645.

Klarman, H. E. *Hospital Care in New York City.* New York: Columbia University Press, 1963.

Klarman, H. E. *The Economics of Health.* New York: Columbia University Press, 1965.

Klarman, H. E. "Economic Aspects of Projecting Requirements for Health Manpower." *Journal of Human Resources*, 1969, *4* (3), 360–376.

Klarman, H. E. "Economic Research in Group Medicine." In R. E. Beamish (Ed.), *New Horizons in Health Care.* Winnipeg, Manitoba: First International Congress on Group Medicine, 1970.

Klarman, H. E. "Major Public Initiatives in Health Care." *Public Interest*, 1974, *34*, 106–123.

Klarman, H. E. "The Economic Determinants of Health Care Expenditures." In D. A. Ehrlich (Ed.), *The Health Care Cost Explosion.* Bern, Switzerland: Hans Huber, 1975.

Klarman, H. E. "National Policies and Local Planning for Health Services." *Milbank Memorial Fund Quarterly*, 1976, *54* (1), 1–28.

Klarman, H. E. "Planning for Facilities." In E. Ginzberg (Ed.), *Regionalization and Health Policy.* Washington, D.C.: U.S. Government Printing Office, 1977.

Klarman, H. E. "Some Alternative Approaches to Health Planning and Regulation." *Health Communications and Informatics*, 1979, *5* (5–6), 339–350.

Klarman, H. E. "Health Care Financing." In D. W. Clark and B. MacMahon (Eds.), *Preventive and Community Medicine*, 2d ed. Boston: Little, Brown, 1981.

Kleinman, J. C., Fingerhut, L. A., and Feldman, J. J. "Trends in Mortality." In *Health United States, 1980*. Washington, D.C.: U.S. Government Printing Office, 1981.

Lee, R. I., and Jones, L. W. *The Fundamentals of Good Medical Care*. Chicago: University of Chicago Press, 1933.

McKeown, T. *The Role of Medicine*. London: Nuffield Provincial Hospitals Trust, 1976.

Newhouse, J. P. *The Economics of Medical Care*. Reading, Mass.: Addison-Wesley, 1978.

Roemer, M. I. "Bed Supply and Hospital Utilization: A Natural Experiment." *Hospitals*, 1961, *35* (21), 36–42.

Schwartz, W. B., and others. "The Changing Geographic Distribution of Board-Certified Physicians." *New England Journal of Medicine*, 1980, *303*, 1032–1038.

Shain, M., and Roemer, M. I. "Hospital Costs Relate to the Supply of Beds." *Modern Hospital*, 1959, *92* (4), 71–73 and 168.

Sloan, F. A., and Steinwald, B. *Hospital Labor Markets*. Lexington, Mass.: Heath, 1980.

Stambler, H. V. "Health Manpower for the Nation: A Look Ahead at the Supply and the Requirements." *Public Health Reports*, 1979, *94* (1), 3–10.

U.S. Department of Health and Human Services, Bureau of Health Manpower. *The Current and Future Supply of Physicians and Physician Specialists*. Washington, D.C.: U.S. Government Printing Office, 1980.

White, K. L. "Life and Death and Medicine." *Scientific American*, 1973, *229* (3), 23–33.

Yett, D. E. *An Economic Analysis of the Nurse Shortage*. Lexington, Mass.: Lexington Books, 1975.

# 17

*Julius B. Richmond*
*Milton Kotelchuck*

# Political Influences

## Rethinking National Health Policy

The making of public policy in a pluralistic nation is a complex process. The development of health policy is no exception. American health policy emerges from the workings of both public and private sector organizations, profit and nonprofit; it is intricately tied to a series of professional and institutional associations and their policies. Even within the governmental sector, large health programs are operated by a variety of different agencies, not always congruent in objectives and operations. The American health care system is not a unified system. Indeed, it can be thought of as a series of highly developed but fragmented enterprises, somewhat mechanically connected to each other.

Conscious attention to the development of a national health policy is a relatively new emphasis in public policy formulation. There is as yet no annual public debate on health care funding priorities and goals. Clearly, many people and organizations are concerned with health policy, largely from the vantage point of their specific interests. But there has never been a single locus for the discussion and implementation of something that could be called health policy in the United States.

At the outset, it is important to note that too much of the current discussion about health policy in the United States focuses on funding levels, government regulations, and professional prerogatives. Health promotion and the improvement of health status have dropped into the background; they are appendages to the dialogue. Health and decisions on improving the health of our citizens must take the highest priority in shaping a national health policy.

As can be seen in Figure 1, the shaping of health policy involves three critical areas: the development of a knowledge base, the development of political will, and the development of social strategy. All three must come together for the development and implementation of public policy.

A *knowledge base* provides the scientific and administrative data base upon which to make health care decisions. It is fine to have as a long-term goal the prevention or eradication of cancer, but without a firm knowledge base of the biology of cancer or the epidemiological effectiveness of different preventive strategies, we can only have a policy that proceeds incrementally in many directions. Many areas of health improvement must await basic biomedical research. It is important to point out that we had the technology for eradicating smallpox from the world many decades before we made the commitment to apply it fully. Technology alone will not provide good health, but its absence will, ultimately, limit our health care delivery capacity. Nor is it simply biomedical knowledge that is critical but also knowledge about social and economic factors involved in the delivery of health care services, the culture in which health is defined, physi-

**Figure 1. Three-Factor Approach to Health Policy.**

Development of Public Policy

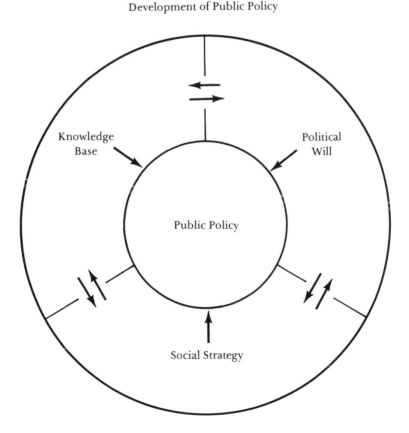

cian behavior, patient satisfaction, and the like. The knowledge base must be broad-gauged and multifaceted.

Second, health policy depends on *political will*. Political will is society's desire and commitment to support or modify old programs or to develop new programs. It may be viewed as the process of generating resources to carry out policies and programs. Often people in the health professions know that there are better ways of dealing with a problem, but they may not succeed because they have not perceived the need to gain the political support for change. Too often the political process is used to inhibit change. In order to effect improvements or changes in the system, it is necessary to develop a constituency. The constituency for change may come from existing professional organizations or institutions that identify problems and help raise consciousness among decision makers, or the constituency may come from the public that makes its aspirations and/or dissatis-factions heard through the legislative process.

Third, and finally, health policy depends critically on the existence of a *social strategy* or plan. Social strategy is a blueprint for accomplishing the worthwhile goals that we have established; it is the plan by which we apply our knowledge base and political will to improve programs. It entails clearly outlined goals and a detailed statement of the means to reach them. However, it is not sufficient simply to articulate a social strategy, for health policy is not the same as the social strategy. A social strategy merely provides the outline and framework of a health policy.

All three components—a developed knowledge base, the political will, and a clear social strategy—are critical in order to bring about any changes in health policy. The inhibition of change in the U.S. health care delivery system can be identified as a result of the lack of one or all three of these factors.

## Role of the Federal Government

Given the complexity of shaping health policy in the United States, it is not surprising that many people look to the federal government for leadership. Indeed, many people often use the words *health policy* to mean government policy in health. While this is obviously not completely accurate, this chapter attempts to provide a historical account of the recent governmental interventions in the health care delivery and health care policy areas, to examine the strengths and weaknesses of these interventions, to assess the underlying political rationale, and then to give some suggestions for future health policy directions. The presentation in-cludes some historical analysis of what the federal government, under both Demo-cratic and Republican administrations, has accomplished and what it has the potential for accomplishing in the future.

*Limited Governmental Role Prior to 1965.* Prior to 1965, the role of the federal government in health was quite limited. Only 3.8 percent of the 1960 federal budget was devoted to health, compared to 12.8 percent in 1980; in 1960, federal expenditures accounted for 9.3 percent of the total U.S. health care expen-ditures, compared to 28.7 percent by 1980 (Health Insurance Association of Amer-ica, 1982). The Maternal and Child Health and Crippled Children's Programs, which were embodied in the Social Security Act of 1935, were virtually the only direct health services the government subsidized outside of the uniformed services' and veterans' health programs. Most other governmental health activities were limited to the promotion of public health practices. In addition, following World War II, the federal government became involved in hospital construction, through Hill-Burton legislation, and in expanded support of biomedical research.

*1965 Federal Health Care Legislation.* By the early 1960s, the long neglect of the American health care system had become apparent. No longer could the platitudes that we had the best health care record in the world be offered without serious challenge. In the late 1950s, infant mortality rates that had declined steadily since the turn of the century leveled out and even began to climb for some minority groups. By 1965, the United States ranked sixteenth in national infant mortality rates throughout the world (Richmond, 1967). Studies demonstrated the higher mortality and morbidity rate among the poor, especially the nonwhite poor (National Center for Health Statistics, 1964; Metropolitan Life Insurance Company, 1967). During this period, physicians were leaving urban slums and rural poverty areas for life in the more affluent suburbs. For example, in one poor, white, working-class section of Boston, there were thirty-nine physicians in 1942 and only nineteen in 1964, despite a rising population (Richmond, 1969). The same phenomenon was apparent in rural areas (Johnson and Cooper, 1982); for example, between 1900 and 1960, the number of counties in Kentucky with an insufficient supply of physicians steadily grew. At the same time, there was a gradual deterioration of the public hospital system. The public outpatient services had undergone little change in decades. Emergency room visits were increasing dramatically (Seifert and Johnstone, 1966). Since most of these people did not need emergency services, their use of the emergency room was a clear indicator that they had no other primary health care resources to turn to. By the 1960s, it was apparent, whether one looked at health status indicators, health professionals, or health resources, that the quality of health care for poorer Americans was declining.

The main reason for the federal intervention into health in 1965 was a change in the national political will. The civil rights revolution of the 1960s played a major role in setting the stage for the war on poverty with its focus on the needs of the poor and the near-poor. Nowhere was the need more dramatic than in the area of health care. Not only the poor but also working-class and middle-class families were feeling hard-pressed. This was particularly true of the aged, many of whom ended their lives in poverty because of the cost of meeting their increasing medical needs. By 1965, a coalition of political forces had developed the desire and the strength to ameliorate some of our national health care deficiencies.

Why was it Congress, rather than the health professional establishment itself, that acted at this particular period? One factor was the failure of the health professional establishment to make any meaningful proposals. The American Medical Association (AMA) was devoting all its resources and energy to an attempt to defeat impending Medicare legislation; public health officers and schools of public health had few proposals; medical center and research establishments, busy pursuing new medical knowledge, seemed generally unconcerned; and the federal health care agencies, particularly the Public Health Service, had virtually no program for providing medical services for the nation's poor. In sum, the professional organizations had abdicated responsibility or were actively resisting proposals that an overwhelming majority of the American people recognized as desirable. In this situation, the political leadership had the political will to do something.

With President Kennedy's death, the substantial victory of Lyndon B. Johnson in 1964, and the initiation of the war on poverty, a political mandate was obtained. Federal efforts were then directed toward overcoming the major health care problems articulated prior to the mid-1960s.

The eighty-ninth Congress in 1965 passed more health legislation than had been passed in any previous session of Congress:

- Medicare (Title 18)
- Medicaid (Title 19)
- Regional medical programs
- Comprehensive health planning assistance
- Health Professions Educational Assistance Amendments
- Maternal and infant care, children and youth projects (Title 5)
- Economic Opportunity Act
  Neighborhood health centers
  Head Start

This cluster can be referred to as the bumper crop of health care legislation (Richmond, 1969). It introduced the federal government, in a major way, into the health care delivery system. For the first time, the federal government was explicitly committed to ensuring equity of access to health care for all citizens. Equity was to be achieved both by providing direct financial support for those without sufficient means and by increasing the availability of health resources through the establishment of neighborhood health centers and through efforts directed at the redistribution of health manpower. The introduction of Title 18 (Medicare) and Title 19 (Medicaid), in particular, has profoundly changed medical accessibility and medical financing in the United States. Today, over 28,500,000 people are covered by Medicare and over 21,500,000 people by Medicaid.

*Origins of Federal Health Policy.* What was the federal health care policy in 1965? While, obviously, certain key ideas—equity of access, federal assumption of health care costs for the elderly, and increased health resources for the poor— were influential as the intellectual concepts underlying the legislation, in fact, it is impossible to find a document or master plan for that time describing what should be done about health care in the United States. No blueprint existed! Indeed, the most obvious fact about the 1965 legislation was that each perceived need was addressed by a separate piece of legislation. Little thought was given to coordination among them.

The lack of a blueprint reflected, in part, the lack of prior governmental experience in the area. No place in government had ever been responsible for conceptualizing the health care system as a totality or the government's role within it. The 1965 legislation injected the government into the health services arena and reflected the strong political consensus of the time about the important public problems amenable to specific intervention. What we think of today as health policy, or federal health care policy, had its beginnings in that period.

*Outcomes of New Federal Health Intervention.* Did these specific federal intervention programs work? In certain problem areas, we believe the answer is decidedly yes. In contrast to what is commonly purveyed these days—a widespread pessimism about the effectiveness of the political process on the delivery of health care—an examination of the evidence indicates that governmental action can help to achieve well-targeted goals. There were some spectacular successes. Let us illustrate by looking at what has happened since 1965.

The Surgeon General's Report of 1979 opens with the sentence "The health of the American people has never been better" (Surgeon General, 1979). It is clear that there has been steady and significant improvement in the health status of the American people since 1965. This is manifest in increased life expectancy (now 73.8 years), the lowest infant mortality rate in our history (now approximately 12 deaths per thousand live births), a reduction of 25 percent in cardiac mortality and of 40 percent in mortality from stroke over the last decade, and a consistent decline in the infectious diseases, particularly those of childhood (National Center for Health Statistics, 1980). Smallpox has been eradicated from the world, and we are close to eradicating measles in the United States. While the federal government may not properly take all the credit for these achievements, the coincidence of major government health care expenditures and improved health status is noteworthy.

In addition to health status improvements, equity of access to health care was one of the main health goals of the war on poverty. Examination of this issue reveals that significant progress has also been made in that area. Recent national data show that people from the lowest income groups are now using health care resources as frequently as higher-income citizens (Aday, Anderson, and Fleming, 1980; National Center for Health Statistics, 1980). In 1964, persons from poverty-level backgrounds were only 82 percent as likely to have had a physician visit as a non-poverty-level person. By 1978, the ratio had reversed and low-income persons now had more (119 percent) health care visits. This ratio should not be surprising, given the greater health needs of low-income persons. Similarly, the number of low-income persons who had made no visits to a physician within the past year declined from 28.2 percent in 1964 to 14.3 percent in 1978, while for the non-poor it dropped from 18.9 percent to 13.9 percent. Whether low-income persons yet receive as many health care visits as their poor health status would necessitate is still a debatable issue, but progress has been made. However, equity of access is now being approached in the U.S. health care system, although some 10 percent of the population still have inadequate access to health care (U.S. Congressional Budget Office, 1979).

## Conceptual Model of the Sixties

The conceptual model legislators and health professionals were operating on in 1965, and generally throughout the present period, is a *deficit* model. This model asserts that the basic problem in health care is the lack of resources or the existence of deficits; for example, the lack of sufficient numbers of hospital beds, the lack of proper distribution of health resources in poor areas, the lack of physicians and other health professionals, the lack of money to pay for health care, and the like. In 1965, the focus was on overcoming these deficits; almost no attention was given to structural changes in the overall delivery system.

**Figure 2. Health Status Graph of Infant Mortality.**

Infant mortality rates by color:
United States, 1940–1979

(Deaths under 1 year per 1,000 live births)

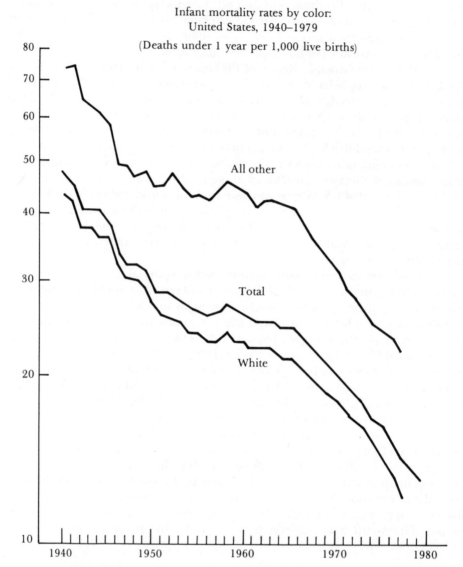

*Note:* Data for total infant mortality for 1973 and 1979 are provisional. Data by color for 1978 and 1979 are not yet available.

*Source:* National Center for Health Statistics, 1980.

However, some perceptive observers of the scene in 1965 saw the need for such change. For example, John Dunlop (1965) on the eve of the enactment of Medicare and Medicaid said: "The real function of the cost increases of the past decade, and those in process, should be to compel vast structural changes in the organization of medical care. Nothing could be worse in our society today than to say we need another three or five billion dollars for medical care and then simply duplicate or multiply the arrangements that we now have. That would get us nowhere" (p. 1325). To this day, the pleadings of special interest groups and of others are still based on the assumption that more resources alone will produce the desired result. Three areas will be examined to show how this deficit model has played itself out: health manpower, hospital beds, and federal expenditures.

*Health Manpower.* As indicated in Figure 3, there have been dramatic changes in the physician/population ratio over this century. The almost 50 percent reduction in the number of physicians in the early part of the century reflects the 33 percent reduction in the number of medical schools that resulted from the improved accreditation process that was introduced following the Flexner report (Richmond, 1969). By the beginning of the 1950s, serious questions were being raised by state health agencies, public and private medical schools, and citizens groups about a shortage of physicians and other health professionals. As late as 1960, there were only a quarter of a million physicians in the United States, for a ratio of 168 physicians per 100,000 population, and only 7,000 new physician graduates per year. The Bane report of 1959 argued strongly for the need to increase the number of new physicians by 50 percent over the next few years (Surgeon General's Consultant Group on Medical Education, 1959). This report was influential in Congress and led to the passage of the Health Professions Educational Assistance Act of 1963, the Nurse Training Act of 1964, and the Allied Health Professional Act of 1966. These acts represented the federal government's effort to overcome the national deficits of physicians, nurses, and other health professionals. Each provided funds, beginning in 1965, for assistance to states to open new professional schools, to increase enrollments in private institutions, and to allow for a substantial increase in the number of foreign-trained physicians entering the United States. By 1980, the federal government had contributed more than $7 billion to medical education (Graduate Medical Education National Advisory Committee, 1980).

The U.S. health education community responded vigorously to these incentives with an unprecedented expansion of U.S. health professional training facilities. Within a decade, forty-one new health professional schools, including twenty-eight schools of medicine and osteopathy, had been opened. The number of medical school graduates has increased by almost 85 percent since 1965; the current physician/population ratio is almost 200 physicians per 100,000 people. It is anticipated that by 1990, there will be almost 600,000 physicians in the United States, compared with approximately 250,000 physicians in the 1950s. In short, the federal programs initiated in the 1960s to deal with the manpower deficit stimulated a dramatic increase in health manpower.

*Hospital Beds.* The number of hospitals and hospital beds symbolizes our limited capital investment in health. In 1946, there were in the United States 3.4 short-term general hospital beds per thousand persons, with that ratio falling as low as 2.0 in some states. This was widely believed to be inadequate, with the inadequacy particularly acute in the South (Institute of Medicine, 1976). Moreover, due to the very limited hospital construction during the Depression and World War II, many of the facilities were in poor physical condition. With the passage of the Hill-Burton Act in 1948, the federal government began to provide direct subsidies for hospital construction. Both state and federal government further subsidized construction costs by insuring hospital construction loans and by allowing hospitals to pass on the cost of borrowing construction money to third-party payers.

Figure 3. Physicians per Population by Time.

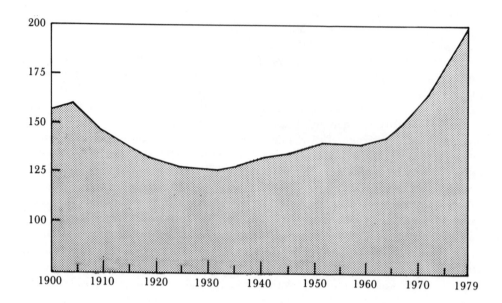

*Source*: Adapted from U.S. Bureau of the Census, 1960, 1980.

These programs were effective in accomplishing their objectives. The number of beds in the United States rose from about 500,000 in 1950 to just under a million by 1980. The ratio of beds per population increased from 3.3 in 1950 to 4.6 beds per thousand population in 1980, far in excess of the generally accepted goal of 4 beds per thousand population (Institute of Medicine, 1976). Although some shortage areas still exist, the 30 percent increase in the number of hospital beds per thousand population between 1950 and 1980 provides another example of the way in which the federal government can develop specific programs aimed at overcoming a well-defined deficit.

*Increase in Expenditures.* Expenditures on health services furnish one measure of the extent of public involvement in the purchase of health care. Since 1935, the states' contributions of all health care costs have remained relatively constant at about 11 to 12 percent, while the federal government contribution has increased steadily from approximately 10 percent in 1965 to approximately 30 percent in 1980. The federal government is now a major purchaser of services and supporter of health care resources. In 1980, the federal government spent over $23 billion for Medicaid and over $35 billion for Medicare. partially as a result, over 90 percent of the American population now has some kind of third-party health care coverage (U.S. Congressional Budget Office, 1979). These federal expenditures have also created a major network of new health care resources. By 1981, 870 community health centers had been established, and 3,000 National Health Service Corps members currently serve in low-income areas. One cannot help but feel that the initial goals of the authors of the 1965 health legislation—to meet the needs of the previously unserved and underserved—have, to a large degree, been achieved.

## Impact of the Deficit Model

In all three areas we have discussed—manpower, hospital beds, and expenditures—the government health programs appear to have been successful, perhaps too successful. Indeed, there is now a growing political and professional perception that national priorities must shift from overcoming deficits to dealing with surpluses and misallocations created as a consequence of recent federal health programs. Changing priorities may be illustrated by examination of the three areas just discussed.

*Health Manpower: Oversupply and Maldistribution.* At the present rate of growth, it is projected that there will be 600,000 physicians, or 239 physicians per 100,000 population by 1990. According to the Graduate Medical Education National Advisory Committee, this will produce a surplus of 25,000 to 50,000 physicians. Morever, there will be serious maldistribution of physicians, both by specialty and by geography. For example, general surgery, obstetrics and gynecology, radiology, and pediatrics will have an excess, while hematology-oncology, preventive medicine, and anesthesiology will still suffer shortages (Graduate Medical Education National Advisory Committee, 1980). Moreover, the Institute of Medicine (1978) has suggested that there are too many medical specialists in general and that 50 percent of all physicians should be trained for primary care. Second, the long-standing historical issue of geographic maldistribution of physicians remains serious. While there have been some modest increases in the number of physicians in poverty areas during the 1970s—from 68 to 74 physicians per 100,000 persons—these areas still do not have adequate health manpower. The majority of physicians continue to settle in the more affluent areas of the country. It is estimated that 16,400 additional physicians are needed in medically underserved areas: 7,500 in rural areas, 5,200 in inner cities, and 3,700 in prisons and mental institutions (Richmond, 1980). These distributional problems do not indicate that recent federal efforts should be abandoned; rather they suggest that the system requires rethinking, with the emphasis shifted from a concern with total numbers to issues related to specialty and geographic distributions.

*Hospital Beds: Too Many.* The Hill-Burton programs and other federal hospital construction supports have resulted in an estimated surplus of approximately 150,000 short-term general hospital beds. This excess tends to obstruct the development of a rational health care system by strengthening the grip of the hospital sector in the determination of national health care priorities. The need to fill existing hospital beds and to be reimbursed for the prior capital investment encourages hospitals to support publicly financed, cost-incurred payment systems, to resist prospective rate setting, to push for more intensive tertiary care, and to oppose less expensive preventive or ambulatory care programs and reimbursement systems.

It is conservatively estimated that about $11 billion per year in health care costs could be saved if excess beds were withdrawn. However, the problem is not so simple. Excess beds are distributed throughout many hospitals. Thus, a reduction in beds cannot be translated into savings unless whole wings of hospitals, or whole hospitals, are closed. Moreover, there still remain problems with respect to the geographic distribution of these resources. Poverty areas are still underserved and are continuing to lose hospitals to more affluent areas (Sager, 1981).

In some respects, federal programs for increasing the national supply of hospital beds have worked too well. Yet, abandonment of federal support for hospital construction would be shortsighted, since prior distributional inequities would soon reemerge. What is required is readjustment of the present construction cost reimbursement systems to address distributional rather than overall quantitative issues.

*Health Expenditures: How Much Is Enough?* Federal expenditures have increased dramatically, up from 5.3 percent of GNP in 1960 to almost 10 percent in 1980. However, the present level of expenditures on health care seems to be increasingly unacceptable to large segments of our population. Three factors seem to have contributed to this rise of expenditures: First, the federal support previously discussed; second, the incremental growth in costs, including federally subsidized coverage of health insurance in the form of tax deductions; and third, the increasing cost attributed to the behavior of health professionals and institutions. The fact that physicians are paid on a fee-for-service basis and that hospitals are reimbursed on a cost-incurred basis means that there is no incentive to keep costs down; almost all expenditures are reimbursable by third-party payment systems.

Reactions to the increasing expenditures take two forms: A rising concern over public expenditures directed at the poorer sections of our population (especially the federal Medicaid program supported in part by state funds) and a growing dissatisfaction with the increasing costs of individual health insurance premiums. Concerns about higher taxes and higher premiums are compounded by widespread perceptions that medical professions are becoming wealthier. No one is proposing total abandonment of federal fiscal involvement in health; even the AMA no longer advocates the abolition of Medicare. Rather, the focus is on determining whether we are getting the most value for the dollars spent and whether we can correct the financial and health inequities built into the original 1965 legislation. Again, refinement, not abandonment, of the federal system is in order.

### Overcoming the Deficit Model: Initial Federal Responses

As a nation, we have made real progress in overcoming some of the perceived health care deficits of the 1960s, but now we must deal with the successful consequences of these programs—surpluses and maldistribution of some resources, and high expenditures. The situation is dialectical; having solved certain problems, we have created new ones that had not been entirely anticipated.

Over the past several years, with increasing recognition of these newer problems, there have been some federal efforts directed at priority setting and resource modulation. The initial federal response has, however, followed a similar strategy to that of the deficit model; namely, one specific health resource surplus, one specific program. Throughout, however, the most pervasive federal concern has been cost containment. The five programs described below represent some of the initial federal efforts to overcome the surpluses and excesses brought about by the prior deficit model programs.

1. The Health Resources and Planning Act of 1974, which may now be phased out, was designed to provide a rational basis for the allocation of resources. Certificate of Need programs for capital construction developed under its aegis. Its orientation has shifted, negatively in our opinion, away from health status improvement to one focused almost exclusively on cost containment. The recent history of health planning efforts in the United States indicates we have not yet developed an appropriate and widely supported strategy.

2. The Professional Standards Review Organizations were developed as a quality control program to monitor the services delivered to federally reimbursed Medicaid and Medicare patients. This program was an effort both to assure quality services and to monitor appropriate utilization and thereby control costs. Monitoring of actual medical practice has met some resistance, and its cost savings have been marginal; its future is uncertain.

3. A national hospital cost containment strategy was developed to control the escalation of hospital expenditures. Capping legislation has been proposed in several recent sessions of Congress. Presently, these proposals have provided the impetus only for the voluntary capping effort of the American Hospital Association (Schaeffer, 1979) that, by and large, has been ineffective.

4. The Center on Health Care Technology was established to assess in a more orderly fashion the introduction of new health care technologies. Quality of care, resource availability, and health care costs were some of the issues to be examined. The center has since been discontinued.

5. A Presidential Commission for the Study of Ethical Problems in Medicine and Biomedical and Biobehavioral Research has been appointed. It has been charged with, among many issues concerning ethics, examining the ethical issues related to resource allocation. For the first time, the federal government, in an explicit way, is facing the ethical issue of how to make choices among competing priorities in health.

These five programs represent some of the initial federal efforts to overcome the surpluses and excesses brought about by the prior deficit model programs. They have had some impact but have obviously failed to solve entirely the problems that brought them into being. Since these are early efforts, it is not suprising that they have been of only limited effectiveness and have led to some disenchantment—prematurely in our view—with federal health policies. Clearly, a new model is required.

## Directions for the Future: Equilibration and Equity—A New Model

In order to deal effectively with the health care problems facing us today, a reconceptualization of health care problems is first required. A deficit model is no longer an adequate theoretical base for national health care policy. For each deficit met, there is a new distortion of the system. It is time that we move our view of policy directions in health care from a deficit model to a model based on equilibration and equity.

A model of equilibration and equity means conceptualizing the health care system as a homeostatic whole, not as a series of discrete pieces. Equilibration means the development of a health care system that has clearly stated unifying health policy goals, with processes that can move us toward these goals. Such a model requires that formal structural programs at national, state, or regional levels be developed to assure rational distribution of limited health resources. It is also a dynamic model that can provide for growth of the health care system; it is not a fixed resource system.

What are some of the programmatic implications of this new health care model? If progress is to be made in improving Americans' health status, the health care system must establish three goals for the immediate future: (1) to reorient the health care delivery system away from acute disease treatment and reimbursement to health promotion and disease prevention; (2) to complete the commitment of assuring all Americans equity of access to health care; and (3) to implement a systematic package of regulatory programs that will assure that health care activities are rationally distributed, of high quality, and cost-effective.

*New Federal Equilibration Programs.* Equilibration requires that an approach to the modulation or regulation of the health care system be initiated. Three types of programs must be established: instituting rate setting and prospective budgeting for hospital costs, rationalizing hospital bed supply through Certificate of Need programs, and establishing quality assurance and utilization review programs. The initial focus should be on federal programs, although this proposal could be developed on a state or regional basis.

Since hospital expenditures constitute 40 percent of total health expenditures, it is clear that some brakes must be put on these costs if efforts to modulate rising expenditures are to be effective. Many observers have commented that the present hospital cost-incurred reimbursement system provides no incentive to keep expenditures down. Effective rate-setting programs can provide one mechanism for forcing hospitals to examine and justify costs before they are reimbursed. The strong rate-setting regulatory programs in Maryland and New Jersey, especially with their emphasis on Diagnostically Related Group (DRG) reimbursements, are being watched with considerable interest by other states to see if they can demonstrate significant savings (Inglehart, 1982).

An alternative proposal to reduce federal expenses by limiting Medicare and Medicaid enrollment simply increases the numbers of non-payers. The added hospital costs are then shifted onto the private sector, particularly to the voluntary health insurance sector. This is not a satisfactory solution to the problem of high hospital expenditures; it is simply an accounting shift among third-party reimbursers. Small wonder, therefore, that the Health Insurance Association of America (which would be expected to be a bastion of free enterprise) has come out strongly for state rate setting.

It is not inconceivable that rate setting could be combined with prospective budgeting for hospitals. Even the American Hospital Association has recently developed a proposal for prospective reimbursement. Such a system must respect the individual differences among hospitals, in order to avoid the mindless comparisons often made between low-cost community hospitals and the necessarily higher-cost tertiary care hospitals. A budgeting system that does not take account of the differential levels of hospital care is destined ultimately to erode quality and to result in failure. A careful program of prospective budgeting should ultimately help reduce the burgeoning national hospital costs.

Other federal equilibration programs deal with the oversupply of hospital beds. Since the financing of hospital construction costs is now incorporated into third-party reimbursement, new construction adds a considerable burden to everyone's health care costs. Small wonder that when public health administrators are asked what one step could do the most for cost containment, they generally respond by saying "a moratorium on the construction of hospital beds."

Certificate of Need programs are the institutional process that has been developed thus far to limit hospital bed supply rationally. They can and do work; however, they are extremely controversial. Today's Certificate of Need regulatory paperwork is pitted against future cost savings. Local politicians are all too well aware of the political issues in communities that have aspirations for hospital construction, but one would hope that the recent high health cost experiences have taught governors and legislators about the heavy long-term financial burden of capital construction. Political will is necessary to have an effective Certificate of Need program.

Unfortunately, Certificate of Need programs are focused only on limiting new construction and have little impact on eliminating hospital beds already in place. Presently, almost the only beds being eliminated are those resulting from financially induced hospital closures in poorer urban and rural areas (Sager, 1981), though many communities are now making efforts to develop rational strategies to reduce the number of existing beds. (See the following chapter by Hadley for a more detailed discussion of this issue.)

The last category of equilibration programs involves establishing quality assurance and utilization review programs. Most recent surveys of American health care attitudes would indicate that, contrary to the federal priorities, the public is much more concerned about the quality of health care than the costs of health care. Yet, until recently there were virtually no governmental efforts to examine medical practices in the light of established standards.

Pressures to develop quality assurance efforts have grown in the last few years. First, the burgeoning of new and potent diagnostic and therapeutic processes makes monitoring of such activities critical. The very potency and specificity of new techniques bespeak the need for careful attention to their application or misapplication. Second, concerns have increased about unnecessary hospitalization, excessive elective surgery, and too lengthy hospital stays. These concerns are not exclusively those of cost. Too much surgery, too many laboratory tests, and inappropriate therapy are serious issues of quality. Third, the public is increasingly concerned over the failure of the medical profession to monitor itself. Too many people believe that health professionals simply protect each other and not their patients.

Certainly, the significant regional differences in hospitalization rates and length of stay, the inappropriate practices of a small percentage of practitioners, and the evidence of profiteering from publicly funded programs are of concern to all providers and consumers. These problems cannot be dismissed by professional organizations as occasional aberrations. A society that invests major resources in health care expects the provider community to be prudent in their management. It does not seem likely that this nation will continue to support expenditures at the present level without some assurance that the funds are being well-spent. Quality assurance and utilization review programs could lead to significant reductions in expenditures.

Recent methodological advances in the evaluation of the quality of health care services make the development of quality assurance programs increasingly feasible. The computerization of hospital and office data as well as the growing professional experience with peer review are suggesting realistic, new approaches. Computer-generated programs can now be devised to serve as the basis for professionally monitored quality assurance programs.

Quality assurance and utilization review need not be a threat to professional integrity but could serve to improve medical practice. The development of computer-based medical care algorithms and protocols, generated through a peer consensus-building process, could become much more valuable to the practitioner than the textbooks of the past. These computer-based protocols could also serve as a baseline for quality assurance programs. Proxies for quality assurance, such as recertification and continuing education requirements, cannot do the job alone.

The three proposals—instituting rate setting and prospective budgeting for hospital costs, rationalizing hospital-bed supply through Certificate of Need programs, and establishing quality assurance and utilization review programs— represent a unified package of regulatory programs to assure that health care activities are rationally distributed, of high quality, and cost-effective. It is critical that these proposals be initiated simultaneously and operate as a coordinated program. A single program alone would serve only to distort the health care system; together, the three proposals should help overcome the excesses brought about by our overly successful prior deficit model programs. They would provide the minimal programmatic basis for operationalizing a health care system based on an equilibration model.

*Equity of Access: A Recommitment.* One of the principal goals of the 1965 bumper crop of health legislation was to provide all Americans equity of access to health care. Progress toward this goal is one of the most positive health care achievements of the recent era. However, it has not yet been fully reached; it was estimated in 1980 that approximately 12 percent of our population were still without access to and/or financing for health services (U.S. Congressional Budget Office, 1979; Dicker, 1983).

Closing the gap between those with adequate service and those without remains a central issue for the financing and delivery of health services today. The problem could be addressed most comprehensively through a national health program; however, because of current economic and political circumstances, this does not seem possible at the present time. In the interim, efforts to provide more adequate services to those still underserved do not call for large-scale increases in expenditures; rather they require extensions of prior programs to areas still in need. A many-pronged approach offers the greatest potential for further reducing inequities in access to adequate health services:

- Extension of Medicaid coverage to those of the poor not currently covered. It is estimated that only 40 percent of the medically needy poor are covered by Medicaid under existing constraints. Urban hospital Health Maintenance Organizations (HMOs) for the working poor are one such innovative program in this area.
- Further extension of health resource programs into areas of continuing poverty. In particular, the continued development of Community Health Centers and Migrant Health Centers and the extension of the programs of the National Health Service Corps still seem warranted.
- Development of state programs to redistribute health care personnel and resources. Various states have made major investments in educational programs for the health professions. It would seem appropriate that states, through adaptations of the National Health Service Corps model, could encourage or even require some repayment by graduates in the form of service in underserved areas.
- Encouragement of professional organizations to play a more significant role in assuring equity. Since the licensed professions enjoy a monopoly, states should consider assigning them a more active role in designing programs for providing health services to the needy.

Achievement of a national goal to provide equity of access to health care for all Americans is within our grasp. We should recommit ourselves to this effort.

## Health Promotion and Disease Prevention

The health needs of the American population today differ from those characterizing the era in which most of our health care delivery practices and institutions developed. The major health problems have shifted from acute to chronic illnesses over the course of this century. As our British colleague, Dr. Archibald Cochrane (1974), has said, we are moving from curing to caring. Unfortunately, our present health care delivery system is still focused too much on the treatment of acute disease and on a system of reimbursement for the treatment of acute disease.

Health promotion and disease prevention are sound approaches for improving health and minimizing the discomforts and burdens of ill health of Americans. Despite the fact that only 4 percent of the total U.S. health expenditures are directed toward prevention, we are clearly achieving improved health outcomes from this limited investment. There has been a remarkable decline in cardiac mortality (25 percent) and stroke mortality (40 percent) in the last decade (Richmond and Kotelchuck, in press). Through immunization there has been a sharp reduction in the infectious diseases of childhood. Indeed, most students of public health would argue that future improvements in health status will come predominantly from programs of health promotion and disease prevention. Prevention clearly works.

Health promotion and disease prevention are beginning to be actively highlighted in recent federal health strategy. Some of these efforts culminated in the publication of the Surgeon General's Report, *Healthy People* (1979). Its emphasis is on public health practices, environmental health, epidemiological surveillance, immunizations, and health and life-style education for prevention and well-being. A critical feature of this publication is the development of concrete, quantitative goals for the nation, and in associated publications, specific programs for reaching these goals. Governmental agencies at the federal, state, and regional levels have important roles to play in refocusing the present health care delivery system to reflect the real health needs of the American people today.

Such a change in orientation has barely begun. Our reimbursement and insurance systems do not yet reflect it, nor are professional organizations fully committed as yet. In many ways, it is the American public that is in the forefront of this movement—a consumer activist movement that can well be designated the second public health revolution. But the fragility of the federal effort in this area is startlingly apparent. Preventive programs, lacking any powerful constituency, are easily targeted for budget cuts. The health needs of tomorrow are being shortsightedly sacrificed for the cost savings of today.

### Delivery of Health Services and the Political Process

It is clear that the public political process has had a tremendous and an increasing influence on the delivery of health care services in the United States. Although the public sector's contribution to health care expenditures is only 40 percent, the lack of unity and clear leadership in the private sector makes the public sector the strongest force in health policy today. In particular, the federal government's control of 30 percent of health care funding allows it to dominate most health care policy decisions. The public, through congressional and presidential elections, has an arena for voicing its desires on how this public sector should operate.

While some of our colleagues fear the intrusions of the public and its concerns into their professional activities, we believe that it is good that health care decisions become more public. The public has a justifiable interest in health care, especially for those members of society who are unable to obtain health care for themselves. Health is a national responsibility. Having a healthy population is critical for the well-being of the country.

A publicly articulated health policy becomes more and more important each year. Yet the formal perception of "a national health policy" is quite recent; prior to the 1965 period, the term itself was rarely used. Today, the public is increasingly conscious of the health care system as a major sector in our society that is strongly influenced by federal action.

### Summary and Conclusion

The principal goals of the post–1965 national health care policy were to provide equity of access to health care for all citizens and public subsidy of medical care costs for the elderly and the poor. Operating on a deficit model, each health resource need was identified and met with a specific federal program. These federal programs have proved to be remarkably successful.

In recent years, however, this original piecemeal approach to health care programs has led to new, unanticipated problems of oversupply, maldistribution of health resources, and high costs. In this chapter, we have suggested that it is time to reconsider the federal approach to health care. We believe that it is necessary to reorient our thinking about health care in the United States, away from a deficit model to a model of equilibration and equity. This model acknowledges that we have met many of the basic health care needs of our population and that we must now bring about a fine tuning of the system to meet the remaining needs and imbalances.

We have suggested that three major agenda items confront health policy today: First, a reorientation of our present health care delivery system away from a dominant concern with the treatment and reimbursement for acute illness to a system focused more on health promotion and disease prevention; second, the fulfillment of the 1965 goal to provide equity of access for all U.S. citizens; and third, the development of new health regulatory efforts, based on an equilibration model, to ensure rational distribution, high quality, and cost-effectiveness of federal, state, and regional health care resources programs.

In spite of the fact that health care policies may seem amorphous, progress has been made in the delivery of health services to the American people. The federal role, in particular, has been a potent force in dealing effectively with some of the major national health care deficits. In recent years, we have learned a great deal about how to shape health care policy. The challenge is not to dismantle, in a mindless way, what we have already done to improve the health of our people and to generate the needed health resources; rather, we are challenged to develop new, creative approaches to build our institutions to be even more responsive to the health care needs of our people.

## References

Aday, L., Anderson, R., and Fleming, G. *Health Care in the United States, Equitable for Whom?* Beverly Hills, Calif.: Sage, 1980.

Cochrane, A. L. "The Value of Epidemiology to Health Services." Presented as one of the Edward K. Dunham Lectures for the Promotion of the Medical Sciences, Boston, Harvard Medical School, April 1974.

Dicker, M. "Health Care Coverage and Insurance Premiums of Families, 1980." In National Center for Health Statistics, *National Medical Care Utilization and Expenditure Survey, Preliminary Report No. 3*. Washington, D.C.: U.S. Department of Health and Human Services, 1983.

Dunlop, J. T. "The Capacity of the United States to Provide and Finance Expanding Health Services." *Bulletin of the New York Academy of Medicine*, 1965, *41*, 1325.

Flexner, A. *Medical Education in the United States and Canada*. New York: Carnegie Foundation for the Advancement of Teaching, 1910.

Graduate Medical Education National Advisory Committee. *Summary Report to the Secretary, Department of Health and Human Services*. Vol. 1. Washington, D.C.: U.S. Government Printing Office, 1980.

Health Insurance Association of America. *Source Book of Health Insurance Data, 1981-82*. Washington, D.C.: Health Insurance Association of America, 1982.

Inglehart, J. K. "New Jersey's Experiment with DRG-Based Hospital Reimbursement." *New England Journal of Medicine*, 1982, *307*, 1655-1660.

Institute of Medicine. *A Policy Statement: Controlling the Supply of Hospital Beds*. Institute of Medicine Publication no. 76-03A. Washington, D.C.: National Academy of Sciences, 1976.

Institute of Medicine. *Report of a Study: A Manpower Policy for Primary Health Care.* Institute of Medicine Publication no. 78–02. Washington, D.C.: National Academy of Sciences, 1978.

Johnson, T. P., and Cooper, J. K. "Physician Shortage in Kentucky, 1930–1980." *American Journal of Public Health,* 1982, *72,* 3.

Metropolitan Life Insurance Company. *Statistical Bulletin.* Vol. 48. New York: Metropolitan Life Insurance Company, 1967.

National Center for Health Statistics. *Medical Care Studies and Family Income, Chronic Illness, and Disability.* Washington, D.C.: National Center for Health Statistics, 1964.

National Center for Health Statistics. *Health United States 1980.* U.S. Department of Health and Human Services Publication no. (PHS) 81–1232. Washington, D.C.: U.S. Department of Health and Human Services, 1980.

Richmond, J. B. "The Gap in Child Health Care." *The American Federationist,* 1967, *74,* 11.

Richmond, J. B. *Currents in American Medicine.* Cambridge, Mass.: Harvard University Press, 1969.

Richmond, J. B. Annual Weiskotten Lecture to Syracuse Medical Alumni Association, Syracuse, New York, September 25, 1980.

Richmond, J. B., and Kotelchuck, M. "Coordination and Development of Strategy and Policy for Public Health Promotion in the United States." In W. W. Holland, E. G. Knox, and R. Detels (Eds.), *Textbook of Public Health.* Oxford, England: Oxford University Press, in press.

Sager, A. "Urban Voluntary Hospitals: Predictable Closure/Relocation Pattern." *Hospital Progress,* 1981, *62,* 46–53.

Schaeffer, D. H. "Voluntary Effort, Best Approach to Containment." *Hospitals: Journal of American Hospital Association,* 1979, *53* (15), 32–35.

Seifert, V. D., and Johnstone, J. S. "Meeting the Emergency Department Crisis." *Hospitals: Journal of American Hospital Association,* 1966, *40,* 55.

Surgeon General's Consultant Group on Medical Education. *Physicians for a Growing America.* U.S. Department of Health, Education, and Welfare Publication no. 709. Washington, D.C.: U.S. Public Health Service, 1959.

Surgeon General's Report on Health Promotion and Disease Prevention. *Healthy People.* U.S. Department of Health, Education, and Welfare Publication no. 79-55071. Washington, D.C.: U.S. Public Health Service, 1979.

U.S. Bureau of the Census. *Historical Statistics of the U.S.: Colonial Times to 1957.* Washington, D.C.: U.S. Bureau of the Census, 1960.

U.S. Bureau of the Census. *Statistical Abstracts of the U.S.* Vols. 1958–1979. Washington, D.C.: U.S. Bureau of the Census, 1980.

U.S. Congressional Budget Office. *Profile of Health Care Coverage: The Haves and Have-Nots.* Washington, D.C.: U.S. Congressional Budget Office, 1979.

*Jack Hadley*

# 18

# Financial Constraints

## Paying for Services and Professional Education

Mies Van Der Rohe, one of the fathers of modern architecture, used the phrase "less is more" to describe his approach to designing buildings. The same phrase has been used to describe the music of Igor Stravinsky and the choreography of George Balanchine. In each case, the esthetic is the same. By stripping away the excessive and unnecessary ornamentation of an earlier period, each was able to reach the essence of his art. The result was a sparer, leaner, more economical creation that communicated more directly and more fundamentally with the user, listener, or viewer.

This chapter is concerned with a more prosaic topic than architecture, music, or choreography. How will changes in the way we pay for health care services affect medical education institutions, medical schools, and teaching hospitals? Thus, the focal point of the chapter will be money. Although deans, administrators, and accountants are not among the nine muses, I believe that one of the challenges facing medical educators and their institutions will be how to achieve "less is more."

*Note:* The research for this paper was supported by Grant no. 95-P-97176 from the Health Care Financing Administration, U.S. Department of Health and Human Services. Opinions expressed are those of the author and do not necessarily represent the views of the Urban Institute or its sponsors.

A period of substantial growth in students and budgets is coming to a close, if not already ended. This was a time of "more and more." While expansion may be chaotic, it generally does not require the hard choices that go with contraction. The next few years may very well see a shrinking of the medical education sector. The immediate problem will be one of "less is less." Meeting the challenges of the new fiscal realities of the 1980s will not be easy. Whether academic health centers succeed in converting "less is less" into "less is more" will depend on innovation, cooperation, and leadership among medical schools and teaching hospitals.

The first question is who pays for medical care? How is total medical care spending distributed among private insurers, governments, and patients' direct expenses? How have these shares changed over time? How will current and potential policy changes influence each party's share of the total? A companion to the question of who pays is how do they pay for medical care? What are the basic approaches to physician and hospital reimbursement? What changes are likely to occur? What will be the effects on physicians and hospitals generally?

The impact of these changes on medical schools and teaching hospitals will depend on how reliant their educational programs are on health care reimbursements. Therefore, what are medical schools' and teaching hospitals' revenue sources? How have they changed in the past? What is likely to happen in the next few years? Given the possible changes in revenue sources, what courses of action are medical schools and teaching hospitals likely to follow? What will happen to medical school tuitions? Will applications to medical schools be affected? What will be the consequences of financing changes for residents' stipends and for the size of graduate medical education programs?

Finally, what strategies can medical schools and teaching hospitals follow to convert "less is less" into "less is more"? While it would be highly presumptuous to claim to have the answers to this question, I would like to conclude with some suggestions for possible courses of action. These suggestions, if implemented, would require medical education institutions to assume greater leadership in issues of health care financing and to risk innovation in seeking ways to solve both the health care and the medical education financing problems.

One caveat before beginning. Although the topic is health care financing, and although the writer is a card-carrying economist with a green eyeshade to prove it, it is important to note that money is not the only thing that matters or that it is even the most important thing in medical education. The assumption here is more modest; namely, money is not irrelevant to the decisions and choices medical schools and teaching hospitals must make. Although almost all such institutions are nonprofit and have goals other than maximizing net income, they cannot repeal the existence of budget constraints. Thus, changes in health care financing need to be considered in planning for tomorrow's health professionals.

## Who Pays for Health Care?

In 1965, the last full year before the implementation of the Medicare and Medicaid programs, payments for health care services were split almost evenly between patients' direct payments, which made up 44.6 percent of the total, and payments by so-called third parties—private insurance and philanthropy, the federal government, and state and local governments. The federal government had the smallest share, 11.3 percent, of the major participants.

Fifteen years later, the picture is dramatically different, as can be seen from the changes summarized in Table 1. The federal government, now the largest source of funds for health services delivery, pays for almost 30 percent of the care provided. Almost all of this growth has been a substitution of federal dollars for patients' direct expenses. Patients are now directly responsible for just over 25 percent of the total bill. The shares paid by private insurance and philanthropy, and state and local governments have remained about the same.

The primary engines generating this shift in payment responsibilities have been the federal Medicare and Medicaid programs. Of course, these programs have done much more than simply shuffle dollars. They've also been the driving force behind a major expansion in access to and the use of health services. In 1965, per capita health care spending was $181 and health care absorbed 6 percent of the gross national product (GNP). After adjusting for inflation, per capita health care spending was $332, and the share of GNP devoted to health care was 9.4 percent in 1980. In other words, by 1980 the average person was consuming almost twice as much medical care as in 1965, and the country as a whole was allocating 56 percent more of its resources to the production of health care than it was in 1965 (Gibson and Waldo, 1981).

Many view these trends as a positive factor in the health and welfare of the nation. Others feel that too much is being spent for medical care in general and that the federal government in particular is spending too much. The argument is made that the federal government is too centralized and too far removed from the actual delivery of services to make prudent judgments about how much and what kinds of care should be provided.

Whatever the merits of these arguments and rationales, the federal government's message, backed up by actions in the budget for the 1982 fiscal year, is clear. Odds are that it is going to spend less for medical care or at least not increase

**Table 1. Percentage Distribution of Health Care Expenses
by Source of Payment, 1965 and 1980[a].**

| Source of Payment | 1965 | 1980 |
|---|---|---|
| Patients | 44.6% | 26.7% |
| Private Insurance, Philanthropy | 31.1 | 29.5 |
| Federal Government | 11.3 | 29.8 |
| (Medicare) | | (16.2) |
| (Medicaid) | | (6.7) |
| (Other) | | (6.9) |
| State and Local Governments | 13.6 | 13.7 |
| (Medicaid) | | (5.1) |
| (Other) | | (8.6) |

[a] Excludes dentists' services, research, and construction of medical facilities; includes prepayment, administration, and government public health activities.
*Source:* Gibson and Waldo, 1981.

its health care spending at as fast a rate as in the past. The most dramatic cuts were made in the Medicaid program. Among the provisions in the Omnibus Reconciliation Act of 1981 (PL 97-35) are the following:

- With some exceptions, reductions in the Medicaid payments states would otherwise be entitled to receive from the federal government by 3 percent in fiscal 1982, 4 percent in fiscal 1983, and 4.5 percent in fiscal 1984
- More flexibility for states to limit coverage of the medically needy
- A repeal of the requirement that Medicaid programs reimburse hospitals, based on the determination of reasonable cost used by Medicare, and the insertion of the looser requirement that Medicaid reimburse hospitals to ensure that Medicaid patients have "reasonable access to services of adequate quality"
- A modification of the provision guaranteeing "freedom of choice" for Medicaid recipients that permits states to use competitive bidding, exclude high-cost or low-quality providers, or limit Medicaid recipients to the use of selected providers

Changes in the Medicare program were not as dramatic but were all in the direction of either increasing beneficiaries' share of the bill or reducing payments to providers. The latter included:

- A reduction in the nursing differential from 8.5 to 5 percent above the average routine nursing costs
- A directive to issue regulations limiting charges for outpatient services
- A ceiling on the reimbursement of hospital inpatient costs at 108 percent of the average cost of providing similar services at a comparable group of hospitals

The third area affected by the reconciliation bill was the large group of categorical grant programs supported by the U.S. Department of Health and Human Services. A number of these were grouped into four so-called block grants, with funding authorizations set at roughly 75 percent of what they would have been as separate categorical grants. Of the remaining categorical programs, health education support is the largest set of grants. These were slated for moderate increases over the next two years, 9 and 4.5 percent, respectively. However, the 1982 authorization is barely more than half of the $409.5 million actually spent in fiscal 1980 (*Drug Research Reports* . . . , 1980). All other categorical programs as a group are budgeted for substantial reductions, almost $340 million by fiscal 1984. Table 2 summarizes the authorizations for the grant programs in the reconciliation bill.

Overall, the message seems clear: Less is less.

The key question with regard to state and local governments is whether they will compensate for cuts made in federal health spending. Unfortunately, many states and cities are caught in financial squeezes of their own. The current recession plus either legal or informal limits on taxes have put sharp downward pressure on revenues. At the same time, high unemployment rates are pushing up demands for unemployment compensation, welfare, and general assistance. Since most state and local governments are legally prohibited from running deficits, the

Table 2. Health Grant Program Authorizations from Public Law 97–35 for Fiscal Years 1982–1984 (in millions of dollars).

| | 1982 | 1983 | 1984 |
|---|---|---|---|
| Health Manpower Programs | $ 218.8 | $ 238.6 | $ 249.3 |
| All Other Categorical Grants | 820.1 | 651.1 | 482.6 |
| Block Grants | | | |
| Preventive health, health services | 95.0 | 96.5 | 98.5 |
| Alcohol/drug abuse, mental health services | 491.0 | 511.0 | 532.0 |
| Primary care | 280.0 | 302.5 | 327.0 |
| Maternal, child health | 373.0 | 373.0 | 373.0 |
| Total, All Grants | $2,277.9 | $2,172.7 | $2,062.4 |

only major option open in many cases is to reduce spending. Medicaid, because it is such a large share of the budget in many states, is one of the primary targets for spending reductions. The actual changes being implemented or proposed across states are too many to list. However, a paraphrase of a *New York Times* survey seems to accurately reflect current trends. States that would like to compensate for federal cuts can't afford to; those that can afford to, don't want to (Pear, 1982).

Changes in the private insurance sector are numerous, diverse, and decentralized. It is fairly clear, however, that the trend is toward less insurance. First, the increase in unemployment is causing many people to lose insurance coverage altogether. Whether this is a short-run or long-run phenomenon still remains to be seen. Second, in order to save labor costs and save jobs, employers and employees are opting for less generous insurance coverage—benefits are being eliminated or limited, coinsurance rates are being raised, and deductibles are being increased. Probably the most striking example of this type of action is the Federal Employees Health Benefits plan. In order to reduce the government's share of employees' health insurance premium costs, the Office of Personnel Management has mandated a sweeping set of changes. For example, the Government Employees Health Association, one of the private insurance plan options available to federal employees, increased the personal deductible from $80 to $200, the family deductible from $160 to $600, and coinsurance rates from 0 to 5 percent (depending on the service) to 20 percent on all services, including inpatient hospital room charges and all ancillary services (U.S. Office of Personnel Management, 1981, 1982).

The third trend that is rapidly picking up steam in the private insurance market is the development of a number of innovative approaches to health care financing and health care delivery. Although the structures of these initiatives vary, they share the common goal of reducing health care expenditures. Some—Health maintenance Organizations (HMOs), individual practice associations (IPAs), and health care foundations—have been around for a while. Others, such as business/labor coalitions, primary care networks, case management plans, preferred provider plans, and stay-well or wellness plans are fairly new to the scene. By changing either patients' behavior, providers' behavior, or simply negotiating lower rates, these schemes aim to economize on health care costs, with one of the primary targets being hospital admissions and lengths of stay.

The general trend and primary consequence of changes in third-party payers' policies, then, appear to be a shift of a bigger share of the cost of medical care back to the patient. Although many may think of the measures I've described as draconian, it is unlikely that the clock will be turned back to the pre-Medicare/Medicaid situation described in Table 1. What does seem clear, both currently and for the near future at least, is that the health sector will be confronted with strong pressures to reduce costs and expenditures.

## How Is Medical Care Paid For?

The previous section described changes in insurers' policies in fairly broad terms, that is, numbers of people covered by insurance, benefits included in insurance plans, and the desire to pay less for care. One of the more subtle, though important and ubiquitous aspects of health care financing is the actual method of payment, typically referred to as hospital and physician reimbursement. Reimbursement is clearly one of the most arcane and complex processes ever invented. A full presentation and analysis would require many more pages than are available here. (The Medicare and Medicaid Guide devotes more than 1,000 pages to reimbursement.) At the risk of being accused of oversimplification, I would like to boil all of the details down to the two basic approaches summarized in Table 3.

Open-ended reimbursement consists of usual-customary-reasonable (UCR) and customary-prevailing-reasonable (CPR) charge methods for physicians' services and reasonable costs, reasonable charges, or percentage of costs or charges methods for hospitals' services. Of course, many, if not most, physicians and hospitals may consider these systems unreasonable, unusual, and unfair. Almost all variations of these systems involve screening charges or costs, basing current payments on a prior period's billings or expenses, and an inordinate amount of haggling over what's included and what's reasonable.

Nevertheless, the key feature of these systems is that the payers say, in effect, "We pay what you charge or spend, or some percentage of that." Consequently,

### Table 3. Health Care Reimbursement Methods.

| Reimbursement Method | Payment to Physicians | Payment to Hospitals |
|---|---|---|
| Open-Ended | Usual-Customary-Reasonable (UCR) Customary-Prevailing-Reasonable (CPR) | Reasonable Costs Reasonable Charges Percentage of Costs or Charges |
| Capped | Fee Schedules (FS) Maximum Allowable Fees Relative Value Schedules and Conversion Factors (RVS + CF) | Rate Setting Prospective Reimbursement Global Budgeting Diagnostic-Related Groups Reimbursement |

these systems have a built-in dynamic that is controlled primarily by providers. Increased charges or expenses lead to increased payments, albeit not necessarily dollar for dollar.

Capped reimbursement, on the other hand, might be characterized by payers saying "You get what we're willing to pay." With fee schedules (FS), maximum allowable fees, and relative value schedules and conversion factors systems (RVS + CF), the maximum, if not the actual, amount the insurer pays the physician is predetermined and cannot be changed without explicit agreement by the insurer. Physicians increasing their charges, either individually or collectively, will have no effect on the amounts they're paid. Similarly, the key characteristic of most rate setting, prospective reimbursement, global budgeting, and diagnostic-related groups reimbursement systems for hospital reimbursement is that the amount the insurer will pay is in some way predetermined and usually also limited. Clearly, increases in costs put pressure on rate setters to increase rates, but there is no automatic "pass-through," as in reasonable costs or reasonable charges systems.

The dichotomy between open-ended and capped reimbursement systems is undoubtedly overdrawn. Reasonable costs/charges systems can be constrained and fee schedules can be altered. The point, however, is that capped reimbursement is typically less generous than open-ended reimbursement.

Data on physicians' fees paid by the Medicaid program illustrate this. In 1979, twenty-five Medicaid programs used a customary-prevailing-reasonable (CPR) method to pay physicians and twenty-five used either fee schedules (FS) or relative value schedules and conversion factors (RVS + CF). (The RVS + CF approach starts with a fixed schedule of numerical values among procedures, that is, their relative values, and then applies a dollar multiplier, for example, fifty cents per relative value unit.) Medicare employs the usual-customary-reasonable (UCR) method nationwide, though it is implemented separately in each Medicare locality. (UCR and CPR systems are conceptually equivalent, even though the terminology differs between Medicare and Medicaid. Medicare localities are states or parts of states that serve as administrative units.) Because Medicare uses a single method nationwide, comparing average fees paid by Medicaid in CPR and FS/RVS + CF jurisdictions to average Medicare fees in those same areas should indicate the relative generosity of the two approaches.

As can be seen in the upper portion of Table 4, in CPR jurisdictions Medicaid fees are only slightly lower than Medicare fees, 97 percent of general practitioners' fees and 92 percent of specialists' fees. In FS and RVS + CF jurisdictions, Medicaid pays only 70 percent of what Medicare pays general practitioners, and 60 percent of Medicare fees for specialists. The lower portion of the table shows similar ratios in selected FS and RVS + CF Medicaid programs. The six states listed accounted for almost 50 percent of total Medicaid expenditures in fiscal 1979. New York, the largest Medicaid program, is the least generous, paying only twenty-five cents for every dollar paid by Medicare.

The impact of capped reimbursement approaches on hospitals is a little more difficult to illustrate because of the diversity of the alternative methods. Early research tended to show little or no impact on hospital costs. More recent studies, however, indicate that once these alternative systems go through a maturation process, they do have a significant impact on hospitals' revenues and costs.

Table 4. Average Ratio of Medicaid to Medicare Fees, 1979[a].

|  | Fee Ratios | |
| --- | --- | --- |
|  | General Practitioners | Specialists |
| CPR[b] States (N = 25) | 0.97 | 0.92 |
| FS[b] and RVS + CF[b] States (N = 25) | 0.70 | 0.60 |
| Selected FS[b] and RVS + CF[b] States | | |
| New York | 0.42 | 0.24 |
| Pennsylvania | 0.45 | 0.28 |
| Missouri | 0.51 | 0.57 |
| Illinois | 0.60 | 0.61 |
| Massachusetts | 0.67 | 0.56 |
| California | 0.69 | 0.54 |

[a]Unweighted average of state ratios
[b]Methods of reimbursement to physicians:
   CPR—Customary-Prevailing-Reasonable
   FS—Fee Schedules
   RVS + CF—Relative Value Schedules and Conversion Factors
*Source:* Holahan, 1982.

Estimates of the impact suggest that a mature, mandatory program (one that has been in place for more that three years) can result in a reduction of from 7 to 20 percent in cost per day (Sloan, 1982). In a study under way at the Urban Institute, we have estimated that if all of a teaching hospital's patient revenues were subject to mature, mandatory rate setting, revenue per patient day would be 16 percent lower than if no revenues were subject to rate setting (Hadley, Lee, and Carlson, 1982).

Figure 1, constructed from data from the American Hospital Association's National Hospital Panel Survey, illustrates the potential impact of mandatory hospital rate setting. It shows that total revenue per patient day in short-term general hospitals grew at an annual compound rate of 14.8 percent between 1975 and 1980, rising from $153 per day to $305 per day. Extrapolating this rate forward to 1985 results in an estimate of $607 per day. If all revenues were subject to mandatory rate setting, the estimates of revenue per day would be between 7 and 20 percent lower.

In the absence of voluntary constraint, it seems increasingly likely that more and more insurers, both private and public, will move from open-ended to some form of capped reimbursement. Less is less.

## Medical Education Institutions and Patient Care Revenue

Changes in health care financing will affect medical schools and teaching hospitals, primarily through their impact on these institutions' revenues. Although there is a natural inclination to focus only on revenues and costs associated

Figure 1. Revenue per Patient Day (Actual 1975–1980, Projected 1981–1985).

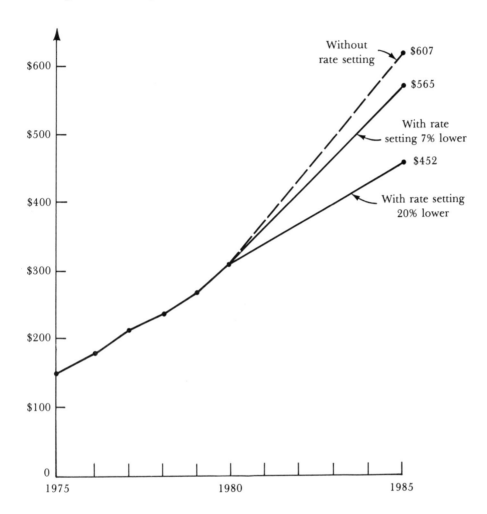

with educational activities, that inclination should be resisted. It is essential that the institution's overall fiscal situation be considered. Even though a large chunk of an institution's income may be earmarked, most of the budget is fungible. Depending on priorities, a revenue loss from one particular source of income may lead to compensating adjustments in other, seemingly unrelated, activities.

How have medical schools' and teaching hospitals' sources of revenue changed over time? Do sources vary dramatically between public and private institutions? Issues associated with tuition levels and stipend funding will be treated tangentially, because they are tangential.

Table 5 reports data on percentage distribution of medical schools' sources of revenue at two points in time, 1967–68 and 1979–80. Separate data are reported for public and private medical schools. Not surprisingly, public schools are far more dependent on revenues from state and local governments than are private schools. Other differences between public and private schools are far less dramatic.

Table 5. Percentage Distribution of Medical Schools' Revenue Sources, by Ownership,
1967–68 and 1979–80.

| Revenue Source | Public Schools | | Private Schools | |
|---|---|---|---|---|
| | 1967–68 (%) | 1979–80 (%) | 1967–68 (%) | 1979–80 (%) |
| State and Local Governments | 26.2 | 34.8 | 2.5 | 3.4 |
| Sponsored Federal | | | | |
| Teaching | 13.3 | 4.7 | 13.0 | 4.4 |
| Other[a] | 35.0 | 19.6 | 43.1 | 30.8 |
| Sponsored Nonfederal[b] | 8.8 | 8.8 | 16.0 | 15.7 |
| Tuition and Fees | 2.8 | 2.8 | 5.3 | 8.7 |
| Professional Fee Income | 5.0 | 13.7 | 3.3 | 17.6 |
| Other Income | 8.9 | 15.6  (7.3)[c] | 16.9 | 19.4  (9.7)[c] |
| Total, All Sources[d] | 100.0 | 100.0 | 100.0 | 100.0 |

[a] Includes research and recovery of indirect costs
[b] Includes recovery of indirect costs
[c] Revenue from teaching hospitals—similar data were not available in 1967–68
[d] May not sum due to rounding
Source: "Medical Education in the United States," 1969, 1981.

Over time, probably the single most important trend affecting medical school revenues has been the decline in sponsored federal support. In 1967–68, sponsored federal funds accounted for about half of all medical school funds. By 1979–80, this source made up less than 25 percent of public school revenues and about 35 percent of private school revenues. These cuts have hit teaching grants proportionately harder than other grants. In both public and private schools, teaching grants accounted for less than 5 percent of revenues in 1979–80, down by about two-thirds from the years of peak federal support. In future years, federal teaching support will be even smaller.

How have medical schools adjusted to declining federal support? First, in spite of all the publicity given to high tuitions, public schools have not increased their dependence on tuitions and fees. It was and remains one of the least important revenue sources for these institutions. Private schools have increased their reliance on tuition and fees, from 5.3 to 8.7 percent of total revenues. Second, public schools have drawn a bigger share of their revenues from state and local governments and other revenue sources, increasing each by about 8 percent. Private schools increased their revenues from these sources only slightly, by a total of 3.4 percentage points.

The most dramatic change, in both proportional and absolute terms, has been the growth of professional fee income. Income from billings for medical care services provided by faculty in 1979–80 accounted for 13.7 percent of public school revenues and 17.6 percent of private school revenues. If revenues from teaching hospitals, which are included in the Other Income category, are added to professional fee income, then the totals increase to 21 percent for public schools and 27.3 percent for private. Thus, direct and indirect patient care revenues are the second most important source of medical school funds after state and local government support at public institutions and sponsored federal funds at private schools.

For teaching hospitals, the key factor, I believe, is not so much changes over time in revenue sources but rather differences across hospitals in both revenues and costs. Table 6 shows revenue sources for hospitals grouped by teaching status and ownership. What is striking is the difference between public teaching hospitals and all other institutions. Public teaching hospitals are more than twice as dependent as other hospitals on revenues from Medicaid, government appropriations, and other nonpatient care sources. They derive smaller proportions of their revenue from Medicare, Blue Cross/Blue Shield, commercial insurance, and self-payment.

Also striking are apparent differences in costs among different types of hospitals. Although a crude measure, differences in expense per admission are suggestive of people's perceptions that teaching hospitals are much more costly than nonteaching hospitals. As the data in Table 7 show, in 1980 the average expense per admission in a hospital that was a member of the Council of Teaching Hospitals (COTH) was 87 percent higher than in a nonteaching hospital. Other teaching hospitals were 29 percent more costly than nonteaching hospitals.

These cost differences are dramatic. They also point up a fairly contentious debate between third-party insurers, especially those that use reasonable costs reimbursement, and teaching hospitals over the reimbursement of hospitals' "educational expenses," primarily residents' stipends and teaching physicians' educational salaries. For a variety of reasons, teaching hospitals consider the salaries of residents and teaching physicians to be educational expenses, rather than costs of providing patient care services. In 1978, these expenses were just under $2 billion, roughly equal to 5 percent of teaching hospitals' total revenues. The great major-

Table 6. Percentage Distributions of Hospitals' Revenue Sources, by Ownership and Teaching Status, 1978.

| Revenue Source | Teaching[a] | | Nonteaching | |
|---|---|---|---|---|
| | Public[b] (%) | Private[c] (%) | Public (%) | Private (%) |
| Medicaid | 17.9 | 7.7 | 7.8 | 7.3 |
| Medicare | 25.4 | 32.7 | 33.5 | 34.9 |
| Blue Cross/Blue Shield | 12.8 | 22.9 | 16.2 | 17.8 |
| Commercial Insurance and Self-Pay | 24.1 | 29.1 | 34.3 | 32.7 |
| Government Appropriations and All Other Sources | 19.8 | 7.6 | 8.2 | 7.3 |
| Total, All Sources | 100.0 | 100.0 | 100.0 | 100.0 |

[a] Hospitals with at least one AMA-approved residency program
[b] Excludes federal hospitals
[c] Excludes for-profit hospitals
*Source:* Hadley, 1981.

Table 7. Total Expenses per Admission, by Teaching Status and Ownership, 1980.

|  | Total Expense per Admission | Average Number of Residents |
|---|---|---|
| COTH Members | $3,203 | 112.7 |
| Private[a] | 3,229 | 109.4 |
| Public[b] | 2,674 | 179.5 |
| Other Teaching[c] | 2,199 | 15.3 |
| Private | 2,225 | 15.2 |
| Public | 1,688 | 19.6 |
| Nonteaching | 1,710 | 0.6 |
| Private | 1,749 | 0.9 |
| Public | 1,436 | 0.1 |
| All Hospitals | 1,841 | 8.0 |

[a]Excludes for-profit hospitals
[b]Excludes federal hospitals
[c]Hospitals that have at least one AMA-approved residency program but are not members of the Council of Teaching Hospitals (COTH)
Source: American Hospital Association, 1980.

ity of these expenses, between 70 and 90 percent, are paid from patient care revenues (Hadley and Tigue, 1982).

As emphasized earlier, third-party payers, both public and private, face mounting pressures to reduce their costs and thus the burden on taxpayers and policyholders. Given the apparently dramatic cost differences between teaching and nonteaching hospitals and the designation of stipends and teaching physicians' salaries as educational expenses, the temptation is great to disallow or exclude these expenses from reimbursements for patient care. After all, physicians are the highest-paid profession in the country. Why should patients pay for their physicians' education?

Unfortunately, appearances are deceiving in this case, and the emotional arguments about who should pay for graduate medical education have made it difficult to see through these appearances. In reality, residents, and to some extent teaching physicians, already pay for most of the costs of graduate medical education by providing services whose value exceeds their salaries (Feldman and Yoder, 1980). This is a difficult point to demonstrate empirically, because salaries can be readily observed while the value of the service provided is elusive. However, the conclusion that trainees who receive general skills (as opposed to firm specific skills) through on-the-job training pay for their own training is a well-established result of economic research (Becker, 1964). It follows then that efforts to disallow educational expenses as non-patient-care costs would not be justified. It also follows, however, that hospitals should not be paid more on the basis of teaching status alone.

By the same token, it is fallacious for insurers to think that they would necessarily save money by not paying educational expenses. To illustrate this, assume that by a wave of the wand all physicians were deemed full-fledged, competent medical practitioners upon graduation from medical school and that there were no such things as residency training programs. Unless residents are totally redundant and contribute nothing at all to patient care delivery, hospitals would have to hire other personnel to provide the services currently provided by residents. These personnel would very likely include salaried physicians, nurses, and technicians. Attending physicians would probably make more visits to their patients. These visits would not be billed as hospital costs, but insurers would nevertheless be expected to reimburse physicians directly. The net result is that unreimbursed educational expenses would be replaced by reimbursable patient care expenses. Thus, insurers would ultimately save very little money, and, according to one estimate of the substitution costs of other personnel for residents, might even pay more (Freymann and Springer, 1973).

The key to solving the puzzle, of course, is that simple comparisons, as in Table 7, between teaching and nonteaching hospitals are inappropriate. These institutions differ by more than the presence of residents and the existence of educational activities. Teaching hospitals are larger. They are more likely to be in cities, which are generally more costly than suburban and rural areas because wage rates are higher. Most importantly, teaching hospitals, especially COTH members, do not treat the same mix of patients or provide the same mix of services as other hospitals. Clearly, one has to control for differences like these in assessing the impact of educational activities on hospital costs.

A recent study has attempted a controlled comparison of this sort, using a variety of hospital data from 1974 and 1977 (Sloan, Feldman, and Steinwald, 1983). The key features of this study are the use of a case mix measure, explicit exclusion or imputation of physician costs, and analysis of costs at the departmental as well as hospital-wide level. The basic result is that when other factors, especially case mix, are taken into account, nonphysician cost per adjusted admission is at most 13 percent higher for a COTH member than for a nonteaching hospital. (An adjusted admission to a weighted average of inpatient admissions and outpatient visits.) Other teaching hospitals are 5 percent more costly than nonteaching hospitals. Furthermore, it appears that at least some of the cost difference occurs in nonclinical departments, such as dietary, plant operations, and housekeeping. It is unlikely that the presence of residents or education per se should have any effect on these types of costs.

What does one conclude from these observations? Changes in health care financing will affect medical schools and teaching hospitals primarily through the consequences for these institutions' total revenues. Changes in the reimbursement of so-called educational expenses, while more visible in terms of their apparent impact on training programs, are likely to be relatively trivial compared to overall changes in patient care reimbursements. Similarly, medical schools are likely to be more heavily affected by changes in physician reimbursement methods than by an end of capitation grants.

## Responses of Medical Schools and Teaching Hospitals to Changes in Health Care Financing

The previous section of this chapter outlined medical schools' and teaching hospitals' dependence on patient care revenues for their educational activities. The two preceding sections described probable changes in insurance and reimbursement. This section will attempt to tie these factors together to focus more specifically on (1) the fiscal pressures medical schools and teaching hospitals are likely to face and (2) possible responses to these pressures in the absence of any major structural reforms in either health care financing or reimbursement.

A major distinguishing feature in institutions' responses will be their ownership. Public and private medical schools are likely to pursue different courses of action that over time may very well narrow some current distinctions between them. Public and private teaching hospitals will also follow different strategies. As a result, there will be an even bigger gap in resources and patient mix than currently exists.

All medical schools will find it more difficult to generate professional fee income. Changes in Medicare and Medicaid reimbursement rules, especially a shift toward limits on increases in fees paid physicians, payments to hospital outpatient departments, and payments to hospital-based radiologists and pathologists will provide one set of revenue constraints. Another source of downward pressure will be increased competition in the privately insured part of the health care market. Competing provider groups such as HMOs and IPAs will attempt to enroll privately insured people at rates below those that would support faculty practice plan fees. At the same time, insurance organizations and beneficiary groups will seek to negotiate lower rates with teaching hospitals and faculty practice plans through approaches like preferred provider arrangements and primary care networks. Third, trends in traditional private insurance plans toward higher cost sharing and more limited benefits will make consumers more generally cost-conscious. If faculty practice plans charge fees toward the higher end of the spectrum, as seems probable, some patients will choose to seek care from lower-cost, office-based providers.

Federal grants to medical schools are likely to continue their downward trend, if not in absolute dollars, then at least in real dollars adjusted for inflation in the prices and salaries of the goods medical schools buy and the staff they hire. These cuts may be more burdensome to private schools because of their greater dependence on federal funds. The most prestigious and most research-oriented schools may be able to replace lost federal research support with private sector research dollars. For most schools, however, this will be a limited option. Furthermore, even where private money is available, it is likely to shift the focus of research activity to more practical and more marketable areas. Whether this is good or bad is an issue beyond the scope of this discussion, but one that clearly needs careful examination.

Lastly, many state governments are going to be reexamining their support for medical education. Faced by their own budget crisis and the need to maintain basic human and public services, appropriations for state-owned medical schools may receive lower priority than in the past. These pressures will be especially strong in those states with the most difficult economic conditions. Many of these states, particularly in the northeast and north central regions of the country, are also losing population. The rapid growth in the number of physicians over the last few years, coupled with projected population declines, will make it difficult to justify additional support for medical schools. States in the south and southwest regions, on the other hand, have reasonably healthy economies and are gaining population. Medical school support in these states is likely to grow. To a large extent, state support of medical education will parallel broader trends in the redistribution of population and economic activity.

How are medical schools likely to respond to these pressures? Raising tuitions is the action that receives the most publicity. As noted earlier, private medical schools have already increased their dependence on income from tuitions and fees. Public schools have not, nor have tuition levels been raised to the range typical of most private schools. For example, in 1979, 93 percent of students at public schools paid less than $4,000 in tuition; 1 percent paid between $6,000 and $8,000; and 1 percent paid more than $10,000. In contrast, 10 percent of students at private medical schools paid more than $10,000, and the modal tuition level, paid by 45 percent of private medical school students, was $6,000 to $8,000 (Lee and Carlson, 1981).

It appears, then, that raising tuitions is probably a feasible option for most public schools. Private schools will find this course less desirable because many already charge high tuitions. Raising tuitions will have two consequences. The first is that some applications will be discouraged. A recent Urban Institute study estimated that a $1,000 increase in tuitions would deter an average of 120 applications per medical school (Lee and Carlson, 1981). Between 1974 and 1980, the total number of applicants dropped by 15 percent. Some of this was due to the 3 percent drop over the same period in the number of college graduates. However, tuitions also increased over this period, by about $500 after adjusting for inflation. Extrapolating the estimates reported above suggests that tuition increases were responsible for about 3 percent or one-fifth of the drop in the number of applicants.

The second consequence of higher tuitions is that students would bear a bigger share of the responsibility for financing their educations. Whether this is fair or desirable is a question beyond the scope of this chapter (Lee and Carlson, 1981; Hadley, 1980). At a minimum, however, medical schools should work to establish an unsubsidized but manageable loan program that will enable medical students to pay for their educations.

If applications continue to fall, either because of increasingly higher tuitions or for other reasons, it is likely that medical schools will reduce class sizes (Hall, 1978). This suggests a second major avenue of response to fiscal pressures, namely, reducing costs. Limiting class size is one way to trim costs. Two other cost-reducing strategies are to reduce faculty-student ratios and limit increases in faculty salaries. For example, between 1965 and 1980, the number of medical students doubled, but the number of faculty tripled. If the number of faculty per student were cut back to its 1975 level, this would reduce expenses for faculty salaries by about $316 million, almost 6 percent of medical schools' total expenses in 1970–80. Limiting the rate of increase in faculty salaries may seem unfeasible at first, but the various trends at work in the health care market will make it an easier goal to achieve over time. The growing supply of physicians, tighter insurance and reimbursement conditions, and growing competition from the organized provider groups will all make the private practice of medicine a relatively less rewarding alternative to a faculty appointment than it has been in the past.

A third option is to expand clinical activities. Tighter reimbursement means that professional fee income will be expanded only by attracting more patients and providing more services. The key to this option, as will be discussed in the next section of this chapter, will be to organize clinical activities more efficiently in order to be able to meet increased market competition.

For teaching hospitals, fiscal pressures will be transmitted through more restrictive Medicaid and Medicare coverage and reimbursements, through leaner budgets at the local government level, and through increased competition from nonteaching hospitals. How hospitals respond to these pressures will depend on the hospital's ownership and mission and where it is located. Many public hospitals, particularly those in urban areas, are committed to treating all patients who need care, regardless of their ability to pay. Private hospitals share this commitment to varying degrees but have only weak obligations to implement it. As a result, private hospitals that face budget pressures are likely to respond by reducing the volume of free or below-cost care provided and by imposing stricter financial conditions on prospective patients in order to reduce bad debts. There are numerous mechanisms by which such a policy could be carried out—reducing hours of operation for outpatient departments and emergency rooms, closing them outright, requesting some payment in advance, or transferring uninsured patients, once medically stable, to public institutions. In general, most private hospitals can follow a strategy of stretching their budgets by reducing activities that do not generate any revenue, or at least not enough to cover a reasonable portion of their cost. Although actions of this type may seem both crass and venal, they may also be necessary for institutional survival.

Hospitals that maintain a standing commitment to provide care to all will find it much more difficult, on both philosophical and political grounds, to adopt such a strategy. In fact, these institutions, many of which are major teaching hospitals, will face the double bind of having to treat more uninsured and non-paying patients but receiving fewer revenues from public sources, especially Medicaid and local government. Traditionally, some amount of free care has been implicitly subsidized through higher charges to charge-paying patients, primarily those covered by commercial insurance or charge-paying Blue Cross plans. As indicated in Table 5, public teaching hospitals derive a relatively small proportion of their revenue from charge-paying patients. Increased competition in the health care market will erode this potential source of internal cross-subsidy even further. First, privately insured groups will be bargaining for "better deals" from hospitals through preferred provider plans and other fixed or reduced payment schemes. Second, teaching hospitals are likely to face stiffer competition from lower-cost, nonteaching hospitals. This competition will be keenest for those people who are covered by charge-paying insurance plans and whose own out-of-pocket liability is directly related to the hospital's charges.

What implication will these trends have for teaching programs? An Urban Institute study has been examining the impact of economic factors on the size of hospitals' graduate medical education programs (Hadley, Lee, and Carlson, 1982). By economic factors, we mean residents' stipends, hospitals' revenues (per patient day), and the volume of hospitals' outputs, measured by average daily census and outpatient visits. Teaching program size is measured by the total number of residency positions offered. Our results suggest that other things held constant, increases in revenue per patient day, average daily census, or the volume of outpatient visits would result in more positions offered. However, the magnitudes of the effects are not equal. A 10 percent increase in outpatient visits would lead to about

9 percent more positions offered. A 10 percent increase in either revenue per day or average daily census would increase offers by about 5 percent.

The scenario just outlined implies that private hospitals on average would reduce their patient care loads, particularly in the outpatient area. This strategy will attempt to preserve revenues, so that revenue per day may be unaffected. According to our model, this should create incentives to reduce teaching program size. Teaching hospitals whose mission includes caring for all will face different and conflicting incentives. To the extent that there is patient shifting, especially for outpatient care, these hospitals will be prompted to expand teaching activities. If these hospitals are also confronted by reduced revenues because of lower payments from Medicaid and smaller government appropriations, they will simultaneously encounter fiscal pressure to cut teaching program size.

It is here, I believe, that the crisis in graduate medical education financing will occur. Reimbursement of residents' stipends and other so-called education expenses is the "tail of the dog." Its "body" is the payment for care provided to teaching hospital patients. Where that body is disproportionately composed of uninsured and partially insured patients, then the issue of its sustenance and survival will dominate grooming the tail. If new ways of financing that care cannot be developed, then the alternatives are either to reduce the volume of care or its quality to a level consistent with available revenues.

### Future Strategies

The prognostications of the previous section were premised on the absence of any major structural reforms in how medical care is paid for. One clear consequence of past expansion that perhaps went too far and of the current desire to reduce health care spending is that some contraction in both undergraduate and graduate medical education is probably inevitable and perhaps appropriate. Whether the process of change will also lead to a better way of doing things, that is, "less is more," will depend, I believe, on medical schools' and teaching hospitals' willingness to cooperate and to innovate.

The goals to be attained are not new, but remain elusive: maintaining an adequate flow of funds to support quality medical education, providing quality medical care to those who need it, and keeping the costs affordable. This chapter concludes with an outline of some possible strategies for doing things differently in the pursuit of these goals.

*Community-Based Medical Practice Plans.* Professional fee income generated by medical school faculty has become the second most important source of medical school revenues. In order to deal with tighter reimbursement policies and increased competition, faculty practice plans should be organized more efficiently and marketed more aggressively. This means active enrollment of capitation and preferred provider beneficiaries, practicing in off-site facilities with lower overhead rates and more convenient patient access, and restructuring internal incentives for physicians so that they provide care in a more cost-conscious fashion. For example, a faculty practice plan could experiment with the concept of a primary care case manager, a physician who shares with the patient some of the fiscal responsibility and consequences of specialty referrals and inpatient hospitalizations. Changes of this sort probably mean that some faculty will have to change how they practice. Establishing and implementing such innovations will not be easy, but the alternatives, outright reductions in the number of faculty or establishing a private practice in an overdoctored, highly competitive environment, may be worse.

Community-based practice plans also offer some advantages in addition to revenue generation. They could provide an excellent alternative to the hospital as a place for training both medical students and residents. These settings will probably offers more contacts with primary care medical problems. They would also provide an opportunity to teach cost-conscious medical practice by doing it, rather than by hiring pedants, economic and otherwise, to lecture about it. Finally, the environment would be fully controlled by the medical school faculty and the medical trainees would not be adjuncts to a practice that is not primarily education-oriented.

*Broader Local Financial Support for Indigent Care.* For teaching hospitals that provide large amounts of charity care or have substantial bad debts, the key issue is how to maintain revenues in the face of shrinking support from Medicaid and direct government appropriations. Although this is predominantly a public teaching hospital problem, it is not exclusively so. Even hospitals that do no teaching, have few bad debts, and provide little charity care cannot ignore the problem of financing care for the medically indigent. In the extreme case, some of these institutions of last resort may be forced to close, but the people they treat will not disappear. Thus, all hospitals should have a clear stake in finding a solution.

In the past, hospitals and local governments had looked primarily to Washington to provide fiscal sustenance. The Reagan administration's policies and philosophy as well as the general mood of the country as a whole have turned off the federal spigots. It is also unlikely, in the next few years at least, that state government will come to the rescue by expanding Medicaid eligibility. If anything, the trend is in the opposite direction.

Hospitals that provide substantial amounts of charity care talk about attracting more privately insured, charge-paying patients as the answer. This, too, is looking into the past. Increased competition among insurers and patients' greater cost-consciousness will continue to induce them to seek care in lower-cost institutions. Cost shifting or internal cross-subsidies loaded onto charges may have worked well enough when charity care was distributed fairly evenly among hospitals. When it becomes concentrated in only a few institutions, however, the implicit charity markup becomes too large for charge-paying patients to bear. Many simply go elsewhere.

What is left then, I believe, is the development of broad-based local solutions to expanding the financial support for indigent care. This means explicit, cooperative agreements among hospitals and local governments in an area to determine how much money is needed to pay for indigent care, how that money is to be raised, and how its use is to be administered and monitored. Although the problem of health care for the poor is a national problem, it is one that is localized in areas that differ in political structure, political philosophy, economic resources, and structure of the health care delivery system. Because the nature and magnitude of the problem are also likely to vary across areas, the solutions should be permitted to vary as well.

Two examples of local solutions already exist—the statewide rate-setting systems used in Maryland and New Jersey (Office of Research Demonstrations and Statistics, 1980). Although the specific methodologies in the two systems are quite different, both incorporate allowances for bad debts and charity care. Another possible approach is the establishment in specific areas of financial pools earmarked to pay for unreimbursed care. Such pools could be supported by contributions from local governments and/or a mandatory tithe on hospitals' net revenues. Draws from the pool by hospitals could be related to the volume of unreimbursed care, while their contributions could be based on the margin of revenues in excess of costs. A third possibility is the establishment of broad hospital districts that span several political jurisdictions, for example, a city and its surrounding towns and counties. The hospital district might function much like a transit district in terms of its ability to appropriate and spend money.

Regardless of the specific approach developed, it is essential that strict financial monitoring and controls be included. It is in this area that local approaches are probably more workable than a national system. Using local money to underwrite a substantial share of the cost of locally provided care for the indigent increases the odds that effective oversight mechanisms will be developed, through either the political process or private management. Hospitals and/or local governments that contribute to such a pool have an obvious stake in insuring that its funds are spent efficiently and prudently. Teaching hospitals and medical schools, because of both their prestige in the medical community and their potential dependence on such funds, should lead efforts to develop broader local financial support for health care for the poor.

*Prospective, Patient-Based Reimbursement.* In exchange for any broadening of the financial support for hospital care, the hospital industry in general and teaching hospitals in particular, because the latter appear to be so much more expensive than other hospitals, need to give serious consideration to means of reducing the inflation in hospital expenditures. There are many possible approaches, ranging from the American Hospital Association's Voluntary Effort to the Carter administration's proposed Hospital Care Containment legislation. My feeling is that the best approach from the perspective of the teaching hospitals is a prospective, patient-based reimbursement system—in other wo.ds, a system in which the amount paid for a patient's care is (1) determined and known in advance and (2) based on the cost of treating patients of similar diagnosis, complexity, age, sex, and any other factors thought to be relevant.

Probably the best-known method of this type is the one used by the state of New Jersey, which pays hospitals on the basis of diagnostic-related groups (Office of Research Demonstrations and Statistics, 1980). This is not the only approach that could be used, nor is it necessarily the best. Its key feature from the insurer's point of view is that the payment is fixed in advance, and because it is fixed in advance, it creates incentives for providers to be cost-conscious in choosing treatment regimens. The key feature from the hospital's point of view is that it receives a higher payment for treating more difficult cases. Thus, hospitals that treat a more complex case mix of patients and incur higher costs for this reason should receive higher payments than hospitals that treat a less complex, more routine case mix. At the same time, however, a patient who requires only routine care (for example, a normal delivery by a woman not in a high-risk group) but who goes to an "expensive" hospital would be billed at a rate consistent with the cost of providing routine care, not the cost of care averaged over the hospital's entire, more complex case mix. This feature of patient-based reimbursement systems is critical in a competitive health care market that retains significant patient cost sharing, deductibles, and/or coinsurance. Under this system, high-cost teaching hospitals would face less of a competitive disadvantage in seeking to attract patients who do not require sophisticated, state-of-the-art care.

The mechanics of setting up such a system are obviously not trivial. However, it would be an insult to the hospital management industry to claim that it could not be done. Probably more difficult are the political decisions that trade some hospitals' gains for other hospitals' losses. Here again, there is a clear need for educational institutions to play a visible leadership role.

*Restructured Hospital Insurance.* How hospitals are paid is only one side of the hospital insurance coin. The other is how responsibility for that payment is split between patients and insurers. As noted earlier, patient cost sharing is likely to become more, not less, prevalent. Under these circumstances, one clear consequence of a patient-based reimbursement system is that sicker patients will face higher charges and higher cost-sharing obligations. This would undermine some of the risk-spreading aspects of the insurance concept.

In order to avoid what might appear to be a punitive reimbursement system, hospitals should lobby for and work towards a universal catastrophic insurance system that places an upper limit on any individual's or family's out-of-pocket liability for medical care. Ideally, this limit would be related to income, since a specified dollar limit would be much more burdensome to the poor than to others. Again, teaching hospitals and medical schools have an obvious interest in this type of insurance structure, since they are more likely to treat the higher-cost, more complex cases.

How can this type of insurance be financed? One obvious approach that could be used is to trade current first-dollar coverage, that is, low deductibles and low coinsurance rates, for coverage that protects against catastrophic expenses. Premium dollars saved by thinning out first-dollar coverage could then be used to finance catastrophic coverage. It has been argued that this approach is "penny wise and pound foolish," because cost sharing defers needed care for conditions that ultimately become more expensive to treat than if they had been caught earlier. This is not a trivial contention, and careful analysis is required to try to settle the issue. (Feder, Hadley, and Holahan (1981) provide more detailed discussions of broad health insurance issues.)

## Concluding Comment

Analyses of this type are risky ventures, since much of what is said is predicated on events that have not yet occurred. Nonetheless, I hope that this discussion will stimulate some additional reconsideration of existing financing arrangements. In making these reassessments, however, one should remember the sage advice of an old dragon: "It is extremely rash to extend conclusions derived from observation far beyond the scale of magnitude to which the observation was confined" (Gardner, 1971).

## References

American Hospital Association. *Annual Survey of Hospitals.* Chicago: American Hospital Association, 1980.

Becker, G. *Human Capital: A Theoretical and Empirical Analysis, with Special Reference to Training.* New York: Columbia University Press, 1964.

*Drug Research Reports: The Blue Sheet.* 1980, *23* (5), 4-5.

Feder, J., Hadley, J., and Holahan, J. *Insuring the Nation's Health: Market Competition, Catastrophic and Comprehensive Approaches.* Washington, D.C.: Urban Institute Press, 1981.

Feldman, R., and Yoder, S. "A Theoretical Analysis of GME Financing." In J. Hadley (Ed.), *Medical Education Financing: Issues and Options for the 1980s.* New York: Prodist, 1980.

Freymann, J., and Springer, J. "Cost of Hospital-Based Education: The Hartford Hospital Study." *Hospitals,* 1973, *47*, 65-74.

Gardner, J. *Grendel.* New York: Knopf, 1971.

Gibson, R., and Waldo, D. "National Health Expenditures, 1980." *Health Care Financing Review,* 1981, *2*, 20, 30, 42.

Hadley, J. (Ed.). *Medical Education Financing: Issues and Options for the 1980s.* New York: Prodist, 1980.

Hadley, J. "Medicaid and Teaching Hospitals: Current Policies and Future Consequences." Washington, D.C.: Urban Institute Working Paper no. 1298-12, 1981.

Hadley, J., Lee, R., and Carlson, C. "Teaching Hospitals' Demand for Residents." Washington, D.C.: Urban Institute Working Paper no. 1302-9, 1982.

Hadley, J., and Tigue, P. "Financing Graduate Medical Education: An Update and a Suggestion for Reform." *Health Policy and Education,* 1982, *3* (2), 157-171.

Hadley, J., and others. "An Economic Analysis of Graduate Medical Education: The 'Labor Market' for Residents and the Impact of Teaching on Hospital Costs and Service Utilization." Project Report no. 1302-9. Washington, D.C.: The Urban Institute, December 1982.

Hall, T. "An Empirical Investigation of Medical Schools' Behavior." Unpublished paper, Department of Economics, University of Hawaii, 1978.

Holahan, J. "A Comparison of Medicaid and Medicare Physician Reimbursement Rates." Urban Institute Working Paper no. 1306-02-04, March 1982.

Lee, R., and Carlson, C. "The Effects of Reducing Federal Aid to Undergraduate Medical Education." Urban Institute Working Paper no. 1439-1, June 1981.

"Medical Education in the United States." *Journal of the American Medical Association,* 1969, *210* (8), 1486.

"Medical Education in the United States." *Journal of the American Medical Association,* 1981, *246* (25), 2929.

Office of Research Demonstrations and Statistics. *National Hospital Rate Study.* Vols. III and VI. Washington, D.C.: Health Care Financing Administration, U.S. Department of Health and Human Services, 1980.

Pear, R. "Few States Seek to Ease Effects of Cuts for Poor." *New York Times,* January 12, 1982, p. 1.

Sloan, F. "Regulation and Hospital Costs." *Review of Economics and Statistics,* 1982, *64,* 484.

Sloan, F., Feldman, R., and Steinwald, B. "Effects of Teaching on Hospital Costs." *Journal of Health Economics,* 1983, *2* (1), 1–28.

U.S. Office of Personnel Management. *Government Employees Hospital Association Benefit Plan.* Washington, D.C.: U.S. Government Printing Office, 1981, 1982.

*Warren Winkelstein, Jr.*  **19**

# Demographic Changes

---

## Responding to New Population and Disease Patterns

Population patterns are today changing in many ways, and most of these changes are likely to affect health needs and problems. Concentration on the population dynamics of the United States at this time will serve to illustrate the challenge and the possibilities of the study of population in relation to health care delivery. Consider, for example, that the proportion of the population living in the West continues to grow, and with the probable industrialization and urbanization of the more than one million square miles of the intermountain plateau of New Mexico, Colorado, Wyoming, and Montana, this geographical trend is likely to be accelerated; that the increasing proportion of single-parent families is now approaching 20 percent among whites and over 40 percent among blacks; or that increasing proportions of the population are members of ethnic minorities. All of these changes are quite likely to produce profound effects on health and disease. However, each has a limited or circumscribed set of effects. The change of overriding importance during the two last decades of this century is the increasing size of the population in the age group over 65 years. Consideration of this subject will show the impact that changing population patterns might have on our health care system and, by implication, on the education of health care professionals.

Preliminary figures from the 1980 census indicate that, at present, approximately 25.5 million persons are 65 years of age or older. A conservative estimate of the size of this segment of the population in the year 2000 is 30.6 million, an increase of 20 percent. Since most chronic disease morbidity, bed disability, and restricted activity occurs in this age group, the increase has serious implications. However, before discussing these implications, a brief examination of the age and sex composition of the population is in order, as outlined in Figure 1.

**Figure 1. U.S. Population According to Age and Sex, 1978.**

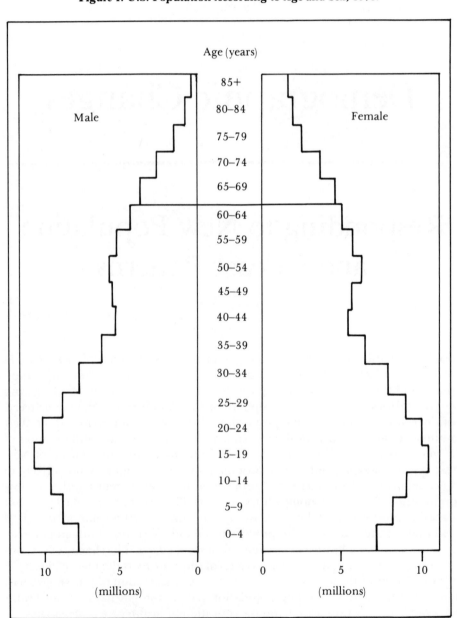

*Source:* U.S. Bureau of the Census, 1978, pp. 6 and 24.

At all ages under 45, men outnumber women by a small margin. After 45, however, women outnumber men, and among those over 65, the female-to-male ratio is three to two, 15 million women to 10 million men. With respect to age, the distributions are somewhat more complicated. If over the past century the birthrate had been constant or rising and the death rates had increased with age, as they have, these data would appear in the shape of a pyramid with the widest span at the base and a variable but continuously narrowing width as age increased. However, the birthrate has fluctuated in such a way that the population pyramid has been constricted at certain ages. The constriction at ages 40 through 49 reflects the low birthrates during the Depression, and the current constriction reflects the declining birthrate since the postwar "baby boom" that began in the mid-forties. The bulge in the population pyramid between the ages of 15 and 25 is partially the result of the maturation to reproductive ages of the population cohort born during the aforementioned "baby boom." It should now be apparent that the population pyramid behaves in a dynamic fashion over time, very much like a snake swallowing a mouse, that is, the bulges and constrictions move up and out over time. If the birthrate remains stable, at a level sufficient to replace the population—a desirable objective—then eventually the age distribution will again assume a pyramidal shape. Before this can happen, however, the bulge centered at ages 50 to 54 will augment the over-65 population by 20 percent, as already indicated, and the bulge centered at ages 20 to 24 will provide an even greater augmentation. In fact, it was partially the miscalculation of the dynamics of the population pyramid that produced the current crisis in the finances of the social security system.

### Health and Disease Model

Before proceeding further, a brief consideration of a model showing the relationships of health and disease and their care systems may be in order. The reason for this is that in recent years, there has developed a considerable amount of semantic confusion that has led, in my opinion, to substantial obfuscation of the nature and solution of health problems. This confusion arises from the use of the word *health* as a synonym for the word *disease* in the usual usage of the term *health care*. Thus, when the term *health care* is substituted for the term *disease care* or *medical care*, the expectation that the care will result in *health* is a logical consequence. However, there is little evidence that treating disease affects the health of the population. That is not to say that medical care is not useful but rather that it should be justified on the basis that the relief of pain and suffering and the cure and rehabilitation of the sick are worthy ends in themselves and warrant large expenditures of effort and money.

The assertion that the quantity, quality, and distribution of care are unrelated to the health status of the population is based on a conceptual model of the relationship of health and disease, as shown in Figure 2. Health and disease are viewed as a continuum, varying from optimum health at one end, through altered health and preclinical disease, to clinical disease at the other.

Focusing first on the health side of the spectrum, we know there are various kinds of inputs (antecedent conditions), some purposeful and some not controlled. Some of these inputs lead to optimum states of health. There is some

**Figure 2. The Health-Disease Spectrum Model of Health and Disease Care.**

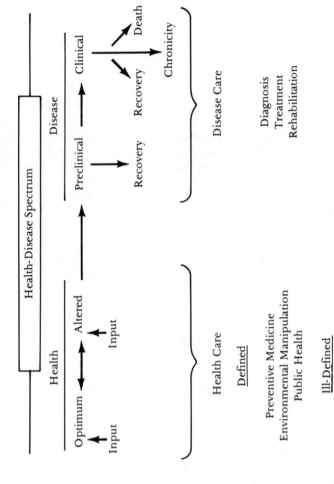

slight tendency for individuals to move to the left on the scale (toward optimum health), particularly early in life and especially in the case of certain specific conditions such as childhood asthma, eczema, and certain types of myopia. However, the general tendency is for individuals to move to the right in the model (toward clinical disease) with increasing age. If the model is generally valid, it is apparent that when an individual moves into the preclinical phase of the spectrum, he or she is already diseased. For many conditions, the subsequent clinical course is predetermined. At best, in these diseases, the individual may be held at the preclinical phase or in chronicity.

The *health care* system, as I see it, has two parts. The first is well-defined and composed of the traditional modalities of public health, preventive medicine, and environmental manipulation. In this part of the health care system, inputs known to produce favorable effects are applied to the population through organized efforts. Sometimes these inputs produce altered health states that increase host resistance, as in immunization or controlled fluoridation of water supplies; sometimes they produce barriers against disease-producing agents, as in selective destruction of arthropod vectors or shielding of sources of ionizing radiation. Unfortunately, however, even in the most developed countries, numerous well-defined inputs are unevenly applied. The second part of the health care system is ill-defined and vague, perhaps usefully referred to as human ecology. A strong case can be made for the position that poorly defined ecological factors remain the most important determinants of the health-disease status of a population (Winkelstein, 1972).

The *disease care* system consists of the organization and delivery of three functional components: diagnosis, treatment, and rehabilitation. Unfortunately, it too is imperfectly and incompletely applied.

If the model is valid, then it is appropriate to consider the health problems consequent to changing population patterns according to whether they are most likely to be amenable to disease care or health care. Let us first turn our attention to the disease side of the health care spectrum. Table 1 shows the changing age pattern of the population expressed as the average life expectancy (remaining years of life for the members of the population who have reached 65 years of age). For each sex, this expectancy has increased substantially during the present century from about eleven and twelve years respectively for males and females in 1900, to about fourteen and eighteen years in 1977. By 2000, male life expectancy at age 65 will approximate fifteen years and female twenty years.

By combining data from the population pyramid and the life expectancy information, it is possible to estimate the person-years of life that may be anticipated for the entire population over the age of 65 in 1980 and 2000. These person-years can also be readily distributed to the appropriate age groupings in order to allow accurate estimates of the actual burden of illness and disability experienced by the over-65 population. However, incidence data are not generally available for such subgroups, and therefore estimates must be tenuous at best. Nevertheless, it will be useful to examine some of the possible trends in the most important indicators.

Table 2 shows the estimated deaths in 1980 and 2000 among the over-65 population due to heart disease and malignant neoplasms—the two leading causes of death—and for all other causes together. The estimates were obtained by

**Table 1. Life Expectancy at 65 Years of Age in United States.**

| Year | Males | Females | Total |
|------|-------|---------|-------|
| 1900 | 11.5  | 12.2    | 11.9  |
| 1950 | 12.8  | 15.0    | 13.9  |
| 1977 | 13.9  | 18.3    | 16.3  |

*Source:* U.S. Bureau of the Census, 1978, pp. 6 and 24.

**Table 2. Estimated Deaths by Major Cause in United States.**

| Major Cause | Number of Deaths | |
|-------------|------------------|------------------|
|             | 1980             | 2000             |
| Heart Disease | 595,000 | 381,000 |
| Malignant Neoplasms | 252,000 | 302,000 |
| All Other | 512,000 | 614,000 |
| Total | 1,359,000 | 1,297,000 |

applying the 1977 cause-specific rates (the most recent available) to the 1980 and 2000 population estimates. However, one important adjustment was required. Heart disease mortality has been decreasing by almost 2 percent per year during the past decade, even among those over 65. Thus, by 2000 it is anticipated that the death rate from this cause will be substantially reduced, so that the total of expected deaths will be actually smaller at the turn of the century than it is today. This is also reason for predicting an increase of more than 10 percent in life expectancy over 65 by 2000. Of course, since everyone must eventually die and since the over-65 population will be substantially augmented by 2000 and even more so for the four decades thereafter, the total number of deaths will rise rapidly during the early part of the twenty-first century.

Despite an increasing concern with the care of the dying, manifested during the past decade by the rapid development of the hospice movement, very little information is available with respect to the actual circumstances characterizing the death process in the United States. A recent search of the medical literature by one of my colleagues did not produce a single article that systematically reviewed a series or sample of deaths in this regard. Such research is urgently needed in order to provide a basis for planning services, identifying problems, and indicating educational needs.

### Care for the Aged

Most biologists consider the natural life span of *homo sapiens* to be in the neighborhood of 80 years. The present life expectancy for U.S. males is close to 70 years, increasing at about 0.4 years annually; for females, it is almost 78 years, and increasing at about the same rate. Thus, the natural life span will probably be reached by 2000 for the population as a whole. The implications of this phenomenon are numerous but certainly include the need to place more emphasis on improving the quality of life and of the death process, as well as simply concentrating on the prolongation of life. At the same time, it must be emphasized that, at present, all segments of the population do not fully share these favorable trends. The poor and several ethnic minorities have substantially lower life expectancies.

*Disease.* To estimate the impact of disease on the quality of life of the over-65 year age group, I have selected two indicators. Obviously, there are many more available, but the two selected should be sufficient for this discussion. They are days of restricted activities caused by acute conditions (Table 3), and numbers of persons with activity limitation due to chronic disease (Table 4). A day of restricted activity is defined as "one on which a person cuts down on his or her usual activities for the whole or part of the day because of an illness or injury" (National Center for Health Statistics, 1981, p. 13). The data shown in Table 3 report restricted activity due to acute conditions; they do not include restriction caused by the acute phases of chronic illnesses. The number of days of restricted activity is huge, more than 400,000,000 or close to 17 days per year per person. It is important to note that almost half, 48 percent, of this burden is attributable to two conditions, influenza and injuries. Respiratory illnesses, taken together, account for 42 percent of all the days of restricted activity. As we shall see, a substantial part of this category of illnesses may be preventable. However, unless important breakthroughs are achieved in knowledge of how to prevent injuries and in delivering the presently known preventive procedures to the population, the burden of acute illness will probably be the same in 2000 as it is today, more than half a month of restricted activity per person per year among those 65 and older.

The burden of chronic disease in the over-65 population is indicated in Table 4. The definition of activity limitation used in the National Health Survey (National Center for Health Statistics, 1981, p. 24) is subdivided into four categories of severity. For the purposes of this discussion, they are irrelevant, since I have used the designation only for the purpose of identifying cases. The data reveal that 40 percent of those over 65, a total of 10.2 million people, suffer some activity limitation due to chronic disease. Of these, almost 25 percent, 2.5 million, have heart

Table 3. Estimated Days of Restricted Activities According to Selected Acute Conditions, United States, Ages 65 and Over, 1980.

| Condition | Days Restricted | Days Restricted Per Person Per Year |
|---|---|---|
| Infective and Parasitic | 28,990,000 | 1.1 |
| Respiratory | 178,069,000 | 7.0 |
| Upper Respiratory Infection | 49,459,000 | 1.9 |
| Influenza | 96,690,000 | 3.8 |
| Other | 31,920,000 | 1.3 |
| Digestive | 20,962,000 | .8 |
| Injuries | 108,636,000 | 4.3 |
| All Others | 88,337,000 | 3.5 |
| Total | 424,994,000 | 16.7 |

*Source:* National Center for Health Statistics, 1981.

**Table 4. Estimated Number of Persons with Activity Limitation by
Selected Chronic Conditions, United States, Ages 65 and Over, 1980.**

| Conditions | Number of Persons | Percentage |
|---|---|---|
| Heart Disease | 2,448,000 | 9.6 |
| Arthritis and Rheumatism | 2,448,000 | 9.6 |
| Essential Hypertension | 816,000 | 3.2 |
| Impaired Back or Spine | 408,000 | 1.6 |
| Lower Extremity or Hip | 612,000 | 2.4 |
| All Other | 3,468,000 | 13.6 |
| No Limitation | 15,300,000 | 60.0 |
| Total | 25,500,000 | 100.0 |

Source: National Center for Health Statistics, 1981, p. 1077.

disease; the same proportion and number suffer from arthritis and rheumatism. In addition, another 4 percent, more than a million, have orthopedic problems of the back, hip, or lower extremity. You will note that neither cancer nor stroke is listed explicitly in this tabulation. The reason for this is that the prevalence of cancer is relatively low due to its generally short duration, and stroke has become increasingly less prevalent as its incidence has declined. Nevertheless, stroke still produces a serious burden of disability, particularly among the extremely old.

If, as expected, the incidence of heart disease continues to decline, it is quite probable that by the turn of the century, chronic diseases of the musculoskeletal system will dominate as the most common cause of chronic disability among those over 65. At present, these diseases receive relatively little attention as subjects for either research or study by medical scientists, students, or residents. Such neglect may be due to the fact that these conditions are less often fatal and are not usually treated on an inpatient basis in the university medical center hospitals that still serve as the principal loci for the training of medical care practitioners. For many years, forward-looking medical educators have argued ineffectively that the primary teaching model should not be the secondary or tertiary care medical center but a community-centered multifaceted primary care center. The disease burdens of the enlarged over-65 population may finally generate the impetus to achieve this objective.

*Health and Prevention.* With respect to the health care side of the health-disease spectrum, far too little attention has been given to health care for those over 65. There is a degree of semantic confusion about preventive medicine as well as a general lack of interest and concern by most physicians. Furthermore, epidemiologists and other medical scientists have directed relatively little effort toward the investigation of risk factors in the over-65 age group. Nevertheless, there already exist some preventive strategies that, if more widely applied, might provide substantial benefits.

First, let us return to a consideration of acute conditions. As noted earlier, respiratory conditions taken together constitute the most important cause of restricted activity in the over-65 age group; influenza alone is responsible for almost 100,000,000 days of restricted activity or 23 percent of all days of restricted activity.

Despite problems of diagnosis, I think it can be assumed that most of this reported illness is, indeed, the result of influenza virus infection. For at least a decade, we have had available a multivalent influenza vaccine with effectiveness measured in clinical trials as high as 83 percent. The data show that for the latest reporting period, 1977–78, less than 25 percent of the eligible at-risk population was reached. We would certainly not accept such a low rate of immunization against such childhood diseases as diphtheria, tetanus, whooping cough, measles, and poliomyelitis, even if it were shown that together they caused less activity restriction, disease complications, or death. Cost is among the many reasons given for the low rate of coverage in the case of influenza vaccination. In a report on the cost-effectiveness of influenza vaccine recently released by the Office of Technology Assessment (OTA) of the U.S. Congress (1981), the health benefits of full coverage of the over-65 population were estimated to be two million years of healthy life gained at a cost per year of healthy life of about $790. A breakdown of the costs is shown in Table 5. The OTA is now evaluating the new pneumococcal vaccine that has considerable promise of making an additional favorable impact on other parts of the acute respiratory groups of illnesses. With respect to injuries—the other major contributor to restricted activity from acute conditions— very little is known concerning risk factors and very little investigation is under way. It is an area crying out for attention.

Let me now turn to the issue of prevention of chronic diseases. As noted earlier, 40 percent of the over-65 age group suffer some degree of restricted activity due to chronic disease. We generally assume that the genesis of much of this burden occurs earlier in life and that it is unlikely that preventive measures will be effective in this age group. As evidence to support this view, consider the data reported in Table 6 regarding relative risks for the major risk factors contributing to the development of ischemic heart disease. The data show clearly that the strength of the predictive value of each major risk factor decreases as age increases. This means that modification of these risk factors after age 65 is unlikely to affect the incidence of ischemic heart disease in this population group.

However, not all diseases have the same natural history. For example, Figure 3 shows trends for lung cancer incidence according to age in upstate New

Table 5. Effect on Medicare Costs of Annual Influenza Vaccination for Persons 65 Years and Older, 1971–72 Through 1977–78.

|  | Per Vaccination | For Population |
|---|---|---|
| *Costs* | | |
| Cost of vaccination and side effects | $ 6 | $ 145,000,000 |
| Cost of treating Guillain-Barre syndrome | —— | 296,000 |
| Reduced influenza treatment costs | –4 | –103,800,000 |
| Medical costs in extended years of life | 60 | 1,541,800,000 |
| Total costs | $ 62 | $ 1,583,226,000 |
| *Health Benefits* | | |
| Healthy life gained | 28 days | 2,003,000 years |

Source: Office of Technology Assessment, 1981.

Figure 3. Incidence of Cancer of the Trachea, Bronchus, and Lung Among Males, New York State (Exclusive of New York City), 1950–1972.

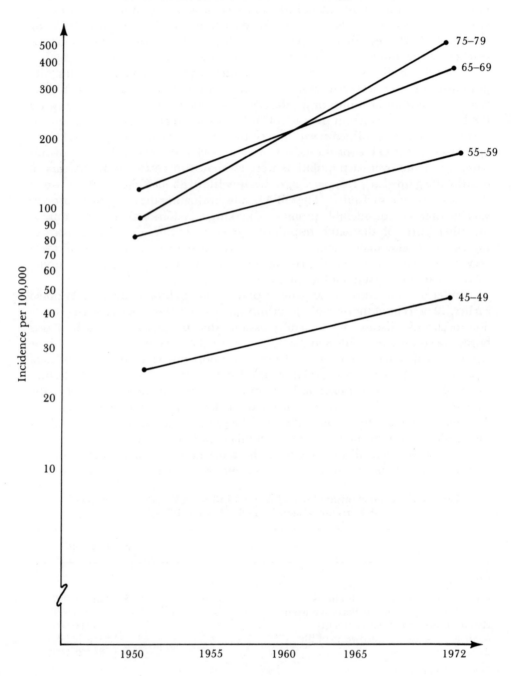

*Source:* Greenwald and others, 1976.

Table 6. Relative Risk of Developing Ischemic Heart Disease in Twelve Years
According to Age and Sex, Framingham Study.

| | Males | | | Females | | |
|---|---|---|---|---|---|---|
| Age at Entry | Blood Pressure | Serum Cholesterol | Smoking | Blood Pressure | Serum Cholesterol | Smoking |
| 35–44 | 3.6 | 3.5 | 4.8 | 4.7 | — | 4.3 |
| 45–55 | 1.2 | 3.9 | 1.7 | 1.7 | 10.4 | 0.5 |
| 55–64 | 1.0 | 1.4 | 1.5 | 1.4 | 0.6 | 0.9 |

*Note:* For high blood pressure (150–159 mm Hg systolic/120–129 mm Hg diastolic), high cholesterol (250–264 mg/100 ml/096–189 mg/100 ml), and smoking (20 cigarettes per day/non-smokers).

*Source:* Winkelstein and Marmot, 1981.

York from 1950 to 1972 (the latest year for which data are published). The increase in incidence over time has been relatively greater in the very old, 75 to 79, than in younger ages. The cause for this is not known and, as far as I know, has not been investigated. It is, however, consistent with the possibility that other risk factors, in addition to cigarette smoking, have affected this population group. Again, it cannot be overemphasized that clinical and epidemiological research among the over-65 is a high-priority need.

Finally, no discussion of health care should be completed without some mention of the most important environmental risk factor presently known. Cigarette smoking is now recognized as the attributable cause of at least 30 percent of all malignant neoplasms and a substantial proportion of chronic respiratory disease, as well as chronic heart disease. However, its specific effects in older ages have not been studied. Fortunately, only about a quarter of the males and half of the females who smoked at any time in their lives continue smoking after age 65. Nevertheless, 25 percent of all men over 65 and 17 percent of all females over 65 are current smokers.

Clearly, the expanding population over 65, their extended life expectancy, and the concentration of morbidity and mortality among them pose a great challenge to those concerned with the cause and prevention of disease, to those responsible for educating the providers of care, and to those responsible for the organization and delivery of care. The relative neglect of that population group should not continue and, indeed, is unlikely to be tolerated as their numbers grow.

## References

Center for Disease Control. *Immunization Against Disease.* Washington, D.C.: U.S. Department of Health and Human Services, Public Health Service, 1980.

Greenwald, P., and others. *Cancer Incidence Mortality in New York State (Exclusive of New York City).* Albany, N.Y.: Bureau of Cancer Control, New York Department of Health, 1976.

National Center for Health Statistics. *Current Estimates from the National Health Interview Survey: United States, 1980.* U.S. Department of Health and Human

Services Publication no. (PHS) 82-1569. Washington, D.C.: U.S. Department of Health and Human Services, 1981.

Office of Technology Assessment. *Cost-Effectiveness of Influenza Vaccine.* Washington, D.C.: U.S. Government Printing Office, 1981.

U.S. Bureau of the Census. *Current Population Reports.* Series P25, No. 800. Washington, D.C.: U.S. Government Printing Office, 1978.

Winkelstein, W., Jr. "Epidemiological Considerations Underlying the Allocation of Health and Disease Care Resources." *International Journal of Epidemiology,* 1972, *1,* 69–74.

Winkelstein, W., Jr., and Marmot, M. "Primary Prevention of Ischemic Heart Disease: Evaluation of Community Interventions." In L. Breslow (Ed.), *Annual Review of Public Health.* Vol. II. Palo Alto, Calif.: Annual Reviews, 1981.

*Raymond R. Suskind*

# 20

# Environmental Problems

## Understanding and Controlling Ecological Impacts on Health and Disease

The original concept of ecology as introduced by Haeckel (1870) defined ecology as "the body of knowledge concerning the economy of nature . . . the investigation of the total relations of the animal, both to its inorganic and to its organic environment." This chapter is concerned with man's interaction with components of his ecosystem. It attempts to provide a historical perspective of environmental problems and issues, as related to social consciousness and assignment of responsibility from which one can derive and define educational needs and objectives.

To determine what issues and problems need to be addressed in the education of health professionals over the next twenty years, as well as what body of knowledge and what new skills must be provided, it is appropriate to understand the role of ecological factors in health and disease. These include the changing chemical, physical, and biological environments in which man lives and works and with which he interacts, particularly those environments that have the potential for adversely affecting health and well-being. To understand ecological impact, we need to examine:

- Changing community environment: urban, metropolitan, and rural environments; those factors that affect health and well-being, such as the contamination of air and of bodies of water and water sources used for drinking, industrial use, and recreation; hazards in living space, including housing; transport hazards recreational area problems
- Occupational environment, industrial as well as agricultural: chemical, physical, and biological agents, including psychosocial stresses
- Consumer goods: food, drugs, wearing apparel, cosmetics, recreational equipment
- Use or abuse of land: soil contamination, ecological damage through land and water use and misuse
- Climatic factors
- Environmental influences on behavior and mental health
- Life-style, one of the most significant but the most difficult factor to control due to influence of personal, cultural, and economic considerations: most obvious environmental factors that influence health and well-being are nutrition, hygiene, cigarette smoking, and substance abuse

## Historical Perspective

The history of attempts to understand and to cope with man-made hazards dates back several thousand years (Rosen, 1958). One of the earliest records appears in the Edwin Smith papyrus dated approximately 3000 B.C. in which the injuries sustained in building the step pyramids of Sakkarah, at Memphis in Egypt, are described and their prognoses with respect to survival are indicated. Hippocrates in 460 B.C. wrote about the relationship between the environment and health in an essay entitled "On Air, Waters, and Places." He also clearly described lead colic in miners. Pliny the Elder discussed the danger of handling sulfur and zinc. He also described the use of animal bladders as masks to prevent inhalation of dust. Galen wrote about acid mists on copper miners and diseases found among chemists, tanners, and cloth handlers. George Bauer, a sixteenth century physician known as Agricola, in his distinguished treatise *De Re Metallica* [*Concerning Metal*] (Agricola, 1950) recorded the dread lung diseases of the Carpathian Mountain miners before they were recognized as cancer of the lung. From these mountains in 1898 came the pitchblende from which Madame Curie extracted radium. There were two sides of these mountains in which there were mining operations. On the Bohemian side was the uranium-containing Joachimstahl mine (arsenic, radium, cobalt) from which in the 1920s and 1930s numerous cases of lung cancer were reported. On the neighboring side of this range, from the Schneeberg, 400 cases of lung cancer were described in the period from 1869 to 1939. Arsenic and dust containing ionizing radiation were suspected.

It was not until the latter part of the seventeenth century that the first comprehensive treatise on occupational diseases was published. This was the classical work of Bernardino Ramazzini, *De Morbis Artificum Diatriba* [*Diseases of Workers*] (1940). It was Ramazzini who insisted that the only effective way to study occupational diseases was to study them in the work environment itself.

In industrial England of the late eighteenth century, it was Percival Pott who first described cancer of the scrotum in chimney sweeps overwhelmingly exposed to soot. In nineteenth century England, Thackrah and Percival made that country aware of the very special health problems of the workplace. It was the work of one of them, Dr. Thomas Percival, that resulted in the initial Factory Act in England—the first attempt in that country to control occupational hazards.

In the United States, the indefatigable investigator of environmental and occupational illness and injury was Dr. Alice Hamilton, who first learned of the health problems of impoverished workers through her efforts at Hull House in Chicago. In this country, it is only within the twentieth century and especially in the past twenty years that the rapidly developing awareness and spreading concern about environmental health have been translated into effective legislative action.

There is an obvious ecological component to technological growth. The surge in technological and industrial development between World War I and World War II produced new and significant physical and chemical hazards that were reflected in the increase in industrial accidents and occupational diseases. In the United States, it was the industrial achievement of World War II, characterized by unprecedented production levels, that curiously enough created a new climate of safety alertness on the part of the federal government. In this climate, stricter regulations were implemented requiring the testing of new processes and chemicals to determine their health hazards and their safe levels of use.

By the end of World War II, it was obvious that within the industrial and professional community, skilled persons were needed for professional practice and research in environmental and occupational medicine, environmental and industrial hygiene, occupational safety and occupational health nursing, toxicology and environmental epidemiology. The country became aware of the need for a new breed of skilled health scientists and practitioners to determine the nature and level of hazards and their effects on human health; to develop programs of human assessment, surveillance, diagnosis, and treatment; and to develop techniques of medical and environmental control of such hazards. A few training programs were set up at medical schools and schools of public health. The concentration was on graduate, postgraduate, and continuing education in those fields. Certifying boards were created in occupational medicine, industrial hygiene, and occupational health nursing.

## Recent Progress

Less than twenty years ago when René Dubos (1980) presented his Silliman lectures at Yale, he reflected with concern that "like the lay public, the scientific community has paid little heed to the fact that the diseases characteristic of our time are to a large extent the consequence of changes in the ways of life and in the environment. The search for the environmental determinants of disease is not a fashionable topic and carries little scientific prestige" (p. 357). When Congressman John Fogarty was chairman of the Subcommittee of Labor, Health, and Education of the House Committee on Appropriations, a plea was entered for greater support for environmental health research and training. He said to the then Surgeon General "environmental health doesn't seem to ring a bell with people. . . . To the average person if you start talking environmental health they are just not interested" (p. 358).

We have moved quite a distance since then. Witness the enormous surge of scientific activity in this country and the support by both the federal health science establishment and regulatory agencies responsible for the study and control of such problems. In the sixties, there was a slow but definite mobilization of scientific interest within federal agencies and universities to carry out fundamental studies about environmental hazards and their effects on humans. In 1965, university-based centers for environmental health research were created under the sponsorship of the then Division of Environmental Health Sciences. There are now nine comprehensive centers and six specialized centers. They include centers in which the scope of effort ranges from the molecular basis of adverse biological effects of chemical and physical agents to epidemiological and clinical studies of populations at risk. Other centers focus on laboratory studies of specified toxicological phenomena, on mechanisms of mutagenesis and carcinogenesis, and the like. In 1968, Congress created a National Institute of Environmental Health Sciences. In 1969 and 1970, the Environmental Protection Agency and the National Institute of Occupational Safety and Health came into being, with specific mandates to support research and training for their respective areas of scientific and professional concern.

It has already been pointed out that among the important legacies of World War II were the awareness of need and the commitment to carry out toxicological and safety studies necessary to identify and quantify health hazards. It took several years, however, for the community to recognize that the total human environment and the ecosystem on which we depend and in which we live required urgent attention and that the responsibility and accountability for solving and controlling these problems required some tangible definition. These concerns were translated into law, through federal statutes and regulations. Notable among these acts were:

- Clean Air Act of 1963 and its many amendments, including the Ambient Air Standards Amendment
- Clean Water Act of 1972, amended in 1977
- Safe Drinking Water Act of 1974, the basic authority for the water supply program
- Resource Conservation and Recovery Act of 1976, the authority for our solid waste program
- Occupational Safety and Health Act of 1970, creating Department of Labor and Health, Education, and Welfare segments—Occupational Safety and Health Administration (OSHA) and National Institute of Occupational Safety and Health (NIOSH)—to fulfill its important functions
- Mine Safety and Health Act of 1969 and its several amendments: 1972, 1979, and 1980
- Federal Insecticide, Fungicide, and Rodenticide Act, amended in 1972, 1975, and 1978
- Toxic Substances Control Act of 1976
- National Toxicology Program, an attempt to avoid overlap and assign priority
- Comprehensive Environmental Response, Compensation, and Liability Act of 1980 (Super Fund)

### Implications for Education of Health Professionals

It is largely these statutes that deal with ecological matters of environmental pollution and environmental hazards; all have implicit public health objectives and thus a significant impact on health care needs and the education of health professionals. Together they have created an enormous demand for specialized professional and scientific manpower to fill the new positions in government, industry, and academia that were developed to implement the regulatory mandate. Federal support for training health professionals in the environmental and occupational health disciplines has been available for over fifteen years. However, the training support peaked for a major segment of this group—physicians, nurses, safety engineers, epidemiologists, and biostatisticians, hygienists, and environmental toxicologists—about 1980.

In 1970, the Massachusetts Institute of Technology (1970) sponsored a Study of Critical Environmental Problems in preparation for a United Nations Conference on the Human Environment. Work groups met for almost an entire month, but nowhere in their roster of considerations was there any discussion of health issues. In 1972, the World Health Organization (WHO) prepared a survey of environmental hazards to human health, for health authorities concerned with environmental policies. This survey admitted that the field was so vast that the document could provide only a synoptical view of highlights, consisting of little more than a list of hazards and of some methods for their identification and control.

The most comprehensive and well-conceived documents on environmental health issues and recommendations for research were those reports (1970, 1976) prepared for Congress by task forces of the National Institute of Environmental Health Sciences (NIEHS). In the 1976 report, there is a section on education that refers only to the training of toxicologists. The NIEHS recognizes the need for clinical scientists and professionals and now offers career development awards for clinical investigators in the field of environmental health.

Legal remedies for society's problems are often slow to emerge and lag far behind the development of knowledge about such problems. This is not now the case for environmental health problems. The statutes enumerated above have encouraged the development of new knowledge and have made a decisive impact on social and professional attitudes regarding responsibility for maintaining a livable environment. This is particularly true with respect to hazards in the workplace, the use of hazardous chemicals in the home or in agriculture, and processes involving physical agents. Some of the statutes have not only created a need for great numbers of trained professionals but have actually assigned responsibility for providing support for training professionals and scientists to cope with such hazards. Training scientists and professionals is now a mandated responsibility of NIOSH, OSHA, NIEHS, and the Environmental Protection Agency (EPA). For example, the Occupational Safety and Health Act of 1970 (PL 91–596) requires the Secretary of the Department of Health and Human Services to "conduct directly by grants or contracts, education programs to provide an adequate supply of qualified personnel" to protect the health and welfare of the American worker. Although this agency had begun to support training programs shortly after the passage of the act, it was not until 1977 that training centers were created at universities to provide specialists in the field of occupational medicine, industrial hygiene, occupational safety, and occupational health nursing. There are now fifteen such centers.

There is still a serious shortage of trained scientists and professionals in all the occupational health disciplines: medicine, nursing, industrial hygiene, safety, toxicology, and related environmental science disciplines. The need for trained personnel in all these fields far outstrips the supply of available qualified persons. Manpower deficits are acknowledged and recognized by all segments of the community. In environmental toxicology, graduate training programs were started in the mid-sixties by the NIEHS and have grown substantially since then. However, it was not until 1970, when NIOSH was assigned the responsibility for developing and supporting training programs, that federal initiatives were undertaken to remedy general deficits in the occupational health disciplines. Initially, single training projects for individual disciplines were supported. The real breakthrough came in 1977 when the Education Resource Centers (ERCs) for Occupational Safety and Health were created. The centers have enhanced and expanded training in all disciplines, including such special areas as pulmonary medicine and dermatology. The centers provide a unique educational setting in which trainees in all the occupational health disciplines work together as they must when they fulfill their roles in the workplace.

The development of the ERC program represents the most important event in the field of occupational health in the past thirty-five years. When one examines the increases in numbers of trainees since the initiation of the ERCs, the accomplishments are impressive. In 1969 there were 2 full-time physician trainees in occupational medicine in the United States; in 1981 there were 119. In 1969 there were no nurses in full-time training in occupational health; in 1981 there were 90. In 1969 there were 30 full-time trainees in industrial hygiene; in 1981 there were 846. The figures for continuing-education trainees are quantitatively even more impressive. In 1981 there were 1,680 in occupational medicine, 1,965 in occupational health nursing, 3,060 in industrial hygiene, and 2,028 in occupational safety. The largest part of these increases has come from the NIOSH-supported Educational Resource Centers. Although the ERCs have been in existence for only a few years, their impact has been substantial. Despite impressive gains, industry requirements are so great that significant deficits continue to exist. Even if the output of trainees were to be maintained at the present level, it will be many years before these scientific and professional needs will be satisfactorily met. Fulfillment of that goal is likely to be further delayed by the attitudes of the Reagan administration.

Parallel to the development of the Educational Resource Centers for Occupational Safety and Health, attempts have been made to insert occupational and environmental health into the curricula of medical and nursing schools. The penetration has been slow, but with the development of quality graduate training programs at several universities, a few medical and nursing school faculties have recognized the need for experiences at the undergraduate level. Limited numbers of federal grants have been awarded to develop model occupational health training programs for medical students. While the quality and effectiveness of such programs are still to be validated, curriculum committees at medical schools continue to resist the introduction of such programs as part of the required curriculum. What is even more disheartening, however, is the fact that despite the presence of preventive medicine and public health in the undergraduate curriculum for so many years, the preventive aspects of medical practice are given no prominence whatsoever in many medical schools. The ecological issues and the environmental health problems that are identifiable, measurable, and wholly preventable are barely mentioned in most medical schools.

What are some of the human illnesses resulting from ecological factors that need greater attention? At the top of the list is cancer and the potential for genetic injury. It is estimated, though not well-documented, that 50 to 90 percent of all cancers are from environmental sources. The elimination of cigarette smoking would, by itself, reduce the incidence of cancer by 30 percent. Smoking also increases cancer risk from exposure to such other agents as asbestos and uranium. While carcinogens in the workplace account for a modest fraction of all environmental cancer, workplace-induced cancer is of particular significance because it represents a small group of workers in whom the incidence of cancer is high. The workplace agents are identifiable from laboratory experiments and epidemiological studies. The list of such agents is a long one and now includes some heavy metals, beryllium, nitrosamines, urea formaldehyde, and a variety of other uncured polymers. The pesticides and herbicides suspected of carcinogenicity have been more or less eliminated from use. Initiating and promoting factors are found in fossil fuel sources, fossil fuel process streams, and utilization of their products. We are now engaged in producing energy from sources such as oil shale, coal liquification and gasification, synthetic fuels, and nuclear fuels. All have components potentially toxic and carcinogenic.

We are now alert to the fact that common agents such as lead and a variety of organic solvents, even at low levels of exposure, will result in neurobehavioral problems. Other ubiquitous metals such as cadmium produce lung, liver, and kidney damage and compete with such essential metals as copper to produce cardiovascular injury. If one looks at the number of new chemical and physical agents introduced annually—a thousand or more chemicals each year used in industry and consumer goods—and if one then looks at the backlog of chemicals, there are probably 30,000 to 35,000 presently used that have never been adequately tested. The task of assessment for toxicity and standard setting is astronomical.

In determining where our investments in research and education should be, it is necessary to consider the most critical health problems of chemical or physical origin that require environmental assessment, especially those problems with high mortality and disability rates. Cancer and cardiovascular disease lead the list. There are any number of clues that indicate that environmental factors play an important role in the origin and the severity of coronary disease, atherosclerosis, stroke, and hypertension. A third area of common concern is pulmonary disease, particularly obstructive lung disease and emphysema. The latter is related not only to smoking but also to such dusty trades as coal mining, cotton mill operations, and the like. Of high priority are those nutritional problems that can be considered ecological and the influence of nutrition states on chronic diseases.

Chemical waste dumps, which have multiplied enormously during the last twenty-five years, constitute another major area of concern. They can have a major effect on the human ecosystem, the food chain, the water supply, and even the home environment. High priorities in this area include the identification of health effects, the determination of the biological effects of chemical interactions, and the development of strategies of decontamination.

All these issues must be reflected in the construction of proper curricula and training programs for the health professions. For the undergraduate professional student in medicine and nursing in the 1980s and 1990s, new types of educational experiences will be required to provide an understanding of ecological hazards and their health effects. In addition to the traditional forms of teaching—lectures, conferences, and patient care in a hospital setting—students must be allowed to identify and quantify the health hazards in the workplace and in community environments. They must be allowed to determine the relationship between the environment and specific diseases and injuries. Their experience must include opportunities to participate in epidemiological studies, in hazard identification, and control efforts in the field. They should engage in clinical studies of populations at risk, in environmental and population surveillance, and in laboratory investigations, both problem-oriented and mechanism-oriented. Faculties with clinical and research expertise must be assembled. Futhermore, commitments must be made to include attention to this field in the curriculum. For example, at the University of Cincinnati, despite the existence of a critical mass of research scientists and professionals in environmental health for more than half a century, the required curriculum includes only about twenty hours of course work in environmental health; all other experiences in this field are limited to elective time.

## Summary

The impetus provided by social concerns, by legislation, by federal health agencies, by pioneering universities, and by the private sector has resulted in substantial gains in both graduate education and continuing education in the environmental health disciplines. In undergraduate professional training programs, however, the impact of ecological issues has been limited. Effective training in the health professions in the 1980s and 1990s must recognize the significance and importance of such ecological factors as the chemical and physical environments and the health problems that are induced by such environments. These concerns and the management of both environmental and clinical problems should be incorporated into the fabric of the undergraduate curriculum of physicians, nurses, and engineers.

## References

Agricola, G. *De Re Metallica [Concerning Metal].* Translated by H. C. Hoover and L. H. Hoover. New York: Dover Publications, 1950.
Dubos, R. *Man Adapting.* New Haven, Conn.: Yale University Press, 1980.
Haeckel, E. "Ueber Entwicklungsgang und Aufgabe der Zoologie" ["On the Development and Contribution of Zoology"]. *Jenanische Zeitschrift fuer Medizin und Naturwissenschaft [Jenanische Journal for Medicine and Natural Science],* 1870, 5, 358–370.
Massachusetts Institute of Technology. *Man's Impact on the Global Environment: Assessment and Recommendations for Action.* Cambridge, Mass.: M.I.T. Press, 1970.

National Institute of Environmental Health Sciences. *Man's Health and the Environment—Some Research Needs.* Washington, D.C.: U.S. Department of Health, Education, and Welfare; Public Health Service; National Institutes of Health, 1970.

National Institute of Environmental Health Sciences. *Human Health and the Environment—Some Research Needs.* U.S. Department of Health, Education, and Welfare Publication no. (NIH) 77-1277. Washington, D.C.: U.S. Department of Health, Education, and Welfare: Public Health Service; National Institutes of Health, 1976.

Ramazzini, B. *De Morbis Artificum Diatriba [Diseases of Workers].* Translated by W. C. Wright. Chicago: University of Chicago Press, 1940.

Rosen, G. *A History of Public Health.* New York: MD Publications, 1958.

World Health Organization. *Health Hazards of the Human Environment.* Geneva, Switzerland: World Health Organization, 1972.

# 21

*Duncan Neuhauser*

# Technological Innovations

## Revolutionizing Information Management and Decision Making

Medical technology has and will continue to transform the way health workers relate to patients, as well as the organization of medical care. Currently, medical technology calls forth the need for health insurance, and both fuel the fires of rising medical care costs. A core and continuing question of this technology is its effect on the health of patients. Although speculating about the future is a chancy business, we will do so with one technology—computers in support of medical decision making.

### What Is Medical Technology?

For most people, the words *medical technology* conjure up visions of expensive, modern machines such as computerized axial tomography (CT) scanners and operating room equipment. However, this narrow definition has been broadened to consider not only such very expensive machines but much less costly things used many times over, such as the relatively inexpensive drug cimetidine, sold worldwide at the rate of half a billion dollars a year. Furthermore, it is not just these *things* but also the way in which they are employed (technique) and the

448

decision rules that are used to decide when to apply them (Office of Technology Assessment, 1982). From this perspective, medical care can be seen as a set of routines or programs, such as coronary artery bypass surgery or a stress test. Each of these technology programs raises a number of questions: When is it used? For what kind of patients? Does it do any good? For whom? How sure are we of this? How much does it cost? What is its cost-effectiveness?

### Historical Overview of Medical Technology

As medical technology has changed, the doctor-patient relationship has changed. The 1800s saw the physician as no longer dependent solely on the patient's word but dependent on his own technology-aided observations. The 1900s saw the growth of diagnostic technology and chemical analysis, as well as the challenging of the physician's perception of the patient unaided by laboratory and x-ray. Today technology intervenes between the physician and patient, to the sacrifice of the doctor-patient relationship.

*1700–1880: The Doctor.* Professor Stanley Reiser (1978) has developed the thesis that technology was new to medicine in the early 1800s. Medicine in 1700 was university-based and the European physician—unlike the barber-surgeon, midwife, or apothecary—did not lay hands on the patient. This physician was dependent on visual observation of the patient and the patient's verbal description of the history of the disease. Like the other university-based professions of law and theology, knowledge was based on the classics written in Latin.

In 1761, this pattern was broken by Morgagni's idea of pathological anatomy, stating that the pathology observed at autopsy should be related back to prior symptoms. In the 1820s, the stethoscope was created by Laennec, allowing the physician to listen to heart sounds; it was thus the first important technology for the European physician. This technology was soon in widespread use and was followed by other diagnostic technology, including the ophthalmoscope, the blood pressure cuff, and the microscope, and culminating in Roentgen's x-rays of 1895.

*1880–1920: The Hospital.* In 1873, there were 178 hospitals in the United States (Toner, 1873). By 1915, there were over 5,000 hospitals. In 1980, there were 7,000 hospitals (U.S. Bureau of the Census, 1975). At the turn of the century, the hospital became indispensable to the practicing physician for the first time. Aseptic surgery required a controlled environment, and the x-ray machine was not transportable to the patient's home. The 1910s saw the creation of private pavilions for the prosperous associated with voluntary general hospitals, which had previously been devoted to the poor and the working class (Rosenberg, 1979).

The first fifteen years of this century saw the Pure Food and Drug Act of 1906 create the class of drugs obtainable only by the prescription of a physician, thus defining the economic organization of the pharmaceutical industry (Wilson and Neuhauser, 1982). This era saw the introduction in the United States of research-based medical education at Johns Hopkins; the transformation of medical education by Abraham Flexner; the beginnings of institutionalized medical specialization, with the creation of the American College of Surgeons in 1913 and the American Board of Ophthalmology in 1917; and the fixing of the hierarchic relationship between physicians and nurses, who in turn were affected by the Nightingale reforms. The public health movement crested with the massive engineering efforts to create pure city water supplies and sanitary reforms. This era saw the basic organization of medical care defined around hospital-based medicine.

*1920–1965: Insurance.* The one major change that took place after 1920 was the development of health insurance (Anderson, 1975). Although various schemes had been tried prior to 1927, that year saw the initiation of the Blue Cross movement at Baylor University in Texas. In 1942, the Kaiser Permanente Health Plan was created. However, the major growth of health insurance occurred after World War II, culminating in the landmark passage of Medicare and Medicaid in 1965.

Health insurance was necessary only to the degree that medical care became expensive through the application of technology. The increase in research funding through the National Institutes of Health (NIH), in the context of growing health insurance, facilitated the development of medical technology.

The rate of growth was not unidirectional. True, there was a decline in infectious disease mortality, from puerperal fever to polio. However, this era also saw the great growth and then the near disappearance of the tuberculosis hospital; improved living conditions at the beginning, and effective drugs at the end, led to outpatient care for a few tuberculosis patients, compared to years of hospitalization for many patients. The peak in the numbers of patients in mental hospitals was 1955; effective drugs and the community mental health movement created a mental health revolution, whose consequences are still being played out today.

*1965-Present: Inflation.* Figure 1 shows the cost per patient discharged alive from the Massachusetts General Hospital, controlling for inflation in the general economy from 1828 to 1975. (These figures are based on 1967 adjusted dollars and therefore exclude the effect of overall inflation.) "Discharged alive" attempts to control for the quality of care, however approximately. Teaching and research have been part of this hospital's activities from its inception but have taken on a greater role in recent decades. In spite of the difficulties of comparison over 150 years, the message is clear. The exponential growth in costs has come just before and after the introduction of Medicare and Medicaid. It created the need for such health insurance that, in turn, made more technology possible.

In many other industries, new technology and the associated division of labor have been seen as cost saving. Adam Smith pointed this out in 1776, and Henry Ford's assembly line restated it in practice. The robotics revolution is once more transforming the assembly line. In medical care, technology is seen as adding personnel to the hospital payroll and as increasing costs. Why?

There is *one* overriding goal for today's hospital manager—keep the beds filled with patients whose bills are paid. Because only physicians can admit a patient, their goodwill is essential. Full beds and paying patients can generate revenue in excess of expenses. In business, this could result in lower prices under competitive conditions, greater costs, or dividends to stockholders. In hospitals, health insurance has largely eliminated price competition, and the nonprofit status of 90 percent of U.S. hospitals precludes stock dividends. The largely female labor force of hospitals has probably resulted in a low level of unionization and less pressure to increase employee pay than is the case in the automobile and steel industries, although this could change.

**Figure 1. Cost per Patient Discharged Alive in 1967 Inflation-Adjusted Dollars, 1828–1975, Massachusetts General Hospital.**

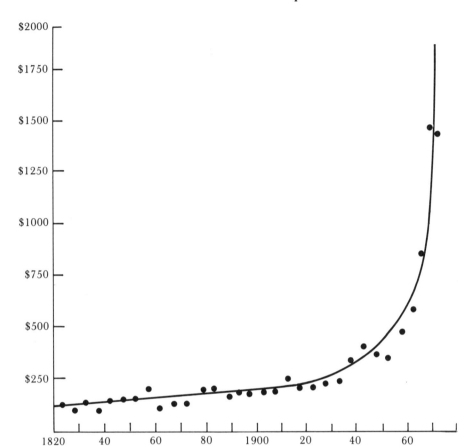

The result is that hospitals tend to spend on technology to attract physicians and to present to the world an image of scientific breakthroughs, wonder drugs, and the best medical care in the world, so satisfying to patients, doctors, and home town chauvinists. The response by payers has been regulation to control costs. Professional Services Review Organization (PSRO), Certificate of Need (CON), Health Services Agency (HSA), rate regulation, and prospective budgeting are only a few of the jargon words of regulation.

The Republican ideology of the Reagan presidency, combined with a widespread unhappiness with existing regulation, has led to the rise of competitive theories as an alternative way to make medical care efficient (Enthoven, 1980). Whether a regulatory or competitive future awaits us is anyone's guess.

### Does Medical Technology Work?

There are several reasons why it is difficult to decide whether a particular medical technology is beneficial:

- The market test is not considered an adequate measure of benefit. In the absence of a competitive market resulting from health insurance coverage, "Does it sell" is not necessarily the same as "Does it benefit."
- The placebo effect results from the doctor's and patient's belief that a treatment will work. In the 1950s, Beecher estimated that a third of the benefits to be derived from medical care come from the placebo effect (Beecher, 1955; Frank, 1973). The real therapeutic effect must be measured in a way that controls for this effect. Double-blind studies are the best way to do this. Neither the patient nor the doctor knows whether the pill is real or just sugar. This technique can only (with rare exceptions) be used to test the effect of drugs and injectables.
- Patients differ. What works well for one type of patient may work less well or not at all for other types of patients. This is a major problem. There is a strong tendency to use a technology that is effective for some for the many, with the hopes it will benefit. The cost implications of this technology creep are very large.
- Controlled studies are expensive. A multicenter, randomized clinical trial can easily cost over ten million dollars.
- Clinical trials using human subjects are fraught with ethical problems. Hospital-based human subject research committees are required in all hospitals using federally funded research. This is one response to the ethical issues in human experimentation.
- Research on efficacy is a form of behavior change. Presumably, physicians are to change what they do on the basis of scientific evidence and to a remarkable degree they do, given that they are human beings. There can be, and are, examples of too rapid adoption of new technology (gastric freezing—Fineberg, 1979), and too slow adoption of others (limited surgery for breast cancer—Schachter and Neuhauser, 1981b). There are also numerous technologies that have never been carefully evaluated (episiotomy—Banta and Thacker, 1982).

The problem of the evaluation of medical technology is as old as America. In 1630 in Boston, one Nicholas Knopp was fined five pounds or whipped for selling a cure for scurvy of "no worth nor value" (Young, 1961). How did the magistrates know it was of no worth?

In 1721, the combined talents of Onsemus (a black man from Senegal), Cotton Mather (the Boston Puritan clergyman), and Zabdial Boyalston (the apprentice-trained doctor), resulted in the introduction of smallpox innoculation during an epidemic and the evaluation of its efficacy using a comparison of death rates between patients innoculated and not innoculated. It is believed that this was the first use of numbers to evaluate a medical treatment (Winslow, 1974; Beall and Skyrock, 1953).

In 1753, the British naval surgeon, James Lind, carried out a controlled trial, believed to be the first, of treatment for scurvy on six sailors and showed the efficacy of what was later to be shown to be vitamin C. Only after decades was lime juice accepted by the British navy as preventive therapy for scurvy—thus the slang term "limey" for the English. This was a necessary change that allowed the British fleet to stay at sea for months to blockade Napoleon's Europe, making the naval battle of Trafalgar possible (McNeil, 1976). In July 1776, American revolutionary soldiers at Boston were ordered to be innoculated for smallpox. This too may have changed history (Blake, 1959). After Jenner's discovery of the safer smallpox vaccine, Napoleon required this for his army, thus allowing his large armies to take to the field year after year. These were the first examples of medicine changing history.

Lemuel Shattuck, in his 1850 Report of the Sanitary Commission of Massachusetts, published a cost-benefit analysis to justify the creation of a state public health department. Shattuck was one of the founding members of the American Statistical Association.

The public demonstration of ether anesthetic at the Massachusetts General Hospital in 1848 was a clinical trial of one patient without a control, but the effect was so dramatic that ether and later chloroform anesthesia rapidly spread all over the world. Lister's statistical analysis of the value of antiseptic surgery was dramatic, but it took decades for its acceptance in the United States (Truax, 1968). Roentgen's x-rays were used within days of the arrival of his paper on American shores. So rapid was this adoption that at least four different communities lay claim to the first American use, although it was only by the 1940s that the risks of radiation exposure to radiology workers were fully brought under control, and we still debate the harmful effects of low-dose radiation exposure.

Advances in laboratory chemistry in the late 1800s in Germany made possible for the first time the chemical analysis of patient nostrums and were a necessary precondition to their effective regulation in 1906, in spite of numerous testimonial letters from patients and doctors as to their wondrous curing powers (Young, 1967). This is an example of replacing patient opinion and unaided physician observation with laboratory test analysis at the turn of the century.

The first known randomized clinical trial was reported in the United States in 1931 (Amberson, McMahon, and Pinner, 1931), but the systematic application of this research method came about in England under the guidance of Sir Austin Bradford Hill after World War II. Even today, outside of drug therapy, the number of randomized trials can be counted in the hundreds.

The excitement in academic medicine has been in tracking down rare, unusual, and exotic diseases. The great aspiration was to be a Dr. Smith of Smith's disease. Routine problems have too often been ignored in the absence of methods to approach them systematically. Such methods have arrived under the general title of clinical decision analysis, which combines aspects of statistics, evaluation methods, economics, clinical epidemiology, the branching logic of decision analysis, the psychology of problem solving, signal detection theory, and computer-based modeling (Weinstein and others, 1980).

Historical points in time are misleading, because they hide a long series of partial effects behind these changes. The historical date I would like to choose for the new era of careful medical reasoning is July 28, 1975. On this date, an entire issue of the *New England Journal of Medicine* was devoted to clinical decision analysis applied to real medical problems. This journal has continued to publish decision analysis and cost-benefit analysis studies of medical problems ever since. The techniques of clinical decision analysis could for the first time make the routine problems of medicine—the workup for hypertension, abdominal pain, the periodicity of Pap smears, routine preoperative chest x-rays, the appropriate number of dental x-rays—academically challenging. This was coupled with a new interest in evaluating the efficacy of frequent or new medical procedures under the title of medical technology assessment.

Medicine has gone through several cycles of enthusiasm over efficacy. In 1794, doctors like Benjamin Rush believed they could work wonders. By the 1840s, the widespread introduction of *numbers* to medical evaluation, promoted by Professor Louis of France, challenged such procedures as bloodletting. The result was an era of "clinical nihilism" best reflected in the homeopathy of Dr. Hahneman's microscopic doses (Kaufman, 1971). The introduction of x-rays, aseptic surgery, wide use of hospitals, and the control of drugs brought on a new era of enthusiasm cresting with penicillin and other "wonder drugs." Medicine was declared a right, insured, and overused. We are in a new era of clinical nihilism resulting from such evaluation techniques as the randomized clinical trial (Cochrane, 1972). In combination with clinical decision analysis, there is a new questioning of the efficacy of many frequent procedures, such as coronary care units, tonsillectomies, and routine surgery. This nihilistic cycle will probably be somewhat shorter and less deep than the cycle of the 1800s.

Thus far, I have tried to demonstrate the historical interplay between medical technology, its evaluation, and the economic and organizational context of medical care. These forces define medical care as it is today and are at the center of the questions about often unclear benefits and clearly rising costs of medical care. These forces will continue into the future.

In some ways, the hospital is remarkable for its organization that allows for the easy adoption of such new technologies as bypass surgery, CT scanners, and nuclear magnetic resonance (NMR) imaging. Such technologies easily fit into existing departmental and hierarchical organization. Reimbursement policies make introduction financially viable, and the fear that a competing institution will get there first all stimulate rapid change. Because of this facile ability to take on new technology, it is not very useful to speculate on specific new technologies of this sort that are on the horizon. The history of NMR will probably be similar to CT scanning in the enthusiasm generated, rapid adoption, and, only afterward, a beginning understanding of its efficacy, if any, in patient care. New drugs are, if anything, more rapid in diffusion, once they have met Food and Drug Administration approval. The costs of this approval to the manufacturer are so large that only drugs with a high hope of marketability are pushed forward. Only very large drug manufacturers can play this game, and they have the wherewithal to advertise heavily, thereby encouraging rapid adoption.

In Europe, the countervailing force to this enthusiastic adoption will be the budgetary control by governments of the hospital systems they own and operate. Whether this approach or a competitive alternative will evolve in the United States is anyone's guess. Those European governments and the United States, as well, are caught in a dilemma: On the one hand, they would like all the world to purchase the medical technology their native manufacturers make and export; on the other hand, they want to limit the costs of their own national health services.

The technology that is of more interest to the observer of health services is not the one that easily fits in but rather the one that compels a restructuring not only of organizational form but of the world view of providers, particularly physicians. Such changes—like the germ theory of disease—take a long time to occur.

One such change is the role of computing in support of clinical reasoning. For this reason, let us focus on this one technology and consider its potentially widespread impact.

## Some Futures

Predicting the future is a doubtful activity. Basically, I believe it cannot be done. I am one of those people who believe you can do quite well choosing stocks by posting the newspaper page of stock quotations on the wall and choosing your stock by throwing darts blindfolded. History is basically a random walk. It can be explained but not predicted. The best prediction of the state of affairs one year from today is what things are like today with a 5 percent random change. Computing in a .01 yearly probability of a nuclear apocalypse does not make prediction easier. That's a 50 percent lifetime probability and, therefore, is the most likely future. At best, we can spot a few long-term trends already in place and consider their implications, knowing that these trend lines are also subject to random fluctuations.

*Communication.* One of the basic principles of good management is the careful analysis of present and future trends in the environment, relating this to the present and possible future position of one's organization. If your grandfather invested in 1910 in a factory to make automobiles or buggy whips, it would make a lot of difference in your life. If he had invested in the former, he might be hailed as a captain of industry; if the latter, he would just be your grandfather.

Let us start with newspapers. Newspapers are undergoing a technological change that is so rapid, it makes medicine seem barbaric and sluggish by comparison (much of what follows about newspapers is based on material from *Goodbye Gutenberg* by Anthony Smith, 1980). We are familiar with Ben Franklin's kind of hand press, producing one page at a time using drawers full of carved letters. Then in the 1890s came the linotype machines, high-speed printers, and large urban areas (Tunstall, 1977). The modern newspaper was born in the New York press war between Hearst and Pulitzer ninety years ago. This technology held until recently: reporter to typewriter, to rewriter, to compositor, to layout, to lead plates, to printer, to collator, and on to trucks, to newsboys, and finally to the reader.

Now computers have come. The reporter's word processor feeds directly to the same computer used by the editors. The computer does the layout and controls the printing machines directly. All those human links between reporter and the delivery trucks have gone. The newsboys remain. Computers control the production process, eliminating workers and automating a complex system. So far these changes have had little observable impact on the reader of a paper, except to increase economies of scale massively and thereby to create local monopolies (one-newspaper cities). This technology promotes national newspapers, the *Wall Street Journal* being the best-known example.

The next round of changes may be even more extraordinary. Computer printing will allow variation in newspapers. Urban and suburban, east side and west side, local and national editions are now in existence. The next step will be individual newspapers. However, this will require doing away with newsboys as we know them. The problem is that they cannot be counted on to deliver a particular unique paper to a particular unique house. This requires more skill. Now consider the fact that nearly every newspaper gets one million words a day over the wire services and only uses a few thousand of them. With individualized newspapers, this could change. My neighbor, the internist, could get a unique paper addressed directly to him. His wife, the social worker, could also get a unique insert. Think what that would do. A large amount of the paper is now ignored by him and his family. He is not interested in the real estate section. It could be replaced with medical news—state, local, national, scientific, and otherwise.

Here are some implications. There are now hundreds and hundreds of reporters constantly at the White House, but none at the Veterans' Administration (VA) headquarters three blocks away. Why? Under the present system, a 10,000-word VA article would be one of the 990,000 words ignored by newspapers. Not so in this future. A new chief of VA nursing research would be readable news by several hundred thousand people. It would be printed in their paper. This would give an incentive to greatly improve reporting at middle government levels. Such a limelight is *desperately* needed at such places as the VA or for our local county health services. Secondly, it would wipe out a lot of the 7,000 medical journals. Drug advertising could shift to such specifically targeted daily newspapers.

Why have newspapers in the future? Now your home computer plus a telephone to "The Source" (Source Telecomputing Corporation, a subsidiary of the Reader's Digest Association, Inc.) can get you the contents of five famous newspapers and potentially lots more when they become fully computerized in their operations. You dial up, get the contents of the *Los Angeles Times* listed, and choose your article. Your printer can produce hard copy. There is no technical reason why you could not get the *Lancet* in the same way. Computer production of newspapers makes this feasible. However, it now costs $5 an hour in off time and three times that in prime time to use such services. My internist's newspaper will be free. The reason is targeted advertising. Now, my newspaper has ads for west side stores, even though I am on the east side. With targeted newspapers, ads can be targeted. It will be worthwhile for my favorite specialty wine and tea store to advertise directly to me, a proven customer, without paying for all that newsprint space for two million people who will never use that store. Thus, it is economics that will keep newspapers alive. I can be forced to look at ads in a local newspaper but not in the *New York Times* as displayed on my home computer screen.

This has been a long digression about newspapers, but not without reason. First, it may be that technology changes in such other areas may affect the quality of care and medical learning more than changes within health care. Secondly, I have tried to show, on neutral ground outside of medical care, that it is the interplay between technology and economic factors that is important in combination. Thirdly, changes are likely to take bizarre and unexpected directions. Finally, it is to point out how primitive things are in medical care.

*Medical Care and Medical Education.* We are now starting the third "boom-and-bust" wave of enthusiasm about computers in health care. I observed the first wave as it occurred for Chicago community hospitals in the mid-1960s when quite a few hospitals bought fancy computers to process patient accounts.

They were costly, and by the late 1960s, many were removed in favor of cheaper time-sharing. After this bubble of high expectation burst, there has been a steady, slow growth of business office computer use. The second wave came with Larry Weed and Octo Barnett's computerized medical record systems—the former at Vermont, the latter at the Harvard Community Health Plan. Such systems were to spread everywhere, but again the bubble burst. They have not spread; however, there is a quiet, steady, slow growth of medical uses of computers to report laboratory and x-ray test results and to store patient demographic and appointment data. The time when more than 50 percent of hospitals have more than 50 percent of their medical records computerized is over two decades away. The third wave of enthusiasm for computers in medicine will be associated with careful thinking, and like the first two, it will be oversold at first and leave a residual impact.

Computers will also have an effect on medical education. American medical education is in deep trouble, and it has to change. For me, as an outsider, medical education, in contrast to graduate education in law, engineering, or management, has several distinctive features. First is its authoritarianism. Second is its emphasis on rote memorization, and third is its lack of emphasis on problem solving. In the absence of analytic techniques for problem solving, medicine has tolerated an authoritarian hierarchy based on the seniority of years of clinical judgment. The senior physician need only refer to "my long clinical experience" to carry the argument. Clinical decision analysis should change that, allowing the junior doctor to pull apart the logic of the more experienced physician.

Some large amount of rote memorization will always be required of physicians; however, some of this burden could be reduced by computer support. For example, it is said that patients in tertiary care hospitals receive, on the average, fifteen different drugs. If we assume that there are 1,000 drugs in use, the potential number of combinations that might result in harmful drug interaction side effects is (1,000) (999) (998). . . . That number of potentially different interaction effects is more than you or I can remember. To think that physicians are to memorize this is ridiculous. A central national or international data bank could do a better job, using the same combination of telephone tie lines and the home computer that can get the *New York Times* to you or me now. There are hundreds of thousands of chemicals in the workplace, and tens of thousands of new ones each year. How are doctors, pharmacists, or nurses to remember their possible hazardous effects? A central computerized data bank could do this. Other examples are a cross-index of diseases associated with symptoms, current listings of the nutrition content of brand-name foods, and an index of laboratory tests—their uses, costs, error rates, sensitivity, and specificity.

Quick access to this kind of information is such an obvious need that one wonders why it has not been developed. The reason is economic. The Medical Literature Analysis and Retrieval System (MEDLARS) and the MEDLARS on Line (MEDLINE) system exist because of the reward system in medical research and the economics of medical libraries. Now there is too little pressure to promote the development of other kinds of data banks. The American Medical Association (AMA) is, I understand, actively working on this kind of central data bank on drug reactions. Tufts now employs a user-friendly MEDLARS system that has greatly increased MEDLARS' usage. There is even rumbling that physicians and nurses who fail to consult such data bases will be subject to malpractice suits. That kind of incentive might stimulate change. Another way change might be stimulated is for nurses to insist on their professional rights and refuse to administer medications that are not clearly demonstrated to be cost-effective for that patient. It is a continuing wonder to me that nurses fail to use the power they have to create a medical care revolution. But that's another story.

It has been observed at my medical school (Case Western Reserve University) that the recall decay of a fact for second-year medical students is about 90 percent after three months. A 90 percent loss of recall implies that such medical education runs at 10 percent efficiency, perhaps an unfairly low measure of efficiency if one assumes retention without recall will help with future recall after reinforcement. Such factual learning is inefficient but perhaps once justified. With access to computer memory banks, it is now less than ever justified.

In the past, teaching clinical reasoning could not be justified in the absence of a scholarly basis for good reasoning. This has changed. Increasing numbers of medical schools are developing courses in clinical reasoning. In 1980, after an extensive review of the problems of the second year, the faculty at Case Western Reserve University voted to have a committee develop a course in clinical logic. The committee proposed such a required course in June 1981, and this proposal was unanimously accepted by the faculty. Groups of nine students meet every other week for two hours throughout the year with one instructor who is an internist, pediatrician, or family physician. The course is taught by the case method, using written cases for problem solving. In the middle of the year, there is a sequence on clinical decision analysis, including some use of computers for clinical decision making. It is hoped that this course will be part of a complete rethinking of our medical curriculum. Case problem solving has been taken to its logical or illogical conclusion at Maastricht Medical School in Holland, which has nearly eliminated the lecture as a teaching device. (For a history of the case method of teaching, see Schachter and Neuhauser, 1981a.)

*Computer Dissemination of Medical Information.* How many of you have spent half an hour with your twelve-year-old son or daughter in an arcade, playing the new generation of electronic games: Pac Man, Space Invaders, Caterpillar? Did you know that this is a five billion dollar-a-year industry, and at the rate it is going, it could surpass medical care's percent of gross national product (GNP). These ingenious games are available for home computers. As such, they can easily replace television watching as the preferred occupation for twelve-year-olds. When this current cohort of twelve-year-olds reaches graduate school, they will expect their own microcomputer, and if your school does not provide one, you will have no students. Suppose one took the same extraordinary creativity that has gone into creating Pac Man and developed a computer-based model for decisions related to periodicity of Pap smear screening, to diagnosis and treatment of gastric and duodenal ulcers, to hernia surgery, and so on. All this is technically feasible but utterly ignored. Why is it medicine is becoming increasingly retarded in this area? The reason is that the reward system is not now in place.

The decision models such as the various decision trees or the David Eddy–American Cancer Society screening models are not well-presented in print, which unfortunately is how they now appear (American Cancer Society, 1980; Eddy, 1980). They appear in print because of the academic reward system that gives an academician credit and glory for an article in print, but none for creation of a disk that could be used in the thousands of home computers now being widely purchased by physicians. Such models on floppy disks would allow the physician to change variables, probabilities, and outcome values to fit their preferences and their patients' characteristics, and they could include sensitivity analysis. Such disks could be regularly updated and could be fine teaching tools. However useful this approach, there is no reward system providing the impetus for its wide adoption. Not yet anyway.

These gaps in appropriate innovation point out a real failure of the grant-funded medical research system now in place. The NIH system has a lot to recommend it, but it leaves major gaps—gaps that will become, I believe, more apparent with time. If one looks at the standard Apple microcomputer software list, it is hundreds and hundreds of pages long, and only two pages are devoted to medicine. Of the few medical programs, one sells for $1,500. Someone who tries to sell software at this price is a blooming idiot. Even $30 is too high. The twelve-year-olds in my neighborhood have a thriving system of software piracy of game disks. It is estimated that 30,000 Pac Man disks have been sold for home computers at $30 each and that there are a million copies in existence. The traditional copyright controls do not work. The economics of home computer software is that programs should sell for $7 or $8 and reach a very wide market. This price will defeat piracy by making it not worth the trouble and will create a mass market, a mass market that should exist very soon for medical decision models. In the future, academic rewards in medicine will not come from publishing the lead article in the *Journal of the AMA* but rather by creating and selling a million copies of a software disk—in popular music jargon, a platinum disk. Such clinical researchers will be almost as rich as rock stars and drug dealers.

If war is too important to be left to the generals, and health is too important to be left to nurses and physicians, then this future in medical computerization is too important to be left to the computer experts. The computer experts all too often have that all-American bias: the love for bigger and fancier technology. It's like the generals who want those $25 million dollar tanks that go from zero to sixty miles per hour in twenty seconds. If you leave it to the computer experts, they will spend your money like peacetime generals under Ronald Reagan. A decision model for an Apple computer for the cost-effective treatment of hypertension of the same level of sophistication as Pac Man and selling for $8.95 would do more for medical education than anything I can think of.*

### Future Organization of Medical Care

The coming abundance of doctors is a worldwide phenomenon. Sweden, Denmark, Iceland, and Israel have a lot of doctors. Mexico City is said to have hundreds of underemployed physicians. The impact in the United States will result in the following:

---

*In fact, there is a simple program for an Apple II+ computer that analyzes two problems: what to do about sore throats and whether an elderly person should have elective inguinal herniorrhaphy or wear a truss. This disk is available from Biomatrix, 2401 Queenston Road, Cleveland, OH 44118 or Eriksbergsgatan 36, 114 30 Stockholm, Sweden.

- The high level of medical student debt will not be as easily recovered, as physician incomes fail to hold their relative place.
- Banks will be more reluctant to loan money to doctors wanting to start practice.
- An economically profitable private practice will be increasingly expensive to start, have high fixed costs, and result in more grouping of doctors.
- Existing medical practices will once again be sold.
- The high costs of malpractice insurance will make starting a practice more difficult.
- Physicians will become more docile organization members.
- Hospitals will have more power.
- Staff privileges will be fought for.
- Contracts between pathologists or radiologists and hospitals will either be replaced by employment or be renegotiated regularly by periodic open bids.

*Growth of Medical Care Conglomerates.* All these phenomena make our coming era one in which physician office practices will be controlled by hospitals and, as hospitals form conglomerates, by large groups of hospitals formed into entrepreneurial corporations. It makes good economic sense for a hospital to buy a home computer for referring doctors so they can get patient data at 2:00 a.m. at home and thereby lock them into admitting patients to that hospital.

In short, doctors' offices will be franchised like the Colonel Sanders' fast-food fried chicken restaurants. Vertical integration will link hospitals and doctors' offices to assure the flow of patients. The satellite clinics of the Henry Ford Hospital in Detroit are one example. The signs of hospitals grouping together are now very obvious, whether it be the Veterans' Administration, the Hospital Corporation of America, Kaiser Permanente, the Fairview Hospital System, or the Sisters of Mercy, to list some widely divergent examples. The grouping of hospitals around medical schools provides another example (Brown and McCool, 1980).

The issue of the supply of doctors is an economic and political one. All these large corporations need abundant, cheap, docile physician labor. These corporations, backed by political power, have reason to enjoy the coming abundance of physicians. They will also preempt the control of clinical education from academic institutions and recast it to their own economic concerns. My current medical care parallel to Colonel Sanders is Professor Jack Myers of the Pittsburgh Medical School. He has been spending ten years developing an artificial intelligence, computer-based, diagnostic decision model called Internist (Miller, Pople, and Myers, 1982). It starts with a symptom and asks further questions in three stages—verbal and physical examination, routine tests, and then rare or invasive tests—to separate out alternative diagnoses and come to a conclusion. When it is finished, every medical, pharmacy, and nursing student should be required to use it or a similar program. Once such an expensive system is developed, it would be technically easy to have it available in your local doctor's office, franchised like Colonel Sanders. At the same time, a marketing entrepreneur could create a TV soap opera with Professor Jack as hero. Your local doctor with a direct wire to Professor Jack could drive everyone else out of business. If the franchise compels its physicians to refer all patients to Pittsburgh instead of Chicago, then Chicago medical schools will either go out of business or have to be sold as sort of triple-A farm clubs to the Pittsburgh major league team.

This takes a probable future to its most illogical extreme, but the trends are there. Many medical schools engrossed in their local tertiary care monopolies and their petty internal academic squabbles will one day wake up to discover the world out there has changed.

Perhaps there will be several competing conglomerates, as medical care belatedly makes the same transformation as the automobile industry did between 1900 and 1925. This transformation was stalled in medicine by the independence of the medical profession (which may be ending), by the only recent development of high technology and therefore high fixed costs, and by the voluntary ownership of hospitals that excludes the possibility of stock market capture—but that too is changing. The future General Motors, Ford, and Chrysler of medical care will have all the good economic incentives to pay to update their decision models, their information networking, and their marketing efforts. Thus, the academic apathy of today may well be replaced by vast efforts at developing computer-based decision support systems in order to maintain a competitive edge by these few giant, vertically integrated, medical care conglomerates.

*Humanism in Medicine.* This revolution in careful thinking in medicine is far enough along that I doubt it will reverse itself and go away. Whether it pushes the kind of change as far as my speculative mind takes it, only time will tell. The emphasis on decision modeling and computer-supported data banks will move physicians and other health professionals in two opposite directions. Those with left-sided brains will happily be developing these mathematical models, allowing those with right-sided brains to free themselves from this kind of mathematics and rote memorization to concentrate on providing understanding and compassionate, humane support to worried patients with long-term illness. One of the good things about clinical decision analysis is its repeated demonstration that patient preferences are usually critical to the choice of treatment options. This concern for patient preferences is not a bad goal for all of us to aspire to. And if we don't aspire to it, the competing doctor and the medical conglomerate across the street will force us to do so. In any case, medical care will never be the same again.

## References

Amberson, J. B., McMahon, B. T., and Pinner, M. "A Clinical Trial of Sanocrysin in Pulmonary Tuberculosis." *American Review of Tuberculosis*, 1931, *24*, 401–435.

American Cancer Society. "Guidelines for the Cancer-Related Checkup: Recommendations and Rationale." *CA: The Cancer Journal for Clinicians*, 1980, *30*, 194–240.

Anderson, O. W. *Blue Cross Since 1929*. Cambridge, Mass.: Ballinger, 1975.

Banta, D., and Thacker, S. "The Risks and Benefits of Episiotomy: A Review." *Birth*, 1982, *9* (1), 25–30.

Beall, O. T., and Skyrock, R. "Cotton Mather, First Significant Figure in American Medicine." *Proceedings of the American Antiquarian Society*, 1953, *63*, 37–274.

Beecher, H. K. "The Powerful Placebo." *Journal of the American Medical Association*, 1955, *159*, 1602–1606.

Blake, J. B. *Public Health in the Town of Boston, 1630–1822*. Cambridge, Mass.: Harvard University Press, 1959.

Brown, M., and McCool, B. *Multihospital Systems.* Germantown, Md.: Aspen, 1980.

Cochrane, A. L. *Effectiveness and Efficiency.* London: Nuffield Provincial Hospitals Trust, 1972.

Eddy, D. *Screening for Cancer.* Englewood Cliffs, N.J.: Prentice-Hall, 1980.

Enthoven, C. C. *Health Plan.* Reading, Mass.: Addison-Wesley, 1980.

Fineberg, H. "Gastric Freezing—A Study of Diffusion of Medical Innovation." In *Medical Technology and the Health Care System.* Washington, D.C.: National Academy of Sciences, 1979.

Frank, J. D. *Persuasion and Healing.* Rev. ed. Baltimore, Md.: Johns Hopkins University Press, 1973.

Kaufman, M. *Homeopathy in America.* Baltimore, Md.: Johns Hopkins University Press, 1971.

McNeil, W. H. *Plagues and Peoples.* New York: Doubleday, 1976.

Miller, R., Pople, H., and Myers, J. "Internist-1, an Experimental Computer-Based Diagnostic Consultant for General Internal Medicine." *New England Journal of Medicine,* 1982, *307* (8), 468–476.

Office of Technology Assessment. *Strategies for Medical Technology Assessment.* Washington, D.C.: U.S. Government Printing Office, September 1982.

Reiser, S. J. *Medicine and the Reign of Technology.* Cambridge, Mass.: Cambridge University Press, 1978.

Rosenberg, C. E. "Inward Vision and Outward Glance: The Shaping of the American Hospital, 1880–1914." *Bulletin of the History of Medicine,* 1979, *53,* 346–391.

Schachter, K., and Neuhauser, D. "A Short History of the Case Method of Teaching." In A. Kovner and D. Neuhauser, *Health Services Management: A Book of Cases.* Ann Arbor, Mich.: Association of University Programs in Health Administration (AUPHA) Press, 1981a.

Schachter, K., and Neuhauser, D. "Surgery for Breast Cancer." In Office of Technology Assessment, *Case Studies of Medical Technology.* Washington, D.C.: U.S. Government Printing Office, 1981b.

Smith, A. *Goodbye Gutenberg.* Oxford, England: Oxford University Press, 1980.

Toner, J. M. "Statistics of Regular Medical Associations and Hospitals of the United States." *Transactions of the American Medical Association,* 1873, *24,* 287–333.

Truax, R. *The Doctors' Warren of Boston.* Boston: Houghton Mifflin, 1968.

Tunstall, J. *The Media Are American.* New York: Columbia University Press, 1977.

U.S. Bureau of the Census. *Historical Statistics of the United States: Colonial Times to 1970.* Vol. 1. Washington, D.C.: U.S. Department of Commerce, 1975.

Weinstein, M., and others. *Clinical Decision Analysis.* Philadelphia: Saunders, 1980.

Wilson, F., and Neuhauser, D. *Health Services in the United States.* 2d ed. Cambridge, Mass.: Ballinger, 1982.

Winslow, O. E. *A Destroying Angel.* Boston: Houghton Mifflin, 1974.

Young, J. H. *The Toadstool Millionaires.* Princeton, N.J.: Princeton University Press, 1961.

Young, J. H. *The Medical Messiahs.* Princeton, N.J.: Princeton University Press, 1967.

*Tamas Fülöp* **22**

# International Needs

## Educating for
## Primary Health Care

The accumulated experience in international collaboration in general and in the health field especially, the conquest of smallpox, the decision of the United Nations to set into motion a program of action for the establishment of a new international economic order, and the increasing realization of the great and growing inequities in the health field were among the main factors that conditioned a historic resolution of the 30th World Health Assembly (WHA) in May 1977. This resolution, after saying that "faced with the magnitude of health problems and the inadequate and intolerably inequitable distribution of health resources throughout the world today" and "considering that health is a basic human right and a worldwide social goal, and that it is essential to the satisfaction of basic human needs and the quality of life" and, "reaffirming that the ultimate constitutional objective of WHO [the World Health Organization] is the attainment by all people of the highest possible level of health," declared that "the main social target of governments and WHO in the coming decades should be the attainment by all citizens of the world by the year 2000 of a level of health that will permit them to lead a socially and economically productive life" (World Health Organization, 1981b, p. 1).

This epochal decision, affirmed unanimously by all 152 countries that were members of WHO at that time (referred to as member states), accepted the greatest challenge in the health field in the history of humanity: to remove the inequalities that the resolution so rightly calls "intolerable" and to ensure "health for all by the year 2000."

## New International Economic and Health Order

What are then those truly intolerable inequalities that have nevertheless been tolerated so far and have even grown? First, it is clear that the origins of health inequalities are deeply rooted in socioeconomic inequities. Between 1971 and 1975, the average annual growth rate of domestic product, taking median values for each group of countries, was 2.9 percent for low-income countries, 6.0 percent for middle-income countries, and 3.2 percent and 3.9 percent for industrialized and planned economy countries, respectively. However, there was a group of forty countries, with roughly 1.2 billion population and a per capita product of less than U.S. $200 in 1970, where the annual rate of growth between 1971 and 1975 was only 1.1 percent. From these data, it is clear that a few rich countries are becoming even richer, and the many poor ones even poorer; this is reflected in the health field.

A recent WHO publication provides some striking figures on health and related socioeconomic indicators, as shown in Figure 1. Based on data for 1980, weighted averages were computed for three groups of countries: the least developed group, other developing countries, and developed countries. The difference between the least developed and developed countries in infant mortality rates is over 8-fold; in life expectancy, twenty-seven years; in premature births (those born with a birth weight of 2,500 grams or less)—over 4-fold; in coverage by a safe water supply, 3-fold; in adult illiteracy rates, 36-fold; in per capita gross national product (GNP), 37-fold (coinciding beautifully with the difference in the illiteracy rate); and finally, in per capita public expenditure on health, 143-fold! These are differences in averages; if we take the extreme values, the differences become even more excessive.

Thus, for example, in the late 1970s, about one-quarter of the countries and territories of the world had ten or more physicians per 10,000 inhabitants, whereas another quarter (23.4 percent) had one or less than one physician per 10,000 inhabitants (World Health Organization, 1980a, pp. 2–8). The difference between physician ratios for the African region and the European region of WHO is 22-fold. Again, such figures represent averages; country differences are even greater. For example, at one end of the scale are countries like Ethiopia with 0.1 physicians per 10,000 inhabitants and Burundi, Chad, Malawi, Niger, and Upper Volta with 0.2 physicians per 10,000 population; at the other end of the scale are the United Arab Emirates with 41.2, the U.S.S.R. with 34.6, and Czechoslovakia with 25.3 physicians per 10,000 inhabitants. In the least developed countries, of which there are now thirty-one, one health worker (including practitioners of traditional medicine and all other categories of health personnel) serves an average of 2,400 people, while in the developed countries this one health worker serves 130 people.

Today nearly a billion people, living mainly in rural areas and urban slums, exist in a state of social and economic poverty. This pernicious combination of unemployment and underemployment, economic poverty, scarcity of worldly goods, a low level of education, poor housing, poor sanitation, malnutri-

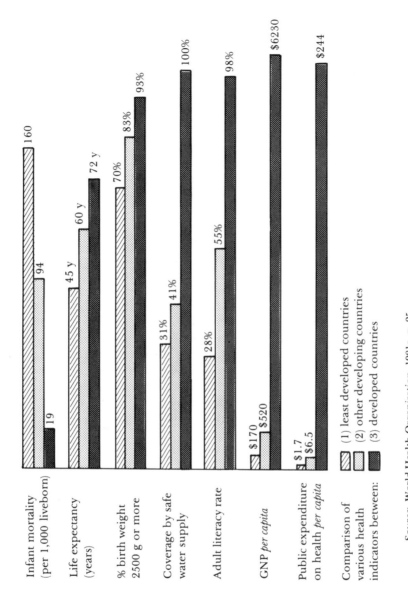

**Figure 1. Health and Related Socioeconomic Indicators.**

Infant mortality
(per 1,000 liveborn) — 160, 94, 19

Life expectancy
(years) — 45 y, 60 y, 72 y

% birth weight
2500 g or more — 70%, 83%, 93%

Coverage by safe
water supply — 31%, 41%, 100%

Adult literacy rate — 28%, 55%, 98%

GNP *per capita* — $170, $520, $6230

Public expenditure
on health *per capita* — $1.7, $6.5, $244

Comparison of
various health
indicators between:
(1) least developed countries
(2) other developing countries
(3) developed countries

*Source:* World Health Organization, 1981a, p. 25.

tion, affliction by disease, social apathy, and lack of will or initiative to make changes for the better constitutes a vicious circle. Improvement in any one of these conditions could contribute to improvement in all of them.

The New International Economic Order (NIEO) and, closely related to it, the New International Health Order were conceived to rectify this situation by or if possible before the end of this century. The declaration on the establishment of a NIEO calls for a more equitable relationship in the sphere of international economic exchange and in the sharing of the wealth of the world among the nations. It calls for the development of "a new international economic order based on equity, sovereign equality, interdependence, common interest, and cooperation among all states, irrespective of their economic and social systems, which shall correct inequalities and redress existing injustices, make it possible to eliminate the widening gap between the developed and the developing countries, and ensure steadily accelerating economic and social development and peace and justice for present and future generations" (United Nations, 1974, p. 3).

The very concept of socioeconomic development has undergone a profound change. In a basic reorientation of thinking and action, development goals are no longer defined exclusively in terms of economic growth. Development has been reinterpreted, as Dr. H. Mahler, Director-General of WHO says, "as a process aiming at the promotion of human dignity and welfare and at the radical elimination of poverty as the greatest obstacle to national and international progress and peace. Developmental policies and priorities are currently being reformulated so as to meet basic human needs for all mankind within the shortest possible period and to promote social and economic equity and the attainment by all of fundamental rights" (World Health Organization, 1980b, p. vii). In brief, it could be said that socioeconomic development has one main goal, that of improving the quality of life.

In this concept, health is one of the main components of quality of life, itself contributing to and benefiting from socioeconomic development. Thus the "main social target" of "health for all by the year 2000" is an aspect of the New International Economic Order, declaring in fact a New International Health Order. This order stems from a recognition of the fact that health and socioeconomic development are inseparable and that health development can no longer be considered as the affair only of the traditionally defined health sector but should be the concern of all other interested development sectors; thus, concern for health is of a truly intersectorial character.

### Health for All

With this background in mind, it is easy to understand the enthusiasm with which countries and people of the world greeted the prospect of "health for all by the year 2000." It is more and more clearly understood that health for all is *not* a single, finite target; it is rather a process leading to progressive improvement in the health of people. The concept of health for all will be interpreted and adapted differently by each country in light of its unique social, economic, and political characteristics, the health status and morbidity patterns of its population, and the state of development of its health system. "Health for all" is a moving target; as a certain health status is reached, people will set a target to reach a higher level.

However, it is now a common understanding that "there is a baseline below which no individuals in any country should find themselves" and that "by the year 2000, *all* people in *all* countries should have a level of health that will permit them to lead a socially and economically productive life" (World Health Organization, 1981a, p. 31). What does this imply? "The level of health of all people should be at least such that they are capable of working productively and of participating actively in the social life of the community in which they live" (p. 31).

Health for all is certainly not an unrealistic concept. The World Health Organization (1981a, pp. 31–32) states that it

> does not mean that in the year 2000 doctors and nurses will provide medical care for everybody in the world for all their existing ailments; nor does it mean that in the year 2000 nobody will be sick or disabled. It does mean that health begins at home, in schools, and in factories. It is there, where people live and work, that health is made or broken. It does mean that people will use better approaches than they now do for preventing disease and alleviating unavoidable disease and disability, and that they will have better ways of growing up, growing old, and dying gracefully. It does mean that there will be an even distribution of whatever resources for health are available. It does mean that essential health care will be accessible to *all* individuals and families in an acceptable and affordable way, and with their full involvement. And it does mean that people will realize that they themselves have the power to shape their lives and the lives of their families, free from the avoidable burden of disease, and aware that ill-health is not inevitable.

In essence, it implies freedom from avoidable suffering, pain, disability, and death for all people by the year 2000. It represents a new approach whereby health is considered in the broader context of its contribution to and promotion by social and economic development.

*Primary Health Care.* In September 1978, an International Conference on Primary Health Care was held in Alma Ata, U.S.S.R. The conference declared solemnly that "health for all by the year 2000" is a main social target and "primary health care is the key to attaining this target as a part of development in the spirit of social justice." The Alma Ata conference defined primary health care as being the "essential health care based on practical, scientifically sound, and socially acceptable methods and technology made universally accessible to individuals and families in the community through their full participation and at a cost that the community and the country can afford to maintain at every stage of their development in the spirit of self-reliance and self-determination. It forms an integral part both of the country's health system, of which it is the central function and main focus, and of the overall social and economic development of the community. It is the first level of contact of individuals, the family, and community with the national health system, bringing health care as close as possible to where people live and work, and constitutes the first element of a continuing health care process" (World Health Organization, 1978, p. 3).

The essential elements of primary health care were also defined by the Declaration of Alma Ata as "education concerning prevailing health problems and the methods of preventing and controlling them; promotion of food supply and proper nutrition; an adequate supply of safe water and basic sanitation; maternal and child health care, including family planning; immunization against the major infectious diseases; prevention and control of locally endemic diseases; appropriate treatment of common diseases and injuries; and provision of essential drugs" (World Health Organization, 1978, p. 4).

This concept of primary health care represents a different approach to health development. It implies community involvement or, as somebody has expressed it, "health as if people mattered." Such community involvement can have a broader influence than the local organization of health care. It can be instrumental in bringing about the commitment of community leaders to support the health reforms required, and through them, it can stimulate the political commitment of their government to introduce and sustain these reforms.

This concept of primary health care development requires that health resources be more evenly distributed and that top priority be given to the socially underprivileged. This requirement applies both within and between countries, since the more fortunate countries will have a double responsibility—to their own people and to those in countries in less favorable circumstances.

Finally, in this view, development of primary health care is seen as multisectorial in nature. Promotion and protection of health are certainly not only a matter of health services. Government decisions and popular insistences are also necessary to ensure that many sectors in addition to the health sector take the necessary action to promote health. For example, the education of the masses on health matters, the provision of safe drinking water and adequate sanitation, an adequate supply of the right kind of food, and housing that shelters against excessive sun, rain, and wind and gives protection against insects and rodents usually depend on actions in other sectors, as well as in the health sector. The involvement of people in ensuring this action is just as important as their involvement in action within the health sector.

*Global Strategy.* In 1979, the Health Assembly endorsed the Alma Ata Report and Declaration and invited member states to act individually in formulating national strategies and collectively in formulating regional and global strategies. In response to that invitation, member states of WHO formulated their national strategies for "health for all by the year 2000" as broad lines of action required in all sectors to give effect to the new health policy. Based on these national strategies and in support of them, regional and, finally, global strategies were worked out. The Global Strategy for Health for All by the Year 2000 was discussed and adopted by the 34th World Health Assembly in May 1981 (World Health Organization, 1981a). It reflects the national and regional strategies, as seen from a global perspective. It is not a separate "WHO strategy" but an expression of individual and collective national responsibility and a statement of a plan of action for WHO support. The strategy assumes the importance of health as a fundamental right, an equitable distribution of health resources, community involvement, political commitment of the state, national self-reliance, intersectorial cooperation, and technical and economic cooperation among countries. It applies equally to *developed* and *developing* countries. It explicitly recognizes the serious health problems of developed countries, such as cardiovascular diseases, cancer, accidents, environmental health problems (due to industrialization and urbanization), mental disorders (to the extent that vast numbers live on tranquilizers), social pathology (such as alcohol, nicotine and drug abuse, and high suicide rates), lung cancer and other chronic diseases due to smoking, obesity due to overeating, and chronic diseases and other sociomedical problems related to old age—all of which are growing.

Even health services are not free of problems. The overwhelming proportion of resources for the delivery of health care is concentrated in the large cities. These resources are devoted to expensive, highly sophisticated technology, unduly emphasizing the curative element, more often than not useful only to a very small fragment of the population. There is undue emphasis on secondary and on tertiary care, to the detriment of the often quite rudimentary primary care. Health care is deeply fragmented and provided mainly to the individual, to the neglect of the community and the goal of improving the health of the entire population. There is no well-formulated health policy or plan, and there is insufficient coordination both within the health sector and with other sectors of socioeconomic development. In sum, the health system lacks coherence and institutions now function in a more or less unrelated way with a failure to involve the community, that is, the "consumers," in the planning, provision, and evaluation of health services. The explosive costs of health care make it impossible, even in the most highly developed countries, to provide a complete range of health technology to the whole population, despite social pressures to do so even when such technology is unnecessary.

It is quite evident, therefore, that developed countries as well as developing ones need to strive for "health for all" and that they too stand to benefit from international cooperation in their struggle. The strategy adopted encourages intensified cooperation in such areas as the assessment of clinical, laboratory, and radiological technology and of the usefulness of selective health screening for early detection of disease; research on prevalent noncommunicable diseases and mental health; control of environmental hazards, including the long-term health effects of chemicals in the environment; accident prevention; and the care of the elderly. To this list could be added the development of adequate measures to combat smoking, overeating, alcohol and drug abuse, environmental pollution, personal stress, and alienation of people living in urban areas. Further consideration should be given to abandoning the attempt to provide everybody with every type of medical technology currently in vogue, a goal that even the richest countries cannot afford and that would not be of real benefit to the people, even if they could afford it. Finally, collaboration in the field of health services and health manpower development to promote critical analysis and exchange of experiences could also be added to the list. The Health Assembly, adopting the strategy in its resolution WHA34.36, also invited member states "to enlist the involvement of people in all walks of life, including individuals, families, communities, all categories of health workers, nongovernmental organizations, and other associations of people concerned" (World Health Organization, 1981a, p. 8).

## Problems in Health Manpower Development

It is evident that to achieve the goal set for the year 2000, there is a need to plan, train, and deploy health manpower in response to specific needs of people as an integral part of the health infrastructure. This involves both qualitative and quantitative considerations. As identified by the member states of the World Health Organization, the problems in achieving the goal may be grouped into three main areas: problems related to the quantity of personnel, those concerning the development of primary health care, and finally, those related to the promotion of social relevance of the health manpower development process.

The shortage of health personnel has remained a major problem throughout the post–World War II period. This problem is complicated by a serious maldistribution of trained health personnel. In many countries—both developing and developed—there are many times more doctors, nurses, dentists, pharmacists, and even medical assistants in the cities than in rural areas. In many countries, there is also a serious imbalance among the different categories of health personnel. It is not a rarity to see a country where there are three, and in some cases five, times as many doctors as nurses. The migration of trained health personnel is often a reflection of the relative overproduction of one or another category of health personnel.

The problems of quantity have become much more complex than they were in the period when there was an acute shortage of all categories of health personnel everywhere. Today, not only developed countries but also many of the developing countries, especially in Latin America, are more and more concerned about the specter of a plethora of physicians. No doubt the quantitative problems are, at least in part, due to failure to develop and implement consistent health manpower policies and plans responsive to the needs of society. They also reflect difficulties in the deployment and management of health personnel. Often there is no appropriate incentive or career scheme that would stimulate health personnel to work where they are most needed.

The second group of problems is those related to the provision of primary health care. These include the newly identified problems of training and utilizing practitioners of traditional medicine and traditional birth attendants, as well as the old but as yet unresolved problem of training and utilizing all categories of auxiliary personnel; the need for a team approach in health manpower development and, correlated with it, the problems of the university centers of health sciences. Finally, the "old" problem of nursing and midwifery education may also be assigned to this problem group. It is increasingly evident that the provision of adequate health care for all makes necessary the introduction of new policies, both in health services and health manpower development. New categories of health workers may have to be envisaged, while the orientation and training of "old," "classical" groups may have to be radically changed.

The third group of problems relates to the social relevance of the health manpower development process. Until recently, these problems were overshadowed by the so-called quality issues, which represented a largely misdirected concern with the scientific comprehensiveness and sophistication of education. The relevance issue is the heart and essence of the need for an integrated development of health services and personnel; that is, the need for orientation of the health manpower development process to serve the development of health services (see next section on HSMD concept), for community orientation and adaptation of curricula to local conditions, for teacher training, and for taking account of worldwide comments and criticisms of medical education.

The problems outlined above grow out of another set of deficiencies. First and foremost is the lack of coordination in the health manpower development process. Training institutions often fail to take account of health manpower policies and plans, even when they exist, and health workers' activities are not monitored to provide a basis for adjusting planning and training. Second, health manpower policies that do exist are rarely integrated with development policies in other sectors of the national economy; this problem is exacerbated by the low status of health in the allocation of national budgets. Third, insufficient efforts are made to strengthen institutions so that they will be able to fulfill the national requirements for basic and advanced training and continuing education; nor is there adequate support of the educational process through provision of teacher training and of adequate teaching/learning materials. However, the underlying problem is again the irrelevance of curricula to the real needs of health services and populations, resulting from the lack of coordination between educational institutions and health services. In addition, in most countries, there is virtually no system of continuing education to maintain and upgrade the competence of practicing health staff.

Finally, there are those problems in the health manpower field that arise from the absence or weakness of community involvement in decision making and evaluation of health workers' performance, the inadequate political commitment to a coherent long-term policy and plan for developing health manpower to meet the needs of health systems, and insufficient professional commitment to the major social goal of "health for all."

## HSMD Concept

The new health manpower development policies, principles, priorities, objectives, and targets are all based on the concept of integrated health services and health manpower development (HSMD). This concept has been actively promoted since the mid-1970s. It implies that the quality and quantity of health manpower must be planned in response to the specific requirements of the national health system, and these requirements must in turn be derived from the health needs and demands of the population. Training of health personnel should place "at the disposal of the system the right kind of manpower in the right numbers at the right time in the right place." This training should also "ensure that health workers are socially motivated and provided with the necessary incentives to serve communities" (World Health Organization, 1981a, p. 45). Further, the utilization and management of health personnel should be such as to ensure that personnel will be efficiently deployed to meet the needs of the system and that they will obtain job satisfaction by meeting the health needs and demands of people they are meant to serve. An effective monitoring system should be put in place to provide feedback as a basis for adjusting the planning and "production" of health personnel. The monitoring system should check whether the health workers are being properly utilized at the tasks they were trained for, whether they are ready and able to cope with these tasks, in what fields their competence requires updating, their job satisfaction, their contribution to consumer satisfaction, and their living and working conditions. Thus, the self-directing, cybernetic cycle of the health manpower development process (planning, "production," and management of health personnel), created in this way would be entirely geared to, and in fact integrated with, the process of health services development (Figure 2).

    *Mechanism for Implementation.* To effect this type of integrated HSMD process, a permanent national mechanism is needed. This will, of course, take different forms in different countries. However, it should in each case promote the functional integration of health services and health manpower development. This means fostering a permanent dialogue between relevant groups; ensuring efficient collaboration and coordination between the various governmental and nongov-

**Figure 2. National Activities in Health Services and Manpower Development (HSMD) and Some of Their Interrelationships.**

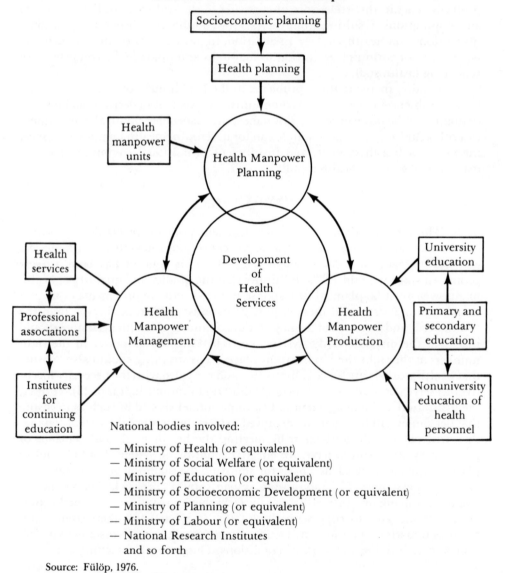

National bodies involved:

— Ministry of Health (or equivalent)
— Ministry of Social Welfare (or equivalent)
— Ministry of Education (or equivalent)
— Ministry of Socioeconomic Development (or equivalent)
— Ministry of Planning (or equivalent)
— Ministry of Labour (or equivalent)
— National Research Institutes
   and so forth

Source: Fülöp, 1976.

ernmental departments, institutions, and other bodies responsible for the different aspects of developing health services and health manpower; and bringing them together for the purposes of planning, management of, and decision making in HSMD. Such a mechanism should include representatives from the following sectors: health, general education, universities, economic planning and development, social welfare, labor, agriculture, communications, sanitation, water supply, housing, professions, and the community.

The mechanism should permit the most effective planning, "production," and utilization of health personnel, as a part of the managerial process for national health development (World Health Organization, 1981c), taking into account the national political framework and integrated with socioeconomic, cultural, educational, and labor (manpower) policies, plans, and development activities. It should facilitate specification of present and predictions of future requirements of a national system of health services, based on the present and foreseeable future health needs and demands of the entire population.

In order to foster intersectorial action, the global strategy envisages several different mechanisms, such as "the establishment of multisectorial national health councils comprising personalities representing a wide range of interests in the fields of health and of political, economic, and social affairs, as well as the population at large, to explore jointly policy questions affecting health and socioeconomic development" (World Health Organization, 1981a, pp. 42–43). These national health councils, which are being established in an increasing number of countries, can very well play the role of the HSMD mechanism at the national level. However, these decision-making national bodies need a strong secretariat that can prepare the decision alternatives, based on sound research data, and then see through and monitor the implementation of the decisions made. Again, the form of this secretariat is country-specific; however, in several countries a network of already existing institutions is being created, most recently in Ethiopia under the name of "national health development network," to fulfill the task of the HSMD secretariat. These national networks are created to bring together and make better use of existing resources, to coordinate often rather disparate activities, and to harness them so that they all contribute to the same goal—health for all by the year 2000.

In addition to HSMD mechanisms at the national level, a great variety of solutions has emerged at local and regional levels in many countries. However, whether at the central or a subnational level, the establishment and functioning of an HSMD mechanism is not an end in itself. Where effective, it will facilitate the provision of primary care services to the entire population, to meet their preventive, promotive, curative, and rehabilitative health needs and demands. These services will be staffed in sufficient numbers by health personnel whose skills have been developed to deal with the relevant health problems of the country.

*Policy and Planning Implications.* To implement this view of HSMD, it is necessary to formulate national health manpower policies as part of national health policies that, in turn, are an integral part of national socioeconomic development policies and are based on the overall national political framework. Health manpower planning in this concept consists in identifying and defining the categories, numbers, and ratios of health workers required and the composition of the health teams, striking the balance among health team members that is best-adapted to local conditions. Health manpower plans prepared on that basis will define not only the numbers, categories, and types of health personnel to be trained but will also indicate the knowledge, skills, and attitudes, and the areas and level of competence needed to carry out the tasks to be performed by each of them. On the basis of functional analysis, the definition of job patterns for the different types of worker within the health team will then lead to the specification of requirements and the translation of such requirements into learning objectives and, subsequently, into educational programs, curricula, and methods (including evaluation instruments) to assist the learners in achieving those objectives.

*Training Implications.* Clearly, the recommended global strategy has serious implications for the training component of the health manpower development process and provides for guidance to curriculum planners. In fact, it is stipulated in the strategy that a policy should be introduced whereby health manpower will be prepared "to perform functions that are highly relevant to the country's priority health problems, in contrast to accepted practice in many countries . . . (and countries) will review the functions of health personnel throughout the health system, and will take the necessary measures to ensure their reorientation as necessary" (World Health Organization, 1981a, p. 44).

If we agree that health workers, including physicians, should be socially motivated to be able and willing to serve where they are needed and in such a way as they are needed, then the learning experience provided to each of them should be planned not only to *allow* them to acquire the necessary knowledge, skills, and especially attitudes but also to *stimulate* them to do so. If graduates of our programs are to meet the real health needs and demands of people and to obtain job satisfaction through this type of service, then it will be necessary to revise many of our present programs that were not devised with such objectives in mind.

Graduates of programs designed in accord with the HSMD concept should be able to:

- Respond to health needs and expressed demands of the community, as well as work with the community so as to stimulate self-care and a healthy life-style
- Educate the community as well as their co-workers
- Solve and stimulate the resolution of both individual and community health problems
- Orient their own as well as community efforts to health promotion and to the prevention of disease, unnecessary suffering, disability, and death
- Work in and with health teams
- Provide leadership to such teams when necessary
- Continue learning throughout life so as to maintain and improve personal competence

An educational program designed to develop such competences (including the necessary awareness, attitudes, values, and sense of responsibilities) will need to rely not only on tertiary care in teaching hospitals but also, and perhaps primarily, on experience to be gained in the community in primary health care. Education that emphasizes health promotion and disease prevention will need to be both community-oriented and, especially, community-based. (Community-oriented education is defined here as one focused on both population groups and individual persons, taking into account the health needs and demands of the community concerned. Community-based education, on the other hand, is defined as one that involves the use of the community throughout the entire educational experience as an important environment in which learning takes place.) It will also need to be multiprofessional, that is to provide experience with interprofessional health care teams. If we want our graduates to be able to work in the community, in and with teams, obviously the learning experience that we provide them should give them ample opportunity to do so. Equally, if we expect them to be able to solve and stimulate the solution of problems relevant to the health of individuals *and* of collectives, their learning experiences should provide them with ample opportunity to practice the solution of individual and community health problems. In this sense, a program built on problem-based integration is preferable to a discipline-oriented program. Furthermore, graduates can be expected to continue lifelong learning only if, as students, they are given full responsibility for their own learning. Student assessment in such a program should concentrate on the valid measurement of learners' problem-identification, problem-solving, and decision-making skills, as well as their attitudes toward and competencies in dealing with community problems and in working as members of health care teams. Such a system of student assessment should be designed to provide both immediate feedback and long-term follow-up of trainee performance in relation to the health care required by the community.

In summary, it appears that the "health for all" movement gives clear guidance to those planning curricula for all categories of health workers. Programs planned with this most important social target in mind and aimed at developing competencies relevant to its achievement, will tend to be:

- competency-based and job-oriented
- community-oriented
- community-based
- multiprofessional (team-based)
- integrated on a problem-solving basis
- student-centered and oriented toward self-learning
- based on the clear understanding that "you are excellent only if you are relevant"
- adapted to the development of sciences and to local needs and resources

The global strategy as adopted speaks directly to curriculum planners in expressing the hope that all efforts will be made "to introduce the necessary reforms in faculties of medicine, health sciences, and other relevant training institutions so that in addition to their technical training, health personnel will become imbued with the philosophy of health development as defined in the Declaration and Report of Alma Ata and in this Strategy" (World Health Organization, 1981a, p. 45). It then speaks about stimuli to be given "to medical, nursing, and other health sciences schools, to include in their educational programs the philosophy of health for all, the principles of primary health care, and the essentials of the managerial process for national health development, and to provide appropriate practical training in these areas" (pp. 58–59).

*Utilization Implications.* Efforts to plan and train health manpower lose much of their value if the trained personnel is not used to best advantage by the health services. Indeed, shortage of personnel may in some instances be related to the fact that existing manpower is not being properly employed. Not even developed countries can afford to waste their highly trained health manpower, but the economic use of personnel is particularly urgent in less developed countries. The Alma Ata Report explicitly recognized the importance of management of health personnel. It recommended that "governments give high priority to the full utilization of human resources by defining the technical role, supportive skills, and attitudes required for each category of health worker according to the functions that need to be carried out to ensure effective primary health care" (World Health Organization, 1978, p. 26).

Optimal utilization of health personnel requires that available health manpower be distributed within the country and within the different sectors of the health services in direct relation to the needs of the population; that no member of the health team carry out activities that could be performed by less qualified personnel (on the principle of using the smallest volume of skill or group of skills with the necessary related knowledge to perform a specified job); and that all health activities be undertaken at the most peripheral level of the health services as is practicable, by the workers most suitably trained to carry out these activities. It is equally important that the interests of each member of the health services be stimulated by a system of motivation and incentives. These incentives will need to include provisions for giving the worker a feeling of responsibility and a consciousness that his/her work is useful, effective, and contributory to the general development of the community; for an appropriate system of social security, which includes moral and financial recognition of achievement, based on systematic review of living and working conditions and of achievements; for a system of continuing education, with opportunities for each member of the health team to maintain and improve his/her performance in relation to the health needs of the population; for job satisfaction and security of tenure for all staff within a properly organized career structure, with vertical and horizontal mobility, that provides opportunities for promotion, including access to posts with increasing responsibility; and for each health worker to receive constant technical support and supervision within a participatory system of teams.

If all the above conditions are fulfilled, the prerequisite for the effective management of health personnel will be present. If such a system is properly administered, not only will a sufficient quantity and quality of health personnel be attracted to posts in health services, but they will also be motivated to remain in the service as long as they are needed.

### Lessons in Strategy Development

The implications of the global strategy and the corollary HSMD idea seem to be clear at the conceptual level; however, they must be translated into strategies and through them, into action. For that, some lessons that have been learned may be worth reviewing, before turning to projections for the coming two decades (Fülöp and Roemer, 1981; Fülöp, 1982).

Policies and actions should constantly be monitored, evaluated, and changed as the situation changes. For example, immediately after World War II, the only concern was to increase the number of physicians and nurses and to maintain "quality", that is, to apply the standards of highly developed, usually former colonizing, countries. It was taken for granted that the only solution was to train as many traditional types of physicians and nurses as quickly as possible, wherever it could be done. In the case of newly independent countries, this usually meant sending personnel abroad for training and/or using foreigners to train personnel *in* the country concerned. In both cases, the content, the spirit, the norms, and the standards of the education were alien to the country in question and to the needs of its population.

Secondly, it was gradually recognized that graduates finishing in the very few schools where relevance to local needs was a real concern had no "slots" to fit into in the health services of their country. Thus, it was concluded that planning of health services and of manpower development should go "hand in hand." The HSMD concept that emerged was based on the experiences of the few countries where experiments were made to solve this problem.

Third, we have learned that sometimes the unanticipated side effects of actions may turn out to be more important than the achievement or nonachievement of the main objectives. A good case in point is the relentless pursuit of the "quality objective." Few would deny that pursuit of this objective has contributed significantly to irrelevance of much educational activity. Further, heroic efforts made to increase the number of physicians led, in several countries, to an uncontrolled growth of medical schools that produced a plethora of medical doctors, without improving the care of the underserved masses. Similarly, a teacher training program that is not based on the HSMD concept may and in some cases did asssist teachers to do "better" what they should not do at all, namely, to teach irrelevant things.

Analysis of these and other examples (Fülöp and Roemer, 1981; Fülöp, 1982) discloses the following factors that, among other things, still hinder development:

- The forces of neocolonialism and cultural and professional colonialism try to impose on developing countries patterns that are foreign to them.
- In some cases, small but powerful groups seek to ensure medical schools for their children and health services for themselves in institutions with the most sophisticated personnel and equipment, thus leaving only an insignificant part of the national health budget for marginal services to care for the overwhelming majority of the population.
- Some conservative forces of society and especially of the "classical" professions want to protect their manifold privileges at any cost and are therefore against innovation, which they feel is threatening.
- There is frequently a lack of national political will, a lack of willingness to carry through innovations that would change radically both the health services and, in consonance with them, the health manpower scheme.
- Often there is no appropriate national mechanism to carry out any forward-looking decisions that are taken and no proper mechanism to disseminate the ideas, concepts, recommendations, and resolutions that are discussed and adopted at the various forums of WHO.

These lessons unequivocally point to the fact that if "where to go" and "how to get there" are known, the only question that remains to be answered is "do we really want to go there?" This is the all-important question of the existence of the *political will* for change and of the *political force* to implement that change.

## Main Thrusts in Health Manpower Development

First and foremost, it is essential to foster the development of a national political will to bring about the change in human resources development necessary to achieve health for all by the year 2000. As an instrument of the much-needed changes, national health councils and national health development networks will have to be established and/or strengthened.

With regard to the various subsystems of the health manpower development process, there is general agreement that, in addition to the traditional stress on "production," increased emphasis should be placed on manpower planning (including problems of oversupply and imbalances), management, and utilization. In the production of manpower, provisions will need to be made for training and monitoring health workers in primary care. For this purpose, it will be necessary to develop task- and problem-based, community-oriented education programs for all categories of health workers.

Finally, national research in the human resources field will need to be strengthened. While the technical content and emphasis in the human resources field will be different in each country, the aim in *all* of them must be to create health manpower development policies, programs, and actions that are invariably directed to relevance of the health manpower development process to present and hypothesized future community health needs.

Political decisions are therefore needed so that

- The permanent national HSMD mechanism that is established and/or strengthened defines clear and unequivocal health manpower policies based on the recognition that development of health manpower is only one component in the development of health services, into which it must be properly integrated.
- The "production" of health manpower conforms to the health manpower plans; that is, new training institutions and programs are established and existing ones are geared to "produce" the right types and categories of health personnel in sufficient numbers, able and willing to meet the health needs and demands of the entire population. This requires the development of educational programs with the characteristics listed earlier in this chapter.
- The management of health personnel is such as to ensure that trained personnel are used to the best advantage by the health services, that is, that they are employed and administered properly for maximum effectiveness of health services.
- A procedure is established to monitor the utilization of health personnel and to ensure that the results are fed back into the planning and "production" process, which is then readjusted accordingly.

From this list, it is clear that a new emphasis should be developed so that it will no longer be enough to promote the development and utilization of the "best" methods for teaching and learning. Emphasis will have to be put not only on how to educate but even more fundamentally on the aims of the training program itself. Is it aimed at training, for example, "very highly qualified academicians equivalent to those of country X" or "technically and socially well-prepared, reliable professionals, able and willing to serve their own people and to meet their health needs and demands"? It is clear that while the "how" is a purely technical question, the "what for" is acutely political.

## Conclusion

The key to further progress in the health manpower development field, in terms of the goal "health for all by the year 2000 through primary health care," is *the promotion of national political will to seek out and apply the right solutions to well-diagnosed priority problems.* There seems to be a health challenge here to which a correct political, an unequivocally political, response is needed. It seems, therefore, that priority should now be given, at least for a while, to the stimulation of national political will, and the appropriate technical approaches and solutions should all be subordinated to the clearly set main targets supported by that firm national will.

The key word in the future should be *relevance.* A systematic, integrated, and holistic program approach will have to be applied, with relevance as the main aspect of all activities—relevance to the main social target of health for all by the year 2000 as well as to the health needs and demands of the people. In view of this, the three main output indicators of the health manpower development process for the future might be (1) extension of health coverage with special regard to primary health care, (2) improvement in the quality of health coverage, and (3) community participation and satisfaction.

Health for all by the year 2000 is the biggest health challenge humanity ever set for itself. It *is* a realistic aim, but there is a long way to go to achieve it even in the most developed countries. There is an implication in it for all elements of society and, among them, primarily for the universities and other teaching institutions involved in the education of health professionals. It is my hope that this chapter will provoke discussion that will lead to further clarification of the role of those institutions and to their closer association with the worldwide and ever larger movement that aims at health for all by the year 2000 through primary health care.

## References

Fülöp, T. "New Approaches to a Permanent Problem: The Integrated Development of Health Services." *WHO Chronicle,* 1976, *30,* 433–441.

Fülöp, T. "The Future of WHO's Health Manpower Development Program." *WHO Chronicle,* 1982, *36,* 3–6.

Fülöp, T., and Roemer, M. I. *International Development of Health Manpower Policy.* World Health Organization Offset Publication no. 61. Geneva, Switzerland: World Health Organization, 1981.

United Nations. "Declaration on the Establishment of a New International Economic Order." Resolution 3201 (S-VI). In *Resolutions Adopted by the General Assembly During Its Sixth Special Session, 9 April–2 May 1974.* General Assembly Official Records, Sixth Special Session, Supplement No. 1 (A/9559). New York: United Nations, 1974.

World Health Organization. *Primary Health Care.* Health for All Series, No. 1. Geneva, Switzerland: World Health Organization, 1978.

World Health Organization. *Health Statistics Annual 1980.* Vol. III: *Health Personnel and Hospital Establishments.* Geneva, Switzerland: World Health Organization, 1980a.

World Health Organization. *Sixth Report on the World Health Situation, 1973–1977, Part I: Global Analysis.* Geneva, Switzerland: World Health Organization, 1980b.

World Health Organization. *Global Strategy for Health for All by the Year 2000.* Health for All Series, No. 3. Geneva, Switzerland: World Health Organization, 1981a.

World Health Organization. *Handbook of Resolutions and Decisions of the World Health Assembly and the Executive Board.* Vol. II (1973–1980), 4th ed. Geneva, Switzerland: World Health Organization, 1981b.

World Health Organization. *Managerial Process for National Health Development.* Health for All Series, No. 5. Geneva, Switzerland: World Health Organization, 1981c.

# Part Four

---

## Policy Recommendations for Improving Health Professions Education

# Introduction:

## Educating Tomorrow's Health Professionals: Three Perspectives

## Alan Gorr

After all has been said and done, we return to the focal question: How do the programs that educate health professionals maintain a proper sense of mission or purpose in the face of technological, economic, environmental, and demographic revolutions that can, it seems, undermine even the most established and basic assumptions? The scholars who have examined the past research in the education of health professionals in Parts One and Two of this volume point to vast areas of incomplete or inconclusive findings. The prognosticators in Part Three have elegantly explained why long-term forecasts of the future based upon today's realities are at best chancy and at most likely to be confounded by future events. And this inquiry occurs at a time when the prospects of additional economic resources to help in the search for responses to today's problems are not easy to find.

Yet there is broad consensus on a number of points among the authors of this volume. They all believe that health professionals must be selected from the most appropriate pool of applicants for the profession they are to pursue. Education in their professions must be as good as it can be. The graduates must be certifiably able to perform their functions. The mission of the professions must derive from some triangulation among the scientific possibilities, societal values, and the resources available. Thus, health professions education is a subset of many larger realities and must find a way to be genuinely interactive with the forces that affect it. "What to do" is the subject of Part Four of this volume.

The recommendations in this last section of the book come from three perspectives: from the consumer of health care—Russell Mawby; from the deliverer of health care by academic health centers—Alexander Schmidt; and from the educator of health professionals—Ronald Richards, who endeavors to synthesize the many trends found in the preceding chapters. While the perspectives of these three authors differ, they are united by certain common concerns. They all wish to reemphasize the fact that the health professions are people professions, by and for people. The first and ultimate arbiters of the availability and quality of health care are the people whom it serves. Thus, the research sciences and the health care specialties may not overrule societal desires. It is important, therefore, that the public know what is possible and be able to make informed choices. Society must be given the tools to maintain itself in a healthy state and to minimize its reliance on the health care system. And it must have the wherewithal to help shape the health care system to its own needs. It must not be forced to consume more service than it requires. And when it requires service, the scientific and humane quality of that service must be high.

Russell Mawby believes that a commitment to primary health care is required. Such care would include health teams composed of family physicians and nurse practitioners, whose efforts are well-coordinated with more specialized services, should these be necessary. This primary care organization would treat the whole person and emphasize health promotion. Insurers also have an important role to play in rewarding positive health behaviors.

Alexander Schmidt, speaking from the perspective of large academic health centers, documents the process by which these have become alienated from their original and primary mission—to provide health care services. Their abdication of this role to the community hospitals in favor of basic science research and medical subspecialization has had deleterious effects in the health care services, *as well as* in the fields of research and subspecialization. He calls for a new thrust in research into the delivery of health care as a way to redress this imbalance.

Ronald Richards, writing as an educator, tries to synthesize the insights of the authors of this entire volume. He urges a comprehensive reconstitution of the education of health care professionals. He believes that modification of patient care and educational programs can lead society in achieving the goal of more comprehensive health care for more people at less cost. The academic health centers must become a positive force in health promotion and in influencing public policy.

The authors believe that the academic health centers must act quickly and decisively if their identity and effectiveness are to be maintained. In summary then, health professions educators today need to express their commitment on four fronts:

- Commitment to *questions* of the purpose of the health professions
- Commitment to *processes* of educating students for the actual roles they will have in their professional lives
- Commitment to *investigation* into better ways of delivering health care services

- Commitment to *leadership* in reforming the health care delivery system to better meet the needs of the people whom it serves

The authors in Part Four provide practical recommendations that express these commitments and that will help bring about the needed policy changes in health professions education for the next decades.

*Russell G. Mawby*

# Setting New Goals
# for Health Professions
# Reform

I welcome this opportunity to make a few observations from a layman's perspective on the subject of priorities for health professions educational reform. In reviewing the preceding chapters of this book, I am struck, in particular, by two points. First, the depth and breadth of the topics addressed and the qualifications of the authors who write about them are most impressive. Hopefully, these presentations have challenged your thinking, possibly substantiated some of your own beliefs, and given you pause for thought. It is always a challenge to have discussions such as these make a real difference "back home." But the processes of institutional change, carefully designed to protect us all from hasty decision or impulsive action, can as easily serve to smother a flame of innovation.

Second, I am impressed with the comprehensive framework of this book. At least in the table of contents, *everyone* is represented. Usually, physicians talk with physicians, nurses with nurses, public health specialists with sociologists and political scientists, and dentists with themselves. But all dimensions of the health professions are considered here—the basic sciences, medicine, dentistry, nursing, administration, pharmacy, public health, and the allied health fields. Such an interprofessional approach can assist in moving forward, in tangible and gratifying ways, the concept and genius of the academic health center. At the moment, the academic health center is accomplished in disciplinary scientific contributions, but its potential is unfulfilled in programs for *maintaining health* and *promoting interprofessional education*, benefits which therefore are not yet realized.

### My Perspective

My background and my graduate education are in agriculture. My observations are from the point of view of a layman, albeit an informed layman, whose role as chief executive officer of the W. K. Kellogg Foundation, which each year provides about $25 million for demonstration programs in health education, services, and delivery, obligates me to be aware of issues in the field. I still recall vividly a series of rude awakenings as I first became involved in the foundation's programming in health. I was shocked and disappointed by much of what I learned of the inner workings, both in education and practice. While there is much to be admired, the realities eroded the pinnacle on which the health professions had resided in my mind. I have tried to learn wisely and to place the various components carefully in proper perspective and balance. In so doing, I have had to learn the lexicon of the hospital hallways, the differences between radiology and rheumatology, to recognize a "third-party payer" when I see one, to understand that "four-handed dentistry" doesn't refer to a clumsy practitioner or a carnival freak, and to appreciate a career ladder in nursing (but I must confess I still cannot easily distinguish a nurse practitioner from one who is not).

Actually, I bring more baggage than that to this discussion. I grew up on a farm in west central Michigan, not really "rural rural" because the homeplace is now part of a suburb of Grand Rapids, but a farm nonetheless, and in a family that enjoyed for years the splendid services of a country doctor, Dr. Jay D. Vyn. His wife was his office nurse and receptionist; later his daughter served in that role also. They worked together in harmony (we now call that joint practice), supportive of each other, the patient, and the family. I am not a nostalgia buff, yearning for the good old days—a return to the outhouse, tuberculosis, and "bloodletting"—but there were some things in that pattern that would still serve us well.

But perhaps my best qualification as author of this chapter is not that of a foundation executive but simply a layman—a son, husband, parent, and concerned citizen. I have been blessed with good health, so my personal involvement with the health care system has been minimal. But I have had more than enough opportunity to be deeply involved, emotionally and in every other way, in my responsibilities and relationships with brothers and sisters, parents, and friends. I have spent more hours than I care to remember at a hospital bedside, leaning on the wall of a hospital corridor, and sitting endlessly in a waiting room. I have sought information and assistance by asking, begging, cajoling, and threatening, in order to get a tidbit of information, a glimpse of the truth, a glimmer of understanding. I have experienced triumphs and tragedies, compassion, arrogance, selflessness, insensitive callousness, and both the brilliance and the pettiness of the caring professions. So the perspective I bring is that of a layman—a concerned individual, a grateful beneficiary, a constructive critic, an eager participant in the unending process of making the superb health system and situation we have today even more responsive, effective, and satisfying.

### Ideal Arrangement for Primary Care

Health professions educators are charged with key responsibilities in the preparation of the professionals who design, manage, and conduct the affairs of our health care system in its various components, institutions, and programs. They shape tomorrow. W. K. Kellogg said it well: "Education offers the greatest opportunity for really improving one generation over another." Health professions educators are vital participants in the selection and molding of physicians, nurses, pharmacists, dentists, and other health professionals of the future. They help to determine the criteria by which the tough decisions are made as to who is in and who is out; they shape the pattern of experiences to which·students are exposed and the rigors to which initiates are subjected; and they establish the criteria by which the success or failure of trainees is determined. Thus, ultimately, they influence the shape, the character, the personality, and the morality of what we call our health care system. We are grateful for the degree to which they succeed; we worry about the whys, the hows, and the so-whats of the job they do; and we are the beneficiaries, or the victims, of the consequences of their efforts.

Quite frankly, I have struggled with how I might approach the preparation of this chapter most productively. My first inclination was to approach the task as I always approach doctors and nurses—hat in hand, in awe, and in admiration of those who are privileged to serve and influence so intimately the human condition. Despite many experiences that abuse that idyllic image, to me there is no higher calling than the caring professions.

But I have chosen a different course. Quite simply, I leaned back in my chair and said, "Suppose I were a health professions educator. What would I do?" As a logical first step, I then pursued the question "If I could design it, what kind of a health care arrangement would I like for the Mawby family?" This is neither an idle nor an impulsive question; it is one I have been asking myself, members of our foundation program staff, and leaders in the health professions for a number of years. I have finally concluded that, ideally, I would have the Mawby family affiliated with a small group practice consisting of three or four family physicians, a pediatrician, and an obstetrician-gynecologist, working appropriately and in harmony with nurse practitioners, with a receptionist/bookkeeper, other support personnel in nursing and the allied health fields, and two dentists. This group would have appropriate privileges with community hospitals and referral arrangements with specialists. Philosophically, the group would be committed to a program of health promotion/disease prevention or health maintenance, as well as treatment of illness. Let us consider the implications of this model.

First, the core of the group would be three or four family physicians, concerned with the individual and with the family. When our family physician was away, we would be covered by one of the group partners who would have complete access to our health records. When warranted, these family practitioners would involve appropriate specialists for consultation and/or treatment.

They would be working in harmony with nurse practitioners. Very often my minor complaints do not require the attention or time of a board-certified specialist. I am quite content to be treated by a competent nurse practitioner, with confidence that if a problem is identified that requires further expertise, physician colleagues will be involved. It seems to me deplorable, in fact inexcusable, that the competence of the nursing profession is provided so little opportunity to contribute maximally to human health care. The public, I am convinced, would welcome such modification. The problem lies not with the consumers but in the professions and their working relationships, or lack thereof.

The pediatrician and the obstetrician-gynecologist would, of course, contribute their appropriate specialties to the group enterprise, as would the other health professionals. And the dentists? As a layman, I don't understand why the profession of dentistry is practiced in isolation—perhaps splendid isolation—but nonetheless isolation from the mainstream of the health care system. The problems of my teeth and my mouth are not isolated from the rest of me, and, I believe, can have an impact throughout my body. Thus, the failure of the professions to address this idiosyncrasy in the present pattern of practice is difficult to fathom.

And the emphasis on health promotion/disease prevention? Health professionals have designed a system that compensates them only for the treatment of my illness or injury. I can engage specialists to design and implement a preventive maintenance program for my air conditioner at home, or the elevator or duplicating machine at the office. In such a contractual arrangement, I always have responsibilities that I must fulfill if that contract is to be valid. In similar fashion, I would like to compensate a health care group for the design and the continued monitoring, with my full participation and fulfillment of my obligations and responsibilities, of a maintenance contract for my most precious possession—my health. Why have the health professions been so unimaginative, so uncreative, and so unresponsive in this area?

So that's a brief insight from a layman's perspective of one model of an ideal primary care arrangement. There can and should be many others, to provide primary care to diverse client groups in varied settings. That's as far as I will go here as a layman. Educators, who are the experts, will need to give further consideration to issues involved in providing secondary and tertiary levels of care, which offer the benefits of superb specialization and sophisticated technology and link primary care providers ultimately to the rich resources of research institutions and academic health centers. With modern communications technology, practitioners in even the most remote locations can be in touch with their colleagues for consultation and counsel on a continuing basis.

As a layman surveying today's health care scene, both in education and practice, I see the "bits and pieces" as superb. By that I refer to our professional schools in medicine, nursing, dentistry, pharmacy, administration, allied health, and all the rest; the professions, with dedicated and competent individuals and effective associations; the various practice settings, including solo and group offices, clinics, hospitals, and research and teaching centers. All are superb, without question the finest in the world.

But I have the uneasy feeling that too little thought and effort have been given to rationalizing the whole, with an objective of serving maximally the interests of the ultimate beneficiaries. The "total system" (this phrase sounds tidier, more prescribed, and more restrictive than intended or possible), with multiple alternatives and pluralism in every sense, should be particularly sensitive to the public it serves and by which it is sustained, subjugating the more selfish interests of professions and institutions to the higher purpose. We lack a "grand design" or a series of grand designs that bring together in the most effective ways the expertise of the various health professions and network more efficiently the resources of the health care institutions of our society. Wisely done, building on the terrific strengths of the day but responding objectively and sensitively to the demands and unmet needs of the public, the result surely would be far greater than the simple sum of the parts of which it is comprised.

It is educators who must meet the challenge to fulfill such a vision and goal. It is not enough to be simply a nurse educator or a medical educator. It is necessary to see the larger picture, with its strengths and shortcomings, and to move relentlessly toward the realization of the better situation. Universities, of which the schools of the health professions are a part, are the knowledge reservoirs of our society, established and sustained to preserve, create, and transmit knowledge. An unending challenge is that of mobilizing these knowledge resources in ever more effective ways to deal with the concerns of society.

While there is much in the health care scene in this country of which health professionals can be justifiably proud, there is still much "unfinished business." Hopefully, the health professions, with educators in the vanguard, will provide aggressive and imaginative leadership in addressing issues of concern, lest the responsibility fall by default to those less able.

## Requisites of an Effective Health Care Delivery System

In the health programming of the W. K. Kellogg Foundation, our health program team focuses on five issues: availability and access to health care; comprehensiveness and continuity; quality; cost containment and productivity; and health promotion/disease prevention/public health. Health professionals understand these issues and their ramifications so there's no need to elaborate in detail, but I will comment on each briefly since they relate so clearly to opportunities in education. Because the issues are so interrelated, I will not try to separate them artificially but simply touch on them in a natural sequence.

*Comprehensiveness and Continuity.* It may be appropriate to begin with a problem identified in the writings of Herodotus some 2,400 years ago. The Greek historian perceived a discontinuity of health care and practices, and he lamented, "Each physician treateth one part and not more. And everywhere is full of physicians; for some profess themselves physicians of the eyes, and others the head, others the teeth, and others of the parts about the belly, and others of obscure sicknesses."

Herodotus was correct in his view that a discontinuity of care can result from the trend toward overspecialization. Health care, offered or provided in a fragmented fashion, is difficult to deal with in itself, but the problem goes deeper. Often accompanying such specialized care is the problem of transfer of information between providers of care who unwittingly or worse, knowingly, inhibit the patient's access to comprehensive care.

Let me use a personal example to illustrate what I mean. My mother, by the time she reached her mid-seventies, had several different health problems, including cancer and complications from a series of strokes. In the course of her cancer treatment, she was shunted from one specialist to another, from internist to surgeon to radiologist to oncologist, none of whom really took a comprehensive look at her problems in order to assess her overall condition. The internist who diagnosed the problems initially refused to continue as her primary care physician, so the responsibility for continuity rested with the patient and her family, certainly an unsatisfactory assignment by default. We encountered another stumbling block—a great reluctance, and at times, refusal on the part of several physicians to transfer medical records of the care they gave my mother to other physicians who also were treating her. Consequently, examinations, tests, and procedures were duplicated unnecessarily, at inconveniences, discomfort, and cost. I understand the reasons given, but I do not accept the final result as adequate or defensible. There must be better ways. This example is not an isolated one. Friends and associates have told me similar stories, and everyone can surely add personal anecdotes of a similar nature.

Overspecialization and a lack of continuity in care are not problems confined to the practice of medicine. Specialization, some observers contend, has resulted from the implementation of technology in almost every field, forcing the individual to deal with an ever-increasing number of providers of service. The specialization of health education and health services is, in many ways, an achievement in America that we can be proud of. But at the same time, we must manage it so that it does not become an end in and of itself. If such specialization results in frustration and fragmented, incomplete patient care, it needs rethinking and rearranging.

What does this mean in terms of health professions educational reform? It means we must consciously and with determination move toward making the academic health center the focus for comprehensive, interprofessional education —education that begins to remove professional barriers that stand in the way of more effective, patient-centered health care. And it means encouraging student receptiveness to the kinds of joint practice arrangements that can ultimately bring improvements in clinical settings.

In the absence of an integrated approach such as might be provided by an academic health center, the responsibility keeps coming back to the individual schools that prepare dentists, nurses, physicians, allied health personnel, administrators, and public health professionals. These schools generally give their students only cursory exposure and limited sensitivity to health problems and care from the viewpoint of the patient. There are exceptions, of course, but too often related professional studies abruptly leave off with the important but limited process of taking a patient's personal history "for the record." This problem should be addressed by all health professional schools, and particularly by the medical school. The medical school has the responsibility of educating the key member of the health care delivery team. The physician is the quarterback, the chief executive officer (CEO), the guardian, and the gatekeeper, largely determining in what manner and with what emphases patient care is provided. Thus, the medical school plays a particularly crucial role in determining exactly what health care delivery is today and what it might be tomorrow. Even when academic health centers become well-developed in health professions education, the medical component will continue to be of special significance. Is it too much to hope that these schools and their graduates will increasingly pursue a statesmanship role of leadership, setting the highest of professional standards for patient-centered care and simultaneously encouraging and permitting other health professionals to contribute maximally?

As a part of the improvement of health care, attention must be directed at learning how new specialties in medical practice can be created to treat *human* problems, as well as defining society's needs to make the best use of those specialties once they are in place. An orderly system of limiting, monitoring, and coordinating specialty practice must be established. Certainly, the same responsibility falls on the other health professions schools, as we see more and more emphasis on new specialties within nursing, allied health professions, pharmacy, and dentistry.

My physician friends tell me that in many educational institutions, the social analysis aspects of health care are in the schools of public health. But they also admit that usually there is little relationship between what the schools of public health are seeing and what is happening in the medical, dental, or nursing educational process. Very few universities have, for example, what can be called a "Center for Health Services Research" that has a relationship to or an effect upon education of health professionals. This is linked to that grand design I mentioned earlier that should be a backdrop for professional education if care is to be comprehensive and continuous.

*Availability and Access.* Let me use a true story, slightly dramatized, to illustrate the issue of availability of and access to health care. Not long ago, on a visit to a county seat town in southern Michigan, I met with a group of young physicians. I asked them: "If the Mawby family moved to this area, could any of you take us on as new patients?" There was a quick consensus, "Oh, yes, Russ Mawby, president of the Kellogg Foundation, of course we will get you in."

"No, no," I said. "Russ Mawby, with a wife and three kids, living on forty acres south of town." Again there was quick agreement, "None of us is taking any new patients. You'll just have to go to the emergency room at the hospital."

I don't believe that is a satisfactory answer to primary care for families; emergency room care should be for emergencies, not serve as a usual point of entry for primary care.

Experts keep telling me that access to health care is a serious problem only for the urban poor and for people in remote, rural communities. But that simply is not true, if the measure we apply for adequacy goes beyond the most primitive or basic standard. In communities of all types, urban and rural, without regard to economic circumstances, many families have real difficulty in gaining access to satisfactory primary care on a continuing basis.

As a layman, I have observed that health professionals—in particular physicians, but to a degree all health professionals—have no problem gaining access to the health care system. If their child or mother or good friend needs to see a doctor, even a specialist who is booked six months in advance, there is no problem of access. I suspect this may be a fringe benefit that also extends to health professions educators. But don't let this lull you into a belief that this is therefore no problem for the rest of us, regardless of geographic, cultural, or economic circumstance.

While many medical schools believe they are addressing the problem of access to and availability of good medical care by increasing the numbers of graduates, simply increasing numbers does not go far enough. In simplistic terms, there are two problems: preparation of physician specialists in appropriate proportions and the geographic distribution of practitioners. Each needs to be addressed creatively and forthrightly. Part of the distribution problem may correct itself as numbers increase, but there are certainly further options. For example, of more direct benefit is the effort by some medical schools to expand residency experiences in small communities for graduate physicians.

Certain medical schools have also established agreements with incoming students that require that they, upon graduation, practice for two or three years in an underserved area in exchange for repayment of a student loan. Models such as the student loan program that the University of Illinois College of Medicine has had since 1950 with the Illinois Agricultural Association and the Illinois State

Medical Society must be continued and promoted. In addition, better information systems must be created that log data on those areas that need physicians, where physicians migrate upon graduation, and what kinds of things communities can do to attract doctors.

I can't help but think that the very pressing problems of maldistribution, and some would say actual shortage, of nurses also relate directly to health professions educational issues, specifically medical education. As a layman, I cannot understand, nor do I sympathize or have patience with, the kinds of "professional snobbery" that separate the health professions in both educational and clinical settings. For example, I do not understand the reluctance of the medical profession and the medical schools to take a more enlightened view toward recognizing the unrealized potential of nurses and other nonphysician health professionals in meeting the health care needs in this country. I suspect the elitism and separation that still characterize too much of physician education and care will not be tolerated much longer. This would seem particularly true as the public becomes more and more aware of how such parochialism is affecting the quality, availability, and cost of care in their communities.

Innovative approaches to encouraging physicians, nurses, dentists, and other health professionals to practice together more efficiently and effectively, including the provision of care in underserved areas and to unreached clientele, must continue to be supported so that all people, whether they be affluent or poor and whether they live in the city or the country, have access to *quality* health care.

*Quality Health Care.* Notice I said *quality* health care, certainly a persistent and basic concern of all. In recent years, not just in the practice of medicine, quality increasingly has come to be defined in terms of the application of high technology. We pride ourselves on making use of the latest equipment, procedures, and systems, whether in medicine, the auto industry, or communications. In the health field, this emphasis on technology can contribute to a failure by the professions to recognize that actual *practice* as an indicator of quality for common health problems may be just as good or better in the small, modestly equipped clinic as in the major medical center.

Medical schools have taken the lead in applying high technology to practice (as well they should), but they must not rush so far ahead that they forget the human dimension. The patient's perception of quality often hinges on how the physician treats the *person*, not just the medical *problem*. Despite statements by individual faculty members that they recognize this patient perception of the quality of care as contrasted with the physician's perception of care, most observers are unable to note much evidence of that recognition.

When someone has a coronary, the spouse does not walk into the hospital and ask, "What's the average length of stay?" But that yardstick has been valued too heavily as a primary measure of quality in hospital reviews. Instead, a loved one is likely to ask, "Is he (or she) in pain? Is he being kept comfortable? Is someone with him? May I see him?" Physicians and hospital administrators tend not to worry enough about those humanly critical gauges that are so significant, both to the patient and the family and to the patient's ultimate recovery.

There is a definite need for educators to give as much consideration to the patient's perspective on quality in practice as they give to health science and research. Many respected authorities have long called for increased attention to the humanities and social sciences as a means for instilling a concern for humane care in the budding physician, dentist, nurse, or pharmacist. Several schools now do this, but it is usually on an elective basis.

Just as concern for the whole human being is important to quality in the practice of health care, so too is concern for preventing illness, rather than solely responding to it after the fact. There is a good deal of talk about the benefits of jogging, careful diet, decreased smoking, reduction of stress, and so on. These actions, it is said, can lower the risk of heart attack or other health problems and improve overall well-being. But one expert says one thing; another says something else, even the opposite. People think they want to take responsibility for their own health, but they don't know what to believe and what to do.

*Health Maintenance.* Who's minding the store as far as *health promotion* and *disease prevention* are concerned? Is there an appropriate emphasis on preventive medicine in health professions schools today? My best information is no. Programs abound on preventing the common infectious diseases, but if one thinks of prevention in terms of heart disease, cancer, and similar serious concerns, it appears that we aren't making much headway in medical education.

For example, I am told that most departments of preventive medicine deal with community health problems having to do with the transmission of disease—sewer systems, infestations, and the like. Their actions focus broadly on the population rather than on the individual. For the most part, I understand that physicians are informed about nutritional requirements of infancy, with a goal of correcting of specific diseases and preventing contagious diseases from birth to about age fifteen. But educational emphases on adult nutrition and adult disease prevention, including that of the elderly, are weak at best. Our whole health care system, including patterns for reimbursement, needs rethinking if we intend to stress health maintenance as well as treatment of illness.

*Cost of Care.* Another question the public has begun to fire at the health professions with increasing intensity is: Why has the cost of health care outpaced almost everything else?

Each of us has an answer, but each may have a different answer. Undoubtedly, part of this increase can be attributed to the use of sophisticated, costly new technology in diagnostic, therapeutic, and supportive health care. Another portion must be attributed to the aggressive organizations of professional hospital staff and support workers seeking improved wages and working conditions. Still other causes are inflation's effects on the entire U.S. economy and precautionary reactions to the threat of malpractice litigation.

But the health care provider, specifically the physician, is a cause for part of the increased cost of care. The initiation of expenses to be incurred in health care rests with the physician. Some, in a position to know, claim too many patients are being admitted to the hospital for the convenience of the doctor. Though physicians cannot control the daily room cost once a patient is hospitalized, they do have control over the number of x-rays, the number and types of diagnostic or surgical procedures, the extent of rehabilitative measures ordered, the amount of medications prescribed, and the length of stay.

So what is called for? Two things, as starters. First, medical schools must work cost awareness and cost containment into their curriculum so physicians are prepared to make careful, discriminating choices among the various procedural tools available to them. This means learning to weigh benefits against costs, costs against personal convenience, and convenience against the patient's well-being. In turn, the physician must be convinced (and convincing) that these actions will provide good, appropriate care to people. Second, all health professionals must maintain the highest personal standards of self-discipline and conscientious execution of their assigned responsibilities in an atmosphere of cooperation. The physician is the key catalyst in the delivery of appropriate health care. Therefore, he or she must be educated and prepared to take the lead in cooperative and cost-effective approaches to delivery of health care.

Further, the physician can help overcome territorial possessiveness and "turf rivalries" in the delivery of quality care. The opportunities today are becoming more plentiful for teamwork that can vastly improve the efficiency and quality of care, as well as contribute positively to cost containment. A legion of new health professionals has joined the field: physicians' assistants, geriatric nurse practitioners, physician specialists in new areas, skilled nurses, and others. New practice opportunities exist in group practice, joint practice, and varied team approaches in delivering health care. Medical education should take the lead in grooming students to view cooperatively, not territorially, their responsibility as care providers. Quality care should be defined to include the patient's perspective, not simply the professional's own preferences or conveniences.

An attempt to set up working models for team practice experience at the undergraduate level might be premature because each student is overwhelmed with learning the basic knowledge and skills of that profession. But the establishment of good working models, mentorships, and practice experiences in cooperative care delivery in clinical education would seem well-advised. By then, the student has matured in skills, self-concept, and readiness; can integrate this team practice experience; and can enter professional practice freed of territorial constraints and attitudes. Such team skills can also be reinforced through carefully planned continuing education programs.

## Prime Responsibilities of the Privileged

Health professionals are a privileged group, compensated by society to an extent matched by few other professions or occupations. No one denies that health professionals have worked hard to enter their professions. However, we must also remember that while the medical or nursing or dental or pharmacy student pays a high price in terms of time, energy, and dollars, the overall education of the health professional is heavily subsidized by the people of this country, both from public sources via tax dollars and from private benefactors. Estimates on the financial contribution of students to their medical or dental education vary from about 5 percent to 50 percent of the total cost, depending upon whether the school attended is public or private and whether the experience does or does not include a broad range of practice experiences in a large medical center. Additionally, the health professional's primary *workplace*, the hospital, is most often subsidized by the public to a degree unmatched by any other profession. This arrangement implies an obligation by the health professions to use that setting in a judicious, responsible, and equitable manner for the benefit of all people, not a select few.

It remains the physicians' responsibility to practice their ageless, revered, and respected work in ways that will assure the perpetuation of such respect. The same can be said about the responsibility of all who choose the health professions.

## Priorities for Reform

In summary, let me suggest four topics that, from this layman's perspective, would have priority in health professions educational reform.

First, I would call for a comprehensive conceptual framework for health care delivery at all levels, including primary, secondary, and tertiary care, incorporating a major role for the teaching and research institutions. The most appropriate and productive roles for all health professionals—physicians, dentists, nurses, pharmacists, public health specialists, allied health personnel, and administrators—would be clarified. The vital contributions of the various specialties would be fully utilized but would not be permitted to distort the system. Educational programs, both in broad terms and in curricular detail, would then be made consistent with society's goals and needs as represented by this overall concept. It would not be a single national plan but a broad statement of purposes, principles, relationships, and roles.

Second, emphasis throughout the educational process would be related to the ultimate goal, that being a healthy population. The population would have health care services available and readily accessible, comprehensive and continuous in character, of appropriate quality, and with attention to cost and productivity. Emphasis would be placed on health promotion/disease prevention for the individual and public health programs for the community. The educational process, from its philosophical approach through tangible clinical experiences, would be patient-oriented.

Third, the curricula of the various health professions would be dramatically revised to provide for maximal interaction between faculty and students in both classroom and clinical settings, focused upon ways in which various members of the health care team should work together. A part of this curricular review process would also address the issue of appropriate training for specific roles, so that individuals are neither underqualified nor overcredentialed for the services they perform.

Finally, a lifelong pattern of learning, most likely in the form of continuing professional education, would be designed and implemented for all the health professions. The knowledge explosion that continues to accelerate in the health fields mandates this. As this concept is fully realized, the preprofessional and professional curricula would be more finely tuned, recognizing that everything known need not be squeezed into a four-, six-, or eight-year framework but could be addressed systematically over a longer period of time, as an individual practitioner's goals and responsibilities change. Such continuing education should be based on individualized professional needs and measured in terms of performance behavior, not simply units of lecture time before golf or on a cruise ship. Perhaps this development of a comprehensive approach to continuing professional education offers the greatest promise for addressing our society's health care concerns more effectively.

And now to return to my first observations: While there is much in our health care system in this country of which we can be proud and while, in fact, it is unequaled in the world, improvement is possible. There are shortcomings that need to be imaginatively addressed, and it is the health professions educators who will visibly shape tomorrow.

In most areas of human concern, "we *know* better than we *do*." Certainly this is true in the education of professionals for health care. A great deal more is known about what good health care could be—and should be—than is generally put to use. The unending challenge to educators is to move reality closer to the vision of what ought to be.

# 24

*Alexander M. Schmidt*

# Challenges to
# Academic Health Centers

The title of Part Four, "Policy Recommendations for Improving Health Professions Education," could hardly be more appropriate to this time of transition and change at the health sciences center from which I come. I find it interesting, even a bit ironic, that our College of Medicine at the University of Illinois is celebrating its centenary in part by conducting a major study of its function and form. One might think that after a hundred years, we would have that right! In addition, the recent decision by our board of trustees to consolidate the Medical Center and the Chicago Circle campuses of the University of Illinois is causing all of us, or at least those of us in university administration, to reexamine closely the relationships between our health sciences center and the other parts of our parent university. As if these studies were not enough, the current downward trend in the financing of health care for the medically indigent is forcing us to consider, once again, the difficult and complex questions of why a university is in the health care business and how a university should obtain the dollars and patients necessary to the successful operation of a large, university-owned hospital and clinic. Of all these issues, perhaps the last is the most serious in the short run; it is the one on which attention will be focused in this chapter.

Given so widely encompassing a topic as "the institutional setting in which health professions education occurs and the need for change in organizational, managerial, and decision-making structures and processes within that institution," the natural inclination is to range far too widely, treat too many aspects of the subject, make too many overly general declarations, and so conclude nothing of specific value. After several tentative forays into the subject during which I could see no boundaries, I finally decided arbitrarily to limit myself to one area wherein lies one of the most important and, I think, obligatory changes that health sciences centers must make in order to survive and be relevant to the coming two decades. The subject I chose is the health care activities of a university—how they have been changing in the past couple of decades, what purposes they should serve, and what they should be in the future.

## Health Sciences Centers and Health Care Delivery

In discussing a university's involvement in the delivery of health care, I intend to reflect the views of an administrator who worries daily about some rather mundane problems of a health sciences center. I worry, for example, about having enough money to make the next hospital payroll. I worry about whether we can afford to fund our Center for Educational Development at its current level. And I even worry about whether there is any connection between our affording our hospital payroll and how faculty in the Center for Educational Development spend their time. Authors of preceding chapters have addressed a wide range of social, scientific, and technical developments that have had an impact on health care in recent years and that will necessitate change in the future. Our concern here is that our future educational programs must respond to these developments by producing new and different kinds of health professionals, capable of working in different practice settings, trained to do new and different things so as to be able to function effectively in the eighties and nineties and to be more successful in improving the public's health than they have been in the past.

I believe that most academic health sciences centers, even those recognizing the need for change, are ill-equipped to respond to the need for certain changes in our educational system. We can respond effectively in most of the purely scientific areas. For example, we are doing well in molecular biology because we have faculty with the requisite knowledge and interest and we have the laboratories in which faculty can work. Faculty enthusiastically recruit students to the field, so that the coming decades will see continued advances in this area. In the health care arena, however, the picture is different. We are not responding well to the need for significant changes in the delivery of health care. As just one example, we seem to know neither how many health professionals of what kind we should be producing nor what effect on health care costs our decisions about health manpower production might have. Our laboratories for studying such issues, the university owned or operated hospitals and clinics, are in serious trouble. What is worse, we have very few faculty in those laboratories engaged in health services research or recruiting students to the field. We rarely apply the results of the health services research we do to the educational process so that our students can become better practitioners than we are today.

My thesis, then, is that health sciences centers are not responding too well to our nation's need for a critical examination of our health care system, in part because we are not doing very well in the business of health care, but mainly because we do not have a cadre of faculty studying how to improve our delivery of health care and, from that knowledge, influencing our educational system.

## University Hospital vis-a-vis Community Hospital

The reasons for our health sciences centers being in this undesirable position are worth a brief review. I would like to begin with a discussion of our principal clinical "laboratory," the university hospital. During the past twenty years, the most notable development in health professions education has been the dramatic expansion of our educational programs. We have increased greatly the numbers of students graduating from our health sciences centers and, significantly, the numbers completing specialty training. In so doing, we have expanded our campus facilities; in addition, we have gone off our traditional campuses to establish regional "mini–health sciences centers," such as the University of Illinois has done in Rockford and Peoria. Also, we have affiliated with many privately owned community hospitals, assisting them to become teaching centers in their own right. This has been a most significant development, with consequences hardly anticipated fifteen to twenty years ago. We did not realize that we were creating our future competition, institutions that soon would outdo us in the delivery of health care (Cluff, 1982; Frank, 1980; Shapiro, 1981).

The numerous graduates of our expanded medical school classes became, in turn, our residents, fellows, and clinical trainees. Then, in large numbers, having become superbly trained in their specialties, they went to our affiliated hospitals—the large, private community hospitals—where they established excellent medical and surgical services. In a relatively short time, academic health sciences centers trained and sent out across the nation tens of thousands of very fine practicing specialists who could do for their patients in private hospitals everything that could be done for the patient's benefit in a university owned or operated teaching hospital. Often, they could do better, and they could do more. Further, the orientation of the private hospital to the efficient delivery of health care, combined with skillful marketing of their health services, made the modern private community hospital attractive to patients who could get the best of health care in a pleasing setting from an accommodating staff.

The rapidly increasing costs of in-hospital care in modern, private settings were borne largely, and relatively cheerfully it seemed, by the government, by employers, and by private insurers, who were at the same time seemingly reluctant to pay for outpatient care. As a result, physicians freely admitted their patients to hospitals, and patients began to expect to enter hospitals for practically any diagnostic, therapeutic, or even restful purpose. As a result, a number of private hospitals became rich. The policy of reimbursing hospitals for costs or charges has provided hospitals having a large percentage of insured patients the ample funds with which to expand, modernize, and, recently, lead in the acquisition of technology. Given this reimbursement policy, it is not surprising that hospital costs account for the largest fraction of our health dollar and that inflation of hospital costs has exceeded that of most other parts of the economy, far outstripping the general price indexes.

All this time, medical, nursing, and other schools on health sciences campuses, needing to expand and regionalize their educational programs and wanting their students to learn in a variety of settings, have been affiliating with these private community hospitals. We have provided faculty appointments for qualified members of private hospital staffs, who, after all, were our former students, residents, and fellows. We have sent our students, residents, and fellows to the private hospitals, to be taught by the clinical faculty in the "private setting." In a relatively short period of time, some of these private community hospitals have indeed become teaching hospitals, equaling or exceeding university owned or operated hospitals in their ability to care for patients and teach the practical aspects of health care.

But the inevitable result of the growth, development, and enrichment of private community hospitals has been the decline of many university owned or operated hospitals as referral centers. University hospitals, not long ago the models of the best and the latest in medical practice, can no longer be assumed to be on the "cutting edge" of health care. Now, often, larger private community hospitals are the first to obtain the expensive new technologies, and many of them do more tertiary care and do it better than the nearby university hospital. Several private hospitals in Chicago had CT scanners before either the University of Illinois or Cook County Hospitals because the private hospitals had either the necessary cash or the ability to borrow it, and we did not. Several private hospitals in the Chicago area already are planning the purchase of a nuclear magnetic resonance imager, waiting only to be reasonably certain that they will not waste a million dollars on a useless technology. In most large cities, there now are one or more private community hospitals that do more cardiovascular surgery, more organ transplants, and more radiation therapy—to name but a few examples—than the nearby university hospital.

More recently, we have seen another important development. Many private community hospitals, having modernized and expanded their facilities, having acquired the newest equipment for their staffs, and having developed teaching programs, still have sufficient capital financing to enable them to acquire or build such other health care facilities as ambulatory care centers or surgicenters, to form consortia, and even to "spin off" conglomerates of various kinds. Many private hospitals have been able to finance the planning and initiation of their own Health Maintenance Organizations (HMOs). Many now employ advertising agencies, market research firms, and even real estate developers to help maintain or expand their health care domains. By taking such steps, the hospitals have begun actually to control their markets and thus insure their future, while endangering ours.

Some university hospitals, but only a very few, have kept pace with these developments. By and large, those that have are teaching hospitals owned by private colleges and universities or public universities in smaller cities, where by tradition, the teaching hospital has been self-supporting via referred "paying patients," and where substantial support for the educational program has had to come from health care dollars. Even these few university hospitals are suffering from increasing competition for patients and referrals and are having difficulty staying solvent. Most publicly owned university hospitals in large cities, having a tradition of caring for indigent patients and being supported by tax dollars, have not kept pace with these developments and so are in varying degrees of financial programmatic difficulty. By programmatic difficulty, I mean not having the right numbers or types of patients needed for clinical teaching and research, not having the resources to deliver the most advanced care, and not supporting needed health services research.

## New Research Role for Health Sciences Centers

Invariably, at this point in discussions such as this, someone offers the suggestion that perhaps, then, the private community hospitals have become and should be the teaching hospitals of the future. My answer to that is "No, they shouldn't, and they can't be." It is true that private, community hospitals have become an important teaching resource and partner to the academic health sciences center. They can be great places to teach and learn the current mode of health care and to learn the art of medicine from expert practitioners. But, to return to the question of our ability to respond to future health care needs, most private hospitals will not and cannot perform one of the necessary functions of a university: research—in this instance, clinical research and health services research. For a private community hospital to do such research would often run contrary to their operating principles and would require the presence of faculty not often found in the private setting. In fact, such faculty are found all too seldom in the university setting.

In the clinical sciences, we have traditionally expected faculty to sit on the three-legged stool—to teach, to do research, and to practice their profession. Research done by clinical faculty, for the most part, is either preclinical work in the basic science or animal laboratory or else it is clinical research directed at elucidating disease mechanisms and modes of therapy. We have very few faculty in health sciences centers engaged in health services research.

The clinical practice of most full-time faculty consists of caring for the patients who present themselves or who are referred to the medical center. Often that care is given more by house staff than by faculty. This incidental type of practice is about all that many faculty want to do, have time to do, or can be expected to do, given their other activities. This limitation of faculty who engage seriously in the practice of medicine and while practicing study the delivery of health care presents the academic health sciences center with a serious problem. The absence of such faculty means that the academic health sciences center cannot contribute much to the solution of the many problems surrounding the organization and delivery of health care, such as rapidly escalating costs. The lack of such faculty means that the university hospital will have a hard time gaining in the competition for patients with private community hospitals.

The scarcity of faculty engaged in the systematic study of the organization of health care, its delivery, and its effects on patients, families, and the health status of the American people is not new. Probably it has always existed, but it has not mattered quite so much. I know from personal experience, however, that it has existed for more than twenty years, as I can easily illustrate with two brief stories.

Around twenty years ago, during the early days of the Great Society programs of Lyndon Johnson when there seemed to be lots of money for health programs, someone conceived the idea of starting a new national institute within the National Institutes of Health. The new institute was to be the National Institute for Health Services Research and Development. Just as the existing institutes supported the science of health care, the new institute would investigate the caring part of health care—how health could be maintained, how people could be convinced to care for themselves better, how sick people could be cared for more efficiently and effectively and at lower cost, how health professionals should be educated and trained, in what numbers, for what health-related professions, and so on. President Johnson, by nature an enthusiast, loved the idea; shortly there were plans to start the new institute and to make it as important to the delivery of health care as the other institutes were to the science of health care. It was intended that, eventually, the new institute would be funded at a level equal to all the other institutes combined, if you can believe that. Perhaps most important of all, the new institute was to fund training programs for faculty interested in health services research. Ample funds were provided for start-up, the institute was begun, and a search was launched for a director. In a short time, the institute became the National Center for Health Services Research and Development, a name perhaps familiar to you. But whatever the name, the program never really got off the ground, for a very interesting reason that I will outline shortly. Similar circumstances impeded the growth and development of my other example, Regional Medical Programs (RMP). Originally, it was intended that RMP would have a far greater impact on the health services system of this country than on universities and continuing medical education. However, the early promise of RMP was lost, just as with the National Center for Health Services Research and Development.

While explanations of such program failures are obviously complex, involving politics, competition for power and money, and so forth, I think it fair to say that both RMP and the National Center for Health Services Research and Development suffered from a fatal inability to find worthy people and projects in the health services area to support. I can remember clearly when RMP had $150 million with which to support improvements in the delivery of health care, and we couldn't identify projects worth spending it on. I can remember the first Director of the National Center for Health Services Research and Development making a similar complaint. Finally, both RMP and the National Center for Health Services Research and Development began to fund such expensive technology as cobalt machines for cancer therapy, in part so as to have something to show Congress for the money appropriated to the programs. If these two programs were initiated again today, I think that the end result might well be the same, as we still don't have faculty interested in or capable of studying the delivery of health care.

### Implementing the New Agenda

In the immediate post-*Sputnik* period, we need a new generation of physicists, doing a different brand of physics. So this nation first produced a new breed of physics teachers who, in turn, produced a new generation of physicists capable of putting a man on the moon. I suspect we need to do a similar thing in medicine today if we are to solve any of the health care problems we all are so familiar with and about which we have been hearing so much. What our new breed of faculty should do is well-described in the last chapter of George Miller's latest book (1980). In discussing the future of health education research and future directions for that research, Miller quotes from a provocative paper written by Richard Magraw and his colleagues (Magraw, Fox, and Weston, 1978), in which Magraw suggests a research agenda for the future. The agenda includes several items of obvious great importance:

• Study of the relationships between what is learned in health professions education and the effect of professional intervention on the care of individual patients and the health status of the American people
• Studies of the effects of educational programs aimed at diminishing profes-

sional and disciplinary insularity on practice patterns and, subsequently, on the health status of the population served

- Analysis of the lack of attention given to preventive health measures in health professions education, in professional practice, and by the public
- Studies relating financing and reimbursement policies for education and practice to the educational system, practice patterns, and health status
- Analyses to provide a better understanding of how health services research can influence changes in education practices, health status, and relief from discomfort

This, of course, is an awesome agenda, but if health sciences centers had had the faculty to begin such studies twenty years ago, then the National Center for Health Services Research and Development and Regional Medical Programs would have funded the work. Certainly, if that had been the case, our health sciences centers today would differ from what they are, and our hospitals would most likely be more competitive than they are now.

To me, then, a major change in health sciences centers needed for the future is first to develop significant numbers of faculty who can and will use their professional practice and the university hospital as their laboratory, studying how they can better practice, how to better assure the health of the public, and how our curricula can reflect that knowledge.

Whenever I get this far in a discussion, I am usually asked how I would reward such faculty, the reward system in academia being related to productivity in more basic scientific research. My answer always is "I'd pay them well." Such faculty would, undoubtedly, more than earn their keep, and if academic traditionalists deny them traditional academic rewards, then money should make up for that loss. It goes without saying that universities will have to be both imaginative and flexible in fostering the development of various kinds of service plans, using the service money earned to reward practicing faculty and support their health services research. To return full circle, universities will have to provide the clinical facilities—the laboratories—in which these faculty can work.

Obviously, universities have much to learn right now from their affiliated private community hospitals, including such basics as how to care for patients and get paid for doing it, how to tap financial markets, how to market services, how to diversify, and all the rest of what now is necessary to be in the business. Beyond simple emulation, however, I believe universities should renegotiate their affiliation agreements, forming alliances that go beyond the sending out of medical students, to include the exchange of clinical faculty and clinical programs. We probably should develop health service partnerships that would include both the community and the university hospital in a health care consortium. Staff memberships and admitting privileges in university hospitals can reward part-time faculty, who may well bring to the university hospital patients whom they would not previously have sent there. Our affiliated community hospitals could become part of the research base of our new full-time faculty, who might practice part-time in the community hospital, thus learning about health care as it is practiced in community hospitals and then, subsequently, improving upon that practice. Such faculty, in time, ought to be able to tackle Magraw's research agenda and, in the process, improve the university's teaching and health care programs.

This is the direction in which academic health sciences centers should move. Their centers for educational development should assist in developing new faculty, to foster the conduct of the needed research.

## References

Cluff, L. E. "Medical Schools, Clinical Faculty and Community Physicians." *Journal of the American Medical Association,* 1982, *247* (2), 200-202.

Frank, D. J. "Developing Marketing Strategies for University Teaching Hospitals." *Journal of Medical Education,* 1980, *55,* 574-579.

Magraw, R. M., Fox, D. M., and Weston, J. L. "Health Professions Education and Public Policy: A Research Agenda." *Journal of Medical Education,* 1978, *53,* 539-546.

Miller, G. E. *Educating Medical Teachers.* Cambridge, Mass.: Harvard University Press, 1980.

Shapiro, A. P. "Universities, Medical Schools and Hospitals—Can They Coexist?" *Perspectives in Biology and Medicine,* 1981, *24* (2), 169-188.

# 25

*Ronald W. Richards*

# Challenges to Health Professions Educators

Health professions education is but a subsystem of our larger society and world. It is at any moment like a rowboat, being swept along by turbulent, larger waves that are a cauldron of multidirectional, smaller waves. It is possible, however, to grasp a sense of direction from contradictory currents and to seek to influence the swirling societal forces that comprise the larger context. Fully aware of the frequent admonition that only fools try to predict the future, the purpose of this chapter is, nonetheless, to make some observations about health professions education in the 1980s and 1990s, as the basis for offering recommendations regarding policy directions for academic health centers.

In recent decades, the public mood in the United States supported the improvement of health care through improved access to the health care system. The means to this goal consisted in a removal of the cost barriers and an expansion of the system—expansion of research capabilities, expansion of the knowledge base, expansion of health care facilities, expansion of the number and types of health professionals. Our economic wealth was considered sufficient to expand the health care system, with little or no regard for financial cost. The outcome of this frenetic governmental activity has been a larger, more costly, but fundamentally unchanged system for delivering health care. The legacy that this expansionary period has left is an oversupply of hospital beds, indiscriminate use of high-cost technology, and a perceived oversupply of health professionals. At the same time, there are indications that we are a healthier population. Infant mortality rates, for example, have steadily decreased, and our life expectancy has increased. Whether there is a cause-effect relationship between the expansion of the health care system and the improvements in the state of societal health remains a matter of conjecture. Nonetheless, our health care system is larger, more entrenched, and more expensive.

For the most part, the recent history of health care has been guided by the "inner" demands of medicine. During the last half century, the progress of medical knowledge formed a scientific juggernaut that took its directions from what might be done. The nature of our health care system in the future will be hammered out under the influence of many forces, interacting with the interests of the educational and health care institutions. This concluding chapter presents a review of those societal forces, followed by an analysis of the health professions and their educational institutions as they face the future. Some recommendations for directions for health professions education are then offered.

## Influences of Society

Certain societal forces are considered to be particularly important in affecting the environment within which health professions education must respond and to which it must adapt. For convenience, these forces have been categorized as demographic, technological, sociopolitical, or economic, though it is clear that such categories are by no means discrete.

*Demographic Forces.* The most significant demographic change affecting health care in the United States for the next twenty years will be that of the increasing age of the population. By the year 2000, more than 20 percent of the population will be over sixty-five years of age. Heart disease, arthritis, and rheumatism will be the predominant chronic diseases of this more aged population. Chronic diseases of the musculoskeletal system will increase if the incidence of heart disease continues to decline as is expected (Winklestein, see Chapter Nineteen). Therefore, the health care system will have greater demands for both acute and chronic care placed upon it to meet the needs of elderly patients.

*Technological Forces.* There has been and will continue to be dramatic progress in science and technology. New knowledge about biophysical processes, as exemplified by the advances in genetics, has the potential to modify significantly the approaches to diagnosis and treatment. Technological improvements in such areas as computerized axial tomography and nuclear magnetic resonators for use in body imaging will continue to influence health care systems. Technological breakthroughs in information processing and transmission via such systems as microcomputers, random access videodiscs, and interactive television, all at lower costs, will sooner or later significantly change the way health care and education are provided.

Accomplishments in science and technology as well as belief in the benefits to be derived from them have been, in part, responsible for the specialization of health care. This American commitment to, and fascination with, high technology should be expected to continue and so too will the pressures for further specialization and subspecialization of health care and health professions education.

*Sociopolitical Forces.* Public policy is influenced by those values about which there is a broad-based consensus. In the post–World War II period, the question of equitable access to basic living and educational standards became fused with the liberal concept of society. For the first time, it seemed that resources would be sufficient to satisfy need. This belief was transformed into policy in the health care sector, perhaps more than in any other sector of society. Today, the vision of unlimited economic wealth has been largely supplanted by one of contracting financial and other resources. The values, therefore, concerning equity of access to health care will need to take account of this economic picture.

As always, the nature of our health care system will be heavily influenced by the magnitude of the consensus about how much we want to spend and in what ways. The likely answer to this question is not discernible. The direction of our changing societal value consensus—if it is changing—is far from apparent at one moment. Our American dependence on government as an instrument of distributive justice seems to be moderating. Evidence might be the deregulation of various sectors of business, industry, and health care, and the reductions in governmental expenditures for human services program. There is emphasis on the high cost of health care, a problem that is seen by some as soluble by unleashing the forces of competition, thus treating health care as a commodity. The concern for equity, social need, and health care as a right has been tempered. Some warn that "our fragmented specialization and our reliance on ad hoc pragmatism (endangers) the consensus on basic values which binds our fragile civilization together" (Overholt, 1983, p. 2). Whether this shift is temporary or indicative of a permanent trend remains to be seen. There is evidence to suggest, however, that it may be temporary and *not* based on fundamental shifts in our value consensus. Rather, it may be a phase of reaction and political opportunism. Navarro (1982) reports that several independent public opinion polls do not support claims of a broad-based public mandate against the general provision of health care and other services. Our speculation is that the public is taking a more sophisticated stance than simple rejection of the underlying fundamental values. Instead, there appears to be acknowledgement that choices must be made, realizing that not all people can indiscriminately receive all that is available. Secondly, the conclusion has been reached that existing health care structures are inefficient and unnecessarily costly. People have simply concluded that they should expect more for their money.

Aside from the question of what will be the value consensus upon which public policy in health care will be formulated, another sociopolitical factor will be the relative political influence of the proportionately greater number of aged voters and the proportionately smaller number of wage earners who, obviously, also will be voters. In the United States, politicians are very pragmatic, for the most important objective is to be elected and then reelected. This objective can generally be achieved by taking as much credit as one can for things the voters like, while at the same time avoiding responsibility for things they don't like. Such political tightrope walking is never easy, but it may become more difficult. The continuing debate over the long-term fiscal viability of the social security system in the United States exemplifies the problem. Politicians will need to support the demands for more health care as well as for other human services. At the same time, the wishes of wage earners as reflected in such constituent groupings as industry, commerce, unions, and consumer groups will continue to modulate the political process as they always have. Thus, the increased needs of the aged, combined with their growing influence in the political system, will lead to greater demands that will have to be met. At the same time, there will be fewer wage earners to pay the bills.

*Economic Forces.* Under the general rubric of economics, there are three factors that appear likely to have considerable impact on health care and health professions education. They are the increasingly higher costs of health care, the resulting massive size of the health care system, and changing manpower needs. The health care system in the United States now consumes approximately 10 percent of the gross national product (GNP), compared to less than 5 percent in the early 1950s (Gibson and Waldo, 1981). The important question that must be—indeed, will be—answered is: How much are we willing to spend? Certainly in relative terms and perhaps in absolute terms, the amount expended for health care can be expected to be less in the next twenty years than it was in the past twenty years. In Hadley's (see Chapter Eighteen) phraseology, we have moved from "more is more" to "less is less." Whether we move on to "less is more" remains to be seen. Nonetheless, an increasing demand for health care services and a decreasing willingness to pay will bring about changes in the health care system.

Any enterprise that consumes 10 percent of the U.S. GNP is, simply put, gigantic. Its power and influence are formidable. Obviously, the character of health care in the future will be affected by the inertia of this massive existing structure. As has been pointed out in Part One of this book, the character of social reform in the United States has been conservative. Existing social structures have not been regarded as in need of major revision. Any significant structural modification in the health care system would require a coalescing of public mood that it should be changed and a reconfiguration of political power structures so that it could be changed.

One popular approach to determining policy directions for health professions education is to prepare manpower projections. The first step is usually a determination of the health care needs, followed by a derivation of the numbers and types of health personnel required to fill those needs. There are serious limitations to the use of the concept of health care needs as a policy-making tool, including its "reliability, validity, and feasibility of implementation" (see Klarman, Chapter Sixteen). Need in the abstract is probably less useful than the economic concept of demand, an operationalization of need that includes the costs people are willing to pay. Factors to be considered in predicting supply are the balance of pecuniary and nonpecuniary rewards of a particular health profession, tuition costs relative to long-term financial returns, and changes in third-party insurance structures and reimbursement formulas. All things considered, it is expected, for example, that there will be no increase, and possibly a decrease, in the number of dentists. There will be an increase in the number of physicians. Depending on the general economic situation, there may be a shortage of practicing nurses. If so, it will not be because of limited nursing school capacity; rather, the nursing shortage will be the result of continued turmoil within the profession. Wages are too low, stresses are high, and nonpecuniary rewards are minimal. The extent of nursing's control over its own profession and its general professional status are in question. If it turns out that there is a continued shortage of nurses, the expansion of nursing education does not appear to be the preferred solution (see Klarman, Chapter Sixteen).

The accuracy of such projections is not of as crucial concern as the recognition that projections will not influence policy as much as they did in the past.

There are two factors associated with this conclusion: (1) manpower projections, based upon perceptions of needs and how to meet them, are fundamentally subjective in nature; and (2) projections of manpower needs will have different effects on public policy under contracting, as opposed to expanding, circumstances. Manpower projections serve more to rationalize policy decisions than to provide the independent and rational basis for judgment that they claim to furnish. In decisions regarding increasing or decreasing enrollments or the addition or elimination of programs, it is seductively simple to turn to quantitative statements of over- or undersupply. However, the essentially subjective nature of such estimates cannot be escaped. In expansionary periods, the logic that certain health care problems are seen to be due, in part, to manpower shortages and that, therefore, more health manpower should be produced serves the interests of health professions educational institutions. The reverse logic, perceived as not being in the best interests of health professions education and the health professions, is likely to be more of a problem, especially in nonexpansionary periods. That is, if such health care problems as high costs are seen to be due, in part, to manpower surpluses and, therefore, less health manpower should be produced, it obviously does not follow that the various health professions educational institutions and the professions will line up for self-sacrifice.

## Health Professions and Their Educational Institutions

Several of the important forces that will be at work in influencing the future character of the health care system and, therefore, health professions education have been noted. These forces will interact with the internal dynamics of each health profession and its educational institutions, as well as with the collectivity of these educational institutions and health care delivery systems known as academic health centers.

Health professions educators have been justifiably buoyant over their extraordinary achievements in expanding the output of their schools. Now they face increasingly complex circumstances and some hostility from the public they serve and upon whom they depend. The environment has changed, but for health professions and their educational institutions, the dominant interest continues to be, not surprisingly, the search for and maintenance of professional status and control.

The dynamics of professionalization of the health professions are not unique. They are characteristic of all occupations. Bledstein (1976), for example, contends that democracy and professionalism are mutually supportive. Discussing professionalism in the late nineteenth century, Bledstein states, "Professionalism was also a culture which embodied a more radical idea of democracy than even the Jacksonian had dared to dream. . . . The mid-Victorian as professional person strove to achieve a level of autonomous individualism, a position of unchallenged authority heretofore unknown in American life" (pp. 87–88). The authority of the professional rests in the ability to "release nature's potential and rearrange reality on (scientific) grounds" (p. 90). Professionals thus acquire power through their control of "a magic circle of scientific knowledge which only the few specialized by training and indoctrination are privileged to enter" (p. 90).

Conditions during the past twenty years have provided a field day for further professionalization of health occupations. Professional status and the autonomy, control, and financial security that come with it can be achieved, in part, by the manipulation of the educational system for the profession. Public perception of an unlimited need for more and different kinds of health professionals provided the impetus for the creation of a wide array of new educational programs and the enlargement of the content of existing ones. One consequence was the creation of "magic circles of scientific knowledge," available only to a privileged few. The educational changes that occurred reveal no doubts about the underlying nature of the health professions or of the health care system itself. If an extended period of formal training and a distinctive body of knowledge were the means to more professional control and status, then both could be arranged with relative ease.

The interests of the health professions in acquiring higher status through formalization and specialization of function and training are compatible with the nature of academic institutions in the United States. Quoting Bledstein (1976) again, "the cultural demands upon higher education in America, especially the university, compelled it to be far more flexible and diversified than European systems. Any occupation and any subculture of American life achieved recognition and status when it became deserving of study as a professional and academic science with its distinct theory and intellectual requirements" (p. 125).

The basic organizational structures of higher education lend themselves to specialization because of the reductionist ways in which academicians have come to carry on their work. These work patterns have been nurtured by the professional socialization of academicians in times of generous research support. Reductionism shapes the character of academic interaction and, most importantly, its reward systems. Innovation in a pervasively reductionist academic environment, therefore, is mostly achieved by making subspecialties out of specialties and by creating new specialties. Such is the case whether the desired change lends itself to organizational compartmentalization or not. Primary care, community medicine, and public health are notable examples of the phenomenon. The fundamental structure is not changed; it merely acquires a new appendage, usually a new department, center, program, or even a college. Ironically, then, when societal needs call for integrating the pieces into a whole, the processes of internal differentiation in higher education tend to make the institutions even less socially responsive.

Both the formalization and legitimation of occupations through association with universities and the internal differentiation of academe are in evidence in the case of the health professions. Certainly the natural tendencies of professions for self-preservation and the inclinations of higher education in academic health centers toward specialization will be as strong in the future as they have been in the past, but the conditions have changed sufficiently so as to expect that the outcomes might be different. What will not change is the extent to which the roles of the other health professions are determined in the end by what the medical profession regards as in its best interests. As in the past, the future of the other health professions depends, for the most part, on what the physicians want it to be. The challenge for the health professions and their educational systems will be role redefinition, especially in relation to each other. For some, it will be a matter of fighting hard to preserve the level of status and control achieved in recent years. For others, it may be a matter of survival.

## Directions for Health Professions Education

Public opinion, as it affects policy directions, is usually clearer about what are perceived to be the problems than about what solutions should be pursued. With regard to health care, our analysis suggests that the perceived problems are that the present health care system is too costly, that the health care needs of our increasingly aging population are not and will not be adequately met, and that our present system is unnecessarily fragmented. There is no consensus evident regarding how these problems should be addressed. To complicate things further, medicine has changed and has yet to accommodate itself to those changes. There has been extraordinary achievement in the diagnosis and treatment of disease, so much so that medicine must now face more extensive problems of chronic illness. Regrettably, medicine and the health care system have not fully realized the implications of their own success.

Human, organizational, and societal behavior are based upon some set of values or beliefs about what is good or what is right. "Whether induced by internal or external circumstances," says Callahan (1977), "every major social change in a society forces a confrontation with its values. Nowhere is this more evident than in the changes that have been wrought in medicine" (p. 23). We are again being influenced by major social change and, therefore, confronting our values regarding health care. The kind of health care system we have, its accessibility, its equity, and the proportion of our resources it receives are all a reflection of basic values about what we regard as right. Many ethicists, humanitarians, health professionals, and academicians muse about the need to have panels of "experts" systematically determine our health care–related values. Doing so is seen to be a prerequisite to achievement of a rational health policy and, ultimately, a more rational health care system. Examining and establishing our societal values regarding health care must be done, but doing so by way of a tribunal of our greatest thinkers gathering to reach judgment is simply not the way our sociopolitical system works, and it will not be cajoled by criticism into working that way. There is a value-based rationality to the way our society establishes public policy. It is a rationality of pragmatic political realities, not of academic abstraction and linear decision analysis. Our collective value consensus is a perpetually renegotiated compromise among multiple value positions of a myriad of interest groups.

Academic health centers constitute one of those groups. Academic health centers can and should take a position. As Pellegrino (see Chapter Fifteen) points out, considering the extent of the present policy shifts regarding all of society and, certainly, health care, "notably absent are the voices of the academic health centers . . . . Academic health centers have a responsibility that goes beyond mere adaptation and compliance." They must reexamine the values that underlie policy decisions in health and take a stand. At a minimum, that stand must include a reaffirmation of our belief in the value of every human life and of our concern for the quality of that life; it is this belief that leads academic health centers to speak out in total opposition to the escalation of the nuclear arms race as a threat to the safety of the human race. In addition, academic health centers must reemphasize their belief in the right of all people to equal access to health care and health professions education.

In the cumbersome process of representative democracy, sooner or later American society will determine what it will do about the acutely felt health care problems and who should do it. How academic health centers and, more broadly, all of health professions education will respond to these changing societal expectations is not at all clear. Health professions education may opt to take a leadership role in a major restructuring of the health care system. If it does, it is hard to imagine these institutions being denied the opportunity to take such leadership. On the other hand, it would be less surprising if health professions educators chose a more reactive mode, watching from the sidelines as the changes take shape. Either way, accomplishment of new public policy directions in health care, regardless of what they are, would be difficult without the participation of academic health centers.

Either by action, reaction, or inaction, the many components and, therefore, the whole of health professions education will acquire a direction. I will now make some recommendations regarding what that direction should be. These recommendations derive, in part, from analysis of the past and the potential determinants of the future. Many of the sources of these ideas are found in previous chapters. In addition, these policy recommendations are heavily influenced by conclusions reached at a special working conference on directions for health professions education in the 1980s and 1990s, to which leaders from all health professions education contributed. The recommendations are presented in two categories, in answer to two fundamental questions: How should the health professions educational model be changed? What should health professions educators do to influence public policy regarding health care?

*Changing the Approach to Health Professions Education.* All health professions education is strongly influenced by the prevailing biophysical paradigm of medicine, by the priority that must be given health care services in the settings used for clinical training, by the economics of health care delivery, and by the prominent role of the hospital in health care delivery and education.

For over a century and a half, perceptions of health care in the United States and other developed as well as developing countries have been increasingly influenced by constructs of the biophysical sciences and by forms of technological intervention. Engel (1973, p. 129) has labeled the two dominant characteristics of this prevailing paradigm as "physiochemical reductionism" and "technologic primacy." Physiochemical reductionism is a dogma that "assumes all activities of the living organism are ultimately to be explained in terms of its component molecular parts," while technologic primacy holds all human problems to be "amenable to technologic solutions" (Engel, 1973, pp. 129, 130). Medicine and the health care system, therefore, have searched for cures for diseases and for sophisticated technologies of diagnosis and treatment. One of the products of scientific exploration has been increasingly more subtle systems for classifying groups of related symptoms as diseases and finding appropriate treatments for them. While such an approach often is effective for many problems, it creates considerable difficulty for other medical problems that are not easily classifiable as disease, such as pregnancy or admission to a long-term care facility (Richards, 1981).

A distinguishing feature of health professions education is that much of it occurs in health care settings and is thereby heavily influenced by the character of those settings. It is more in the hospital environment than in the standard classroom that students acquire a conception of their professional role (Richards, 1981). The system of procedures, communication patterns, hierarchical structures, and reward patterns in the delivery setting are important determinants of the education received by health professions students. But it is exceedingly difficult to exercise enough control over this health care environment to accomplish certain specified educational ends and probably impossible if those educational ends are in conflict with the local patient care process. Even in university-based academic medical centers, where ostensibly the patient care system exists to serve an educational purpose, the forces that shape the system and to which the system must respond are more those of patient care and the personal interests of practitioners than they are of education.

In recent history, most health professions education has occurred almost exclusively in hospitals. Hospitals, especially those in academic health centers, have come to be paragons of technology and subspecialization. It is inevitable, then, that education occurring in such hospitals is an education in specialized, technologized, and interventionist medical care.

There is no escaping the fact that the way health professionals are educated is a significant contributor to many problems—the unnecessarily high costs of health care in the United States, the inaccessibility of health care to many segments of our population, the overemphasis on curative and episodic medical care, and the fragmented and generally uncoordinated character of medical services. Therefore, minimizing these problems requires substantial changes in health professions education. The changes must proceed along two dimensions at the same time: in the health care settings used for the education of health professionals and in the curricula of health professions schools. Attempting to modify the latter without changing the former is an exercise in educational self-deception. Health professions education must lead in developing alternative health care delivery approaches more suited to health promotion, comprehensive and coordinated care, and ambulatory chronic care, all at lower costs than the existing system. Educational curricula must be adapted so that students spend a significant portion of their educational experience in these modified clinical settings and so that the preclinical education prepares students for such experiences.

In order to change the health care delivery system, the health professions educational model should be changed to support a health promotion comprehensive, coordinated, ambulatory, chronic care model of lower cost by

- Developing alternative "comprehensive conceptual frameworks for health care delivery at all levels" (see Mawby, Chapter Twenty-three), including redefinition of health professional roles
- Implementing one or more of these conceptual frameworks as central components of the health care delivery system of academic health centers and related community health care agencies
- Using these alternative health care settings extensively to provide primary and secondary health care experiences to students
- Modifying curricula to increase psychosocial emphases of training; to stress education related to the development of principles, values, and ethics; to focus

on problem-solving models of learning as opposed to rote memorization and recall of facts; and to increase the student's experience with patients of various cultural, social, economic, and age groups

- Conducting educational research and development on the interface between health services and education, on public policy formulation and its influence on health professions education, on the processes of successful implementation of innovations at academic health centers, and on the development of better social-psychological indicators of health status

- Modifying the academic and practice reward systems in educational institutions to support the recommended innovations

*Influencing Public Policies.* Academic health centers are obliged to interpret their external and internal environments and to adapt to changing conditions. Academic health centers must take a value stance and redirect their patient care and educational programs accordingly. In addition, academic health centers must be aggressive in attempting to change public policy for health care.

Not only are academic health centers influenced by their environment but they can, if they choose, be a significant influence on that environment. Most public policy initiatives have their origins outside of government. The proposals of such associations as the American Dental Association, the American Medical Association, the National League for Nursing, the Association of American Medical Colleges, and various foundations and expert panels find their way into legislation in some form. What is needed of academic health centers is painfully difficult for them to do. They must seek to change the health care system in controversial ways that will force change upon themselves. Academic health centers should put forward proposals for restructuring both the health care system and health professions education. It is consistent with the mission of academic health centers that these proposals for change place academic health centers as central to the implementation of these reforms. To do so is to act on the premise that for society and for themselves, academic health centers should strive to put their future under their own control.

To reiterate, the growing perception of the problem in health care is its high cost for the benefits received, combined with the growing need for more health care of all kinds. There are many causes for the high costs—societal expectations, unhealthy living, unhealthy environmental conditions, the availability of more and higher-cost diagnostic and therapeutic options, and the education of health professionals (especially physicians) to expect to have all technology available for their use (Fuchs, 1975). It is the way we finance our health care system, however, that exacerbates the problems and works against our finding acceptable ways of solving them.

The educational processes for health professionals are heavily influenced by the economics of generating revenue. This is the case of hospitals of all types, whether profit or nonprofit, university or community, public or private. Two factors influence significantly the health care system in the United States: a fee-for-service pattern of paying most health professionals, particularly doctors, and a pattern of paying for hospital care by the day. As Richards (1981) points out, "hotels with swimming pools, saunas, and golf courses charge more for a room than hotels without such amenities, and hospitals with open heart surgery teams, rehabilitation services, and elaborate dining rooms charge more than those without" (p. 7). It is to be expected that the educational activity tolerated within such settings will depend in large measure on its effect on the economics of doing business; there is little tolerance for educational activity that negatively affects revenues.

For academic health centers, such a reimbursement system will eventually, if it has not already, lead to a disaster because of their high costs and loss of uniqueness in the marketplace and because of the declining governmental support for medical care. Academic health centers offer a distinctive combination of research and education, in conjunction with two kinds of patient care—primary, general medical care to the indigent and highly specialized tertiary care. The academic health center of the 1980s is no longer unique, as was its counterpart, the teaching hospital of earlier years. Community hospitals can now provide nearly the same range of general and specialty services at lower costs. An increasing proportion of the costs of health professions education, especially medical education, is being borne by patients. Overall, governmental support for education and research has actually declined. Governmental support for patient care services is declining as well. The net effect is a developing financial crisis for health sciences centers.

Academic health centers are reacting to this financial crisis in two general ways: (1) by arguing with third-party payers that academic health centers should be reimbursed for their services at a higher-than-average cost because of the unique and more costly character of what they do; and (2) by attempting to compete with private community hospitals through cost reductions and shifts in patient mix, to include a greater percentage of private paying or self-paying patients. The argument that academic health centers are justifiably higher in cost because they are different, when taken together with their financial survival strategy of acquiring a patient mix that results in their becoming more similar to community hospitals, makes for a curiously contradictory picture, indeed.

Unfortunately, for academic health centers, it is more than merely curious; it has regrettable consequences. In the first place, it is very unlikely that the competitive strategy will work. Hadley's analysis (see Chapter Eighteen) makes this point very clear. Several strategies are now being adopted by private and public hospitals to respond to the decreasing governmental support for medical care, combined with the more deregulated and more highly competitive economic climate. They are trying to cut costs by reducing the volume of "free or below-cost care" and to increase activities that generate revenue. For political, functional, and philosophical reasons, public academic health centers will have great difficulty in adopting such a strategy. As noted earlier, what academic health centers offer is frequently available elsewhere at less cost for those who can afford it. Private insurers are unwilling to continue to subsidize the higher charges of teaching hospitals when good alternatives are available. The political consequences for academic health centers, especially public ones, of turning their backs on the lower-paying or nonpaying indigent in order to court the paying patient are serious; such a strategy is likely to be regarded as an unacceptable shirking of public responsibility. The dissatisfaction of lawmakers can be expected to be reflected in appropriations decisions regarding support for health professions and the privileged status of academic health centers in reimbursement for patient care services.

Perhaps more important than the probable failure of the strategy of attempting to be simultaneously both different from and the same as community hospitals is the fact that academic health centers are being drawn into becoming more integrated with, and dependent upon, the existing system for paying health care costs. And that system is itself the major problem. The net effect is to render academic health centers unable to carry out a historically fundamental responsibility—contributing to the solution of society's most perplexing and important problems. The painful fact is that academic health centers are, in many respects, anachronistic. Academic health centers are victims of what Riesman (1958) has called "the stalemate of success," moving toward the future as if guiding a speeding car forward, with eyes firmly fixed on the rearview mirror. The fee-for-service system and hospital charges by the day, combined with declining financial support for health professions education, will lead to the elimination of academic health centers as a societal mechanism for achieving the needed restructuring of the health care system. This trend might be reversed by reducing the dependence of academic health centers on fee-for-service and by creating a direct appropriations system, designed especially for academic health centers, to provide incentives for educational and patient care innovations leading to improved care at lower costs per unit.

The subject of this book has been health professions education. A review of its recent past and the factors that in some way may influence its future has led to the acknowledgement of what is perhaps the obvious—the system of educating health professionals is inextricably related to the health services delivery system. If, therefore, fundamental change is called for in health professions education, it cannot be accomplished without changing the health care delivery system. Further, it is the responsibility of health professions education, to society and to itself, to pursue ways of reforming that system so more can be equitably provided for less cost, by first changing academic health centers. It is our view that the public, acting through government, especially state governments, would be willing to appropriate large amounts of funds directed toward this goal if there were clear evidence that academic health centers intended to undertake the research, development, and piloting of alternative health care delivery systems that could and eventually would affect their own health care structures. It is not within the scope of this chapter to make specific recommendations as to how the medical care system and its financing should be changed; that is the province of other experts. More importantly, the point is not to take a position on how the system should be changed but rather to emphasize the need for academic health centers to accept responsibility and be funded for finding and demonstrating alternative ways of delivering care at more reasonable cost. In summary, it is recommended, therefore, that academic health centers take the initiative in aggressively seeking to influence public policy associated with needed health care reforms by

- Encouraging modification of the reimbursement system in order to be more supportive, generally, of health promotion, health maintenance, and the like, and, specifically, to reduce the extent to which academic health centers are dependent upon fee-for-service and hospital daily occupancy rates for their financial survival
- Urging establishment of a comprehensive governmental agency at the state level, with broad powers to direct and control the activities of existing de-

partments of public health, environment, licensure, Medicare/Medicaid, and the funding of higher education associated with health professions education. Such a comprehensive agency would provide direct financial support for the development and implementation of coordinated, alternative health care systems in academic health centers, to include the redefinition of the roles of health professionals, especially in relation to each other; seek to eliminate fragmentation in the delivery of health care services; and reduce the overall costs of care.

## Conclusion

The recommendations in this chapter can be briefly summarized as (1) changing the health professions educational model, (2) modifying the reimbursement system for medical care, and (3) establishing a comprehensive agency at the state level to coordinate governmental activity relating to health care and health professions education. These recommendations are not new ones. Such directions have often been articulated, and yet little has been accomplished. Many factors will militate against the achievement of these goals in the future, as they have in the past. Self-interest will motivate the health professions, as it does all professions, to modify proposals for fundamental structural changes until the objectionable elements are minimized or even turned to advantage. Academic health centers will be inclined to accede only to those modifications in the status quo that are necessary for self-preservation. The restructuring of health professions education that is called for will precipitate intense, interprofessional warfare within academic health centers, for the requisite changes will pose a threat to the long-term survival of some of the professions.

In the face of these and other difficulties, the easier path for academic health centers may be seen to be that of acquiescence—to regard health care as a commodity and to do whatever is necessary to compete successfully in the marketplace. But it is also the case that these circumstances offer an unusual opportunity. There is much to be gained if academic health centers are prepared to take the risks of innovation.

One way or another, society will find alternatives. For example, corporate involvement in health care for profit is increasing and will create new options. More informed and assertive consumers will make choices for themselves. There is growing intolerance by consumers of the dysfunctional competition among the health professions. Increasingly, people seem to know what they want and what they feel they deserve. They want ready access to comprehensive, good-quality health care for themselves and their families. They want the health professionals to make caring for people in need their main concern. They want a system that treats patients with dignity and recognizes their right as well as their responsibility to live a healthful life and to make decisions about the care they should receive. They want the various health professionals to work together in a coordinated way. They want the many compassionate health professionals that comprise the health care system to see to it that the system itself is more compassionate.

Modification of the basis for funding academic health centers would make it possible for them to take the leadership in the necessary restructuring of the health care system and to educate health professionals to be willing and able to work effectively in that reformed system. Such societal responsiveness on the part of academic health centers would be comparable to their responsiveness in the past, when these centers met the then perceived needs for providing specialty care unavailable elsewhere, for expounding education and research regarded as urgent, and for increasing the numbers of health professionals seen to be in short supply. The issue, of course, is whether academic health centers will remain captives of their own and their professions' narrowly drawn interests. The irony is that their ultimate self-interest—survival—will be served only if academic health centers respond to society's emerging needs according to prevailing political and economic rules. In Mawby's words (see Chapter Twenty-three), "the unending challenge to (health professions education) is to move reality closer to the vision of what ought to be."

## References

Bledstein, B. J. *The Culture of Professionalism: The Middle Class and the Development of Higher Education in America.* New York: Norton, 1976.

Callahan, D. "Health and Society: Some Ethical Imperatives." In J. Knowles (Ed.), *Doing Better and Feeling Worse: Health in the United States.* New York: Norton, 1977.

Engel, G. L. "The Best and the Brightest: The Missing Dimension in Medical Education." *The Pharos of Alpha Omega Alpha,* 1973, *36,* 129–133.

Fuchs, V. *Who Shall Live?* New York: Basic Books, 1975.

Gibson, R. M., and Waldo, D. R. "National Health Expenditures, 1980." *Health Care Financial Review,* 1981, *3,* 1–54.

Navarro, V. "Where Is the Popular Mandate?" *New England Journal of Medicine,* 1982, *307,* 1516–1518.

Overholt, W. A. "Exploring Ethical Guidelines to Public Policy." Paper presented at the Ninth Annual Distinguished Lecture Series on Ethics for the Health Professions, University of Illinois at Chicago, February 1983.

Richards, R. W. "Defining the Nature of Primary Care Education." In H. J. Knopke and N. L. Diekelmann (Eds.), *Approaches to Teaching Primary Health Care Education.* St. Louis, Mo.: Mosby, 1981.

Riesman, D. *Constraint and Variety in American Education.* New York: Doubleday, 1958.

# Name Index

# Subject Index

## A

Academic health sciences centers: allied health education in, 115, 116, 121; analysis of challenges to, 498-505; background on, 498-499; and community hospitals, 499-501, 504, 516-517; and delivery system, 499; evolution of, 143; first, 142; future of, 512-513; graduate programs in, 141-161; implementing agenda for, 503-505; new model development by, 370-371; public policy impact for, 515-518; research role for, 501-503; and value systems, 359, 365

Access, equity of, in health care policy, 400-401

Accountability, and continuing education, 323-324

Accreditation: for allied health programs, 120, 122-123; of graduate programs, 145-146, 157; of medical education, 145-146; of pharmaceutical education, 69, 73-74, 77, 78, 80, 81, 82, 85, 86-87; for public health, 134

Adjective Checklist, 214

Administration, of graduate programs, 143-146

Administrative sciences, in pharmacy curriculum, 79-80

Admission: analysis of, 202-233; clinical criterion measures for, 222; in dentistry, 54-55; and grade point average, 207, 208, 211-212, 213, 214, 216, 217, 218, 219, 220, 221, 222; implications and recommendations for, 222-226; major findings on, 220-222; and

manpower projections, 223-224; overview of, 202-203; research directions for, 225-226; selection methods in, 206-211; and selection related to outcome measures, 211-220; and self-selection, 224-225; and student characteristics, 203-206

Advanced Instruction in Medical Settings (AIMS), 300

Africa, needs in, 464

Aged persons: care for, 432-437; and curricular change, 179-180, 184-185; and disease, 433-434; health and prevention for, 434-437; and values, 508

Allied health: alliances and, 122; analysis of trends and priorities in, 113-126; concepts of, 113-114, 153; evaluation of competence in, 257, 258, 261, 271; federal government impact on, 116-118, 121-122; funding of, 121; issues in, 120-121; journal in, 119-120; planning in, 123; professional organization in, 119-120; research in, 123-124; summary on, 124

Allied health education: accreditation for, 120, 122-123; admission to, 220; age of students in, 203; applicants to, 202; development of, 116-120; faculty evaluation and development in, 296, 303, 307, 308; grade point average in, 211-212, 213; graduate programs in, 153-154; learning styles in, 245; manpower training in, 114-116; program review in, 157; selection methods for, 207, 208, 221;

## L

Latin America, plethora of physicians in, 470

Learning: lifelong, acceptance of, 320; principles of, and research needs, 249; research on types of experiences in, 198-199; styles of, research on, 244-247

Learning Preference Inventory (LPI), 245-246

Learning Style Inventory, 245

Lectures: in continuing education, 332; research on, 240-241

Liaison Committee on Medical Education (LCME), 145-146, 157

Licensure: and dental education, 53-54; public involvement in, for pharmacy, 84-85

London Hospital Medical College Dental School, 167

Louisiana State University, School of Dentistry at, 303

Lysaught report, 104-105

## M

Maastricht Medical School, case method at, 458

McGill University, Kellogg Center for Advanced Studies in Primary Care at, 303

McMaster University: evaluation at, 260, 283-284; faculty development at, 307; medical curriculum at, 175, 185, 241, 243

Macy Foundation, Josiah, Jr., 42n

Malawi, needs in, 464

Manpower needs: and admissions, 223-224; in allied health, 114-116; and auxiliary workers, 376; and dental education, 52-54; and economic trends, 373-385; formulation of, 374-375; and health care policy, 393, 395; and international needs, 469-471; and planning in public health, 137-139; projections of, 509-510; specialized, and allied health, 114; thrusts in development for, 478-479

Markle Foundation, John and Mary R., 164

Maryland: public health in, 135; rate-setting regulation in, 398, 423

Massachusetts General Hospital: costs at, 450-451; ether anesthetic at, 453

Massachusetts Institute of Technology: and public health, 139; Study of Critical Environmental Problems by, 443, 446

Maternal and Child Health program, 388, 390

Medicaid: and economic trends, 378, 379, 381, 450; and financial constraints, 406, 407, 408, 409, 410, 411-412, 415, 418, 420, 422; and health care policy, 390, 392, 394, 396, 397, 398, 401; and medical education, 23, 35; and social reform, 13, 17

Medical audits, and continuing education, 326-329

Medical College Admissions Test (MCAT), 163, 208-209, 213-214, 216, 217, 221, 242

Medical College of Virginia, 167, 168

Medical economics, and curricular change, 179

Medical education: accreditation of, 145-146; admission to, 220; age of students in, 203; basic sciences in, 28-34, 151; clinical experience in, 26, 35-38, 271-274; computers for, 456-458; curricular changes in, 24-25, 28-38, 163-164, 170, 175, 180-181, 183, 184; curricular concerns in, 38-42; curricular goals changed in, 24-25; curriculum length in, 27-28; and delivery system, 491; faculty for, 148; faculty evaluation and development in, 296, 300, 301-302, 303, 304, 305, 306-307, 309-310, 311; grade point average in, 214, 216; graduate degrees in, and tertiary care, 23-24; history of, 142-143; independent study in, 242-243; learning styles in, 245; lectures in, 240-241; minority students in, 204; peer teaching in, 241-242; physician-researchers in, 155-157; problem-based learning in, 243; program review in, 158, 159; selection methods for, 207, 208, 210-211, 221; selection related to outcome measurs in, 213-217, 222; self-instruction in, 240; simulation in, 235-236; special interest topics in curriculum for, 41-42; student personalities in, 204, 205; televised instruction in, 236. *See also* Continuing medical education; Medical schools

Medical laboratory science: minority students in, 204; skills measure needed for, 222

Medical records: learning styles in, 246; minority students in, 204; student personalities in, 205, 206

Medical schools: applicants to, 202; attrition from, 214; clinical activity expansion at, 419-420; community-based, and clinical teaching, 36; community-based practice plans of, 421-422; cost awareness in, 494-495; cost reductions at, 419; expansion of, 23; and faculty, 164; and patient care revenues, 412-417; responses of, to financial constraints, 418-420; sex distribution in, 203; sources of revenue for, 413-414; tuition raising by, 419

Medical technology: analysis of, 448-462; as career choice, 206; computers for, 455-459; concept of, 448-449; and conglomerates, 460-461; evaluation of competence in, 261; future of, 459-461; history of, 449-451; and humanism, 461; impact of, 451-455; and inflation, 450-451; selection related to outcome measures in, 212; student personalities in, 205

Medicalization, process of, 14-15